DRUG DESIGN

Basics and Applications

DRUG DESIGN

Basics and Applications

Editor

MUKESH DOBLE

Professor, Department of Biotechnology
IIT Madras

Tata McGraw Hill Education Private Limited
NEW DELHI

McGraw-Hill Offices

New Delhi New York St Louis San Francisco Auckland Bogotá Caracas
Kuala Lumpur Lisbon London Madrid Mexico City Milan Montreal
San Juan Santiago Singapore Sydney Tokyo Toronto

Tata McGraw Hill

Published by the Tata McGraw Hill Education Private Limited,
7 West Patel Nagar, New Delhi 110 008.

ISBN (13): 978-1-25-900574-9
ISBN (10): 1-25-900574-7

Vice-President & Managing Director—Asia Pacific: *Ajay Shukla*
Executive Publisher—Professional: *R Chandra Sekhar*
Assistant Sponsoring Editor—Science, Technology and Computing: *Simanta Borah*
Sr. Production Executive: *Rita Sarkar*
AGM—Sales and Business Development: *S Girish*
Deputy Marketing Manager—Healthcare: *A. Rehman Khan*
Controller—Production: *Rajender P Ghansela*
AGM—Production: *B L Dogra*

Typeset at Le Studio Graphique, Guru Shivir, 12, Sector 14, Gurgaon 122 001, and
printed at Gopsons Papers Limited, A-2 and 3, Sector 64, Noida 201 301

Cover Design: Kapil Gupta, New Delhi

RXBCRRQGLXDRL

The McGraw·Hill Companies

To

My parents

Preface

The global pharmaceutical business is about \$750 billion (2009) and has grown at more than 6% over the last five years. North America is the biggest pharmaceutical market—a share of almost 48%—followed by Europe (30%) and Japan(9%). Some of the leading pharmaceutical companies across the world are Merck & Co., Glaxo Wellcome, Novartis, Bristol-Myer Squibb, Johnson & Johnson, Pfizer, American Home Products, Smithklein Beecham, Hoechst, and Eli Lilly.

Drug discovery and development is a time consuming and expensive process. It takes 12–15 years and about \$1.2 billion to launch one drug molecule in the market. The costs are spiraling upwards at an annual rate of ~11%, while the number of new chemical entities developed by the top 20 pharmaceutical companies has continued a steady five-year downward trend. Large number of 'blockbuster' drugs has been withdrawn due to safety concerns, and so, pharmaceutical companies are facing serious challenges. It has been estimated that as many as 50% of all new molecular entities (i.e., new chemical entities and new biological entities) that enter preclinical animal testing fail to proceed to human trials. About 30% of all drugs that enter clinical testing, are terminated. Also, animal trials are not foolproof, since they predict in the range of 10–70% of all human adverse effects. These tests predict adverse gastro-intestinal, cardiovascular, and hematological toxicities. However, they cannot predict drug-induced adverse immune reactions, dermatological reactions, or central nervous system adverse effects.

The advances in technology, instrumentation, and computational techniques have made modern biological research easy and simple. A lot more diseases have been discovered during the last 50 years, and the current technology helps us in understanding the etiology of these diseases better, with a goal to find a cure as quickly as possible. All this has helped the drug discovery process in developing from a 'trial-and-error' approach to a much focused and directional process. The field of drug discovery has seen remarkable changes that have helped automate the process for a speedy drug discovery. Some of the modern methods of drug discovery include proteomics and bioinformatics, natural products screening, high-throughput screening, combinatorial chemistry, molecular diversity and compound library designing, protein 3D-structures, NMR-based screening, *in silico* screening, 3D-QSAR, physico-chemical properties, and computer-aided prediction of drug toxicity and metabolism.

Inspite of all these, new drugs entering the market are still dismal, mainly due to several failures during the clinical trials because of side effects, toxicity, poor bioavailability, etc. An early understanding of these phenomena could reduce the discovery time as well as the cost of the discovery process.

This book, titled *Drug Design: Basics and Applications*, is meant to address several of these issues with suggestions and solutions focused towards important diseases such as cardiovascular, diabetics, inflammation, TB, etc.

The first four chapters of this book discuss the fundamental concepts such as target and lead identification and *in vitro* assessment methodologies, which are generic to any discovery process, irrespective of the disease. The remaining seven chapters focus on specific diseases, describing the targets involved in the disease, currently available commercial drugs, their mode of action and recent developments. The subject areas covered are TB, diabetics, cardio vascular diseases, inflammation, cardio tonics, Inositides, G protein coupled receptors, and human hepatic drug metabolism. Each chapter is written by a domain expert from industry, academia, and/or research institution from India and abroad.

Drug discovery is a highly inter disciplinary field, and it needs support from medicinal chemist, organic chemist, analytical chemist, pharmacologist, pharmaceutical chemists and technologists, biologist, molecular biologist, biochemist, and systems biologist. This book will be useful for scientists, researchers, teachers working in the area of drug discovery and design.

MUKESH DOBLE

Contents

1

The Science of Drug Discovery

***Lavanya Madhuri Balivada*[1], *Ashif Y. Shaikh*[2], *Srinivas Hotha*[*,2] *Gopala Krishna Aradhyam*[#,1] and *Mukesh Doble*[†1]**

[1]*Department of Biotechnology, Indian Institute of Technology Madras, Chennai, India*
[2]*Division of Organic Chemistry (Synthesis), National Chemical Laboratory, Pune, India*

Drug discovery programs have mostly depended on the engineering prowess of Mother Nature. The traditional knowledge that was transferred between generations with or without scientific rationale became the ground for the discovery of novel small molecules that eventually became drugs after thorough evaluation. Some drugs were discovered accidentally or serendipitously. Keeping that apart, the ambiguity in the process of drug discovery can be compared to that in choosing a winning stock in the stock market or finding a terrorist in a densely populated city. In India, China and some other parts of the world, there has existed for a long time a system of medicine that primarily depends on plants. For example, the famous *Charaka Samhita*, written centuries ago, describes the significance of various flora and fauna of India to many different classes of diseases; it became a good resource for many of the drug discoverers. Later, Alexander Fleming's serendipitous discovery of penicillin during the Second World War opened microbial sources as a new vista for drug discovery. During the late 1990s, Schreiber's small molecule approach to the hit molecule discovery highlighted the significance of large number of synthetic compounds that were available through combinatorial methods. The salient features, merits and pitfalls of the three approaches are shown in Table 1.1.

---

[*]*s.hotha@ncl.res.in;* [#] *agk@iitm.ac.in;* [†] *mukeshd@iitm.ac.in*

Table 1.1 *Traditional and Modern Methods of Identifying New Small-Molecule Inhibitors*

Method Used	*Comments*	*Examples*
Plant/Microbial/Marine Resources		
Predictions from traditional or folk medicine Exhaustive search from soil, air, water, oceans, etc.	Trial and error as it all depends on authenticity of the hypothesis Nature dictated success Structure to be assigned Often synthesis protocol unknown	Paclitaxel Tetracyclines Epothilones Aranorosin Others
Chemical Genetics		
High-throughput screening of combinatorial libraries	Reduced errors as chemical libraries are chosen by humans Human knowledge interfered with success Structure known from chemical libraries Synthesis protocol known	Monastrol HR22C16 Uretupamine Tubacin Histacin Fexaramine

HISTORY OF DRUG DISCOVERY

Since time immemorial, natural flora and fauna have been exploited to maintain health and wellness of the body. The pre-1800 era is known as 'the age of botanicals' or 'the age of herbal medicine' (Somberg, 1996). The first half of the 19th century saw many new diseases being discovered and identified, and the search for a possible cure by administering patients with medicines dominated the second half of the same century. The search for new medicines and advances in homeopathy led to the birth of pharmaceutical industries (Lesney, 2000). The accidental discoveries of natural drugs such as quinine, digitalis, cocaine, anti-pyrine and aspirin were some of the major breakthroughs of that century. Moreover, the 'microbial theory of disease' was one of the key developments in medical science, which states that some or all of the diseases are caused by microorganisms. This developed the need to study microbes and understand their physiology in order to cure the disease. This, in turn, led to the modern drug discovery, which exploits substances found in nature for a probable source of drug. Table 1.2 gives a brief description of the history of the drug discovery process.

Table 1.2 *Timeline of the Drug Discovery Process (Pizzi, 2000; Frey and Lesney, 2000)*

Year	*Development*
1920s–1930s	• Discovery of vitamins and development in Chemistry • Discovery of new vaccines and drugs, for e.g., accidental discovery of Penicillin by Alexander Fleming in 1928 • Merging of Biology, Physics and Chemistry gave birth to pharmacology • Development of new instruments and techniques to study diseases

(Contd)

(Table 1.2 Contd)

Year	Development
1940s	• *'The antibiotic era'* • Discovery of numerous drugs targeted at various diseases, seed for rational drug design concept • New drug therapies for Malaria (Pyrimethamine), Leukemia (6-mercaptopurine and Thioguanine), Gout (Allopurinol), Organ Transplantation (Azathioprine) and bacterial infections (Co-trimoxazole)—George Hitchings, Sir James Black and Gertrude Elion received Nobel Prize for these drugs and Hitchings especially for chemotherapy. These advances later led to the development of major antiviral drugs for Herpes (Acyclovir) and AIDS (Zidovudine)
1950s	• New techniques led to better understanding of human body and hence new drugs, for e.g., Vancomycin, a glycopeptide, was discovered during this phase which later led to its use against methicillin-resistant *Staphlycocci* infections • Elucidation of the structure of DNA by Watson and Crick and later understanding the process of DNA replication, transcription and translation led to a better understanding of the viral replication cycle, thus making it easier for the discovery of new antiviral drugs • Breakthrough in biological instrumentation led to the birth of Biotechnology
1960s	• *'Pharma decade of the century'* • Etiology of diseases led to an increased understanding and subsequent discovery of new drugs • DNA was found to be the genetic material in most of the organisms, except some viruses • Instrumentation and powerful computing techniques led to lab automation
1970s	• Advances in computing techniques and life sciences gave birth to recombinant DNA and molecular cloning during the mid-1970s • Setting up of Genentech Inc. in 1976 marked the beginning of the Biotech sector • Advances in knowledge, instrumentation and powerful computer applications for biology • This era also saw the synthesis of Vitamin B12 by Woodward R B, for which he received the Nobel Prize • Taxol was also discovered during this period, however, it was clinically approved only in 1993
1980s	• Appearance of new diseases, like AIDS, gave birth to Immunology, the science of understanding body's immune system • Computing techniques led to design of new drugs • Increased knowledge on body physiology and medical disorders in conjunction with knowledge about drugs led to directional drug designing and discovery • Commercialization of the drug discovery process • Development of Combinatorial Chemistry- simulation of large sets of chemically similar agents which can be screened for biological activity • Major breakthrough in Biotechnology with the development of the Polymerase Chain Reaction (PCR) by Kary Mullis in 1984 • Recurrence of diseases that were previously cured with drugs
1990s	• Continued recurrence of diseases previously cured • Use of Robotics and automation in drug discovery • Rapid advances in technology and computation techniques • Birth of Molecular Modeling and Bioinformatics

(Contd)

(Table 1.2 Contd)

Year	Development
	• New techniques led to the development of libraries of compounds that would aid in drug designing • Many new and big Biotech companies led to increased competitive pressures, management and financial performance of the organization

MODERN METHODS OF DRUG DISCOVERY

Natural Products

There was a time when natural flora and fauna were used to combat illness of the body. Advances in chemistry later helped identify the active principles of these natural sources of drugs and their uses in the medical field, and also chemically synthesize a few of these natural and medicinally useful compounds like quinine, penicillin G, theophylline, morphine, cyclosporine, to name a few.

With a void in the eras subsequent to the age of botanicals, the current drug market is shifting its focus again toward natural drugs, which can be studied much more easily with respect to their mode of action, side effects and, more importantly, any modifications that need to be done to fit the 'drug-cures-disease' process perfectly. Natural products are now being used more widely as lead molecules in the drug discovery process, since advances in technology have led to a better understanding of their structure. About 50–60% of the modern-day drugs are either natural products or their derivatives or have been inspired by the structure of specific natural products (Newmann and Cragg, 2007).

Natural products can be derived from a wide range of sources, such as plants, marine organisms, microbes and animals. The biological and geographical diversity in nature contributes to the chemical diversity for the drug discovery process and is known as *bioprospecting*. While it was Sertürner who first isolated the first ever natural plant product, morphine, from opium, which came from the poppy plant, the Greek physician Galenus was the first to develop a pharmacopoeia describing the properties of several plants used during his period. Similarly, many more plants and their natural drugs were discovered over a period of time among different parts of the world. Some of the examples include quinine from the bark of Cinchona tree used to treat fevers, coca or cocaine from *Erythroxylum* used for varied benefits, either singly or in combination with dead seashells or dried plants, also later used by Carl Koler as a local anesthetic for eye surgery.

The process of nature-inspired discovery (NID) starts with the authentic information received from traditional medical practitioners or folklore. Identification of the plant material and collection is followed by drying them under the shade to get dried material, which can then be milled to obtain powder. The powder then will be subjected to a variety of extraction procedures in various solvents (organic as well as aqueous) so that the decoction can be obtained in respective solvents. Then the decoction will be evaporated to dryness and subjected to thorough chromatographic fractionation and/or purifications, ideally to get single compounds. Isolated single compounds will be subjected to bioassays to identify the correct component of the whole extract that is responsible for a biological activity (Fig. 1.1). Once the component is identified, it is then time for the identification of the structure of that compound by exploiting various modern spectroscopic tools, such as nuclear magnetic resonance (NMR), infrared (IR), ultraviolet (UV), mass spectrometry (MS) and elemental analysis. The unambiguous structure assignment lets organic chemists to develop a retrosynthetic strategy that facilitates the synthesis of the molecule, which might take a few weeks to many years depending on the complexity of the structure. Several molecules, which are topographically, stereochemically or electronically similar, will be synthesized and checked in order to optimize the pharmocophore. Simultaneous endeavors by process engineers would enable the production of the small-molecule inhibitor in large quantities, so that it would be available in case it passes through a series of stringent safety and toxicology tests.

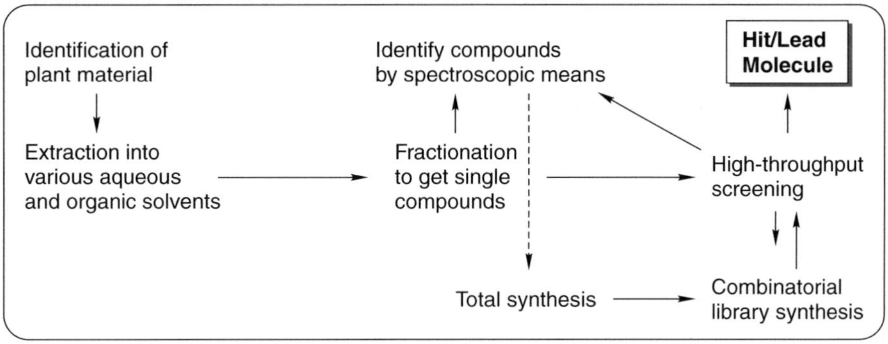

Fig. 1.1 *Nature-inspired Discovery of Drugs*

Contrary to this, in 1990s Schreiber put forward a new method to identify small-molecule inhibitors by the systematic high-throughput screening (HTS) of small-molecule libraries. The HTS devices developed for the successful completion of human genome project were used for this purpose. Before we jump to that, it would be highly appropriate to understand a little regarding the combinatorial way of synthesizing compounds. The last decade has seen the greatest changes in the thinking of drug discovery as two major fields have emerged, viz. combinatorial chemistry and chemical genetics.

Proteomics

Proteomics is the study of the proteome of a cell, a tissue or an organism. A proteome refers to the complete set of PROTEins expressed in a genOME. Proteins form an integral part of a system as they carry out most of the biological functions. The types of proteins present, and their functions, modifications, localizations and interactions aid in a better understanding of cellular functioning. An organism has a single genome but can have multiple proteomes, based on growth conditions and stages of development of life (Anderson and Anderson, 1998). Exploring the local and global patterns of protein content, their functions and how they change during an illness or development of disease forms the baseline of proteomics research. Understanding and correlating the vast posttranslational modifications a protein undergoes to a particular phenotype and then assessing if that modification is necessary for the phenotype forms the rationale for proteomics. A protein can be posttranslationally modified in all or some of the ways—phosphorylation, methylation, acetylation, sulfation, glycosylation, sumoylation, ubiquitination, and so on. Proteomics employs many different techniques for protein mapping and identifying and characterizing specific proteins with their complete structure and functional role (Blackstock and Weir, 1999).

Protein mapping involves the effective separation, characterization and mapping of proteins present in sample mixtures. The most reliable and common technique of protein mapping is two-dimensional polyacrylamide gel electrophoresis (2D-PAGE). This technique is about 40 years old, when innovations in electrophoresis, gradient gels and discontinuous buffer systems were used to increase the sharpness of protein bands. This paved the way for 2D electrophoresis, which can separate thousands of cellular proteins in a single gel (Klose, 1975). This seemed interesting since 2D-PAGE could display all the cellular proteins simultaneously, which means that it was easier to check changes in a proteome under diseased condition. 2D-PAGE separates proteins in two dimensions, based on their charge and mass. In the first dimension, the proteins are separated based on their charge by isoelectric focusing and in the second dimension they are separated based on their mass. Unlike, 1D-PAGE, proteins are visualized as spots instead of bands. The spots in combination with a wide range of proteins that can be separated and analyzed make 2D-PAGE more complicated than 1D-PAGE. Hence, many 2D gel analysis softwares are available in the market, such as Delta2D and MELANIE. Innovations in 2D-PAGE along with protein tagging have helped to study several diseased states (Görg *et al.*, 2000). 2D-PAGE in combination with mass spectrometry has formed the basis for disease-related proteome analysis (Hanash, 2001).

MS, though a relatively new technique in biology, has its 100-year-old roots in physical and chemical studies. MS is a technique that recognizes the chemical composition of a sample based on its charge-to-mass ratio. The sample is subjected to chemical fragmentation to form charged particles called ions, whose charge-to-mass ratio is calculated by passing them through electric and magnetic fields in a mass spectrometer (Sparkman, 2000). Electron spray ionization (ESI) and matrix-assisted laser desorption/ionization (MALDI) are two common techniques used for preparing protein samples for MS (Fenn *et al.*, 1989; Baldwin *et al.*, 2001). Another method of protein sample preparation for MS is by enzymatic digestion of the proteins, which have been separated by 2D-PAGE (O'Farrell, 1975). These proteins/peptides are then identified by peptide mass fingerprinting (PMF) or tandem mass spectrometry (T-MS) (Hernandez *et al.*, 2006; Haqqani *et al.*, 2008). The process of protein identification using the ionization techniques is called the top-down approach while the enzymatically digested proteins subjected to MS and PMF/T-MS is called the bottom-up approach. However, the ionization techniques work well only when the sample mixture has all proteins in equal concentrations. Hence the alternative method of protein sample preparation is preferred, which employs 2D-PAGE, high-performance liquid chromatography (HPLC) or affinity chromatography to separate proteins/peptides (Zhang and Smith, 1994; Liu *et al.*, 2002). Shotgun proteomics refers to this HPLC-employed MS technique, used to characterize proteins/peptides. The mass analysis of proteolytic peptides uses two kinds of instruments—time-of-flight MS (TOF-MS) or Fourier transform ion cyclotron resonance (FT-ICR). The most important application of proteomics is developing disease-specific protein biomarkers (Rathin, 2002). This involves the use of alternative techniques like biomolecular interaction analysis–mass spectrometry (BIA-MS) and surface-enhanced laser desorption/ionization (SELDI) in combination with protein chips (Nelson *et al.*, 1999; Merchant and Weinberger, 2000).

Many databases that store the information obtained from 2D-PAGE and MS have been created and are maintained. GELBANK is one such annotated database of 2D gel electrophoresis patterns of organisms with completed genome sequencing. Similarly, many 2D gel databases exist based on organism (human, *Saccharomyces cerevisiae*, *Acinetobacter radioresistens*, the unicellular cyanobacterium *Synechocystis* sp. strain PCC6803) or tissue/organ type (human and rat hearts, *Arabidopsis* mitochondria, bovine kidney, liver, muscle, plasma and RBCs, hematopoietic cell lines, human lung fibroblast line, TIG-3, mammalian inner ear) or parasite–host cell interaction or plant proteomes (*Oryza sativa* anther tissue, *Medicago trunculata* root).

Target identification and validation is also another important part of the drug discovery process. Disease-causing genes are identified and confirmed and targeted for drug intervention for diseases like cancers and autoimmune disorders. Microarrays are one of the many tools that aid in target discovery and validation at the tissue/cellular level (Wang *et al.*, 2004; Sioud, 2007).

These different proteomics techniques have been employed to study subsets of microbes in an effort to gain a better understanding of the host–pathogen interactions, and differentiate virulent and avirulent strains for vaccine development, changes in expression type and levels of proteins in a diseased state or biomarkers for disease identification such as tumor cells in comparison with non-tumor cells (Schonberger *et al.*, 2001; Jungblut, 2001; Martin and Nelson, 2001; Mattow *et al.*, 2001; Rodriguez *et al.*, 2001; Washburn *et al.*, 2001; Hanash *et al.*, 2002).

Bioinformatics and Molecular Modeling

Using traditional drug development techniques it took nearly 40 years to capitalize on a basic understanding of the cholesterol biosynthesis pathway to develop statin drugs. On the contrary, a molecular-level understanding of the role of the human epidermal growth factor receptor 2 (HER-2) in breast cancer led to the development of the chemotherapeutic agent Herceptin® within only 3 years. HTS, access to databases containing genomic and proteomic information and use of *in silico* (computer-based) techniques have become a part of the drug discovery process. The 1998 Nobel chemistry prize was awarded to Pople and Kohn for their work in computational chemistry and molecular modeling. The 1999 Nobel chemistry prize was awarded to Ahmed Zewail for his work in developing spectroscopic methods for studying reactions, in particular transition states, an essential aspect of molecular modeling.

The ultimate goal is to model a disease process at the molecular level, predict which specific chemical compounds are best suited to treat the disease for a genetically defined patient population, then perform all binding experiments *in silico*, including absorption, distribution, metabolism and excretion and toxicology analysis of the compound. Techniques like quantitative structure–activity relations (QSARs)/quantitative structure–property relations help in predicting properties of the new compounds using computers.

Bioinformatics is the field of science that uses mathematics, statistics, informatics, chemistry and biology to have a better understanding of the biological systems and, thus, aids in solving biological problems through employing computational techniques like data mining and algorithms. It helps study and compare genome and proteome sequences, characterizes genes by predicting reading frames and exons from sequences and expressed sequence tags (ESTs), protein structure prediction and protein–protein interaction (Baxevanis and Ouellette, 2005). In this effort many databases have been created, which are sorted as sequence, domain, structural, mutation comparison and bibliographic databases. With the advances in genomics and proteomics, bioinformatics can be effectively used to exploit, discover and assess drug targets. If not anything, bioinformatics will definitely speed up the process of drug discovery as it uses the combined power and knowledge of structural biology, structure-based drug designing and computational technology (Fauman *et al.*, 2003).

Small-molecule drug design can be performed using a structure or target-based approach (Fig. 1.2). Both have their pros and cons. The former approach involves developing a QSAR between the biological activity and the molecular or structural descriptors. These descriptors describe small molecule/drug shape, size, thermodynamic, electronic, topographic and 3D features. The developed QSAR can be used to predict the activity of new compounds. The second approach needs some knowledge about the target for which drugs are being designed. If the 3D structure of the target protein is not known then homology modeling could be done to arrive at a 3D structure making use of the structure of a similar protein. The binding energy or the energy of interaction between the drug and the target could be determined by carrying out docking studies and a mathematical relation could be developed between these two values. This relationship can be used to predict the activity of newer molecules after estimating the binding energy with the target.

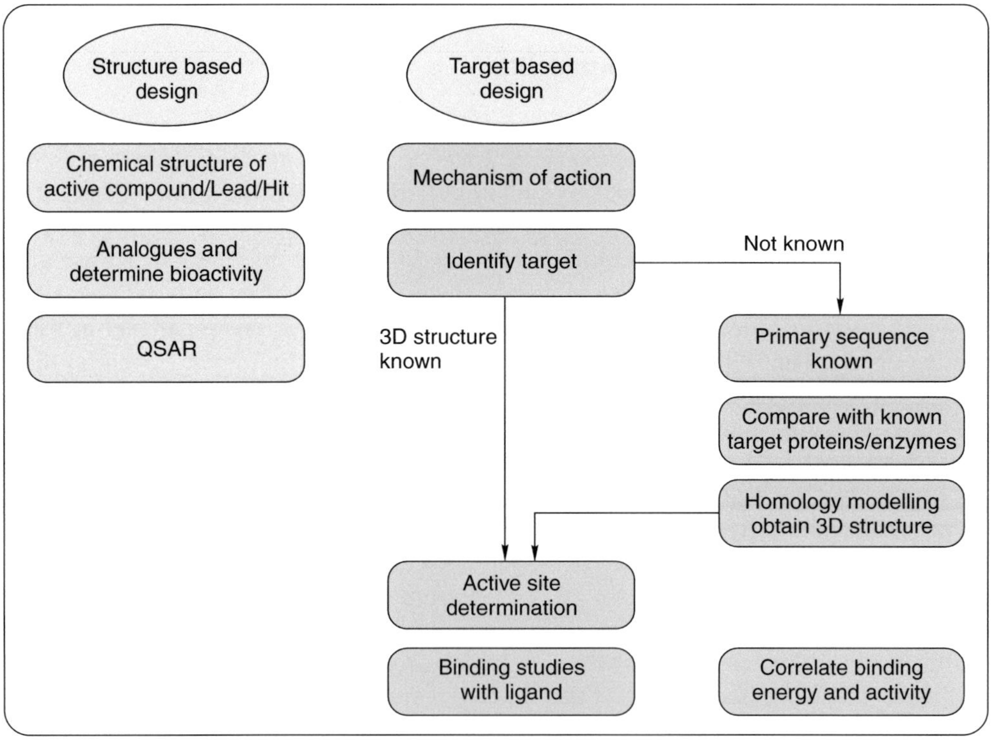

Fig. 1.2 ***Step-by-Step Approach to Structure- and Target-based Drug Design***

Protein 3D structures, either by X-ray crystallography or NMR, can be extrapolated to predict the probable function of the protein. In the case of drug discovery, 3D structures help in assessing the ability, and hence the importance, of the molecule as a potential drug candidate. Structures also help in determining if the molecule is druggable, i.e. if it can be used as a target for small-molecule inhibitors. Moreover, the structural availability also aids in detecting any cross-reactivities that the drug might have with nontargeted molecules (Thornton *et al.*, 2000). Structure-based drug designing goes hand in hand with combinatorial chemistry to design and develop new drugs. NMR-based drug designing can also be used to design compound libraries for NMR-based drug screening.

In Silico *Screening Tools for Leads*

In addition to performing QSAR and ligand protein- (target-)binding studies, several *in silico* techniques are resorted to screen possible lead molecules. They are shown in Fig. 1.3. The possible small molecules can be screened based on: (1) Lipinski's rule of five, (2) their toxicity and (3) drug likeness properties including absorption, distribution, metabolism, excretion, blood–brain barrier properties, P-glycoprotein (Pgp) efflux and membrane permeability.

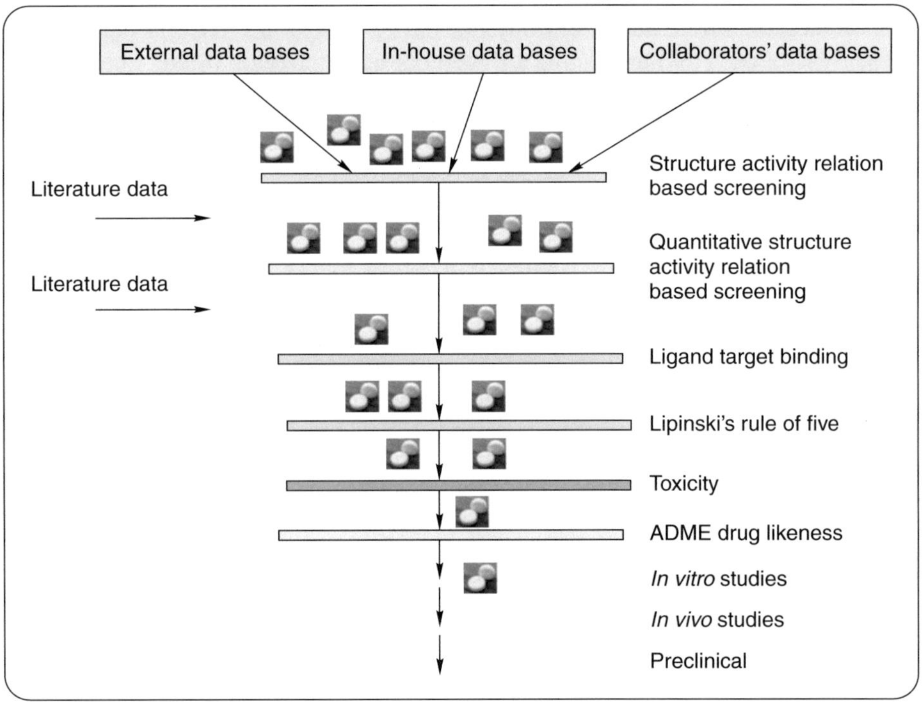

Fig. 1.3 **In Silico *Screening of Possible Lead Molecules (For color figure please see Plate 1)***

Lipinski's rule of five (Lipinski *et al.*, 1997) is a thumb rule to evaluate if a chemical compound with a certain pharmacological or biological activity makes it an orally active drug in humans. The rule was formulated by Christopher A. Lipinski in 1997, based on the observation made on more than 2500 medication drugs. The rule describes molecular properties important for a drug's pharmacokinetic properties in the human body. The rule states that an orally active drug has no more than one violation of the following criteria: (1) not more than five hydrogen bond donors (nitrogen or oxygen atoms with one or more hydrogen atoms), (2) not more than 10 hydrogen bond acceptors (nitrogen or oxygen atoms), (3) molecular weight under 500 Da, and (4) octanol–water partition coefficient, log *P* of less than 5.

This *in silico* approach could reduce the number of drug candidates from possible millions to possible hundreds, which could then be tested in the wet lab using *in vitro* screening before moving onto *in vivo* and preclinical trials.

High-Throughput Screening Techniques

HTS is one of the important aspects of drug discovery that assays a large number of libraries of compounds in an effort to identify the ones that are most likely to bind to a target, which can be a receptor or an enzyme. HTS done *in silico* is known as *virtual HTS*, which screens a large number of chemical structures that might bind to a target more effectively (Rollinger *et al.*, 2008). HTS finds a place for itself in genomics, protein/peptide library screening and combinatorial chemistry. However, for successful screening, it employs different assays and robotic equipment. Standard biochemical assays are used and the results are read out using enzyme-linked immunosorbent assay (ELISA) readers or different reporters employed during the assay. An assay can be homogeneous, where addition of all the components of the assay is done at a time, which is read out directly after a specific incubation time, or heterogeneous, where components are added in a specific order and time. Sometimes heterogeneous assays involve additional steps like centrifugation, washing and the like, apart from the simple addition of components (Hamilton *et al.*, 1996).

Since HTS involves screening of a huge number of compounds simultaneously, automation and robotics are an integral part of it. In addition to speeding up the process, automation helps in accurate delivery of the assay components into microwell plates. Moreover, many second-generation microplate devices automate the centrifugation, washing and filtering steps involved in many heterogeneous assays. Robotics takes automation a step further as they can be programmed to set up microwell plates, assays and the complete process of HTS. Hence, HTS robotics further speeds up the time of drug discovery process (Armstrong, 1997). HTS miniaturization is a recent key development that not only reduces the volume employed for assays (in nanoliters), but by doing so also increases the number of samples that can be screened at the same time. However, miniaturization is limited as it is expensive compared to the conventional methods of HTS (Wallace, 1998).

Combinatorial Chemistry

Combinatorial chemistry dates back to the 1960s when Bruce Merrifield developed the solid-phase synthesis of peptides (Merrifield, 1963). However, it was not until the 1990s that industries started adopting this technique. Combinatorial chemistry is a technique by which a large number of structurally distinct yet related molecules can be synthesized and subjected to pharmacological assays. These molecules can be synthesized or simulated *in silico* (Gordeeva *et al.*, 1992; Feher and Schmidt, 2003). With vast amount of research going into the drug discovery process, combinatorial chemistry finds itself well-placed in the modern-day drug discovery process, leading to the creation of a library of similar yet distinct compounds. Moreover, robotics has helped combinatorial chemistry two fold by speeding up the process of compound synthesis. So far, only one compound developed by combinatorial chemistry, sorafenib (used for advanced renal cancers), has been approved by FDA for clinical use (Newmann and Cragg, 2007). Moreover, many deconvolution methods find widespread applications in combinatorial chemistry-based drug discovery since they remove noises or instability associated with errors relating to pharmacokinetics, such as time taken for a drug to be absorbed from plasma. Also, many commercial software packages used in combinatorial chemistry come preloaded with some or all of the deconvolution methods, such as tagging, positional scanning and iterative deconvolution methods.

Combinatorial chemistry generally employs a divide, couple and recombine (DCR) method or the resin-mixing method for compound synthesis. DCR involves physically dividing and recombining the resins after each coupling step (Furka *et al.*, 1991; Houghten *et al.*, 1991; Lam *et al.*, 1991). In contrast, the physical resin-mixing approach has only one peptide bound to each resin and involves combining many such peptide-bound resins (Houghten *et al.*, 1991; Lam *et al.*, 1991). The chemical synthesis method, known as chemical ratio method, involves the incorporation of equimolar amounts of amino acids to the resins, in order to obtain a peptide–resin mixture library (Geysen *et al.*, 1986).

Combinatorial chemistry can be described as systematic and repetitive covalent connections among a set of different building blocks of varying structures in order to yield a large collection of molecules. This method enables a faster, more efficient and cheaper way to synthesize millions of molecules in a short span of time. Combinatorial libraries can be synthesized by either solid-phase or solution-phase methods. Merrifield's notable contributions for the solid-phase synthesis of peptides and the subsequent developments in polymer-supported organic synthesis significantly changed the combinatorial chemistry landscape (Table 1.3).

Table 1.3 *Comparison of Solid Phase versus Solution Methods*

Solution Phase	*Solid Phase*
Easy mass transfer of reagents	Reagents need to diffuse through polymeric supports
Reaction monitoring easy	Reaction monitoring difficult
Chromatographic purification laborious but achievable	Chromatographic purification not possible
Large excess of reagents cannot be used because of the need to separate them chromatographically	Excess reagents can be easily removed by simple filtration
Incomplete or inefficient reactions can also be carried out due to the enabling purification strategies	Non availability of purification methods is a big limitation
Overall process is sluggish as chromatographic separations are time taking and laborious	Fast. Due to purification by simple filtration
Work-up to remove excess reagents	No work-up but simple filtration
Large scale or scale-up of reactions is possible	Large-scale reactions are not very efficient due to the reduced mass transfer of reagents

In the recent times, combinatorial libraries are routinely synthesized by liquid dispensing robotic systems by two ways: split pool synthesis or parallel synthesis (Table 1.4).

Table 1.4 *Features of Parallel Synthesis and Split Pool Synthesis*

Parallel Synthesis	*Split Pool Synthesis*
Number of compounds produced increases linearly with the number of reactions carried out	Number of compounds produced increases exponentially with the number of reactions carried out
Leads to spatially separated and thus individual compounds	Compounds are not spatially separated and must be screened collectively
Property measurement can be either in solid or solution phase	Assay must be amenable to substrates anchored to solid supports and the assay must give easily interpretable visual readout
Screening results in unambiguous identification of the compound responsible for the response	Screening identifies only the existence of the hit compound but not the exact compound
Quick automation is possible	Can be automated but with difficulty
Suitable for the synthesis of libraries containing 100–1000 compounds	Suitable for the preparation of millions of compounds

Split Pool Synthesis

In the split pool way of synthesis, products at the end of the first reaction are pooled together to get a uniform mixture of compounds and then split again and reacted with a second set of reagents in order to get a mixture of compounds (Fig. 1.4). At the end of the second step, the compounds are pooled again and split to effect a third reaction. The process continues until the completion of the synthesis plan. The split pool methodology is particularly useful when it is required to screen compounds quickly without a particular preconceptualized target. Once a hit molecule is identified, one can identify or characterize the ligand responsible by various spectroscopic and chromatographic methods.

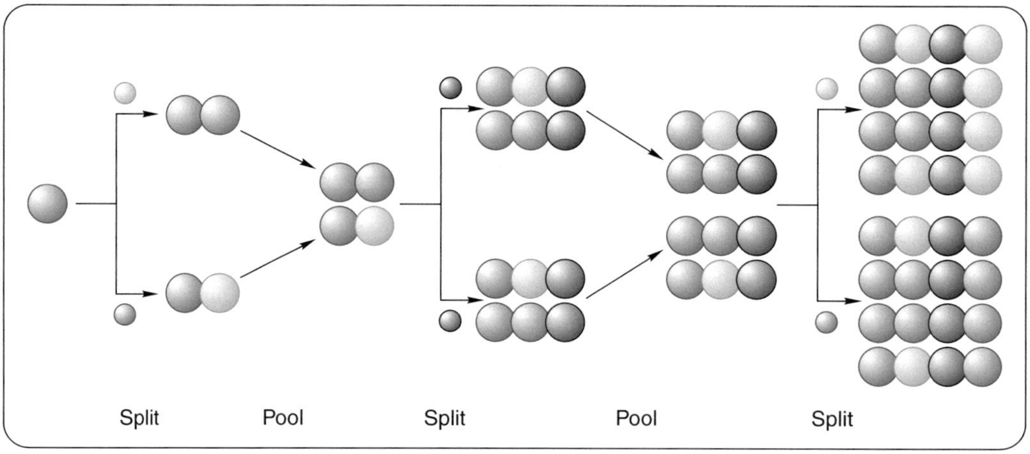

Fig. 1.4 *Schematic of Split Pool Synthesis (For color figure please see Plate 1)*

For example, consider a case where a library of all possible tripeptides needs to be synthesized. The split pool synthesis of tripeptide library begins with the distribution of the polymer-bound first amino acid into two individual vials and subsequent reaction with the second amino acid to get two dipeptides individually. The pooling of these products into a single vessel is followed by redistribution into two individual vials and reaction with the third amino acid to get tripeptides, and then again pooling them up and splitting them into another two fresh vials and then conducting the next reaction to get eight tripeptides. Identification of compounds after the property measurement becomes a bottleneck in this way of synthesis. Individual members of the peptide library can be identified after cleavage of the compound from solid phase followed by peptide sequence analysis, which may not be the case when we want to make small-molecule libraries. In such cases, bifunctional polymeric beads will be useful, where the chemistry at one end of the bead will be orthogonal to the other functional group, thereby facilitating the use of coding methods. One has to cleave the compound as well as the tag that reads the code at the end of the property measurement in order to identify the compound. In this context, one-bead-one-stock solutions using sufficiently larger beads is an important milestone. The split pool strategy is effected normally while performing reactions on solid phases.

Parallel Synthesis

In the parallel synthesis method, products of the first reaction are split into many individual vials and then separately reacted with different reagents and substrates. Then the resulting products of the first set of vials are again split into various second set of vials so that the second set of building blocks can be added. In this way, the synthesis of a large collection of pure compounds can be synthesized in a short period of time. For example, consider a case where a library of all possible tripeptides needs to be synthesized. Initially, a single suitably protected amino acid on solid phase is divided into two different vials and a peptide coupling is conducted using the second amino acid. At the end of the reaction, the products of the first reaction are further split into two more vials (2 × 2), and then the second peptide coupling reaction using the third amino acid is conducted in individual vials (Fig. 1.5), thus resulting in the synthesis of all eight possible tripeptides in individual vials. The parallel synthesis can be effected using either solution- or solid-phase synthesis.

Identification of a small molecule inhibitor that can become a potential drug is a tedious and arduous task. Thus, several different algorithms were developed that would facilitate easy and rapid identification. From the traditional medicinal chemistry of making compound by compound, drug discovery took a quantum jump when the combinatorial methods were applied for compound synthesis. However, the small-molecule inhibitor discovery programs breathed a new life with the introduction of an algorithm popularly called as diversity-oriented synthesis (DOS). The traditional medicinal chemistry facilitates the evaluation of one compound at a time and the later-introduced combinatorial chemistry gives compounds that are complex and similar.

However, DOS allows us to prepare compounds that are complex but diverse in nature, so the chances of obtaining a hit molecule will be very high compared to the combinatorial methodology. DOS can be defined as a deliberate, simultaneous and efficient synthesis of more than one target compound in a divergent route exploiting complexity-generating reactions, which are traditionally practiced in organic synthesis (Fig. 1.6). Such an endeavor requires the use of branch points as well as very efficient regio- and stereochemical reactions.

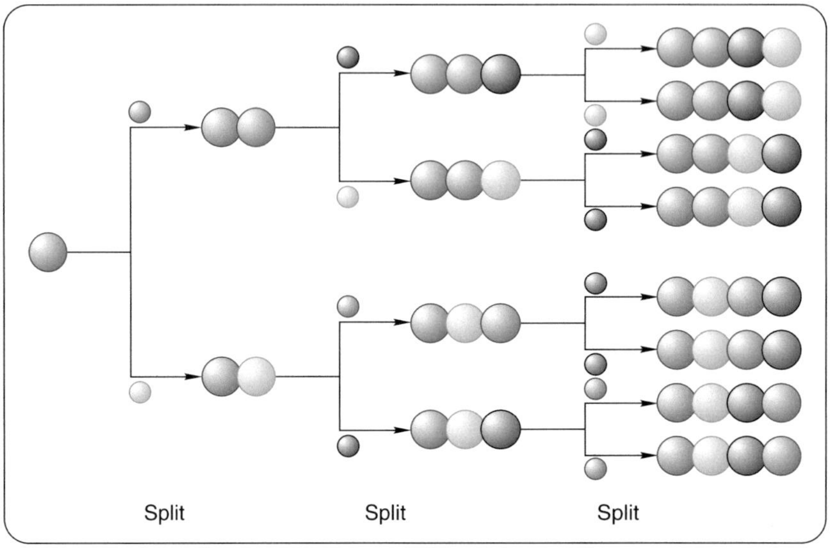

Fig. 1.5 *Schematic of Parallel Synthesis (For color figure please see Plate 2)*

DOS finds applications in a variety of fields from catalysis to HTS for biologically active compounds. The drug discovery process has gained overwhelmingly from the principles of DOS to the lead or hit identification, and hence facilitates the discovery of new chemical entities (NCEs). In this context, there are two types of approaches for lead identification.

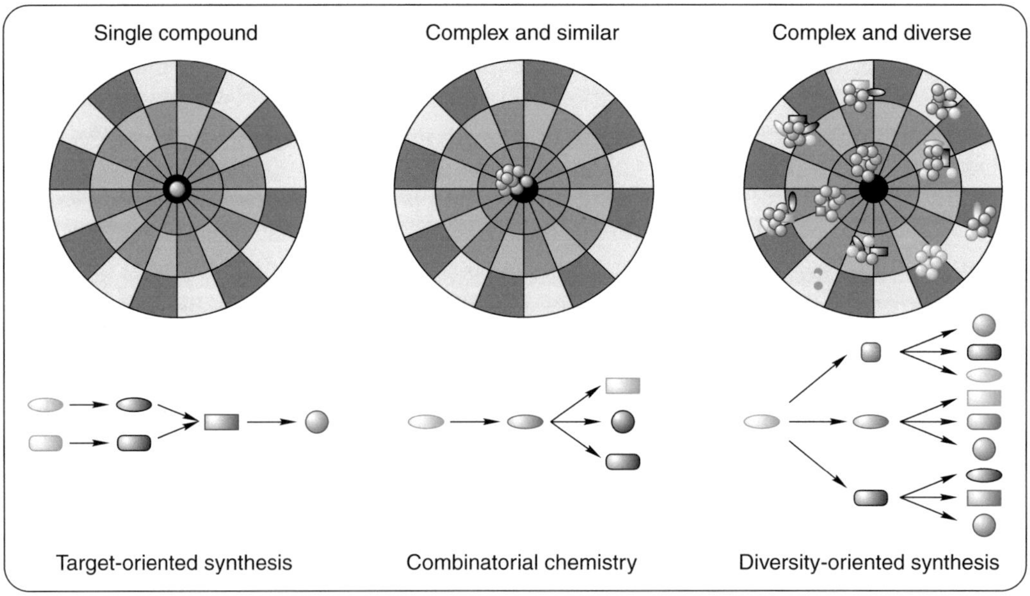

Fig. 1.6 *Target-Oriented Synthesis, Combinatorial Chemistry and Diversity-Oriented Synthesis (For color figure please see Plate 2)*

The first approach looks for a small molecule that causes the desired phenotype, which is subsequently probed for the protein responsible for the phenotypic change. For example, it is well reported that the size and morphology of a cell changes upon its entry into the mitotic phase of the cell cycle. Thus, a simple morphological change effected by a library of 16,000 commercially available compounds was studied in a high-throughput manner to identify a small-molecule inhibitor HR22C16 as an antimitotic agent. Furthermore, the protein responsible for this phenotype was identified as Eg5, a key protein involved in the transportation of DNA from the poles to the middle of the bipolar spindle during the mitosis. The second approach starts with a target such as a typical protein and looks for small molecules that modulate its function. In both approaches, a large collection of diverse small molecule libraries is required for the screening, and these can be effectively synthesized by applying the salient features of DOS.

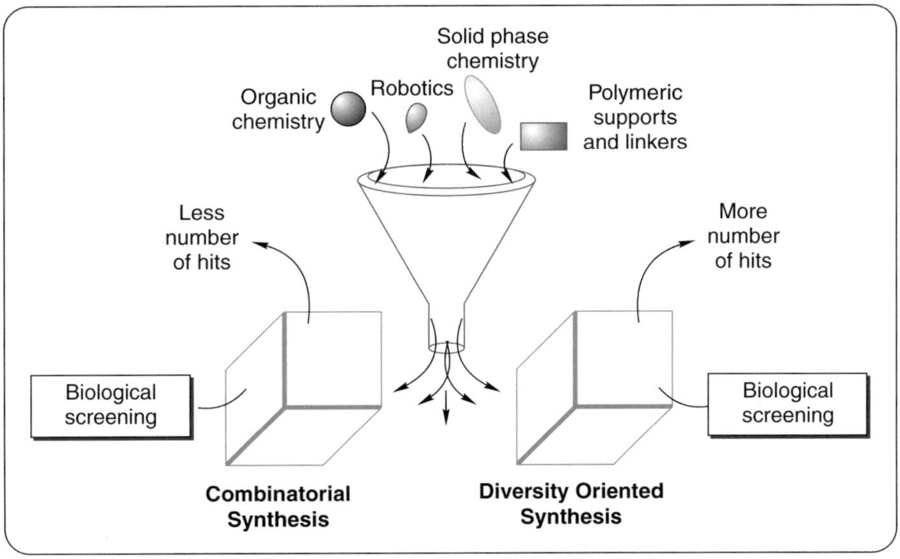

Fig. 1.7 *Combinatorial Chemistry versus Diversity-Oriented Synthesis*

In conclusion, DOS and combinatorial chemistry play a pivotal role in the design, synthesis and discovery of small-molecular probes, which can potentially become drugs of the future. Often drug discovery platforms utilize multiple algorithms while identifying the hit molecule or taking the hit molecule to a lead molecule (Fig. 1.7).

Peptidomimetic libraries are also gaining pace due to combinatorial chemistry. A peptide library is a systematic combination of many peptides synthesized on solid resins. Combinatorial chemistry has taken these peptide libraries a step further by mimicking them or chemically transforming them to create peptidomimetic libraries. While many peptide libraries are limited to the use of L-amino acids, which makes it difficult for these peptides to resist proteolysis, peptidomimetic libraries, on the other hand, employ D-amino acids and unnatural amino acids, making them highly stable to proteolytic digestion (Peng *et al.*, 2006). These peptidomimetic libraries are gaining importance in the field of drug discovery, especially in the field of clinical oncology.

Molecular Diversity

Molecular diversity is the study of structural, physicochemical and biological heterogeneous elements of molecular collection. With the advances in HTS, molecular diversity has moved a step forward and involves studying molecular similarities, structure–activity relationships among molecules, and statistical design. By doing so, it reduces the redundancy and cost of experiments and, hence, increases the chances of discovering a new drug. Various diversity calculations are used to develop appropriate selection strategies, which allow syntheses of the smallest number of compounds.

REFERENCES

Anderson, N.L., Anderson, N.G. (1998). Proteome and proteomics: New technologies, new concepts, and new words. *Electrophoresis* **19**:1853–1861.

Armstrong, J.W. (1997). *HTS and Robotics Implementation: A Critique of Robotics Equipment and Strategies.* HTS Consulting Ltd.: Thousand Oaks, CA, 19–33.

Baldwin, M.A., Medzihradszky, K.F., Lock, C.M., Fisher, B., Settineri, T.A., Burlingame, A.L. (2001). Matrix-assisted laser desorption/ionization coupled with quadrupole/orthogonal acceleration time-of-flight mass spectrometry for protein discovery, identification, and structural analysis. *Analytical Chemistry* **73**:1707–1720.

Baxevanis, A.D., Ouellette, B.F.F., eds. (2005). *Bioinformatics: A Practical Guide to the Analysis of Genes and Proteins*, 3rd ed., Wiley.

Blackstock, W.P., Weir, M.P. (1999). Proteomics: Quantitative and physical mapping of cellular proteins. *Trends in Biotechnology* **17**:121–127.

Fauman, E.B., Hopkins, A.L., Groom, C.R. (2003). Structural bioinformatics in drug discovery. *Methods of Biochemical Analysis* **44**:477–497.

Feher, M., Schmidt, J.M. (2003). Property distributions: Differences between drugs, natural products, and molecules from combinatorial chemistry. *Journal of Chemical Information and Computer Sciences* **43**:218–227.

Fenn, J.B., Mann, M., Meng, C.K., Wong, S.F., Whitehouse, C.M. (1989). Electrospray ionization for mass spectrometry of large biomolecules. *Science* **246**:64–71.

Frey, R.B. and Lesney, M.S. (2000). Anodynes and Esrogens: The pharmaceutical decade. The pahrmaceutical century: Ten decades of drug discovery. Supplement to American Chemical Society, 92–109.

Furka, A., Sebestyén, F., Asgedom, M., Dibó, G. (1991). General method for rapid synthesis of multicomponent peptide mixtures. *International Journal of Peptide and Protein Research* **37(6)**:487–493.

Geysen, H.M., Rodda, S.J., Mason, T.J. (1986). *A priori* delineation of a peptide which mimics a discontinuous antigenic determinant. *Molecular Immunology* **23**:709–715.

Gordeeva E.V., Lushnikov D.E., Zefirov N.S. (1992). COMPASS program–An original semi-empirical approach to computer-assisted synthesis. *Tetrahedron* **48**:3789–3804.

Görg, A., Obermaier, C., Boguth, G., Harder, A., Scheibe, B., Wildgruber, R., Weiss, W. (2000). The current state of two-dimensional electrophoresis with immobilized pH gradients. *Electrophoresis* **21**:1037–1053.

Hamilton, S., Armstrong, J.W., Gerren, R.A., Janssen, A.M., Petersen, J., Stanton, R.A. (1996). An overview of automated biotechnology screening. *Lab Automation and Robotics* **8**:287–294.

Hanash, S. (2001). 2-D or not 2-D–Is there a future for 2-D gels in proteomics? Insights from York Proteomic Meeting. *Proteomics* **1**:635–637.

Hanash, S.M., Bobek, M.P., Rickman, D.S., Williams, T., Rouillard, J.M., Kuick, R., Puravs, E. (2002). Integrating cancer genomics and proteomics in the post-genome era. *Proteomics* **2**:69–75.

Haqqani, A.S., Kelly, J.F., Stanimirovic, D.B. (2008). Quantitative protein profiling by mass spectrometry using label-free proteomics. *Methods in Molecular Biology* **439**:241–256.

Hernandez, P., Müller, M., Appel, R.D. (2006). Automated protein identification by tandem mass spectrometry: Issues and strategies. *Mass Spectrometry Reviews* **25**:235–254.

Houghten, R.A., Pinilla, C., Blondelle, S.E., Appel, J.R., Dooley, C.T., Cuervo, C.H. (1991). Generation and use of synthetic peptide combinatorial libraries for basic research and drug discovery. *Nature* **354**:84–86.

Jungblut, P.R. (2001). Proteome analysis of bacterial pathogens. *Microbes and Infection* **3**:831–840.

Klose, J. (1975). Protein mapping by combined isoelectric focusing and electrophoresis: A two-dimensional technique. *Humangenetik* **26**:231–243.

Lam, K.S., Salmon, S.E., Hersh, E.M., Hruby, V.J., Kazmierski, W.M., Knapp, R.J. (1991). A new type of synthetic peptide library for identifying ligand-binding activity. *Nature* **354**:82–84.

Lesney, M. (2000). Patents and Potions: Entering the Pharmaceutical Century; The Pharmaceutical Century Ten Decades of Drug Discovery. *Supplement to American Chemical Society*, 18–31.

Lipinski, C.A., Lombardo, F., Dominy, B.W., Feeney, P.J. (1997). Experimental and computational approaches to estimate solubility and permeability in drug discovery and development settings. *Advanced Drug Delivery Reviews* **23**:3–25, doi:10.1016/S0169-409X(00)00129-0.

Liu, H., Lin, D., Yates III, J.R. (2002). Multidimensional separations for protein/peptide analysis in the post-genomic era. *Biotechniques* **32**:898–911.

Martin, D.B., Nelson, P.S. (2001). From genomics to proteomics: Techniques and applications in cancer research. *Trends in Cell Biology* **11**:S60–S65.

Mattow, J., Jungblut, P.R., Schaible, U.E., Mollenkopf, H., Lamer, S., Zimny-Ardnt, U., Hagens, K., Muller, E., Kaufmann, S.H.E. (2001). Identification of proteins from *Mycobacterium tuberculosis* missing in attenuated *Mycobacterium bovis* BCG strains. *Electrophoresis* **21**:2936–2946.

Merchant, M., Weinberger, S.R. (2000). Recent advancements in surface-enhanced laser desorption/ionization time-of-flight mass spectrometry. *Electrophoresis* **21**:1164–1177.

Merrifield, R.B. (1963). Solid phase peptide synthesis. I. The synthesis of a tetrapeptide. *Journal of American Chemical Society* **85**:2149–2154.

Nelson, R.W., Jarwik, J.W., Taillon, B.E., Tubbs, K.A. (1999). BIA/MS of epitope-tagged peptides directly from *E. coli* lysate: Multiplex detection and protein identification at low-femtomole to subfemtomole levels. *Analytical Chemistry* **71**:2858–2865.

Newmann, D.J., and Cragg, G.M. (2007). Natural products as sources of new drugs over the last 25 years. *Journal of Natural Products* **70**:461–477.

O'Farrell, P.H. (1975). High resolution two-dimensional electrophoresis of proteins. *Journal of Biological Chemistry* **250**:4007–4021.

Peng, L., Ruiwu, L., Mari, J., Wan, X., Takad, Y., La, K.S. (2006). Combinatorial chemistry identifies high-affinity peptidomimetics against $\alpha_4\beta_1$ integrin for *in vivo* tumor imaging. *Nature Chemical Biology* **2**:381–389.

Pizzi, R. (2000). Salving with science: The roarong twenties and the great depression, The pharmaceutical Century: Ten decades of drug discovery. Supplement to American Chemical Society, 34–51.

Raju, T.N.K. (2000). The Nobel chronicles. *Lancet* **355**:1022.

Rathin, C.D. (2002). Progress and partnerships in proteomics. *American Biotechnology Laboratory* **20**:42–48.

Rodriguez, J.M., Salas, M.L., Santaren, J.F. (2001). African swine fever virus–induced polypeptides in porcine alveolar macrophages and in Vero cells: Two-dimensional analysis. *Proteomics* **1**:1441–1446.

Rollinger, J.M., Stuppner, H., Langer, T. (2008). Virtual screening for the discovery of bioactive natural products. *Progress in Drug Research* **65**:213–249.

Schonberger, S.J., Edgar, P.F., Kydd, R., Faull, R.L.M., Cooper, G.J.S. (2001). Proteomic analysis of the brain in Alzheimer's disease: Molecular phenotype of a complex disease process. *Proteomics* **1**:1519–1528.

Sioud, M. (2007). Main approaches to target discovery and validation. *Methods in Molecular Biology* **360**: 1–12.

Somberg, J.C. (1996). In: Welling, P.G., Lasagna, L., Banakar, U.V. (eds), *The Drug Discovery Process: Increasing Efficiency and Cost Effectiveness*. New York: Marcel Dekker.

——— (1996). The Evolving Drug Discovery and Development Process, In: *The Drug Development Process: Increasing Efficiency and Cost Effectiveness*, Eds. Welling, P.G., Lasagna, L., Banakar, U.V., pp. 1–38, Marcel Dekker, New York.

Sparkman, O.D. (2000). *Mass Spectrometry Desk Reference*. Pittsburgh, PA: Global View.

Thornton, J.M., Todd, A.E., Milburn, D., Borkakoti, N., Orengo, C.O. (2000). From structure to function: Approaches and limitations. *Nature Structural Biology* (Suppl.) **7**:991–994.

Wallace, R.W. (1998). A little too much? Expense versus return in HTS miniaturization. *Drug Discovery Today* **3**:299.

Wang, S., Sim T.B., Kim, Y.S., Chang, Y.T. (2004). Tools for target identification and validation. *Current Opinion in Chemical Biology* **8**:371–377.

Washburn, M.P., Wolter, D., Yates, J.R. (2001). Large-scale analysis of the yeast proteome by multidimensional protein identification technology. *Nature Biotechnology* **19**:242–247.

Zhang, Z., Smith, D.L. (1994). Probing noncovalent structural features of proteins by mass spectrometry. *Mass Spectrometry Reviews* **13**:411–429.

2

Target Identification and Validation in Drug Discovery

***Samashekara, N.*[1] *and C.N. Ramchand**[1,2]**

[1]*Laila Pharmaceuticals Pvt. Ltd., Chennai, India*
[2]*Visiting faculty, Swinburne University of Technology Melbourne, Australia*

The process of developing a new drug involves two main stages, viz. discovery and development. The objective of drug discovery is to find synthetic compounds or natural products that will cure or ameliorate diseases. The discovery stage is the key step, which includes target selection, lead identification and preclinical studies, while the development stage includes clinical trials, manufacturing and marketing of the developed drug and managing the life cycle of the drug.

The resources and time required for new drug discovery are enormous. The discovery has become a costly process on account of the possibility of the end failure of drugs, due to either lack of efficacy or high toxicity. The earlier drug discoveries were either accidental or serendipitous in nature. In contrast, the modern process typically starts by identifying potential targets that participate in the disease process. Rational drug design is aimed at the targeted discovery and optimization of new drugs based on detailed structural and chemical information of the protein. Drug target is the specific binding site/molecule of a drug *in vivo*, through which the drug exerts its action. Selection of the right targets is one of the key decisions in drug discovery. A wrong target will generate a lot of expense without the possibility of finding the required drug. One of the strategies to solve this problem is identification and validation of targets. The identification of suitable target populations can often substantially reduce development times and costs, and this approach holds the promise of identifying more efficacious compounds with fewer undesirable side effects and also reduce the chances of drug

**ramchand@lailapharma.com*

failure during clinical trials. This approach also provides a rich source of intellectual property and can act as a valuable competitive differentiator for companies seeking proprietary positions for drugs that act through novel mechanisms.

Target identification and validation is a highly complex and resource-intensive process, which requires an integral use of various tools, approaches and information. Reliable technologies for addressing target identification and validation are the foundation of successful drug development. A wide array of target identification and validation approaches and technologies are available, including physiological approach, mechanism-based approach, omics approach, gene expression profiling and proteomics. Biomarkers and metabolomic profiling are the emerging tools for monitoring the biological effects of manipulating a potential drug target. Technologies such as DNA microarrays, protein microarrays, chemical microarrays, genome database mining, bioinformatics, antisense technology, zinc finger proteins, haplotype analysis, chemical genomics and proteomics, directed gene disruption, conditional gene expression by promoter replacement, aptamers, knockout/in, gain-of-function, transgenic models, pathways analysis, chemical knockouts and chemical biology and protein inhibition provide researchers with a multipronged approach to identifying and validating new targets. More recently, RNA interference (RNAi) technology has emerged as an extremely useful and efficient method for drug target identification and validation. With the advances in genomics, proteomics and bioinformatics, there is a great potential for identification of high-quality drugs and also for reducing the time and cost of drug discovery. The most successful approaches combine several technologies to provide a detailed understanding of the biological effects of altering the activity of a single target.

INTRODUCTION TO DRUG DISCOVERY

Drug is "a substance intended for use in the diagnosis, cure, mitigation, treatment, or prevention of disease" or "as a component of a medicine" (The Merriam-Webster Online Dictionary). Drugs generally affect the biological processes and must be present in the body at an adequate concentration for it to act at the specific site, where it can exert its effect. Drug must be easily absorbed, metabolized and eliminated from the body without causing any injury. The process of developing a new drug consists of two main stages, called discovery and development. The objective of drug discovery is to find synthetic compounds or natural products that will cure or ameliorate diseases (Mart *et al.*, 2006). The discovery stage is a key step, which includes target selection, lead identification and preclinical studies, while the development stage includes clinical trials, manufacturing and marketing of the developed drug and managing the life cycle of the drug. Target may be a biomolecule such as gene or protein, which can potentially be affected by a drug molecule. Once the target is identified, a promising lead molecule can be developed, which in turn can be used therapeutically. The lead is optimized by further analyzing and screening through *in vitro*, *ex vivo* and *in vivo* techniques to get the drug molecule, which will further go for preclinical development to access the pharmacokinetics, pharmacodynamics and toxicity. Once the preclinical studies are over, the drug will go through Phase I, Phase II and Phase III development programs. After starting with thousands of compounds, only a few drug candidates continue into the development stage for clinical trials and manufacturing (Lifeng *et al.*, 2008).

CLASSICAL/TRADITIONAL DRUG DISCOVERY PROCESS

Earlier drug discoveries were either accidental or serendipitous in nature (Ratti & Trist, 2001; Sweeny, 2002). In the past, people have been found to cure diseases through trial and error, with berries, roots and barks used for medicinal purposes to alleviate the symptoms of illness (Boa, 2003). Drug discovery has been a product of trial and error, guided as much by intuition as serendipity of chemists, biologists and physicians (Papanikolaw, 1999). However, the later variants of these drugs were synthesized by analogizing to produce drugs with better pharmacokinetics, fewer side effects and better efficacy, and this approach proved to be very successful in the discovery and development of new drugs (Sweeny, 2002). For example, the willow bark, which contains salicin, was used as a fever reducer in the same vein as the cinchona bark from which quinine was discovered (Boa, 2003). Both digitalis and aspirin, used to treat dropsy, brought about by congestive heart failure, and willow bark for arthritis were described and used hundreds of years before the isolation of their active components. In a similar way, willow bark (*Salix alba*) was an antipyretic drug known to the ancients; in the early 19th century a glucoside of salicylic acid was isolated from it, and this was followed shortly by the isolation of salicylic acid, which was shown to be antipyretic. Later, widespread use followed the recognition of its analgesic activity. The drug discovery process would continue to be by trial and error until the early decades of the mid-20th century, when the pharmacological basis of diseases and drugs began to be defined (Boa, 2003). Many successful drugs such as chlorpromazine, meprobamate and benzodiazepines were discovered by trial and error (Ratti & Trist, 2001). However, this approach at that time suffered from a lack of sufficient molecules with high enough structural diversity (Sweeny, 2002). The compounds from which these variants are made were initially discovered by a combination of accident and luck, but became increasingly based on systematic attempts to exploit the increasing knowledge base of chemistry, biology and medicine. Over time, companies and research groups developed large libraries of compounds, which could be tested for effect against the disease of interest (Sweeny, 2002).

SERENDIPITY AND DRUG DISCOVERY

Serendipity was sought in the 1950s and 1960s in the pharmaceutical industry by screening known compounds or randomly testing any molecules that were at hand, to a large part in *in vivo* models. Serendipity has always played an important role in science, especially in the search for new drugs (Kubinyi, 1999). The earlier approach to drug discovery focused more on the efficacy of drugs than their toxicity. Traditional pharmacological drug discovery approaches involve the incorporation of a large number of hypothetical targets into cell-based assays and automated high-throughput screening (HTS) of vast chemical compound libraries. Lack of predictive models often leads to failures in drug development due to toxicity and/or lack of efficacy (Kubinyi, 1999) in drug discovery.

The discovery of *Penicillium* strain by Alexander Fleming was serendipitous in nature (Moulay, 2007), which led to the development of penicillin and its synthetic derivatives. The discovery of chlordiazepoxide, which is a potent tranquillizer, resulted from an unexpected chemical rearrangement (Kubinyi, 1999; Ratti and Trist, 2001). The hallucinogenic activity of lysergide (LSD) is another well-known serendipitous discovery. Albert Hofmann, while synthesizing lysergic acid diethylamide, inhaled minute amounts of the vapor that escaped from the flask containing LSD and he experienced hallucinations (Hugo Kubinyi, 1999; Moulay, 2007). Acetylsalicylic acid, a known irreversible cyclooxygenase (COX) inhibitor, preventing blood coagulation by the inhibition of thrombocyte aggregation, was originally designed as a prodrug of salicylic acid to treat headache, fever and rheumatic diseases (Kubinyi, 1999). The potent antitumor compound cisplatin was discovered when biophysicists investigated the effect of electric current on the growth of *Escherichia coli*. The observed cytotoxic effect led to the surprising result that it was due to the cisplatin in the electrolysis medium (Sneader, 1996; Kubinyi, 1999). Cyclosporin, an immunosuppressant drug that is used to prevent the rejection of organ transplant, is a serendipitous discovery by Sandoz, which had observed it to be an immunosuppressant while doing other experiments (Roberts, 1989; Sneader, 1996; Kubinyi, 1999). Phenylbutazone and valproic acid were designed as solubility enhancers for other drugs. However, both compounds turned out to be valuable drugs on their own (Kubinyi, 1999). Discovery of quinine, an antimalarial drug, is serendipitous. Its therapeutic application was discovered when an Indian suffering from fever ingested water from a pool that was nearby a cinchona tree. Vaccination was discovered serendipitously by Edward Jenner, who was told by a milkmaid that the person who caught cowpox (a harmless disease caught via contact with cow) never got smallpox (Moulay, 2007).

TOWARD RATIONAL DRUG DISCOVERY

Drug Discovery in the 1950s and 1960s

Drug discovery during this period was serendipitous. The lead molecules were found by chance or by screening available chemicals, and the molecules were later optimized by medicinal chemists to produce candidates, which were moved to the development phase and marketed (Fig. 2.1). However, the approach at that time suffered from a lack of sufficient molecules with high enough structural diversity, and the common use of animal models meant that other factors such as absorption, metabolism, brain penetration and pharmacokinetics had profound effects on the number of active molecules found. Many chemicals that showed activity in the animal models were of unknown mechanism. This greatly impeded the drug development process, particularly when the lead failed due to toxicity or poor pharmacokinetics during clinical trials because of lack of information on mechanism of action of tested drug (Ratti and Trist, 2001).

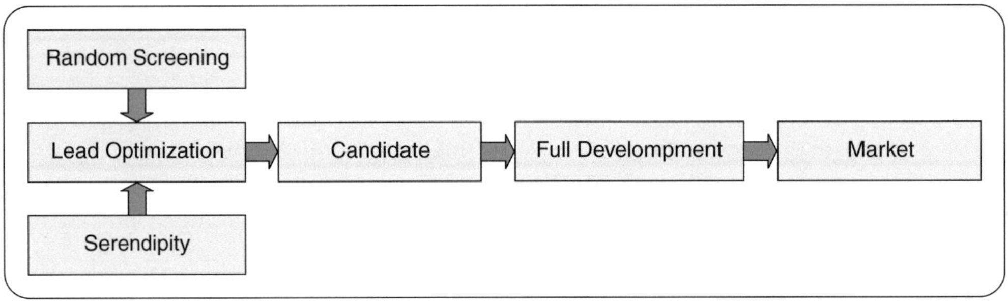

Fig. 2.1 ***Drug Discovery in the 1950s and 1960s***

Source: Ratti and Trist (2001).

Drug Discovery in the 1980s

The process of discovering drug by a serendipitous approach was improved to a more rational approach. In this improvised approach, which became mainstream in the 1980s, *in vitro* assays using animal tissues (rather than previously used *in vivo* methods) became central in the process for giving valuable information on structure–activity relationships, for a widely used study in the refinement of pharmaceutical agents and in the identification of the structural alerts for toxicity (Michael *et al.*, 2003) and eventual pharmacophore construction. In this way, if the lead molecule fails there is sufficient information around the structure and activity to allow the cause for failure to be extricated from the molecule (Fig. 2.2).

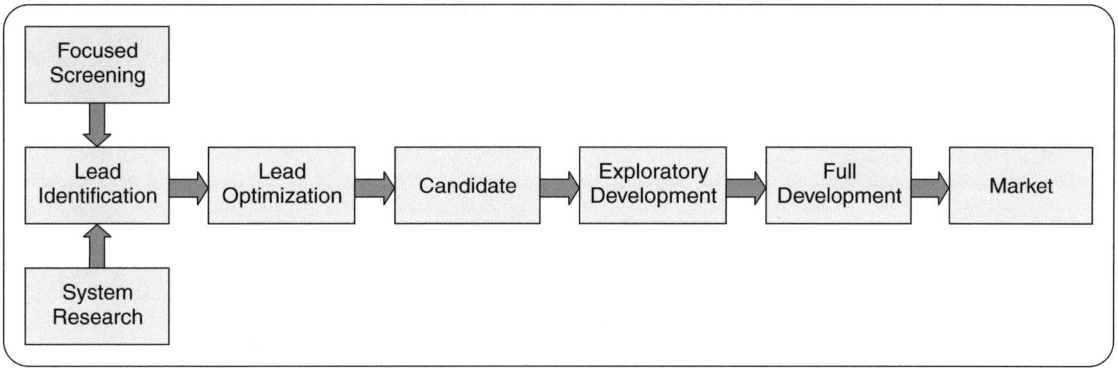

Fig. 2.2 *Drug Discovery in the 1980s*

Source: Ratti and Trist (2001).

Advances in synthetic organic chemistry led to the identification of many key chemical molecules that offered more opportunities to develop novel compounds. Many new drugs emerged through this route, particularly those now being used to treat infections, infestations, cancers, ulcers and heart and blood pressure conditions. Many drugs were developed through random screening of thousands of chemicals synthesized as dyestuffs and the like; many others resulted from serendipity (Patwardhan *et al.*, 2004).

Drug Discovery Today (1990s and Beyond)

A different approach to drug development was to use the body's own biological molecules for disease treatment. Antibodies, cytokines and other immune system substances can be produced in the laboratory for use in disease treatment. This approach had already been pioneered in the 1920s by companies such as Lilly, which developed injectable insulin for the treatment of diabetes, but is most closely associated with the rise of biotechnology companies over the past 30 years. These companies sought to identify which naturally occurring biological molecules are associated with disease and to use newly discovered biotechnology methods to manufacture these compounds (Sweeny, 2002). Thus, the traditional drug discovery strategy based on experience and serendipity was no longer able to meet the needs of pharmaceutical companies. A shift from serendipity to rationality in drug discovery happened. Rational drug discovery based on knowledge of the biological system being investigated allows highly specific selective antagonists and agonists to be developed (Fig. 2.3). These molecules can then be developed as lead compounds, drug candidates and even drugs (Chen and Du, 2007).

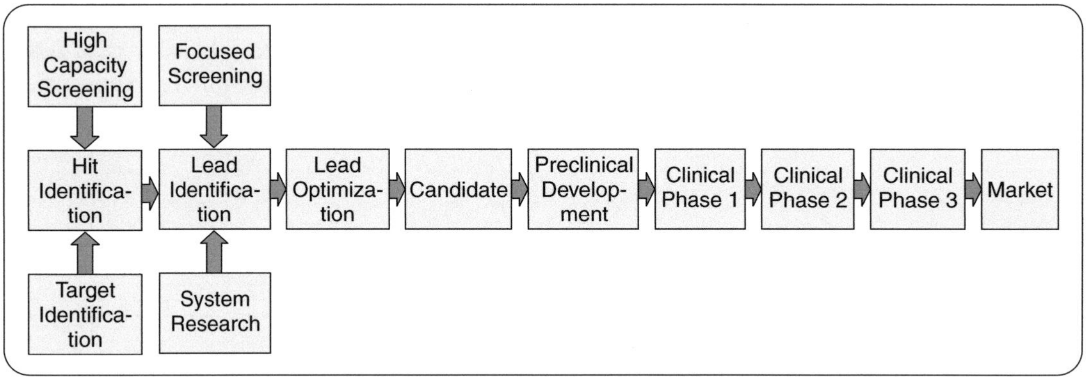

Fig. 2.3 ***Drug Discovery Today (1990s and Beyond)***

Source: Ratti and Trist (2001).

RATIONAL DRUG DISCOVERY

Rational drug design (RDD) is a method for developing new pharmaceuticals that typically involves the elucidation of fundamental physiological mechanisms. RDD is aimed at the targeted discovery and optimization of new drugs based on detailed structural and chemical information of the protein. Unlike the earlier approaches to drug discovery, through trial-and-error testing of chemical substances on animals, and matching the apparent effects to treatments, RDD begins with a knowledge of specific chemical responses in the body, and tailoring combinations of these to fit a treatment profile. It thus combines the quest for a scientific understanding of natural phenomena with the design of useful technology and hence integrates the epistemic and practical aims of research and development. The rational method usually involves a theoretical understanding of which protein is targeted by the drug, how the drug acts on it and which mechanisms lead to the desired therapeutic effects (Adam, 2005).

This approach is based on the very reasonable assumption that if one knew the structure of a natural ligand and that of its receptor, one should be able to say something useful about the kind of molecules that might mimic or antagonize the activity of the natural ligand (Adam, 2005). It would be easier to find molecules that would interact more efficiently in an active protein site once the three-dimensional (3D) structure was known because chemists then would be able to see how to design more efficient drugs (Sinskey and Finkelstein, 2002). In this approach much reliance is placed on X-ray crystallography, very high field nuclear magnetic resonance (NMR), computer-assisted molecular modeling, quantum-mechanical calculations, cloning and expression of receptors and peptidic ligands (O'Connor, 1993). RDD programs have not, as yet, many successes to point to, but interesting and potentially useful applications have been described for inhibitors of renin, HIV-1 protease and the carbonic anhydrase associated with glaucoma (Adam, 2005).

Several factors such as rapidly increasing costs and longer development times have contributed to the growth of rational approach to its current significant size. RDD has gradually become more popular in drug development since its first instances in the 1950s, and triggered by a number of impressive successes such as the development of the cholesterol-lowering drug lovastatin or the antihypertensive drug captopril in the 1970s, RDD acquired the status of a professed methodological ideal in the 1980s (Gambardella, 1995). This is also evidenced by the awarding of the Nobel prize for medicine or physiology of 1988 to the pharmacologists Sir James Black, Gertrude B. Elion and George H. Hitchings, three pioneers of RDD (Nobel Assembly, 1988) and (Adam, 2005). However, this approach initially did not deliver the results because crystal structure does not always accurately depict how a molecule will behave *in vivo*. Also, medicinal chemists often found it difficult to develop new structures for the "rational" approach. This led to the development of combinatorial chemistry to provide large, diverse libraries for drug discovery (Sinskey and Finkelstein, 2002). The best example for RDD is that of imatinib, a tyrosine kinase inhibitor designed specifically for the bcr-abl fusion protein that is characteristic for Philadelphia chromosome-positive leukemias (chronic myelogenous leukemia and occasionally acute lymphocytic leukemia). Imatinib is substantially different from previous drugs for cancer, as most agents of chemotherapy simply target rapidly dividing cells, not differentiating between cancer cells and other tissues (BambooWeb dictionary).

DRUG TARGET

Drug target is a key molecule involved in a particular metabolic or signal transduction pathway that is specific to a disease condition or a specific disease (Chen and Du, 2007).

From a pharmacological viewpoint, a drug target is either inhibited or activated by drug molecules (e.g. small organic molecules, antibodies and therapeutic proteins). Drug target is the specific binding site of a drug *in vivo* through which the drug exerts its action. Drug molecules can physically attach to a drug target, triggering a cascade of intracellular biochemical reactions, followed by a cellular reaction (Wissenbach *et al.*, 2004).

A specific drug target might have the following characteristics:

1. The drug target is a biomolecule(s), normally a protein that could exist in isolated or complex modality.
2. The biomolecules have special sites that match other molecules (commonly small molecules with special structures). These molecules could be endogenous or extraneous substances such as chemical molecules (drugs).
3. The biomolecular structure might change when the biomolecule binds to small molecules and the changes in structure normally are reversible.
4. Following the change in the biomolecule's structure various physiological responses occur and induce regulation of the cell, organ, tissue, or body status.
5. The physiological responses triggered by the changes in biomolecule structure play a major role in complex regulation and have a therapeutic effect on pathological conditions.

6. The expression, activity and structure of the biomolecule might change over the duration of the pathological process.
7. Small molecules binding to the biomolecules are drugs (Chen and Du, 2007).

The targets especially include those belonging to protein families that are targeted with currently marketed drugs—specifically G protein-coupled receptors, ion channels, nuclear receptors, proteases, phosphodiesterases, kinases and other key enzymes besides ion channels (Figures 2.4 and 2.5) (Brueggemann *et al.*, 2004). Ribosome, a synthesis machine of 2.3 MDa molecular weight formed by three long RNA chains and about 55 proteins, is the target of half of the antibiotics characterized so far (Vicens and Westhof, 2003). Targets for large molecule drugs are the secreted proteins, both those expressed on the cell membrane and those secreted into extracellular fluids. Cell surface receptors are targets for development of monoclonal antibodies (Mabs) and recombinant fusion proteins that carry protein ligands for the receptors (Haberman, 2005).

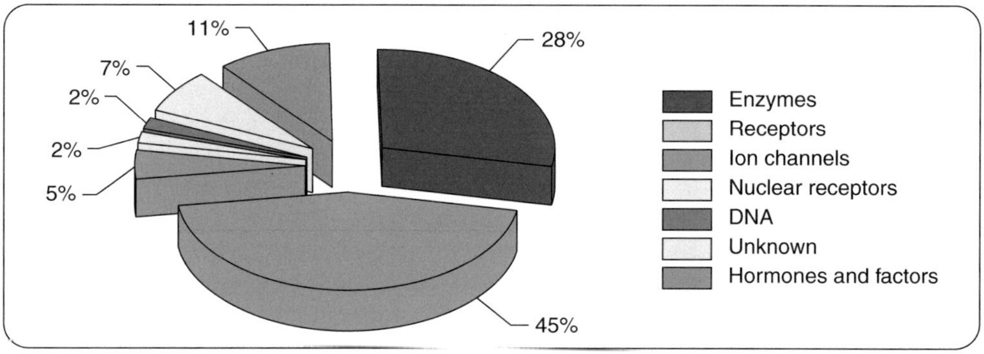

Fig. 2.4 ***Distribution of Targets by Biochemical Criteria (For color figure please see Plate 3)***

Source: Potential Drug Target Database.

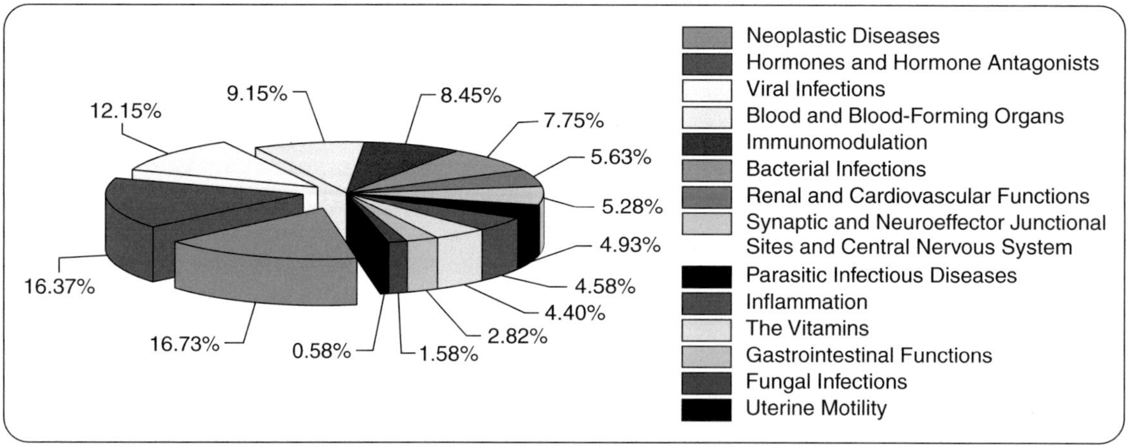

Fig. 2.5 ***Distribution of Targets in Therapeutic Areas (For color figure please see Plate 3)***

Source: Potential Drug Target Database.

Many drugs share the common target and one drug may have more than one target. When a new drug target is discovered and validated, researchers usually hope to identify more specific drugs to target. However, a key understanding to keep in mind is that the body is a subtle organism and a more specific drug might disrupt the homeostasis of the body (Chen and Du, 2007). Multitarget lead discovery, a newly developed combination therapy, is a promising tool for the identification of unexpectedly novel effects of drug combinations. This approach is increasingly used to treat many types of diseases, such as acquired immune deficiency syndrome (AIDS), atherosclerosis, cancer and depression (Borisy *et al.*, 2003). Traditional medications often contain multicomponent extracts of natural products which act by attacking multiple targets (Rollinger *et al.*, 2006; Shafikhani, 2006). Memantine, a drug used to treat Alzheimer's disease and other multitarget noncompetitive NMDA receptor antagonists, shows that low-affinity, multitarget drugs might have a lower prevalence and a reduced range of side effects than high-affinity, single-target drugs (Csermely *et al.*, 2005).

High-Quality Targets and Hard Targets

High-quality targets are those that are expected to give rise to large-selling drugs. However, determining the true value of a target depends on extensive research, including both laboratory and clinical studies (Haberman, 2005). The completion of the human genome project in 2004 revealed many putative proteins that could transform modern medicine. Now, the challenge lies in translating the wealth of genomic information into new therapeutics. A critical step in this process is separating high-quality drug targets from futile ones and developing safe and effective drug compounds (Lum *et al.*, 2004).

Targets that cannot be addressed with currently available medicinal chemistry are called hard targets, such as intracellular signaling proteins involved in protein–protein interactions such as those between signaling proteins and those between cytokine or growth factor receptors and their protein ligands. It is very difficult to develop small-molecule agonists or antagonists to these target proteins as protein–protein interactions involve interactions over large surface areas, which is expected to make inhibition by small-molecule agents difficult. However, a few natural products have been developed that disrupt protein–protein interactions. For example, Ariad discovered small-molecule, non-peptide compounds that target the interaction between SH2 domains in many signaling proteins and their recognition sites, which are specific phosphotyrosine-containing amino acid sequences in proteins (Haberman, 2005).

Target Identification and Validation

The resources required for new drug discovery are enormous. The time to bring a drug to market averages 14–15 years and at the same time the average cost to bring a drug to market is \$1 billion (Dimasi, 2001). The early drug discovery was based on observation of the pharmacological properties of compounds and did not require knowledge of the molecular identity of the drug target. In contrast, the modern process typically starts by identifying potential targets that participate in the disease process (Belfield and Delaney, 2006). The discovery of new therapeutics often ends in costly failure. More than 60% of the drug failure is accounted for by lack of efficacy in Phase II (~53%

of compounds fail during Phase II) and/or Phase III trials and toxicity, including mechanism-based toxicity (European Patent EP1756304). Significant proportions of failures are due to unanticipated system-wide effects. Reducing failures early in development of drug is far more important than filling a pipeline with poorly chosen late-stage products that are likely to fail. Drugs fail in the clinic for two basic reasons—they either don't work or they prove to be unsafe—and both of these are often the direct result of faulty early target validation (Smith, 2003). Starting with the wrong target will generate a lot of expense without the possibility to make a drug in the end. Therefore target identification and validation is critical step of the modern discovery and careful selection of drug target would minimize the drug failure during clinical trials. Even the very first stages of drug discovery are expensive and no organization can afford to spend its resources on targets that have little association with the disease (Aberg, 2005). The major difficulty in drug discovery is understanding the complex chemical pathways involved in the disease process in order to find the most appropriate drug target, and then to discover or design a compound that modifies the chemical process at that point (Sweeny, 2002).

There is no adequate treatment for many of the 30,000 known diseases or the available drugs exhibit very uneven response rates because of the genetic variability of the patient population. Of the 200 drugs with the largest turnover in 1997, most targeted a 7G-protein-coupled receptor.

Strategies to solve the problems facing the pharmaceutical industry (declining/stagnating number of new molecular entities [NMEs]; increasing R&D costs; widening disparity between turnover and R&D costs) involve the following:

1. Identification and validation of new targets
2. Early identification of drug candidates worth evaluation
3. Optimization of development times
4. Early testing of drug candidates with the aid of biomarkers or surrogate markers
5. Mechanistic understanding of action mechanisms
6. Identification of genetic markers and effects of alleles on the absorption, distribution, metabolism and excretion of active ingredients, as well as the safety and efficacy of active ingredients

The process of target identification and validation has become an established discipline and its objective is to show that the modulation of the function of a given gene product has a potential therapeutic outcome (Belfield and Delaney, 2006). The drug discovery process can be described as the identification and validation of a disease target and the discovery and development of a chemical compound to interact with that target (Belfield and Delaney, 2006). This interaction can be to block, promote or otherwise modify the activity of the target. The history of drug development over the past century has been the accumulation of knowledge and techniques that provide a progressively more detailed understanding of both the target and the compound that could become a drug (Sweeny, 2002). The secret of success is the rapid and accurate identification of drug targets with true potential or high-quality targets (Belfield and Delaney, 2006). In today's drug discovery environment, researchers have access to an enormous amount of data, most of it coming from genomic, proteomic, *in vitro* and *in vivo* animal experiments. The challenge the pharmaceutical researcher faces is how to most efficiently use all these data by analyzing them and by extracting from them the bits of biological insight that will ultimately help to identify a novel, clinically relevant target, i.e. a molecular entity that both plays an important role in a particular disease's pathophysiology and is accessible to exogenous modulation (being a druggable target).

Target identification and validation are essential stages in the drug discovery pathway (Wang *et al.*, 2004; Lindsay, 2005). One of the first steps in the development of new small-molecule therapeutics is the selection of a suitable target whose biological activity can be directly linked to a pathological process (Verhelst and Bogyo, 2005). Target-based drug discovery has become the prevailing paradigm used by pharmaceutical and biotechnology companies and it holds the promise of identifying more efficacious compounds with fewer undesirable side effects. Target identification and validation is a highly complex and resource-intensive process, which requires an integral use of various tools, approaches and information (Wang *et al.*, 2004). These approaches provide a rich source of intellectual property and can act as valuable competitive differentiators for companies seeking proprietary positions for drugs that act through novel mechanisms. Companies have therefore invested significant resources in acquiring and developing technologies for identifying and validating new drug targets. Less than 500 drug targets participate in the mechanism of action of currently known drugs (Van Duin *et al.*, 2003). Using traditional approaches, targets are identified and evaluated using *in vitro* systems such as cell lines or primary cell culture. These *in vitro* systems suffer from the fact that they remove relevant cells from potentially important regulatory controls. In other cases, *in vivo* systems, such as animal models (e.g., knockouts and/or transgenics), are often used for this exploratory research. *In vivo* animal models present significant limitations as well. Typically they represent an artificially induced state meant to mimic the disease they intend to represent (Baillie and Michelson, 2002).

The identification of suitable target populations can often substantially reduce development times and costs. For example, a response rate of 10% would require a clinical study with 7000 patients over 12–18 months and would cost US$70 million, whereas at 50% the number of patients would be reduced to 300, the duration of the study to 3 months and the cost to US$1.5 million (Verlag and Aulendorf, 2002). Post-genomic drug research focuses more on the identification of specific biological targets (gene products, such as enzymes or proteins) for drugs, which can be manipulated to produce the desired effect (of curing a disease) with minimum disruptive side effects (Sridhar *et al.*, 2007).

TARGET IDENTIFICATION

Good drugs are potent and specific to the target identified, i.e. they must have strong effects on a specific biological pathway and minimal effects on all other pathways. Confirmation that a compound inhibits the intended target and the identification of undesirable secondary effects are important tasks in developing new drugs. Unraveling of the cellular pathways involved in a disease and identifying potential targets remain a major challenge in drug discovery (Mart *et al.*, 2006). One of the first steps in the development of therapeutics is the selection of a suitable target whose biological activity can be directly linked to a pathological process (Stevan *et al.*, 2005). Scientists use a variety of techniques to identify and isolate a target and learn more about its functions and how these influence disease. Compounds are then identified that have various interactions with drug targets helpful in treatment of a specific disease, and the appropriate science and technology will help in developing antagonists to a particular target. In the case of small-molecule drugs, druggable targets are those that can be addressed with currently available medicinal chemistry. These targets especially include those belonging to protein families such as G protein-coupled receptors, ion channels, nuclear receptors, proteases, phosphodiesterases, kinases and other key enzymes that are targeted with currently marketed drugs. Ion channels are excellent drug targets as they play a major role in many common diseases (Brueggemann *et al.*, 2004). Cell surface receptors are targets for development of monoclonal antibodies (Mabs) and recombinant fusion proteins that carry protein ligands for the receptors (Haberman, 2005). It is very difficult to interpret one's results, searching the databases, and deriving from them adequate information regarding a potential target's role in a given disease. Thus, validating a target with any degree of predictive confidence remains a major bottleneck for the industry. To understand the physiological implications of a potential target's function, one must know what is known about the role of that target in the disease and its progression.

Selection of the right targets is one of the key decisions in drug discovery. A wrong target will generate a lot of expense without the possibility of finding the required drug. Target can be wrong for many reasons, such as being not relevant to the disease, being different in animal systems compared to human, having different subunit compositions in various cells, or that the assay does not reflect the true situation in the diseased tissue (Aberg, 2005). Comprehensive methods that enable researchers to determine which genes or activities are affected by a given drug might improve the efficiency of the drug discovery process by quickly identifying potential protein targets, or by accelerating the identification of compounds likely to be toxic (Marton *et al.*,1998).

There are many tools and techniques available for the identification of potential drug targets. These new technologies in target identification and validation will greatly facilitate the target validation step of the drug discovery process (Liu *et al.*, 2004). Many putative new therapeutic targets have been identified with the advent of many high-throughput genomic and proteomic techniques, such as DNA microarrays (Schena *et al.*, 1995), differential RNA display reverse transcriptase-polymerase chain reaction (DDRT-PCR), reciprocal subtraction differential RNA display (RSDD), serial analysis of gene expression (SAGE), substraction hybridization, representation difference analysis (RDA), protein microarrays, chemical microarrays, genome database mining and highly sensitive mass spectrometry methods. Antisense and ribozyme technologies have traditionally been used to validate a drug target. Although these knockdown techniques work for some genes, they are not sufficiently reliable for systematic gene silencing in tissue culture. More recently, RNA interference (RNAi) technology has emerged as an extremely useful and efficient method for drug target identification and validation Besides using it as a powerful technique to validate a specific cancer therapeutic target, the RNAi technique has also been used to systematically study cancer-associated genes in tissue culture cell (Varambally *et al.*, 2002). Multigene disruption in single animals is an emerging technology that can augment the data gained from knockout models. Cell culture systems are important for drug target validation but they cannot replace transgenic animal models, which can provide a more accurate prediction of what will occur in humans (Liu *et al.*, 2004).

Different Approaches to Identify Drug Targets

Physiological Approach

As early as 50–70 years back, when drug discovery started on a reasonably rational basis, there was no true method to identify the actual protein drug targets. Thus many times it was dependent on the animal model that exhibits the phenotype of the disease target. In rational drug discovery, it is essential to know the single protein target, its conformation and configuration, its binding site of physiological ligand and its interaction with other proteins, eventually leading to the understanding of the phenotype characteristics. However, the characteristics of the proteins were not known because the protein itself was not identified. Scientists started using the next rational model, which is revel vent disease phenotype in whole animal or studying the cell. Many drugs in earlier stage were screened and developed through animal models, e.g., for metabolic disorders, gastrointestinal disorders, infection, inflammation, allergy and psychiatric diseases.

However such approaches also have drawbacks, as it is almost impossible to predict the side effects associated with the drug treatment as there is no easy way to study the drug interaction with other functional proteins. However, a majority of drugs developed till the late 1980s have been based on this method.

Subsequent to this earlier approach, scientists used a more comprehensive and targeted approach by identifying the biochemical pathway associated with disease process. In this approach, a specific protein target can be assayed in a cell system, e.g. crude enzyme. This approach will give an idea of the inhibitor or the activation of a specific target or drug-binding ability. An example of such an approach was the development of captopril, which inhibits angiotensin converting enzyme (ACE), which controls hypertension. A step ahead of this, a way of studying the target is the use of molecular techniques and subsequently the use of genomics, proteomics, metabolics and transcriptomics in identifying targets.

The physiological approach attempts to identify novel targets through studies in whole organisms because most diseases, including psychiatric, metabolic, cardiovascular and gastrointestinal disorders, are only manifest at the level of the organism (Lindsay, 2005).

Mechanism-Based Approach

A step ahead of physiological approach to identify the novel targets is the mechanism-based approach. The mechanistic approach attempts to identify drug targets by comparing the intracellular pathways that regulate biological responses in primary cells from normal patients with those from diseased patients. The complexity of the interactions and variations between individuals have made it difficult to pinpoint specific targets involved in disease by disease pathway comparison. This task also further hardened because of the rapid biochemical and structural changes that occur in cells *ex vivo* and the experimental difficulties. For example, the investigation of the profile of protein expression in the plasma membrane of endothelial cells showed that of the 450 proteins expressed in rat lungs, 41% were found to be absent in the equivalent cultured cells. The limitations of the mechanistic approach to target identification are best exemplified in oncology. In this area a lot of money has been spent for elucidating the genetic and molecular mechanisms responsible for cell proliferation, leading to the identification of numerous oncogenes, tumor suppressors and repair genes. However, with the exception of some minor success in the treatment of rare cancers, such as the treatment of chronic myeloid leukemia using Gleevec™, this enormous investment has had little impact on the overall patient prognosis (Lindsay, 2005).

Despite these problems, the mechanism-based approach succeeded in making us understand the basic cellular interactions that have been useful for identification of novel targets in infectious diseases. For example, the knowledge of the life cycle of the human immunodeficiency virus (HIV) has resulted in the development of inhibitors of viral entry, reverse transcription and proteolytic processing of the viral proteins. These drugs, when used in combination, have profoundly reduced the AIDS-related mortality. The discovery of an additional isoform of COX, named COX-2, through the mechanism-based approach indicated that it is possible to avoid the gastrointestinal side effects associated with the existing nonsteroidal anti-inflammatory drugs (NSAIDs) using selective COX-2 inhibitors (Lindsay, 2005).

Omics in Target Identification

The final approach to the identification of potential targets has been to compare the differential expression of genes (genomics) and proteins (proteomics) in normal and disease cells and tissues (Table 2.1). A single gene chip can be used to compare the expression of thousands of genes, in diseased and healthy tissue alike, all at once, and informatics technology employed to find follow-up information, on these or related genes, in databases around the world. In general, besides being technically challenging, this approach produces large numbers of potential targets and it has proven difficult to identify those that are causally involved in the disease. Indeed, a recent investigation of different experimental approaches to the identification of genes involved in schizophrenia showed little correlation between data generated by DNA microarrays and other non-microarray-based clinical and biological approaches. This realization has resulted in the increased use of genomics and proteomics approaches for the identification of disease biomarkers rather than novel drug targets. An alternative approach has been to investigate difference in gene sequences and, in particular, to correlate disease phenotype with single nucleotide polymorphisms. As with genomics studies, these genetic association studies only identify correlations and have been difficult to reproduce because

Table 2.1 *High-Throughput Techniques (Omics Platforms)*

	Target	*Analytical Method*	*Conventional Research Equivalent*
Genomics	DNA	microarrays ('gene chips')	gene sequencing
Trancriptomics	RNA	microarrays ('gene chips')	Northern, RNase protection
Proteomics	proteins	microarrays; two-dimensional gel electrophoresis+mas spectrometry	Western, ELISA
Metabolomics	metabolites	NMR-spectroscopy mass spectrometry	HPLC, cellular assays

Source: Editorial (2004), A plea for 'Omics' research in complex diseases such as multiple sclerosis—a change of mind is needed, *Journal of the Neurological Sciences*, 222, 3–5.

they are crucially dependent upon the availability of large, well-characterized patient populations (Lindsay, 2005).

Genomics in Target Identification and Validation

The availability of fully sequenced genomes has enabled researchers to integrate the available genomic information to reconstruct and study the metabolic networks of an organism affected by disease. These studies have revealed important properties of metabolic networks. The potential of an enzyme to be an effective drug target is considered to be related to its essentiality in the corresponding metabolic network. A combination of gene knockout and microarray time course data was used to study the effects of a chemical compound on a gene network (Sridhar *et al.*, 2007).

Metabolomics Approach

Metabolomics is generally accepted as the study of the repertoire of non-proteinaceous, endogenously synthesized small molecules present in an organism (Ryals, 2004). Metabolomics is a powerful and new scientific approach to target identification and will enable faster and more cost-effective processes in target identification and validation by accurately physiological status through biochemical changes. The biochemical fingerprint for a specific enzyme or protein associated with a disease state can be determined in order to identify a specific target (Beecher and Tripp, 2004). Gene deletion will inevitably lead to changes in the concentration of small-molecule metabolites profile, even when phenotypic changes are negligible and identifying the target metabolite will make target identification very easy (Goerge *et al.*, 2005). With metabolomics, it is possible to see the unanticipated secondary effects inherent in a target and thus abandon a target that may carry unacceptable risk and prevent drug failure in clinical trials (Beecher and Tripp, 2004). A powerful benefit of metabolomics is that the individual molecules in the complex mixtures can be identified with certainty both qualitatively and quantitatively. For example, by using a combination of chromatography followed by mass spectrometry, the individual molecules can be separated and identified based on their mass. By using appropriate standards a molecule can be identified with great precision (Ryals, 2004).

Disease Models

Disease model plays a major role in the early drug discovery and more particularly in the target identification. However, ethical implications, as well as expense and technical difficulties, often prevent human-based studies. To overcome this bottleneck, medical scientists have traditionally turned to cell and animal models. Significantly, the advent of molecular biology and the need to manipulate genes has encouraged the widespread use of immortalized cell lines and mouse models. Although these studies are useful for basic mechanistic studies, several issues have emerged that limit their utility as predictive models of human disease (Lindsay, 2005). A widely used organism to study the function of potential drug targets in human disease models is the laboratory mouse because of its high degree of homology in their genetic makeup to humans. More importantly, research over the last 20 years has provided a wide array of tools to manipulate individual mouse genes. The effects of an experimentally manipulated target on a disease relevant phenotype can then be studied (Heck *et al.*, 2004).

Cellular Models

At present, the functional role of a protein is investigated through either overexpression of the wild-type and/or dominant-negative gene or small interference RNA (siRNA)-mediated knockdown. However, because the use of these experimental approaches is dependent upon plasmid and siRNA delivery, this has resulted in the widespread use of easy-to-transfect immortalized cell lines in preference to primary cells. Fortunately, many of the intracellular pathways appear to be evolutionarily conserved and these studies have elucidated important basic mechanistic interactions. Unfortunately, because of the genetic differences between immortalized and primary cells, the difficulty in simulating the *in vivo* milieu and the 'noise' that is inherent in all biological systems, it is virtually impossible to 'model' physiological and pathological responses by extrapolation from cell-based studies (Lindsay, 2005).

Animal Models

Animal studies have provided valuable information on human physiology and pathology. A validated drug target should ideally produce the desired phenotype in several animal models that recapitulate at least some important aspects of the pertinent disease (Artal-Sanz *et al.*, 2006). However, as a result of crucial differences in areas such as immunology, metabolism and anatomy, these investigations were often undertaken in a variety of species (e.g. mouse, rat, guinea pig, rabbit, pig, dog) to identify those that were the most analogous to humans. Today, the ease in breeding and maintenance, the availability of the genome sequence and our ability to produce transgenic and knockout animals mean that mice are almost exclusively employed, irrespective of whether they represent the most suitable species. In addition, unlike earlier investigations that employed 'outbred' and 'wild-type' animals, these mouse colonies are highly 'inbred' and, therefore, genetically homogenous. Although this often means that smaller numbers of animals are required to obtain statistically significant results, the final results are often highly strain dependent. As an example, a recent publication examining the induction of emphysema in five mouse strains, following chronic exposure to cigarette smoke, showed a wide range of responses. Similarly, contradictory results are often produced when using transgenic and knockout mice of different strains to study the role of individual genes. These species and strain differences have brought into question the utility of mouse models even for simple physiological studies. Furthermore, these problems are compounded when developing models of chronic disease, where the long-term environmental factors and the influence of aging need to be modeled. In most cases, the combination of time constraints, expense and experimental complexity means that these important influences are simply ignored (Lindsay, 2005).

The demand for the use of model organisms to validate targets for drug discovery has soared as a result of the high number of candidate genes derived from genomics approaches. The validation of drug targets has traditionally been performed in mammalian models, particularly the mouse.

However, the knockout of specific mouse genes through the use of homologous recombination is a time-consuming process and cannot be performed in a high-throughput manner. To rapidly validate potential targets, many investigators have relied on lower phylogenetic organisms, such as *Caenorhabditis elegans* (nematode worm), *Drosophila melanogaster* (fruit fly) and *Danio rerio* (zebra fish). In these organisms, gene function and pathway analysis can be analyzed in multiple ways, including large-scale mutagenesis, antisense knockdown and chemical genetic approaches. In this chapter, we discuss the use of model organisms for target validation and disease model development, with a particular emphasis on the zebra fish, a vertebrate system that is amenable to higher-throughput validation methods (Doan *et al.*, 2004).

The Network-Based Strategy for Drug Target Identification

With the development of bioinformatics, a number of computational techniques have been used to search for novel drug targets from the information contained in genomics. The network-based strategy for drug target identification attempts to reconstruct endogenous metabolic, regulatory and signaling networks with which potential drug targets interact. Once having this information provided by gene networks or protein networks, the interaction relationships between potential drug targets could be explicitly revealed, so it can be easily determined which one of these potential drug targets is the most proper, or the scope of selecting candidate drug targets could be narrowed down to a great extent; e.g. if a potential drug target participates in many biological pathways, the inhibition of this target may interfere with many activities associated with those pathways, and, therefore, may not be a good candidate for drug target. Along with the development of microarray technology, a large volume of gene expression or protein expression data have been produced, and there have been several models proposed to infer gene networks or protein networks from these data (*Journal of Integrative Bioinformatics*, 2005, http://journal.imbio.de).

Gene Network Strategy for Drug Target Identification

Drug target identification involves acquiring a molecular-level understanding of a specific disease state and includes analyses of gene sequences, protein structures, protein interactions and metabolic pathways. Genetic interactions are central to the understanding of molecular structure and function, cellular metabolism and response of organisms to their environments. If such interaction patterns can be measured for various kinds of tissues and the corresponding data can be interpreted, potential benefits are obvious for the identification of candidate drug targets. It has already been demonstrated that it is possible to infer a predictive model of a genetic network by time series gene expression data or steady-state gene expression data of gene knockout. Using the inferred model, useful predictions can be made by mathematical analysis and computer simulations. In the gene network-based strategy for drug target identification, the estimated gene networks play an important role. The reconstruction of gene networks from gene expression data is gaining popularity as methods improve and as more data become available. In order to draw meaningful inferences from gene expression data and find regulatory relationships between genes, it is important that each gene is surveyed under several different conditions, preferably in the form of expression time series. Such data sets may be analyzed using a range of methods with increasing depth of inference, such as cluster analysis, correlation statistics analysis, weight matrices, neural networks, genetic algorithms and supervised learning algorithms. For the purpose of capturing the interrelated regulatory mechanisms between genes, several genetic network models have been proposed, such as Boolean networks, differential equations and Bayesian networks, which use expression data to trace genetic regulatory interactions. Of these mentioned models, Bayesian networks are promising for learning gene regulatory networks from observed expression data. To discover genes of pharmaceutical interest, various microarray data, such as drug response expression data, time course expression data and steady-state expression data of gene knockout, could be used. With the drug response expression data, a set of drug-affected genes could be collected by differential expression data analysis. The inferences of genetic networks provide insights into the underlying gene interactions and gene regulation of metabolic pathways in the living organisms. These tools helps to readily reconstruct genetic networks based on microarray data without having intimate knowledge of the mathematical models, and can be conveniently used for identification of potential targets for therapeutics (*Journal of Integrative Bioinformatics*, 2005, http://journal.imbio.de).

TARGET VALIDATION

Target validation explains that a molecular target is critically involved in a disease process, and that modulation of the target is likely to have a therapeutic effect. The validation of a molecular target *in vitro* usually precedes the validation of the therapeutic concept *in vivo*; together, this defines its clinical potential. Validation involves studies in intact animals or disease-related cell-based models that can provide information about the integrative response of an organism to a pharmacological intervention and thereby help to predict the possible profile of new drugs in patients (Chen and Du, 2007).

After the identification of a biological target of interest, the next challenge begins with the conversion of the target into a bioassay that can give readout of the biological activity. The range of potential targets is large, from enzymes and receptors to cellular systems, which represent an entire biochemical pathway or a disease process. Developing an assay technique to validate the target is a critical step in target validation and the next key step is the establishment of an HTS method, and then compounds can be tested in the bioassay to see if they inhibit, enhance or do nothing to this activity (Chen and Du, 2007). The basic requirements for HTS assay are that it be sensitive, stable, highly reproducible, robust and suitable for screening thousands or even millions of samples. With sufficient luck, several 'hit' compounds would be discovered by primary screening. The 'hit' compounds must be re-screened to exclude the false positive results. Then, the next step is 'hit' identification, which may include its chemical characteristics, i.e. mainly its stability, its toxicity *in vivo* and *in vitro*, its pharmacological evaluation and particularly its effects in cells and animal models. In summary, target validation should be performed at three levels: the molecular level, the cellular level and the whole animal model level. Small chemicals obtained from HTS provide useful tools for the validation of new drug targets. Most HTS models are at the molecular level, i.e. cell-free systems. There is a significant difference between a cell and a cell-free system. Validation at the cell level provides confirmation of cell-free results. At this level, the pathological significance of the target might be rendered more apparent using small chemicals. The effect of the small chemicals on a cell system will provide a tentative outline of these chemicals. Animal models are used to validate the target at the whole level. At this level, the primary concern is the effect of the 'hit'. If the hit obtained from HTS displays a therapeutic effect in animal models, then it may be promising. However, more often than not a 'hit' displays no effect in an animal model and the result should be interpreted with caution (Chen and Du, 2007).

Basically, the target validation process includes the following steps:

1. Discovering a biomolecule of interest
2. Evaluating its potential as a target
3. Designing a bioassay to measure biological activity
4. Constructing a high-throughput screen
5. Performing screening to find hits
6. Evaluating the hits

Common shortfalls and/or pitfalls that need to be considered during the target validation include the following (Chen and Du, 2007):

1. Wrong animal model
2. Wrong route or dosing regimen
3. Wrong vehicle or formulation of test material
4. Wrong dose level: In studies where several dose levels are studied, the worst outcome is to have an effect at the lowest dose level tested (i.e. the safe dosage in animals remains unknown). The next worst outcome is to have no effect at the highest dose tested (generally meaning that the signs of toxicity remain unknown, invalidating the study in the eyes of many regulatory agencies).
5. Making leaps of faith: Setting dosage levels based on others' data
6. Using the wrong concentration of test materials in screening: Many effects are very concentration dependent.

TOOLS FOR TARGET IDENTIFICATION AND VALIDATION

A wide array of target identification and validation technologies are available, including genomics, gene expression profiling and proteomics. Biomarkers and metabolomic profiling are emerging tools for monitoring the biological effects of manipulating a potential drug target. Technologies such as gene knockouts, RNA interference (RNAi) and protein inhibition provide researchers with a multipronged approach to validating new targets. The most successful approaches combine several technologies to provide a detailed understanding of the biological effects of altering the activity of a single target.

Microarrays

Target identification seeks to identify new targets, normally proteins or DNA/RNA, whose modulation might inhibit or reverse disease progression. Current technologies enable researchers to attempt correlating changes in gene (genomics) and protein (proteomics) expression with human disease, in the hope of finding new targets. Microarrays are a well-utilized tool in both academic and industrial research laboratories. They can be used to assess gene and protein expression (via nucleic acid or protein microarrays) to identify novel targets, and can also be used to validate the found targets at the tissue or cell scale (via tissue or cell microarrays) (Wang *et al.*, 2004). Microarrays have been utilized to address *in vitro* pharmacology and toxicology issues. They are being widely applied to improve the processes of disease diagnosis, pharmacogenomics and toxicogenomics, and these applications (Hardiman, 2003). The application of microarrays to the study of the mechanism of action of antipsychotic drugs, such as clozapine, using animal models, and the interrogation of gene expression in schizophrenic brain tissue have yielded surprisingly convergent results that implicate disturbances in membrane lipid biology and synaptic transmission in this disorder (Hardiman, 2003).

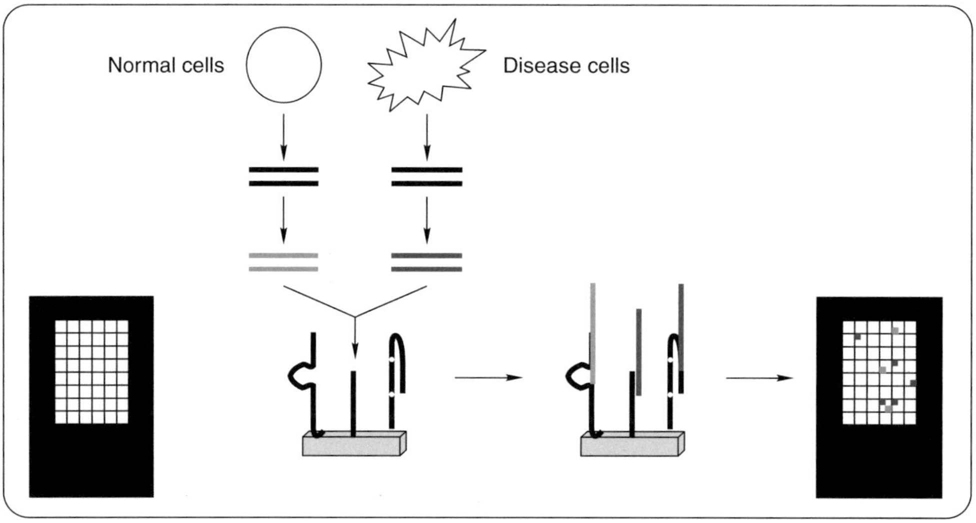

Fig. 2.6 *DNA Microarray Technology (For color figure please see Plate 4)*

Nucleic Acid Microarrays

DNA microarray technology, which permits simultaneous measurement of the expression levels of thousands of genes, provides a comprehensive framework to determine how a compound affects cellular metabolism and regulation on a genomic scale (Fig. 2.6). DNA microarrays that contain essentially every open reading frame (ORF) in the *Saccharomyces cerevisiae* genome have already been used successfully to explore the changes in gene expression that accompany large changes in cellular metabolism or cell cycle progression. In the modern drug discovery, which typically begins with the selection of a single molecular target, the ideal inhibitory drug is one that inhibits a single gene product completely and specifically. Treating cells with such a drug should induce changes in gene expression very similar to those resulting from deleting the gene encoding the drug's target (Marton *et al.*, 1998).

For a known gene sequence, oligonucleotides can be synthesized to hybridize specifically to each gene. This approach obviates the need for management of large clone libraries as it is guided primarily by sequence data (Hardiman, 2003). Today, nucleic acid microarrays, which primarily use short oligonucleotides (15–25 nt), long oligonucleotides (50–120 nt) and PCR-amplified cDNAs (100–3000 base pairs) as array elements, are overwhelmingly dominant because of the relatively easy synthesis and the chemical robustness of DNA. Expression analysis by microarray technology (immobilized DNA probes hybridizing to RNA or cDNA targets) has enabled parallel monitoring of cellular transcription at the level of the genome. The nucleic acid microarrays have made a big impact on the choice of targets for drug design by improving our understanding of normal and abnormal cell biochemistry. The data generated from high-density oligonucleotide microarrays from Affymetrix lead to the identification of 97 genes as physiological targets of the retinoblastoma protein pathway, deregulation of which is a hallmark of human cancer (Wang *et al.*, 2004). Oligonucleotides can be synthesized *in situ* or prefabricated and then printed for the analysis (Hardiman, 2003).

Protein Microarrays

There have been two techniques to characterize proteins in biological samples: 2D gels and mass spectrometry. Both are time consuming and unsuitable for the analysis of low-abundant proteins (Talapatra *et al.*, 2002). Protein microarrays are evolving as useful tools for biopharmaceutical research. Differences in the characteristics of individual proteins have made the development challenging compared with DNA arrays (Kumble, 2007). Because most drug targets are proteins, protein and peptide microarrays are set to have an important impact on drug discovery. Protein arrays, an emerging yet very promising technology, are now being used to examine enzyme–substrate, DNA–protein and protein–protein interactions. By profiling the differential expression of proteins using antibody arrays and correlating the changes to a disease phenotype, putative targets (and biomarkers) to a particular disease can be identified, although to date such microarrays have not been used to their full potential because of difficulties with the technology (Wang *et al.*, 2004). The strategy is based on the mechanism of the reaction between the ligands and proteins, thus demonstrating the approach as an activity-based and high-throughput method. Further application of this method may lie on targeting known drugs or biologically active compounds (Wang *et al.*, 2004).

Protein arrays are comprised of a library of proteins immobilized in a 2D addressable grid on a chip. Protein microarray biochips extract and retain targets from liquid media and remain distinct from microfluidic biochips, which separate and process proteins in a transport medium *in situ* using microfluidic devices. Arrays can be engineered to address protein identification, quantitation and affinity studies (Talapatra *et al.*, 2002).

Bioinformatics

The development of bioinformatics as a result of the explosion of raw data after the completion of the Human Genome Project has added another dimension to the drug discovery process. Bioinformatics was fueled by the need to create huge databases, such as Genbank, EMBL and DNA Database of Japan, to store and compare the DNA sequence data erupting from the human genome and other genome sequencing projects. Besides being used as an essential step in analyzing high-throughput experiments such as DNA microarrays, bioinformatics can contribute to the processes of target identification and validation by providing functional information of target candidates and positioning information on the biological networks. Bioinformatics thus has definite significant advantages over traditionally expensive and time-consuming 'wet lab' research methods because computational tools give the most predictive and accurate information about genes and proteins with regards to mediating aspects of drug action (http://www.hypography.com/topics/Bioinformatics_100147.cfm). Numerous public biological databases are warehousing and providing a great amount of functional information for genes or proteins, and many useful bioinformatics tools are continuously developed. Enriched information and the bioinformatics tools have enabled *in silico* cloning of target candidates. SNAIL3, a potent target of pharmacogenomics in the field of oncology and regenerative medicine, is an example for *in silico* isolation through proper combination of available bioinformatics tools and information. The gene was isolated by a similarity search of a known database, and the characteristics of the sequence, such as chromosomal location, phylogeny and *in silico* expression analysis, were investigated by commonly available tools and databases. In-depth analysis of experimental data using bioinformatics can give new insight into the prediction of target validity in the clinical stage. The supervised machine learning algorithm was applied for the analysis of B-cell lymphoma (DLBCL) array data to select rational targets and to predict DLBCL treatment outcome. The class prediction strategy successfully classified two categories of patients with very different 5-year overall survival rates. The genes involved in B-cell receptor signaling, critical serine/threonine phosphorylation pathways and apoptosis were selected as the featured genes of DLBCL outcome. The application of bioinformatics to single nucleotide polymorphisms (SNPs), one of the key factors for personalized medicine, and systems biology make it possible to investigate the relationship between sequence variation and physiological function *in silico*. The effects of SNPs in the two key enzymes, glucose-6-phosphate dehydrogenase (G6PD) and pyruvate kinase, on human red blood metabolism were assessed through the *in silico* model. In the case of G6PD, the predicted result of overall cell behavior correlated with the severity of the clinical conditions. This kind of study should be useful for the development of personalized drugs and may reduce the time and cost at the clinical stage by pre-investigation of the individual's genotype (Wang *et al.*, 2004).

The traditional process of drug discovery uses synthetic organic molecules, which are then tested in animals or whole organ preparations; however, nowadays with the increased understanding of molecular biology, a molecular target approach is used. Here virtual high-throughput screening (vHTS) is employed. This involves the screening of protein targets against databases of small molecules to determine the ones which fit into the target. The compounds that fit are then further tested, thus allowing researchers to only work with promising leads. This results in cutting costs and time for the research process. vHTS enables millions of compounds to be screened daily. Bioinformatics software tools are used to predict the 3D structure of the target based on the known 3D structures of the templates. Examples of tools used in homology modeling are MODELLER and SWISS-MODEL Repository (Casey, 2005).

Antisense Technology

Natural antisense RNA is known to be involved in the gene regulation in normal organisms (Rayburn *et al.*, 2005). Antisense DNA/RNA is oligonucleotides or analogs thereof that are complementary to a specific sequence of RNA or DNA that binds to the native target to form a double-stranded sequence and thus inhibits its normal function (Eckstein, 2004). Antisense oligonucleotides are single-stranded DNA or RNA or chimeric DNA/RNA that are designed to specifically hybridize to a native mRNA and subsequently prevent protein synthesis (Rayburn *et al.*, 2005), thus achieving knockdown of the target gene. Systems that regulate the levels of gene expression by antisense oligonucleotide production using a highly regulated, inducible promoter would be invaluable tools for studying the function of genes under defined conditions (Fig. 2.7) (Kerstin *et al.*, 2007).

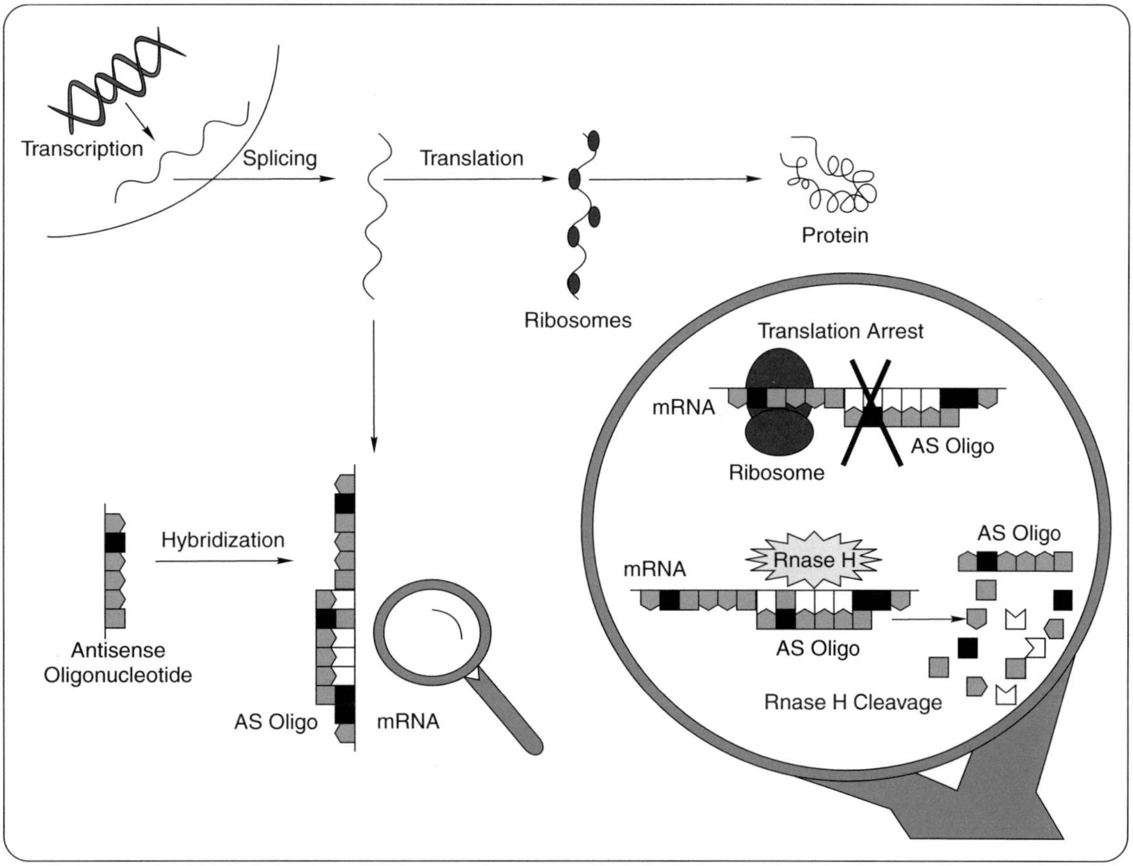

Fig. 2.7 ***Schematic Representation of Antisense Mechanisms (For color figure please see Plate 4)***

Source: Rayburn *et al.* (2005).

Antisense has been widely used to downregulate gene expression in eukaryotes and more recently in some prokaryotes (Bock *et al.*, 2002). It is a key strategy in target validation to determine the changes, with respect to phenotype and/or the expression of other genes in cells or model organisms, if a gene of interest is either deleted or its activity is inhibited. Gene knockout mimics the activity of a drug that completely inhibits the normal function of the gene's product. A temporary knockout, a so-called knockdown, is another popular alternative for real-time analysis of the gene function (Wang *et al.*, 2004).

There are two major approaches to apply antisense RNA into living cells: nuclear expression of RNA by engineered antisense genes and microinjection of artificial antisense RNA. However this technology is limited by the delivery of DNA/RNA into the cells; e.g. RNAs are extremely sensitive to nuclease degradation and also poor cellular uptake. The phosphodiester oligonucleotides (PO-oligos), and their methylphosphonate (MP-oligos) and phosphorothioate (PS-oligos) analogs, are considered the first generation of antisense DNA. Although PO-oligos have high affinity to their targets and the ability to activate RNase H, they have limited practical application due to extreme sensitivity to nucleases and poor cellular uptake. Modified antisense DNA is now being used much more frequently in antisense investigations than antisense RNA, ribozymes or unmodified antisense DNA (highly resistant to nucleases) to overcome the limitation. Almost all of the clinically tested antisense oligonucleotides are modified antisense DNA (Rayburn *et al.*, 2005). Recently, several types of antisense oligomers that inhibit gene expression in a sequence-specific and dose-dependent manner have been reviewed (Kerstin *et al.*, 2007). Recently, an antisense drug for viral retinitis has been approved (Jens *et al.*, 2004). Although initially developed as potential new antituberculous agents, antisense oligomers are proving useful as target validation tools, and a recent study has shown this technology to be a feasible approach to study *in vitro* gene function in *Mycobacterium tuberculosis*. Although antisense oligomers show some promise as target validation tools, there are concerns over their bioavailability and toxicity, and their applications to *in vivo* target validation studies are awaited (Kerstin *et al.*, 2007).

RNA Interference

RNA interference (RNAi), another type of technology involving sequence-specific RNA for use in gene knockdown, has attracted an even greater interest in the scientific community (Wang *et al.*, 2004). In the early 1990s plant geneticists studying pansies noticed an unexpected blocking of expression of color genes, which they called corepression. A similar effect in the nematode *C. elegans* was found to be dependent upon double-stranded RNA. The effect was named RNA interference because the short RNA sequences interfered with normal protein expression by causing the destruction of mRNA (Rayburn *et al.*, 2005). Interfering RNA or RNAi is a gene silencing phenomenon, whereby specific double-stranded RNAs (dsRNAs) trigger the degradation of homologous messenger RNA (mRNA). The specific dsRNAs are processed into small interfering RNA (siRNA), which initiates the cleavage of the homologous mRNA in a complex named the RNA-induced silencing complex (RISC) (Eckstein, 2004). RNA interference (RNAi) is a natural phenomenon where dsRNA induces sequence-specific silencing of genes by degradation of complementary RNA in a cell. This silencing phenomenon is widespread in eukaryotes and has been previously linked to post-transcriptional gene silencing (PTGS) in plants and quelling in fungi. It is an evolutionarily conserved mechanism that inhibits the replication and expression of selfish DNA elements and viruses and hence maintains genome integrity (Owino *et al.*, 2008). Introduction of either dsRNA or siRNA into cells leads to inhibition of the biological function encoded in the targeted mRNA the underlying concept of RNAi therapeutics. For example, this approach is being investigated to silence mutant alleles of tau, APP, ataxin, and SOD1 (Eckstein, 2004).

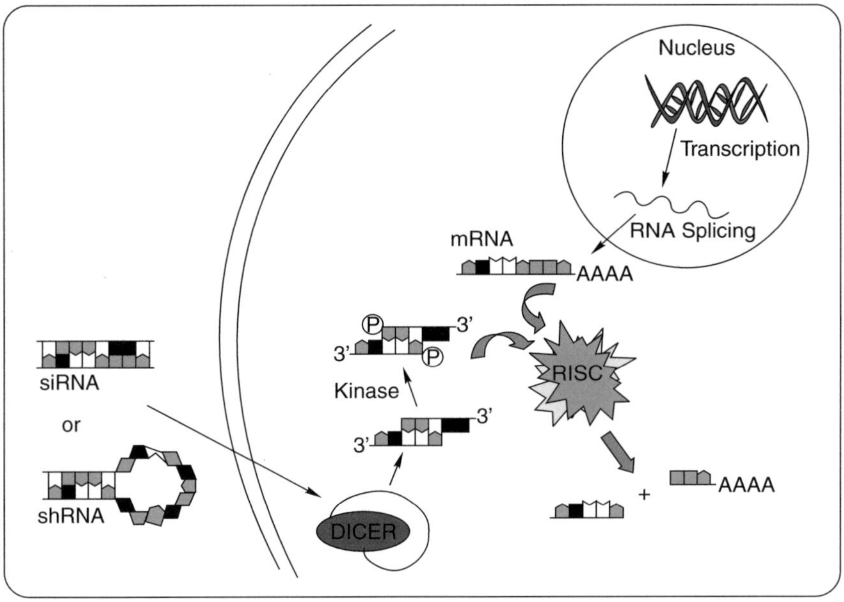

Fig. 2.8 ***Schematic Representation of RNAi Mechanisms. The Interfering RNA Molecule is Processed by the Dicer Enzyme Complex, which Cleaves RNA Strands into Smaller Nucleotide Fragments, which go on to Bind to the RISC. The RISC also Binds the Complementary Target mRNA Sequence, which is then Degraded, Blocking Gene Expression. si/shRNA: Small Interfering/Short Hairpin RNA, RISC: RNA-induced Silencing Complex. (For color figure please see Plate 5)***

Source: Owino *et al.* (2008).

The RNA interference (RNAi) is first introduced in *C. elegans* by feeding bacteria that express copies of dsRNA to worms, which can artificially induce the RNAi response, making this technique highly attractive for reverse genetic screens (Doan *et al.*, 2004). After introduction or expression, these long dsRNAs are cleaved intracellularly by a ribonuclease known as Dicer into short 21–25-nucleotide siRNAs. siRNAs assemble with the protein components of the RISC, unwinding in the process. This activated RNA–RISC complex then binds to the complementary transcript by base pairing interactions between the siRNA antisense strand and the mRNA. The bound mRNA is cleaved and subsequently degraded (Fig. 2.8). This mRNA degradation leads to gene silencing (Kroenke *et al.*, 2004). This guidance of RISC to target mRNA is highly sequence specific and, thus, target specific. RNAi coupled with large-scale cell-based screens holds great promise for target identification (Wang *et al.*, 2004). The knockdown of any targeted mRNA allows a simple, reversible ablation of individual genes to unravel the biology associated with different disease states. The complex biology surrounding most putative drug targets and their pathways can be better understood by knocking down multiple genes within a pathway in multiple cell lines (Kroenke *et al.*, 2004).

RNA technologies are a very useful tool in the identification and validation of genes involved in host–pathogen interactions including host response (Kroenke *et al.*, 2004; Patzel, 2004; Gaither, 2006). The discovery of RNAi in trypanosomes has provided a basis for the elaboration of powerful research tools in reverse genetics studies and utilization of raw and rapidly accumulating information available in the trypanosome genome database. Its ability to specifically ablate the function of individual genes makes RNAi an invaluable tool in drug target discovery and validation (Owino *et al.*, 2008).

Artificial induction of the natural RNAi pathway is now widely used to specifically silence target genes. Applications of RNAi include analysis of gene function, identification of molecules involved in biochemical pathways, lead optimization, toxicological studies and functional genomics. The efficient delivery of siRNA *in vivo* is a crucial step in the RNAi technology. Plasmid/vector-based and chemically synthesized siRNA are mainly utilized. Chemically synthesized siRNAs and vector-encoded short hairpin RNAs (shRNAs) are at present the most broadly used reagents for all scales of RNAi experimentation in human cells (Arts *et al.*, 2003). Direct siRNA transfections have the advantage of high efficiency and immediate initiation of gene silencing when compared to plasmid DNA transfections. Plasmid-based siRNA on the other hand allows storage of trypanosomes with inducible RNAi and is much less expensive (Owino *et al.*, 2008). The inducible RNAi vectors are pZJM (Wang *et al.*, 2000) and p2T7Ti (LaCount *et al.*, 2002); they are widely used because they allow a single ligation of PCR-generated fragments of any target gene between the opposing tetracycline-inducible T7 promoters (Wang *et al.*, 2000; Owino *et al.*, 2008). A number of studies have documented instances of direct off-target effects caused by reagents, including siRNAs, designed to trigger RNAi responses. A second type of off-target effect that has been noted in RNAi experiments is the concentration-dependent modulation of the expression of nontargeted stress response genes, including factors of the interferon response pathway (Jackson *et al.*, 2003; Sledz *et al.*, 2003; Persengiev *et al.*, 2004).

Zinc Finger Proteins

Zinc finger proteins (ZFPs) have a remarkable versatility for recognizing different sequences of DNA, and variations in the amino acid sequence of the C2H2 domains allow them to be targeted to different locations in the genome. Each zinc finger is a short stretch of 30 amino acids, containing two conserved cysteines and two conserved histidines. These proteins have been used as the DNA binding domains of novel transcription factors (ZFP TFs). ZFP TFs can be applied to potential new drug target validation in two ways. One direct way involves designing ZFPs to validate the phenotypic effects of activating or repressing a gene. Alternatively, libraries of ZFP TFs might be used to screen cells for desired phenotypic changes. An example shows that designed ZFP TFs can knock down the mRNA expression of a predetermined target gene, while providing single gene specificity when 16,000 human genes were analyzed. A ZFP TF repressor that binds an 18-bp recognition sequence within the promoter of the endogenous CHK2 gene gives a >10-fold reduction in CHK2 mRNA and protein. Moreover, the extent of repression achieved by this highly specific engineered TF was sufficient to abolish the CHK2 function in two different assays and cell types, while recent data using RNAi or siRNA targeted to CHK2 in human cells reduced CHK2 protein by only 60–75%. Thus, ZFP TFs were demonstrated as precise tools for target validation, and even for clinical therapeutics (Wang *et al.*, 2004).

Haplotype Analysis

Recently, haplotype analysis has attracted an increasing amount of interest. The phenomenon of haploinsufficiency, in which loss of function of just one gene copy leads to an abnormal phenotype, has led to the assumption that, regardless of their frequency, haploinsufficient loci define a set of genes whose dosage and function are critical to the organism. Building on this idea, lowering the dosage of a single gene may result in a heterozygote that is sensitized to any drug that acts on the product of this gene. This haploinsufficient phenotype thereby identifies the gene product of the heterozygous locus as the likely drug target. A genome-wide pool of tagged heterozygotes is used to assess the cellular effects of 78 compounds in *S. cerevisiae*. A mixture of isogenic yeast mutants was generated by pooling 3503 heterozygous deletion strains engineered with strain-specific molecular barcode tags. Competitive growth of the mutant pool was carried out for 20 generations in the presence of selected compounds. Genomic DNA was isolated from cultures before and after outgrowth. Barcode tags were amplified and labeled by PCR and later hybridized onto DNA microarrays. Of the 78 compounds analyzed, 18 resulted in no drug-specific fitness changes, 56 resulted in a small number of significant outliers, and 4 resulted in widespread fitness changes, thus proving this process to be a powerful tool for understanding drug activities and leading to target identification (Wang *et al.*, 2004).

Chemical Genomics and Proteomics

Chemical genomics finds targets for known drugs rather than finding drugs for targets as in the conventional pharmaceutical approach. It aims at discovering the specific molecular targets and pathways that are modulated by particular chemical molecules by using chemical tools to probe the function of specific pathways and networks in human cells (Kim, 2004; Artal-Sanz *et al.*, 2006). Chemical genomics is expected to accelerate the determination of the function and biological role of the gene, through small-molecule interactions with the protein encoded by the gene (Darvas *et al.*, 2001); using simple animal models has the potential to accelerate drug target identification (Mata *et al.*, 2006). Various kinds of chemicals have been used to generate novel chemotypes and once an effect is found, then the biological target will be identified using an affinity matrix made of the immobilized hit compound. However, the synthesis of an efficient affinity matrix without the hit compound's activity loss has been shown to be challenging, or sometimes totally impossible, due to the difficulties of adequate linker attachment. The tagged library approach is giving promising results, in which a tagged library was synthesized through combinatorial methods and screened in the presence of the tag in phenotypic assays. Thus, selected active library compounds were directly connected to the resin beads, or to an affinity moiety, without need for a further structure–activity relationship study utilizing the already-existing tag. This approach dramatically accelerated the connection of the functional screening to the affinity matrix step by reducing the time needed from months to days.

Another way to overcome this problem is by displacement affinity chromatography screening (Wang *et al.*, 2004). The discovery that a small molecule, named FK506, blocks the production of several cytokines that are produced in an immune response was one of the first successful applications of this chemical genetic/genomic approach (Kim, 2004).

Chemical genetics is a multidisciplinary research tool at the interface between chemistry and biology, which has been coined to signify the use of chemicals to determine the function of protein in the same way that mutations are used in conventional genetics (Kwon, 2004). Chemical genetics, using small molecules to selectively disrupt signals or modulate phenotypic changes through interaction with proteins, basically mimics the effect of mutations that lead to the development of disease states (Darvas *et al.*, 2001). Chemical genetics uses small molecules that react with specific molecular targets to define the roles of proteins in cells or whole organisms. The small-molecule approach has advantages over the genetic approach for the identification of targets in terms of saving on time as it does not have to develop genetically modified animals and/or cells. Chemical genetics can also complement mutational studies, providing information about transcriptional, posttranscriptional and posttranslational processes in a cell. Moreover, the chemical genetic approach can be a reversible process; if one removes the drug, the cellular process should revert to normal, thus facilitating the temporal control of gene function. One drawback, however, is that compounds might bind to more than one distinct molecular target. Therefore, it might be difficult to assign a function to a specific gene based solely on the effect of a compound that binds to it. Descriptions of the types of chemical libraries that are available for screening and target validation are reviewed in. For example, one type of library is composed of small organic molecules, which are more likely to penetrate the cell membrane and elicit biological effects. Targets identified from organic molecule screens include G protein-coupled receptors, lectins, proteases, kinases and ligands that bind to SH3 domains. Natural chemical libraries are also available and contain compounds isolated from a variety of organisms, such as plants, microbes and aquatic organisms (http://www.bioscreening.com).

Several proteomic techniques, such as 2D gel electrophoresis and isotope-coded affinity tagging, provide a means to globally monitor changes in protein expression levels (Stevan, 2005). Protein abundance may not directly correlate with protein activity because the activity of proteins is regulated by posttranslational regulation *in vivo*. Thus the methods of activity-based protein profiling (ABPP) is a valuable alternative to conventional abundance variations-based approaches. The chemical probes capable of directly reporting on the integrity of enzyme active sites in complex proteomes might serve as effective activity-based profiling tools. ABPP probes were designed to contain at least a reactive group for binding and covalently modifying the active sites of enzymes and one or more reporter groups (tags), such as biotin and/or a fluorophore, for the rapid detection and isolation of probe-labeled enzymes. Groups such as azides have been used to substitute the bulky tag groups, followed by so-called click chemistry to label the proteins. This method helped in the identification of targets such as a cluster of proteases, lipases and esterases, which distinguished cancer lines across a panel of human breast and melanoma cancer cells (Wang *et al.*, 2004). Additionally, ABPs can be used to develop robust screens for small-molecule inhibitors of a specific enzyme target within a large family of related enzymes (Stevan, 2005). Although the field of chemical proteomics has proven its value in several biologically and pathologically relevant systems, several challenges still remain to be overcome. First, the spectrum of available ABPs needs to be broadened in order to target additional enzyme classes. In addition, the development of high-throughput and non-gel-based assays in conjunction with ABPs will be required to enhance the experimental value of chemical proteomics. It is likely that further development of these methods will improve the applications of chemical proteomics to drug discovery research (Steven, 2005).

Directed Gene Disruption

In order for a protein to be considered a drug target, it is necessary to prove that the gene encoding the protein is an essential factor in the disease process. Isogenic mutants have been widely used to study mycobacterial gene function and essentiality. The generation of targeted gene disruption mutants by allelic exchange is the most powerful tool to study gene essentiality and our ability to create gene-specific mutants has improved the target identification and validation process in the drug discovery. Mutant complementation as a tool for target validation can be laborious and time consuming, but used in conjunction with other mutant generation techniques, such as transposon mutagenesis and specialized phage transduction, it provides vital information of gene essentiality (Kerstin *et al.*, 2007).

Conditional Gene Expression by Promoter Replacement

Conditional gene expression by promoter replacement is another approach to gene regulation in the creation of conditional gene knockouts. There have been two reports using tetracycline-inducible promoters to create conditional lethal phenotypes in *M. tuberculosis*. Essentially the systems use homologous recombination to replace the natural promoter of the gene of interest with a tetracycline-inducible promoter. In the absence of tetracycline, the repressor is bound to the operator sites and transcription of the gene is inhibited. If the gene is essential then bacterial growth is also inhibited and gene functionality can be inferred. Carroll *et al.* have employed the *Staphylococcus aureus* Ptet to create a conditional tryptophan auxotroph of *M. tuberculosis*. Ehrt *et al.* have developed a system based on the *E. coli* Tn10-derived Ptet, to show essentiality for *ftsZ*, and also demonstrated tetracycline-controlled gene regulation in intracellular *M. tuberculosis* (Kerstin *et al.*, 2007).

Aptamers: Multifunctional Tools for Target Validation

Since their discovery in the early 1990s, aptamers have been used as detection reagents, affinity media, pharmaceutical leads and, most recently, drugs. Aptamers are synthetic nucleic acid ligands capable of specifically binding a wide variety of target proteins. They are rapidly isolated from combinatorial libraries by automated *in vitro* selection techniques. They are excellent tools for the identification and functional validation of targets from genomic and proteomic research through their high inhibitory potential and straightforward chemical modification properties. Their potential is proved as substitute inhibitors to streamline identification of small-molecule leads in HTS programs, thus linking target validation with drug discovery. The aptamer technology meets many important criteria required of an effective target validation tool. The complete automation of the *in vitro* selection enables the necessary turnover to produce aptamer inhibitors for a multitude of genomic targets. The high probability of isolating inhibitors of a protein's function makes the process very efficient. A number of studies have shown that aptamers exhibit neither intrinsic toxicity nor immunogenicity, thus avoiding activities that easily perturb the interpretation of validation data. Chemically modified and nuclease-resistant aptamers are normally used to validate the function of extracellular targets (Mayer *et al.*, 2003). The growing number of applications demonstrates that the aptamer approach is both time and cost effective, and especially useful when conventional technologies are insufficient.

Target Validation—Knockout/in, Gain-of-Function, Transgenic Models

Transgenic animals and animal models of disease have allowed for a greater understanding of the pathology of different diseases (James P. Basilion, 2004). Transgenic animals, where the target gene is knocked out, have become an important experimental approach for the determination of the function of targets (genes) in a whole organism. Knockouts of genes that are essential in development are usually lethal. Inducible knockouts, i.e. transgenic models where the transgene can be switched on or off at will in the adult animal, can be used to study the function of such essential genes. Disease models are transgenic animal models that present a phenotype bearing the hallmarks of a certain disease. These can be combined with knockouts to study the effect of modulating or inhibiting the function of the drug target (Jens Eckstein, ISOA/ARF Drug Development Tutorial, Alzheimer Research Forum). In transgenic animals, new genes can be inserted into the animal's genome and a specific target gene knocked out. For example, transgenic mice are most often produced by the injection of a DNA construct, which consists of a promoter/enhancer and the coding sequence of a gene of interest (GOI) into the pronuclei of fertilized mouse oocytes (Heck *et al.*, 2004). Some of the more common transgenic systems include *C. elegans* (roundworm), *Drosophila* (fruit fly), and *Danio rerio* (zebra fish). These non-mammalian transgenic models have several distinct advantages over the transgenic mouse model. These include a short life cycle (equates to short experimental time), easily visible phenotypic changes due to transparent animals, ease of studying large number of animals, being relatively inexpensive, and the less amount of required drugs. Despite these advantages, the transgenic mouse model still remains very important for target validation because it is closer to human. In the last 2–3 years, several investigators have reported the successful silencing of a specific gene in an intact animal by *in vivo* administration of siRNA via a high-pressure hydrodynamic transfection method or through a viral delivery system (Liu, 2004).

Knockins or gain-of-function models reactivate gene expression of the target gene, and often ameliorate or even reverse the disease phenotype. Knockins are also used to create disease models. Knockins or gain-of-function can also be lethal. For example, switching on or restoring the function of cell cycle genes in postmitotic cells often leads to cell death. Selective switching on of genes might present a therapeutic strategy if such restoration of gene function can be engineered in a tissue- or organ-specific fashion. Most neurodegenerative disease models have been generated by introducing mutant genes that cause autosomal-dominant forms of the disease in humans. In these models, the mutant gene (such as APP, presenilin, tau, superoxide dismutase-1 and expanded huntingtin) is assumed to result in a toxic gain-of-function, but the actual mechanisms by which the mutations cause disease phenotypes remain debated (Jens Eckstein, ISOA/ARF Drug Development Tutorial, Alzheimer Research Forum).

Target Validation—Pathways

The action and interaction of genes and their gene products are complex. Research aimed to define pathways that control and regulate processes in living organisms provides valuable information for drug discovery. The knowledge of a pathway allows defining and separate targeting of upstream or downstream targets. Inhibition or modulation of selected targets could lead to the same therapeutics with fewer side effects or better druggability. Knowledge of pathways and their relations to each other helps researchers understand the side-effect profiles. Identification of one disease target can lead to a number of alternative drug targets in the same pathway and increase the possibilities for a novel therapeutic. Examples include the drugs acting on the cholesterol synthesis pathway (Jens Eckstein, ISOA/ARF Drug Development Tutorial, Alzheimer Research Forum).

Target Validation—Clinical Data

The best validation of a target is clinical efficacy and safety data. Second- and third-generation therapeutics often have better efficacy and side-effect profiles based on the clinical trials and track record of first-generation drugs. Efficacy in clinical trials, i.e. amelioration or reversal of disease in human patients, is the ultimate validation of a target. Efficacy in animal disease models does not always predict the outcome in patients. The reliability of disease models for the prediction of human clinical trials varies widely among diseases and needs to be assessed on a case-by-case basis (Jens Eckstein, ISOA/ARF Drug Development Tutorial, Alzheimer Research Forum).

Target Validation—Chemical Knockouts and Chemical Biology

The prevailing approach for target validation involves the study of the biology of a disease. Knowledge of the disease mechanism and the underlying biological pathways leads to the identification and characterization of drug targets. A fundamentally different approach involves using compound collections to screen for phenotypes generated by exposure to molecules; this connects chemical structures to biological effects from the start, irrespective of the molecular targets/pathways that are hit. This "chemical biology" takes a holistic and random approach to drug discovery. It may complement the traditional deductive approaches. In chemical biology, chemical knockouts are a new method whereby the effect of a chemical compound, not a genetic manipulation, knocks out the function of a gene and thus leads to a readable phenotype. Chemical biology and chemical knockouts rely on the creation of diverse chemical libraries of many thousands of compounds. Cornerstone technologies for this new way of drug discovery are combinatorial chemistry and genetic manipulation of biosynthetic pathways in microbes for the production of new compounds (Jens Eckstein, ISOA/ARF Drug Development Tutorial, Alzheimer Research Forum).

REFERENCES

Aberg, A. (2005). Bridging the gap between model systems and human biology. *Daily Biotech Updates* **25(19)**.

Adam, M. (2005). Studies in History and Philosophy of Science Part C: *Studies in History and Philosophy of Biological and Biomedical Sciences* **36**.

Artal-Sanz, M., de Jong, L., Tavernarakis, N. (2006). *Caenorhabditis elegans*: A versatile platform for drug discovery. *Biotechnology Journal* **1**:1405–1418.

Arts, G.J., Langemeijer, E., Tissingh, R., Ma, L., Pavliska, H., Dokic, K., Dooijes, R., Mesic, E., Clasen, R., Michiels, F., van der Schueren, J., Lambrecht, M., Herman, S., Brys, R., Thys, K., Hoffmann, M., Tomme, P., van Es, H. (2003). Adenoviral vectors expressing siRNAs for discovery and validation of gene function. *Genome Research* **13(10)**:2325–2332.

Beecher, C.W.W., Tripp, R. (2004). Metabolomics–Applications in drug discovery and development. *Business Briefing: PharmaTech.*

Belfield, G.P., Delaney, S.J. (2006). The impact of molecular biology on drug discovery. *Biochemical Society Transactions* **34(2)**.

Bock, N.N., Sterling, T.R., Hamilton, C.D., Pachucki, C., Wang, Y.C., Conwell, D.S., Mosher, A., Samuels, M., Vernon, A. (2002). *American Journal of Respiratory and Critical Care Medicine* **165**:1526–1530.

Borisy, A.A., Elliott, P.J., Hurst, NW. (2003). Systematic discovery of multicomponent therapeutics. In: *Proceedings of the National Academy of Sciences USA*, **100**:7977–7982.

Brueggemann, A., George, M., Klau, M., Beckler, M., Steindl, J., Behrends, J.C., Fertig, N. (2004). Ion channel drug discovery and research: the automated Nano-Patch-Clamp technology. *Current Drug Discovery Technologies* **1**:91–96.

Casey, R.M. (2005). Bioinformatics in computer-aided drug design (Published May 10, 2005). Available at http://www.b-eye-network.com/view/852.

Chen, X.-P., Du, G.-H. (2007). Target validation: A door to drug discovery. *Drug Discoveries and Therapeutics* **1(1)**:23–29.

Csermely, P., Goston, V.A., Pongor, S. (2005). The efficiency of multi-target drugs: The network approach might help drug design. *Trends in Pharmacological Sciences* **26(4)**.

Darvas, F., Dorman, G., Urge, L., Szabo, I., Ronai, Z., Sasvari-Szekely, M. Combinatorial chemistry: Facing the challenge of chemical genomics. *Pure and Applied Chemistry* **73(9)**:1487–1498.

Dimasi, J.A. (2001). Risks in new drug development is approval success rates for investigational drugs. *Clinical Pharmacology and Therapeutics* **69**:297–307.

Doan, T.N., Eilertson, C.D., Rubinstein, A.L. (2004). High-throughput target validation in model organisms. *Drug Discovery Today: TARGETS* **3(5)**.

Eckstein, J. ISOA/ARF Drug Development Tutorial, Alzheimer Research Forum.

Editio Cantor Verlag, Aulendorf (2002). Arzneim.-Forsch./Drug Res. 52, No. 12, 922–924 (2002). ECV · Pharmacogenomics PMS-Symposium: Pharmacogenomics Editorial (2004). *Current Science* **87(7)**.

European Patent EP1756304, RNAI-based target identification and validation.

Gaither, A. (2006). Chemical siRNA screens as a tool for drug validation. *Drug Discovery*.

Gambardella, A. (1995). *Science and Innovation. The US Pharmaceutical Industry during the 1980s*. Cambridge, UK: Cambridge University Press.

Haberman, A.B. (2005). Strategies to move beyond target validation. **25(21)**.

Hall, K., Baillie, R., Michelson, S. (2002). Biosimulation: Dynamic modeling of biological systems. *Annual Reports in Medicinal Chemistry* **37**:279–288.

Hardiman, G. (2003). Microarray technologies 2003–An overview. *Pharmacogenomics* **4(3)**:251–256

Heck, S., Qian, X., Velleca, M. (2004). Genetically engineered mouse models for drug discovery: New chemical genetic approaches. *Current Drug Discovery Technologies* **1**:13–26.

Jackson, A.L., Bartz, S.R., Schelter, J., Kobayashi, S.V., Burchard, J., Mao, M., Li, B., Cavet, G., Linsley, P.S. (2003). Expression profiling reveals off-target gene regulation by RNAi. *Nature Biotechnology* **21(6)**:635–637.

Journal of Integrative Bioinformatics (2005). Available at http://journal.imbio.de.

Kang, L., Chung, B.G., Langer, R., Khademhosseini, A. (2008). Microfluidics for drug discovery and development: From target selection to product lifecycle management. *Drug Discovery Today* **13(1–2)**.

Kim, T.T. (2004). Chemical genomics and medicinal systems biology: Chemical control of genomic networks in human systems biology for innovative medicine. *Journal of Biochemistry and Molecular Biology* **37(1)**:53–58.

Kroenke, A., Grabner, A., Hannus, M., Sachse, C., Dorris, D., Echeverri, C. (2004). Using RNAi to identify and validate novel drug targets. *Drug Discovery World.*

Kubinyi, H. (1999). Chance favors the prepared mind–From serendipity to rational drug design. *Journal of Receptor and Signal Transduction Research* **19(1–4)**:15–39.

Kumble, K.D. (2007). *Expert Opinion on Drug Discovery* **2(11)**:1467–1476.

Kwon, H.J. (2004). Chemical genetics/genomics for cancer therapy, 10th Annual Fall Symposium, p. 36 (5th Suppl. 2).

LaCount, D.J., Barrett, B., Donelson, J.E. (2002). *Trypanosoma brucei* FLA1 is required for flagellum attachment and cytokinesis. *Journal of Biological Chemistry* **277**:17580–17588.

Lindsay, M.A. (2005). Finding new drug targets in the 21st century. *Drug Discovery Today* **10(23–24)**.

Liu, R., Hsieh, C.-Y., Lam, K.S. (2004). New approaches in identifying drugs to inactivate oncogene products. *Seminars in Cancer Biology* **14**:13–21.

Lum, P.Y., Armour, C.D., Stepaniants, S.B., *et al.* (2004). Discovering modes of action for therapeutic compounds using a genome-wide screen of yeast heterozygotes. *Cell* **116**:121–137.

Marton, M.J., Derisi, J.L., Bennett, H.A., Iyer, V.R., Meyer, M.R., Roberts, C.J., Stoughton, R., Burchard, J., Slade, D., Dai, H., Bassett, Jr., D.E., Hartwell, L.H., Brown, P.O., Friend, S.H. (1998). Drug target validation and identification of secondary drug target effects using DNA microarrays. *Nature Medicine* **4(11)**.

Mayer, G., Grattinger, M., Blind, M. (2003). Aptamer technology. *Drug Plus International* (Nov–Dec).

Moulay, S. (2007). Therapeutic, tinting, and taste-related molecules: Other facets of serendipity. *Khimiya/Chemistry* **16(6)**.

O'Connor, S. (1993). Rational drug design, medicinal chemistry, planned serendipity and the impact of automation on the drug discovery process. *Journal of Automatic Chemistry* **15**:9–12.

Owino, V.A., Masiga, D.K., Limo, M.K. (2008). RNA interference: A pathway to drug target identification and validation in trypanosome. *African Journal of Biochemistry Research* **2(3)**:66–73.

Patwardhan, B., Vaidya, A.D.B., Chorghade, M. (2004). Ayurveda and natural products drug discovery. *Current Science* **86(6)**.

Persengiev, S.P., Zhu, X., Green, M.R. (2004). Nonspecific, concentration-dependent stimulation and repression of mammalian gene expression by small interfering RNAs (siRNAs). *RNA* **10(1)**:12–18.

Ratti, E., Trist, D. (2001). Continuing evolution of the drug discovery process in the pharmaceutical industry. *Pure and Applied Chemistry* **73(1)**:67–75.

Rayburn, E., Wang, H., He, J., Zhang, R. (2005). RNA silencing technologies in drug discovery and target validation. *Letters in Drug Design and Discovery* **2(1)**.

Roberts, R.M. (1989). *Serendipity: Accidental Discoveries in Science*. New York: John Wiley & Sons.

Rollinger, J.M., Langer, T., Stuppner, H. (2006). Strategies for efficient lead structure discovery from natural products. *Current Medicinal Chemistry* **13**:1491–1507.

Ryals, J. (2004). Metabolomics–An important emerging science. *Business Briefing: PharmaTech*.

Schena, M., Shalon, D., Davis, R.W., Brown, P.O. (1995). Quantitative monitoring of gene expression patterns with a complementary DNA microarray. *Science* **270**:467–470.

Shafikhani S.H., Engel J. (2006). *Pseudomonas aeruginosa* type III-secreted toxin ExoT inhibits host-cell division by targeting cytokinesis at multiple steps. *Proceedings of the National Academy of Sciences* USA **103**:15605–15610.

Sinskey, A.J., Finkelstein, S.N. (2002). Industry watch: Getting to rational drug design–At last. *PharmaGenomics* (Nov–Dec).

Sledz, C.A., Holko, M., de Veer, M.J., Silverman, R.H., Williams, B.R. (2003). Activation of the interferon system by short-interfering RNAs. *Nature Cell Biology* **5(9)**:834–839.

Smith, C. (2003). Drug target validation: Hitting the target. *Nature* 422:341–347.

Sneader, W. (1996). *Drug Prototypes and Their Exploitation*. Chichester, UK: John Wiley & Sons.

Sridhar, P., Kahveci, T., Ranka, S. (2007). *Pacific Symposium on Biocomputing* **12**:88–99.

Sternberg, M.J.E., Muggleton, S.H. (2003). Structure activity relationships (SAR) and pharmacophore discovery using inductive logic programming (ILP). *QSAR and Combinatorial Science* **22**.

Sweeny, K. (2002). Technology trends in drug discovery and development: Implications for the development of the pharmaceutical industry in Australia, Pharmaceutical Industry Project Equity, Sustainability and Industry Development, Working Paper Series.

Talapatra, A., Rouse, R., Hardiman, G. (2002). Protein microarrays: challenges and promises. *Pharmacogenomics* **3(4)**.

Van Duin, M., Woolson, H., Mallinson, D., Black, D. (2003). Genomics in target and drug discovery. *Biochemical Society Transactions* **31(2)**.

Varambally, S., Dhanasekaran, S.M., Zhou, M., Barrette, T.R., Kumar-Sinha, C., Sanda, M.G., *et al*. (2002). The polycomb group protein EZH2 is involved in progression of prostate cancer. *Nature* **419**:624–629.

Verhelst, S.H.L., Bogyo, M. (2005). Chemical proteomics applied in target identification and drug discovery. *BioTechniques* **38(2)**.

Vicens, Q., Westhof, E. (2003). RNA as a drug target: The case of aminoglycosides. *ChemBioChem* **4**.

Wang, S., Sim, T.B., Kim, Y.-S., Chang Y.T. (2004). Tools for target identification and validation. *Current Opinion in Chemical Biology* **8**:371–377.

Wang, Z., Morris, J., Drew, M., Englund, P. (2000). Inhibition of *Trypanosoma brucei* gene expression by RNA interference using an intergratable vector with opposing T7 promoters. *Journal of Biological Chemistry* **275**:40174–40179.

Williams, K.J., Duncan, K. (2007). Current strategies for identifying and validating targets for new treatment-shortening drugs for TB. *Current Molecular Medicine* **7(3)**.

Wissenbach, U., Niemeyer, B.A., Flockerzi, V. (2004). TRP channels as potential drug targets. *Biology of the Cell* **96**:47–54.

3

Development of Screening Assays for Drug Discovery

***Anitha K. Nair*[1]*, Somashekara N.*[1]*, and C.N. Ramchand*[*1,2]**

[1]*Laila Pharmaceuticals Pvt. Ltd., Chennai, India*
[2]*Visiting Faculty, Swinburne University of Technology, Melbourne, Australia*

Drug screening, i.e. the evaluation of the biological activity of candidate drug molecules, is a key step in the drug discovery and development process. A crucial part of drug discovery involves development of an appropriate screening assay for potential drug candidates following target identification. The superiority of an assay depends on its robustness, time consumption, cost effectiveness and automation. Thus, the assay must be developed with utmost accuracy in order to achieve precise results.

Drug screening is performed broadly based on: (1) *in vitro*, (2) *in vivo* and (3) *ex vivo* assays. The *in vitro* methods involve purified or semi-purified protein or cell-based assays. The *in vivo* methods include small animal models for screening. *Ex vivo* refers to experimentation done using live tissue in a simulated environment outside the organism.

Conventional *in vitro* screening assays were mainly based on isolated proteins purified from natural source or cloned cell lines. Enzyme assays were usually carried out using flourogenic/chromogenic/radiolabeled substrates. These are based on the disappearance of substrate, appearance of product or change in the levels of cofactor. Detection involves recording the fluorescent or chemiluminescent signals caused due to enzyme activity on these substrates. The tissue-based methods involve assaying crude tissue lysates containing the protein targets for screening of compounds. Competitive ligand binding assays are used, which can be read using flourogenic/radiometric/chemiluminescence techniques.

[*] *ramchand@lailapharma.com*

Knowledge about signal transduction pathways/effectors being responsible for disease conditions gave rise to cell-based assays. This involves the cloning and expression of specific targets or noncloned targets for screening, e.g. cell surface receptors and ion channels. Cell-based screening normally engages ligand binding assays, which are divided into saturation binding and displacement binding assays, where the efficacy of the drug in binding to the target in the presence of a ligand can be evaluated. This can be studied through radiometric/flourogenic/luminescence assays like reporter construct–based assays. Ion channels in this respect are also interesting drug targets since they are involved in various transduction processes. Traditional screening methods such as fluorescent dye–based, radiometry and ligand binding are indirect assay methods.

In vitro screening results in the generation of lead compounds, which have to be screened further *in vivo* (animal studies). Conventional animal experiments involve rodent models and non-rodent models; however, due to increased cost and time consumption, other models such as zebra fish are gaining importance.

Ex vivo screening methods are adopted to check the efficacy of the lead compound(s) on the target tissue in an artificially simulated environment mainly to test drug sensitivity.

A thorough knowledge of screening assays is essential to carry out a successful drug discovery program.

INTRODUCTION

The high cost of drug development is partly due to the high failure rate of drug candidates in clinical trials. A successful lead molecule needs to be efficacious without any toxicity. One needs to select drug candidates with the most appropriate drug-like properties during drug discovery. Many drugs developed by the pharmaceutical industry fail in clinical trials because of unanticipated toxic side effects. Toxicity may be caused by a compound interacting with a molecular target that is distinct from the target selected for therapeutic benefit, defined as an off-target effect. An example of this is the large number of compounds that interfere with the cardiac potassium ion channel human ether-à-go-go (hERG), which can cause a fatal arrhythmia. Alternatively, severe side effects may result from blockage of a molecular target in a nontargeted tissue, defined as an on-target effect; e.g. nonsteroidal anti-inflammatory drugs (NSAIDS) derive therapeutic benefit from inhibiting cyclooxygenase-1 (COX-1) and/or -2. However, inhibition of COX-1 in the gastrointestinal system is linked to gastric ulcers, and, more recently, specific inhibition of COX-2 has been potentially linked to cardiovascular complications.

Predictive assays for toxicity are a crucial part of drug development to avoid many drugs failing in clinical trials. Testing the compound in mammals is labor intensive and usually toxicity studies are performed relatively late in the development process, after selection of a limited number of compounds. Thus, a need exists for rapid assays that retain the high value of *in vivo* toxicity testing, but can be rapidly performed on a large number of compounds. Advancement in modern drug discovery leads to the early detection of drug failure through screening assays.

The rapid progress in elucidating the mechanisms of different diseases is significantly increasing the number of proteins that can be targeted for potential drug treatment. Parallel to these developments, the number and diversity of compounds that can be tested for activity against their respective targets are also rapidly expanding. The combination of these trends in biology and chemistry has spurred the development of increasingly rapid, selective and reliable high-throughput screening (HTS) assays to be applied in the early phase of drug discovery. These assays allow screening of large numbers of compounds in an automated fashion to identify those that show an activity, either as agonists or as antagonists, on a defined biological target. Most of the assay formats developed to date can be grouped into biochemical or cellular assays.

IMPORTANCE OF SCREENING ASSAYS IN DRUG DISCOVERY

The primary importance of drug screening assays is to understand a new chemical entity (NCE), regarding its pharmacodynamics, pharmacokinetics, metabolism or toxicity. However, in the present context, the importance is mainly given on understanding the pharmacodynamics of a molecule with respect to the target.

Assays are valuable tools in studying the drug absorption, transportation, metabolism, excretion, interaction with ligand and toxicity of the drug molecule. Physical and chemical properties of the compounds can be used for determination of drug-like properties. A study of the interaction between the compound and its biological target has become a very important part of drug discovery. Through genomic and proteomic studies, the potential existence of about 10,000 druggable targets is anticipated; however, <500 of these targets have corresponding existing approved drugs (Ma and Horiuchi, 2006). Therefore, screening a drug candidate against a new target in a quick and economical way has become the most challenging and most important step in modern drug discovery.

Early drug discovery was largely dependent on screenings using whole organisms or cells to evaluate biologically active substances without knowledge of their potential molecular targets. More advancement in elucidating the mechanism of diseases led to a target-based approach of drug discovery, using mechanism-based screening assays. HTS assays have been developed to enable the rapid analysis of large numbers of compounds for their effects on the function of specific targets.

High-quality assays are needed for translating specific biomolecular phenomena into observable parameters to develop meaningful data with the required throughput. Typically this is achieved through the measurements of variety of biochemical phenomena. An HTS assay plays a very important role as the first step in the process of filtering out potential 'hits' to be optimized as downstream drug candidates. Assays will also minimize drug failure at the end of the drug discovery process, which was found to be very costly. These assays need to fulfill several important technical criteria such as being physiologically relevant and at the same time fast and sensitive.

Radioactive methods have become less popular, primarily because of the burden of handling radioactive materials and the availability of non-radioactive alternatives. Assays based on light absorption are commonly used, but they impose limits on assay design and miniaturization because of their low sensitivity. Spectrophotometric assay methods are the dominant assay methodology due to their broad adaptability to biological targets and automation methods, and their ability to deliver the speed, accuracy and sensitivity necessary for successful HTS. In the last few years, cell-based assays using cells and microorganisms have become an increasingly attractive alternative to *in vitro* biochemical assays for HTS in the early phase of the drug discovery process.

TYPES OF ASSAYS

Assays are basically classified into biochemical-based and cell-based assays. The biochemical assays are again divided into assays involving isolated protein and those involving crude proteins. Cell-based assays are classified into mammalian cell-based and microbial cell-based assays.

Biochemical Assays

Biochemical assays are receptor-, protein- or enzyme-based assays using a particular target of interest in a purified form and exclusively rely on a cell-free interaction system. These are broadly used for primary screening of drug candidates and are extremely useful in drug screening. Biochemical assays are not expected to bear the entire burden of hit-to-lead and lead optimization strategies and are normally followed by animal experiments. Many of the biochemical assays are radiometric, colorimetric or fluorescence-based assays. The major draw back is that they do not provide any information on the type of interaction, e.g. whether the NCE screened is an agonist, antagonist or inverse agonist. One needs to do cell-based transduction assay to understand the type of molecular interaction.

Biochemical assays are of two basic types: homogeneous assays and heterogeneous assays.

Homogeneous Assays

Homogeneous assays are one-step assays where the reagents will be added in a single step or in multiple steps and the signals are read in the plate reader. Different detection methods are used for the reading such as chromogenic, radiometric, flourometric, UV-metric, and so on.

Homogeneous assays could be readily converted to HTS by applying detection systems that do not require separation of the reaction product from substrate. For example, fluorescence-based techniques allow detection of enzymatic activities as well as molecular interactions without the requirement of separation, fractionation or purification procedures (Hertzberg and Pope, 2000). These automated assays allow rapid screens of large compound libraries to identify the so-called 'hits', i.e. compounds showing the desired effect on the biochemical activity of the specific target in the isolated *in vitro* system.

Heterogeneous Assays

Heterogeneous assays are multi-step assays involving additions of reagents, incubation, transfers of reagents or intermediate solutions and washings to remove any interference and excess of reagents. Different detection methods can be radiometric, spectrophotometric and fluorescent based. The principle of heterogeneous assays is to use probe molecules bound to solid substrate in order to detect target molecules in a given sample such as immunoassays and DNA binding assays.

Radiolabeled compounds are commonly used in receptor–ligand binding studies due to their high sensitivity and robustness. These assays involve the measurement of radioactivity upon completion of the reaction. A radioactive isotope is mostly linked to one of the reactants, which is released upon the reaction completion. The most commonly used isotopes are ^{3}H, ^{14}C, ^{32}P and ^{125}I. There are various assays based on radioactivity such as precipitation, adsorption, radioimmune and filtration assays.

Bioluminescence and chemiluminescence represent suitable detection techniques for HTS because they allow rapid and sensitive detection of the analytes and can be applied to small-volume samples (Roda *et al.*, 2003). Although assays based on either fluorescence or chemiluminescence can yield high sample throughput, fluorescence has been used more commonly because of its broader familiarity and easier implementation into new assay designs. The main obstacle to the use of chemiluminescence in HTS has been the lack of available assay methods. But new capabilities in chemiluminescence, particularly in bioluminescence, are now changing this. This chapter will focus on the expanding scope of bioluminescence technologies available for HTS and provide some perspectives on future developments.

Bioluminescence is a special form of chemiluminescence found in living organisms. As a class, it is characterized as being an enzyme-catalyzed process, where the high efficiency of photon emission is derived through natural evolution. The enzymes are called luciferases, and the photon-emitting substrates are luciferins. Bioluminescent chemistries have evolved from multiple independent origins, and thus comprise many distinct molecular structures. Of the many natural forms, only three have been widely used in HTS: firefly luciferase, Renilla luciferase and aequorin (Fan and Wood, 2007).

Spectrophotometric assays

Spectrophotometric assays are based on the amount of light absorbed or transmitted by a substance either in the visible, UV or IR range. The assays work on Beer–Lambert law, as per which the concentration is directly proportional to the absorbance and inversely proportional to transmittance. Therefore, if the concentration of a given substance is more, then the absorption of light increases and vice versa.

Every substance has exclusive absorption maxima, i.e. the substance under study will absorb the light at a particular wavelength and transmit it at a particular wavelength. This could be absorbed by specific chemical groups (e.g. reduced form of NAD or NADP) in the substance or chromogenic compounds (e.g. tetrazolium dye in 3-(4,5-dimethylthiazol-2-yl)-2,5-diphenyltetrazolium bromide [MTT] assay) present in the assay mixture. This gives rise to a unique fingerprint for the substance. Thus one can quantify a given substance effortlessly with the amount of light either absorbed or transmitted by the substance.

Spectrophotometric methods are very useful for the determination of psychotropic substances in pharmaceuticals and body fluids (Puzanowska-Tarasiewicz *et al.*, 2009). Table 3.1 shows the different psychotropic drugs and spectrophotometric conditions for measurement (Puzanowska-Tarasiewicz *et al.*, 2009).

Psychotropic drugs such as dibenzoazepines, dibenzocycloheptadienes, thioxanthenes, phenothiazines, fluoxetine, fluvoxamine and trazodone form cations, which react with some organic substances (picric acid, flavianic acid, alizarin S, brilliant blue and triphenylmethane dyes) and thiocyanate or halide anionic complexes (e.g. Co(II), Pd(II), Fe(III), Cr(III), Au(III), Ti(IV), Pt(IV), Mo(V), W(V), U(VI)), forming ion association compounds. These compounds get precipitated from aqueous solutions and can be quantitatively extracted into organic solvents (e.g. chloroform, dichloromethane and butanol). The extracts are intensely colored and stable for 1–3 days. These properties have been applied for the determination of above-mentioned metal ions and active compounds in pharmaceutical preparations. The main disadvantage of direct UV spectrophotometry is the sensitivity to excipients usually present in pharmaceutical formulations (Puzanowska-Tarasiewicz *et al.*, 2009).

Table 3.1 *Different Psychotropic Substances and Spectrophotometric Conditions for Measurement*

Psychotropic Substance	*System*	*Organic Solvent*	*λ (nm)*	*Range of Determination (ppm)*
Levomepromazine (LPZ)	LPZ-[Cr(NH3)2(SCN)4]	Acetone	525	53–427
Chlorpromazine (CPZ)	CPZ-[Cr(NH3)2(SCN)4]	Acetone	520	156–689
Chlorpromazine (CPZ)	Fe(iii)-SCN--CPZ	Chloroform	490	120–300
Levomepromazine (LPZ)	Fe(iii)-SCN--LPZ			140–400
Promethazine (PMT)	Fe(iii)-SCN--PMT			160–550
Chlorpromazine (CPZ)	Co(ii)-SCN--PMT	Ether	620	100–600
Chloracizine (CRZ)	Co(ii)-SCN--CRZ			100–900
Chlorpromazine (CPZ)	Ge(iv)-PCV-CPZ	Cyclohexanone	580	7–70
Chlorpromazine (CPZ)	Sn(iv)-PCV-CPZ	Butanol	580	2–20
Desipramine (DE)	Ti(iv)-SCN--DE	Chloroform	355	5–200
Thioridazine (TR)	Ti(iv)-SCN--TR	Chloroform	417	20–160
Perazine (PZ)	Ti(iv)-SCN--PZ	Butanol (4:1)	360	20–170
Amitriptyline (AM)	Ti(iv)-SCN--AM			3–60
Promazine (PM)	Nb(v)-SCN--PM	Trichloroethylene	400	20–200
Imipramine (IM)	Nb(v)-SCN--IM	Butanol–chloroform (1:9)	350	0.8–8
Doxepin (DX)	Ti(iv)-SCN--DX	Butanol–Chloroform (2:3)	400	5–50
Chloroprothixene (CX)	Nb(v)-SCN--CX	Butanol	362	9–50

Flourescence

Flourometric assays are based on the concept of fluorescence where a given substance absorbs light of a particular wavelength and immediately emits a light of longer wavelength. This light mostly falls in the UV region but can also be in the visible region. The basic principle is that a flourophore at its ground level absorbs light energy as photons and gets excited to the vibrational level. But when the flourophore returns to the ground level it emits the light energy absorbed which is detected as fluorescence.

Bioassays can be performed using this principle as certain substances have an intrinsic fluorescence capability or one can tag the given sample/substrate in the assay mixture with fluorescent tags which can be detected by a flourometer/spectroscope. Therefore this method is considered as far more superior and effective method of detection/quantification over the rest of the available methods.

The various methods that use this principle is polarization, quenching, time correlation, life-time variation and Fluroscence Resonance Energy Transfer (FRET).

Chemiluminescent assay

The principle of chemiluminescence is the light generation produced in chemical reactions without external energy input. This phenomenon was applied in the development of chemiluminescent-based enzyme-linked immunosorbent assay (ELISA) systems. Chemiluminescent-based assays allow increased sensitivity over traditional colorimetric substrates. Horseradish peroxidase (HRP)–based ELISA systems for luminescense assays are among the most common assays. HRP, hydrogen peroxide and luminol react to produce light with an emission maximum at 425 nm, which is also called as chemiluminescent intensity (CLI). Typically an enhancer along with other additives is included with substrate mixtures to increase and stabilize the signal. Because of the increased sensitivity, chemiluminescent assays have been used to replace radioactive-based detection methods and also because chemicals used in chemiluminescent are safe and give researchers an alternative to radioactive assays.

Chemiluminescent assay is also being used for the determination of antibacterial effect of many drugs. One such example is the determination of antibacterial effect of linezolid (LZD) on strains of methicillin-resistant *Staphylococcus aureus* (MRSA). In this chemiluminescent assay, chemiluminescence is based on the generation of hydrogen peroxide by viable cells linking with the bacterial electron transfer system. In this experiment, a bacterial suspension (1.1X109 CFU/l) was made in Rapid-Lumi medium. Then, 45 µl of this suspension was dispensed into each well of a 96-well microtiter plate containing 5 µl of various concentrations of LZD solution (final concentration = 0, 0.5, 1, 2, 3, …, 9, and 10 mg/l). After 3 h of incubation at 37°C, 5 µl of menadione solution (50mg/l) was added. The mixture was incubated further for 1h, and then chemiluminescence intensity (CLI) was measured by the alkaline lucigenin method with a luminescence reader. The CLI directly reflects the metabolic activity of the tested strain. To evaluate the extent of bacterial drug resistance more accurately, the following three parameters can be calculated from the chemiluminescence graphs: (1) ED50: Drug concentration (effective dose) that produced 50% CLI relative to the control activity; (2) ED25: Drug concentration that produced 25% CLI relative to the control activity (i.e., 75% suppression). Chemiluminescence intensity measured in a drug-free medium will be used as a control (100%) (Komatsu *et al.*, 2009). The CLI graph is shown in Fig. 3.1.

The graph show the results of the chemiluminescence assay of LZD for representative MRSA strains. The ordinate of the graph indicates metabolic activity of the bacterial cells (LZD and other agents will not directly interfere with the measurement system). In the graph, except for one strain, the CLI of every strain declined sharply (without tailing or increased baseline activity) as the LZD concentration increased (Komatsu *et al.*, 2009).

Radiometric assay

These assays involve the measurement of radioactivity upon completion of the reaction. Mostly a radioactive isotope is linked to one of the reactants, which is released upon the reaction completion. The most commonly used isotopes are ^{3}H, ^{14}C, ^{32}P and ^{125}I.

An example is a new specific and sensitive lipase assay based on the use of a radiolabeled triglyceride, [^{3}H]triolein. Microbiologists generally assay lipase activities by using synthetic fluorescent analogs related to the coumarin fatty acyl ester family, such as 4-methylumbelliferyl (MUF) fatty acyl esters. One commonly used analog is MUF oleate. However, major drawbacks have been reported concerning this technique. According to Hendrickson and Beisson *et al.*, lipases should

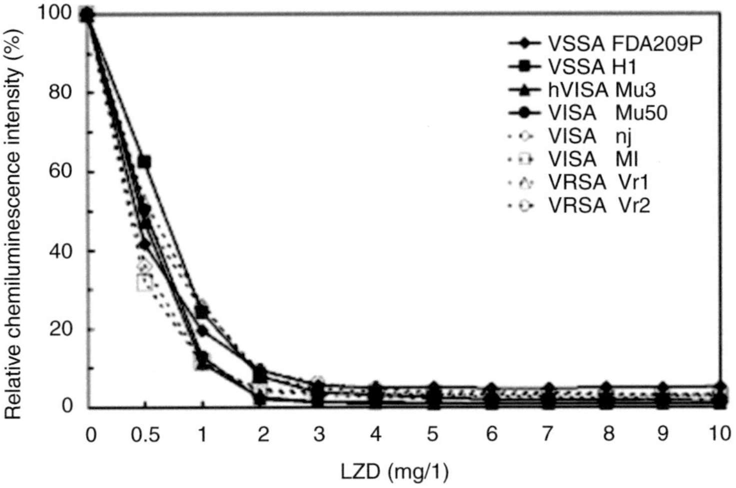

Fig. 3.1 ***Chemiluminescence-based Linezolid Susceptibility Test for S. aureus Strains***

not behave toward triglycerides in the same way as they do toward MUF oleate. Indeed, this analog, being chemically unrelated to triglycerides, is not *a priori* hydrolyzed specifically by lipases and is likely to be nonspecifically hydrolyzed by carboxylesterases (Bourguet *et al*., 2003).

The use of a radiolabeled triglyceride as a substrate for lipase hydrolysis could be an alternative to the conventional methods. Radiolabeled methods are reported to be specific, because lipases cannot distinguish a radiolabeled triglyceride from a natural one, and they are also very sensitive, due to the high specific activity of radiolabeled probes. Therefore, these methods appeared suitable for real lipase activity measurement, particularly in natural seawater samples (Bourguet *et al*., 2003).

[^{3}H]triolein lipase assay

[^{3}H]triolein lipase assay of a new specific and sensitive lipase assay is based on the use of a radiolabeled triglyceride, [^{3}H]triolein (Fig. 3.2). Free fatty acids (FFAs) resulting from its hydrolysis are isolated

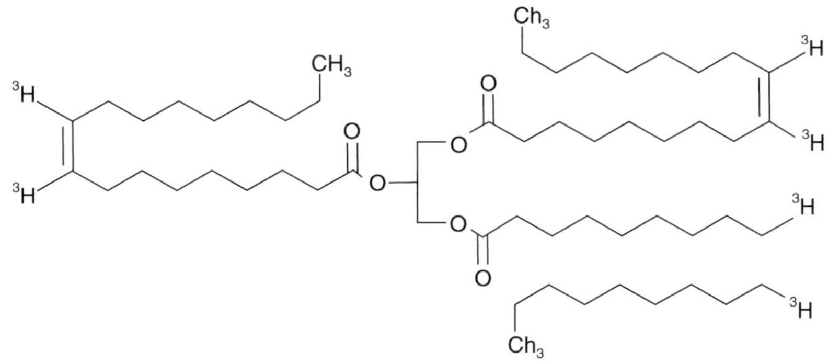

Fig. 3.2 ***Structure of [^{3}H]triolein***

as a function of time in a one-step liquid–liquid extraction and then radioassayed. During the assay, [^{3}H]triolein is hydrolyzed by lipase into free [^3H]oleic acids. The hydrolysis of the [^{3}H]triolein as a function of time is reflected by the appearance of ionized free [^{3}H]oleic acids in the alkaline aqueous phase of the extraction medium.

Chemicals such as [9,10-3*H*(*N*)]oleic acid ([^{3}H]oleic acid, 15 Cimmol^{-1}) and [9,10-^{3}H(N)] triolein ([^{3}H]triolein, 22 Cimmol^{-1}) required for the experiments were available with PerkinElmer—EN. First of all distribute water samples into 50-ml polypropylene centrifuge tubes, and add [^{3}H] triolein (<1 to 60 nM ^{3}H-esterified fatty acid [EFA]) as a solution in ethanol (final concentration, 0.005% to <0.2%). Immediately after vortex homogenization, distribute series (triplicates) of 0.8-ml subsamples into 15-ml polypropylene centrifuge tubes. Stop the reaction in the first series without delay by the addition of 0.5 ml of a 1 M solution of Tris (adjusted to pH 11 using NaOH) and 4.8 ml of a methanol–chloroform–heptane (38.6:34:27.4) solvent mixture, followed by vigorous vortex agitation. Keep the other series in the dark, in an incubation bath (*in situ* temperature, 25 ± 1°C), until the end of their incubation period and then treat as described above. Centrifuge stopped samples (for 3 min at 5445 x g) to allow separation of phases. Transfer a portion (2 ml) of the upper-aqueous phase to polypropylene scintillation vials containing 10 ml of Hionic-Fluor liquid scintillation counting cocktail (available with Packard Bioscience) for radioactivity counting. Estimate the distribution of fatty acids between the two phases at time zero, with the same protocol, using [^{3}H]oleic acid instead of [^{3}H]triolein. No incubation is performed in this case. Finally, calculate the expression of lipase activity from the radioactivity in the total volume of the aqueous phase, the proportion of released [^{3}H]oleic acids contained in this phase, and the specific activity of the radiolabeled probe. It is noteworthy that the transformation products of the [^{3}H]oleic acid (including ^{3}H-fatty acids and $3H_2O$) also end up in the aqueous phase. Autoclaved samples should be used as controls for abiotic substrate degradation (Bourguet *et al.*, 2003). A typical graph from this assay is given in Fig. 3.3.

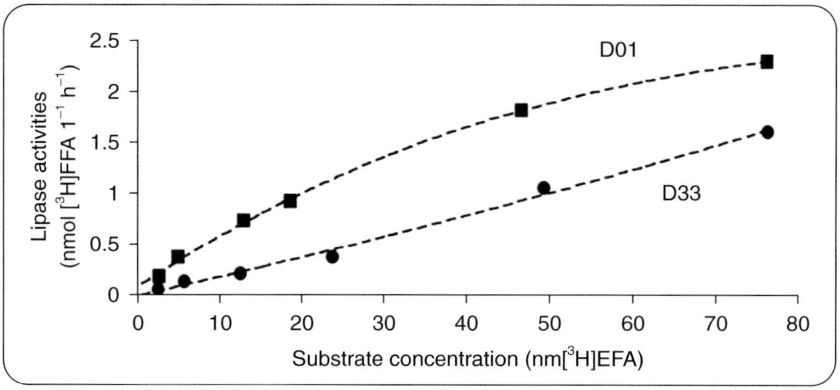

Fig. 3.3

The graphs shown in Fig. 3.3 (Bourguet *et al.*, 2003) show lipase activities at stations D01 (■) and D33 (●), which is determined by using the [^{3}H]triolein lipase assay.

Note that stations along a nearshore-to-offshore transect (D01–D33; depth, 6–23 m) exhibited an increasing gradient of salinity (34.98–35.10 gl^{-1}).

ELECTROCHEMICAL METHODS

Electrochemical techniques have led to the advancement in the field of analysis because of their sensitivity, low cost and relatively short analysis time when compared with other techniques. Moreover, the applications of electroanalytical techniques, including determination of reaction mechanisms, makes them a best choice for analysis. Redox properties of a drug can give insights into its metabolic fate or its *in vivo* redox processes or pharmaceutical activity (Kalanur *et al.*, 2008).

Electrochemical methods of detection generally include three different approaches: (1) measurement of the electrical responses of electrogenic cells, (2) measurement of the conductivity of mechanical contacts between cells and a substrate surface, and (3) measurement of the chemical signals (e.g. pH) resulting from changes in metabolic products (e.g. lactic acid) or substrates (e.g. glucose). These methods can usually provide real-time, dynamic information on cell activities. Toxicity can be detected based on the electrical responses of electrogenic cells and tissues, such as heart muscle and nerve cells. Nerve cells have high-specificity receptors that are sensitive to many neuroactive compounds. Changes in the membrane potential influence the measurable capacity between a microelectrode and axon when nerve cells are grown on a field-effect transistor. Devices using microelectrode arrays, such as multichannel systems, have been developed to monitor extracellular activities for toxicity assays (Ziegler, 2000).

Electrochemical methods have also been used for the study and determination of some psychotropic drugs such as phenothiazines, azaphenothiazines, dibenzoazepines, thioxanthenes and their derivatives. Among the methods, voltammetry (cyclic voltammetry and differential pulse voltammetry) is mainly used. Electrochemical behavior of these active substances in the drug formulation is exploited for using these substances in polarographic and voltammetric analysis (Puzanowska-Tarasiewicz *et al.*, 2009).

Psychotropic drugs are easily oxidized or reduced electrochemically. Chlorpromazine has been determined in urine samples of patients by adsorptive stripping voltammetry in the presence of Triton X-100. Fluphenazine and trifluoperazine were determined by differential pulse voltammetry after pre-concentration at a wax-impregnated graphite electrode. Promazine, chlorpromazine and promethazine spiked in urine samples were oxidized by nitrous acid into the corresponding sulfoxides, which were polarographically active and produce a well-defined diffusion-controlled cathodic wave. The dibenzoazepine derivatives such as imipramine, clomipramine and trimipramine were determined in drug preparations and plasma samples with adsorptive stripping voltammetry. Imipramine and desipramine were analyzed through cyclic voltammetry at glassy carbon and boron-doped diamond electrode and differential pulse voltammetry. Thioxanthene derivatives such as zuclopenthixol were determined quantitatively by measuring the height of voltammetric peaks. The oxidative voltammetric behavior of zuclopenthixol at a glassy carbon electrode has been studied using cyclic, linear sweep and differential pulse voltammetry. Drugs such as chlorprothixene and thiothixene were determined polarographically through the formation of their bromo-derivatives, which manifest well-defined cathodic waves in select supporting electrolytes (Puzanowska-Tarasiewicz *et al.*, 2009).

An example is the determination of human islet amyloid polypeptide (hIAPP) electrochemically by using the oxidized signal of the tyrosine residue in hIAPP.

hIAPP, aggregating into cytotoxic oligomers, polymers or fibrils *in vivo*, has been discovered to be related to cell degeneration and the pathogenesis of Alzheimer's disease. During the aggregation, normally soluble proteins will be converted into an insoluble amyloid, which consists of fibrils rich in β-sheet structures and has characteristic dye-binding properties. hIAPP or amylin is a 37-residue peptide containing an amidated C-terminal and a disulfide linkage between cysteine residues 2 and 7, synthesized in the pancreas and co-secreted with insulin. It has been suggested that hIAPP may play an important role in glucose homeostasis together with insulin. Though hIAPP is itself a soluble polypeptide, its flexible conformation has a tendency to misfold into insoluble, cytotoxic fibrils through a complicated multistep nucleation–aggregation process. An assay of hIAPP and its aggregation is highly required in studying Alzheimer's disease pathogenesis (Zhou *et al.*, 2007).

The previous assay methods are basically based on the techniques of microscopy and spectroscopy, such as atomic force microscopy, circular dichroism spectroscopy and fluorescence assay. Electrochemical techniques are known to be useful to study the oxidation reactions of tyrosine, tryptophan and related peptides. Electrochemical methods have also been adopted to monitor the folding and unfolding of proteins and aggregation of peptides. An intrinsic redox-active amino acid–based detection method has been used to fabricate label-free electrochemical protein sensors (Zhou *et al.*, 2007).

It has been known that tyrosine can be oxidized irreversibly, giving an anodic peak in the corresponding voltammogram. In hIAPP, although it is a 37-residue peptide containing only one tyrosine residue, this residue is at its C-terminal and therefore it may endow the peptide with oxidable properties on an electrode surface. The relationship between the oxidation peak current in the voltammogram and the concentration of hIAPP can be established. Therefore, it is possible to develop an electrochemical method to study the aggregation process of this polypeptide, because with aggregation, less and less tyrosine residues can be oxidized to give an electrochemical signal, so the oxidation peak will be smaller and smaller (Zhou *et al.*, 2007).

A kinetic study of the aggregation process can be carried out according to the relationship between the anodic peak current in the square-wave voltammograms of hIAPP and the incubation period (Zhou *et al.*, 2007). A typical graph of the study is given in Fig. 3.4.

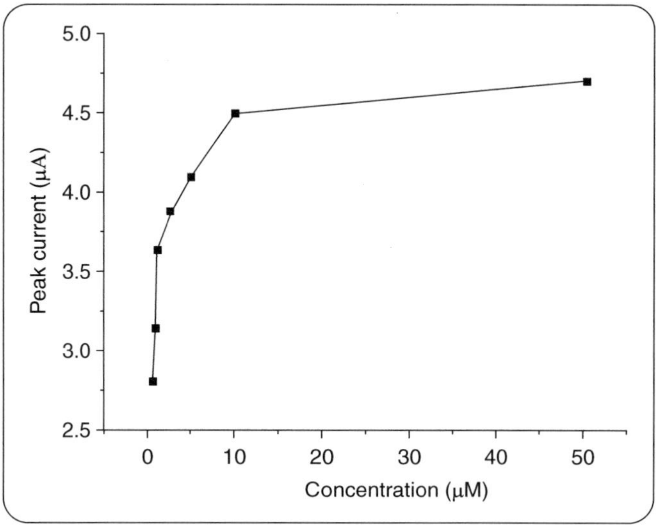

Fig. 3.4

The graph in Fig. 3.4 shows that nucleation starts in the first hour of incubation, and then, during the next two hours, aggregation may occur rapidly. hIAPP can therefore be monitored with a label-free electrochemical method with low detection limit and high sensitivity. This electrochemical method can also be utilized to study the kinetics of hIAPP aggregation, and it may also be employed to study the conformational changes of the polypeptide (Zhou *et al.*, 2007).

ION FLUX ASSAYS

Ion flux assays using nonradioactive ion tracers analyzed in atomic absorption spectroscopy (AAS) have been utilized since the 1950s. Commercial instrumentation for high-throughput AAS screening has only recently become available.

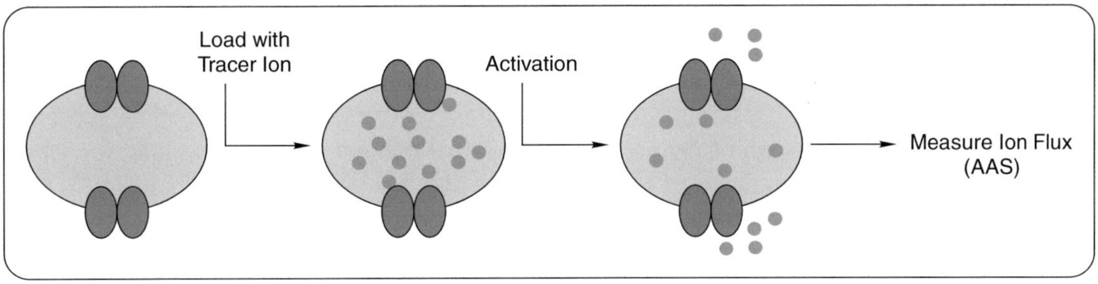

Fig. 3.5

The principal basic AAS assays have been developed for a variety of voltage-gated (Bourguet *et al.*, 2003) and ligand-gated (Zhou *et al.*, 2007) channels. For this assay, nonradioactive tracer ions are loaded into cells expressing the channel of interest (Fig. 3.5). Ion flux is then initiated when channels are activated by a ligand or by depolarizing the cell membrane with a high K^- buffer (50–80 mM). The concentration of the tracer ion in the supernatant and/or within the cells is then measured, and the percentage of efflux (or influx) is calculated. The signal-to-noise ratio of this assay is typically 6–10, and the reagent cost for screening is very low. Both single-channel and multichannel instruments are currently available for 96-well and 384-well screens with moderate throughput. Reports describing the application of this technology for screening assays have been primarily focused on potassium channels such as hERG, KCNQ2 and Ca^2-activated potassium channels where Rb^- is used as the tracer ion (Zheng *et al.*, 2004).

IMMUNOLOGICAL ASSAYS

Enzyme-Linked Immunosorbent Assays

Fundamental Principle

ELISA methods are fundamental tools in the drug discovery process with applications in drug screening, clinical trials and animal studies. ELISA is a simple, rapid and more versatile method used for drug screening. The principal components in enzyme-linked immunoassays are a drug labeled with a specific enzyme, an antibody specific to that drug, a substrate capable of producing a measured optical signal when initiated by the enzyme and the test sample (Tijssen, 1985). In an ELISA, the drug labeled with an enzyme competes with the drug in the test sample for a limited number of antibody binding sites. The principal advantages of using ELISA are its extreme sensitivity and specificity.

Formats of ELISA

ELISAs can be performed with a number of modifications to the basic procedure (Fig. 3.6). The important step, immobilization of the antigen of interest, can be accomplished by direct adsorption to the assay plate or indirectly via a capture antibody that has been attached to the plate. The antigen is then detected either directly (labeled primary antibody) or indirectly (labeled secondary antibody). Sandwich assay is the most powerful ELISA assay format. It is called a 'sandwich' assay because the analyte to be measured is bound between two primary antibodies (the capture antibody and the detection antibody). The sandwich format is used because it is sensitive and robust.

An ELISA can also be performed as a competitive assay. This is common when the antigen is small and has only one epitope, or antibody binding site. One variation of this method consists of labeling purified antigen instead of the antibody. Unlabeled antigen from samples and the labeled antigen compete for binding. A decrease in signal from purified antigen indicates the presence of the antigen in samples when compared to assay wells with labeled antigen alone.

Fluorescent tags to enzyme-based detection can be used for plate-based assays. All of the above-mentioned assays are often called ELISAs despite not involving antibodies.

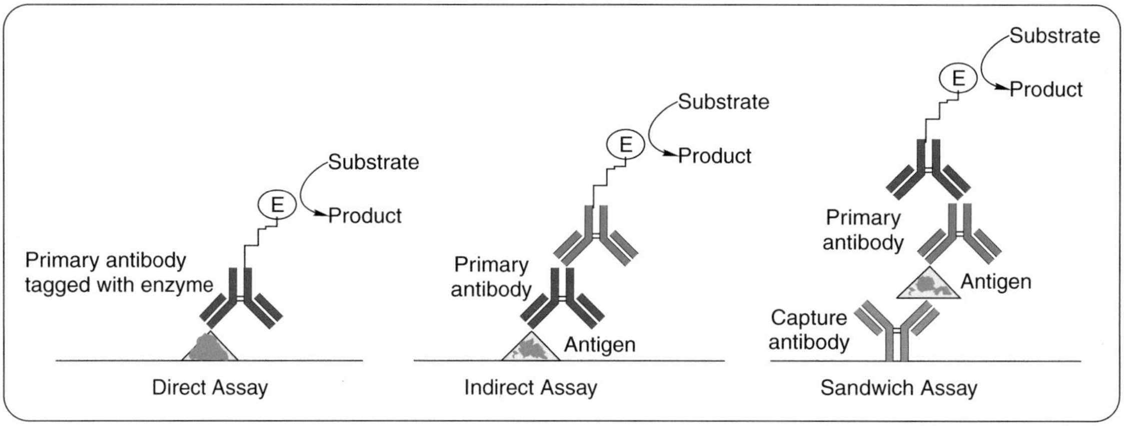

Fig. 3.6 *Formats of ELISA (For color figure please see Plate 5)*

Detection Methods of ELISA

The direct detection method uses a primary antibody (labeled) that reacts directly with the antigen. Direct detection can be performed with antigen that is directly immobilized on the assay plate or with the capture assay format. Direct detection is quite common for the immunohistochemical staining of tissues and cells, otherwise not commonly used.

The indirect detection method uses a labeled secondary antibody, which has specificity for and the primary antibody for detection; this is the most popular format for ELISA. In a sandwich ELISA, it is critical that the secondary antibody be specific for the detection of primary antibody only and not the capture antibody. The antibodies from different host species such as mouse IgG and rabbit IgG will not have affinity to each other. For sandwich assays, it is beneficial to use secondary antibodies that have been cross-adsorbed to remove any antibodies that have affinity for the capture antibody.

ISOLATED AND PURIFIED PROTEINS (ENZYMES)

Enzymes are macromolecules produced by the cells of living organisms that act as biocatalysts driving or facilitating a specific chemical reaction involving only a particular substrate at an increased rate. Substrates are those chemical compounds that are converted into products by the enzymes. These products are involved in various biological processes of the living organisms. The activity of this molecule was first noticed in the 19th century and recorded by Louis Pasteur; later, the molecule was termed 'enzyme' by Wilhelm Kuhne in 1878. Enzymes are proteinaceous in nature. The fact that enzymes are involved in most of the biological processes makes it indispensable for life. This characteristic of enzymes makes the living system more vulnerable to disorders attributed to any dysfunction of these enzymes. Therefore it can be said that enzymes make very valuable drug targets.

Three-Dimensional Protein Structures

One of the most interesting aspects of enzymes is its specificity. As mentioned earlier, enzymes catalyze reactions involving its unique substrate. Thus one enzyme can catalyze only one reaction involving a specific substrate. This substrate specificity has been explained and demonstrated by Fischer's 'lock and key' model and Koshland's 'induced fit model'. This unique feature displayed by enzymes and substrate makes the enzymes more susceptible to inhibition through the use of specific inhibitors. Inhibitors are small molecules that mainly restrain enzyme activity by occupying the active site, thereby not allowing the substrate to enter the active site and bind to the enzyme; or they bind to the enzyme in such a way that it alters the structure of the enzyme, not permitting the substrate binding. For this reason most of the drugs currently in the market are enzyme inhibitors like sulfanilamide of the sulfa drug group.

The inhibitors are of two types:

1. Reversible: Where the binding of the inhibitor and enzyme is reversible due to the non-covalent interactions/weak bonds formed between the two. The binding and detachment of inhibitor and enzyme takes place at a fast rate due to this reason, though the effect is immediate.

2. Irreversible: Where the binding of an inhibitor and enzyme is irreversible due to the formation of covalent bonds usually between the two, resulting in structural alteration and subsequent inactivation of the enzyme. The binding of inhibitor and enzyme is slower in this case due to the formation of covalent bonds, which are stronger but form at a lesser pace.

Reversible inhibitors are of three types: (1) competitive, (2) noncompetitive, and (3) uncompetitive (Fig. 3.7). Competitive inhibitors are those that resemble the substrate structurally and hence compete with the substrate to occupy the active site of enzyme. In the case of excess inhibitors than substrate, the probability of inhibitor binding the active site is high compared to that of substrate and vice versa. Thus reversible inhibition can be overcome by excess of substrate. But in the case of noncompetitive or mixed inhibition the inhibitor binds to either enzyme or enzyme–substrate complex, thereby bringing about the inhibition. In most cases the inhibitor binds to sites other than the active site, which alters the tertiary structure of the enzyme or substrate in a manner not allowing either of them to bind to each other. Substrate concentration does not influence the inhibition. Uncompetitive inhibition is where the binding of the inhibitor is possible only after the formation of enzyme–substrate complex. Even in this case excess substrate cannot overcome the inhibition. This can be quantitatively explained by the use of Michaelis–Menten kinetics.

Inhibition	Km	Vmax
Competitive	⇑	⇔
Noncompetitive	⇔	⇓
Uncompetitive	⇓	⇓

Increase ⇑ No changes ⇔ Decrease ⇓

Fig. 3.7 *Km, Substrate Concentration; Vmax, Rate of the Reaction*

A very simple example can be assaying COX activity in the presence of specific inhibitors such as indomethacin, mecfelminic acid, diclofenac and nimesulide. To start with, a standard curve has to be obtained for COX activity, which is done by taking a known amount of arachidonic acid (substrate), whose concentration is kept constant. Varying concentrations of enzyme are added and incubated for a fixed time frame and then terminated. Following incubation, the release of prostaglandin E2 (PGE2) by varying concentrations of the enzyme is recorded by measuring spectrophotometrically at a wavelength of 610 nm. The conversion of PGE2 from arachidonic acid directly corresponds to the enzyme activity (Fig. 3.8).

For a typical graph the enzyme activity is standardized by assaying the PGE2 synthesized from varying concentrations of the enzyme. From this an optimal concentration of enzyme is chosen and used for the subsequent screening of COX-2 inhibitors. In this the test compound is taken in varying concentrations and incubated with the enzyme and substrate (Fig. 3.9).

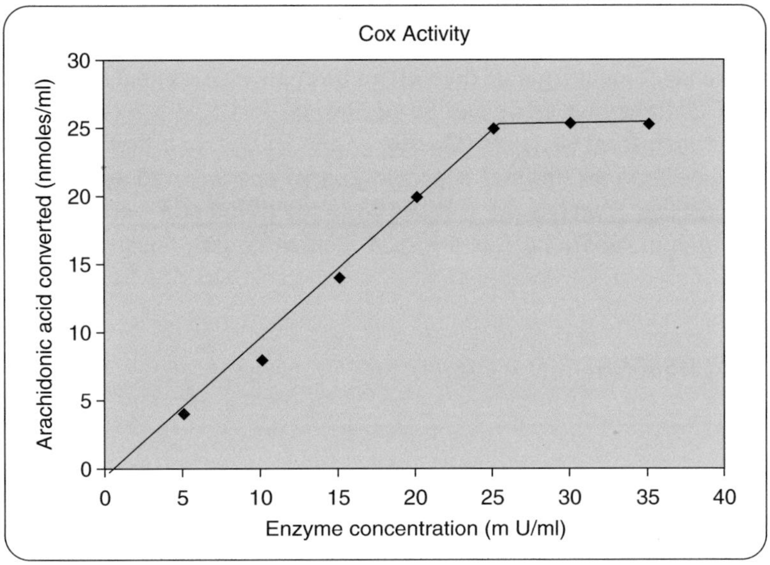

Fig. 3.8

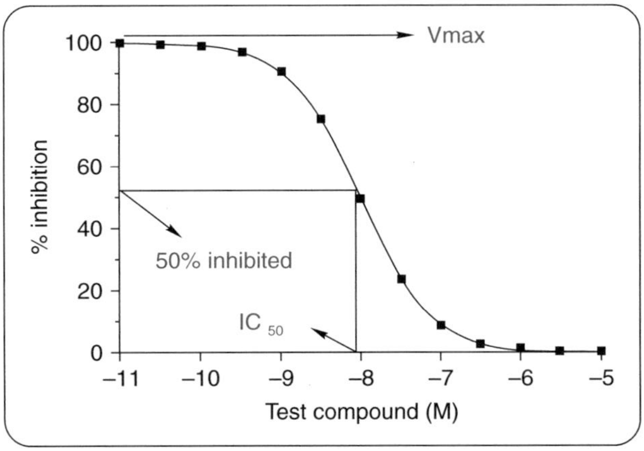

Fig. 3.9 *Vmax, The Rate of the Reaction; 10^{-8} (M), The Concentration of Test Compound Needed to bring about 50% of Inhibition of COX-2*

A radiometric assay (liquid scintillation proximity) can also be done using radiolabeled substrates (14*C*-arachidonic acid) but this will involve a separation step as it is a heterogeneous assay.

CRUDE PROTEIN SCREENING ASSAYS

This type of screening is less complicated than purified protein assays because it does not involve the purification step but only tissue extracts. Assuming that a protein involved in the pathology of a particular condition is present in large quantities in a tissue, then that tissue is taken and extracted with appropriate buffers for the protein of interest. The crude extract is then treated with the test compound to evaluate its efficacy against the protein through various analytical techniques.

For example a COX enzyme assay can be performed just like the one described for purified COX enzyme assay above from platelets (Ouellet *et al.*, 2001). As a first step the enzyme activity is first standardized and then an optimal concentration of enzyme and substrate is chosen for the screening study. In this case platelets are isolated from the blood and washed and separated. These platelets suspended in appropriate buffers are then incubated with the test substance, and IC50 is recorded.

Receptor Binding Assays

Receptors

A receptor is a protein molecule, embedded in either the plasma membrane or cytoplasm of a cell, to which a mobile signaling molecule may attach. A molecule that binds to a receptor is called a ligand. The ligand can be a peptide (such as a neurotransmitter), a hormone, a pharmaceutical drug or a toxin, and when such binding occurs, the receptor undergoes a conformational change, which ordinarily initiates a cellular response. However, some ligands merely block receptors without inducing any response (e.g. antagonists). Ligand-induced changes in receptors result in physiological changes, which constitute the biological activity of the ligands. Receptors play the role of the sensing elements in the wide range of chemical communications that coordinate the function of all the different cells in the body. A receptor binding assay provides a direct approach to the study of receptors in tissue preparations, and their modifications by drugs, disease states, or experimental conditions.

Receptor assays are routinely used for the assessment of the interaction of (new) chemical entities with a given receptor as well as for the quantitation of drugs that exert their action via a particular receptor. Due to the fact that in general the binding of a compound to a receptor cannot be quantitated directly, labeled ligands with high affinity toward the receptor are being used. Competition between the labeled ligand and the analyte for the same receptor binding site will take place in the sample and can be monitored by quantitation of either the free or the receptor-bound fraction of the labeled ligand. Most labeled ligands used in receptor assays are radioligands. The major advantage of using radioligands (mainly tritium and iodine labeled ligands) in receptor assays is that the spatial structure of the ligand is not or only slightly modified by the incorporation of an isotope. Therefore, the affinity of the labeled ligand can be expected to be comparable or even identical to that of the unlabeled compound. Besides, radioligands are chemically stable and can be detected with a high sensitivity and over a wide concentration range. However, there are several disadvantages in using radiolabels, including high costs, radioactive waste, health hazards and the need of special equipment and licenses. Hence the fluorescence-based receptor binding assays are developed to avoid complications associated with radiometric receptor binding assays. Most of the ligands with high affinity toward their receptors will not be having the native fluorescence; fluorescence functionalities will be coupled with the ligand. Many a times, the attachment of a bulky fluorescent moiety will diminish the affinity of ligand to its receptor.

Advantages of Receptor Binding Assays

1. Helps in determining receptor distribution and its subtypes.
2. All substances belonging to a pharmacological class (having affinity to a certain receptor) can be assayed including active metabolites. For enantiomeric substances only the active eutomer will react with the receptor.
3. Potency of drugs can be found with the affinity measurement.
4. Antibodies need not be raised as in the case of immunoassays. Receptors can be isolated relatively simple from animal tissues.
5. Gives a quantitative determination of the amount of an unknown analyte. This is done by comparing the displaced amount of labeled ligand.
6. Screening of new chemical entities and endogenous ligands can be done.

Example: Radioligand Binding Assay

Binding assays were utilized most extensively in the 1980s and 1990s before cell-based functional assays were made available for HTS. The radiolabel ligand binding assay was developed in the 1960s and has been extensively used for the drug screening of many targets, including ion channels. Radioligand binding assays incorporate the use of a ligand that is labeled with a radioactive tracer, such as ^{3}H or ^{125}I. Binding of the labeled ligand to a specific site on a channel protein can be displaced by an unlabeled compound if it binds to the same site on the protein. The activity of the unlabeled compound can be quantified by its ability (IC50) to compete with the labeled ligand. Filtration binding assays utilize a glass fiber filter–mounted 96-well plate to separate free ligands with the ligand–channel protein complex. This assay requires a plate wash step, which limits the screening throughput. The scintillation proximity assay (SPA) uses solid scintillant-containing beads to capture the cell membranes. The labeled ligands bind to these membrane-coated beads, which enables homogeneous detection due to the transfer of energy from labeled ligands to SPA beads in proximity. This SPA binding assay can be miniaturized into 384- and 1536-well formats with a throughput of 50,000–100,000 compounds per day at a moderate cost. Binding assays provide no information about the effect of novel agents on ion channel function. For example, an agonist cannot be distinguished from an antagonist in a binding assay. Additionally, if a compound interacts with the channel protein at a site distinct from the labeled ligand, it will not be detected in a binding assay. For example in hERG ^{3}H-MK-499 binding assay, it has been reported that the potency of certain compounds in the ^{3}H-MK-499 binding assay can differ by more than 100-fold when compared to the potency of the same compounds measured in a functional voltage-clamp hERG assay. Voltage-gated ion channels do not have endogenous ligands, and hence exogenous toxins or compounds are used as the labeled ligands. The structural diversity of hits identified by binding assay-based primary screens for ion channel targets is often limited (Zheng et al., 2004).

Radioactive Ion Flux Assay

Radiotracers can be used to measure the flux of ions moving in or out of a cell via ion channels expressed in the cell membrane. Radiotracers are available for every class of ion channels: $^{86}Rb^{+}$ for potassium channels, $^{22}Na^{-}$ for sodium channels, $^{45}Ca_{2}^{-}$ for calcium channels and $^{36}Cl^{-}$ for chloride channels.

Although these radiotracers have been used for over 20 years in ion channel assays, their application for HTS drug screening has been limited. Tracer assays are heterogeneous and slow, requiring both a tracer loading and wash steps. Only the steady-state function of ion channels can be measured with radiotracers. Signal-to-noise ratio is low because of incomplete removal of extracellular tracer after loading or the continuous leak of tracer out of the cells. Concerns over excessive radioactive waste and safety also limit radioactive flux assay use in HTS[26].

Cell-Based Assays

Biochemical assays have been used with far more frequency than cell-based assays in HTS as these assays are relatively easy to implement with HTS, but important biological issues such as cellular toxicity and the complex cell biology that surrounds the target compounds are often overlooked when using biochemical assays. Cell-based assays in HTS have helped to fill this gap and have enjoyed a rapid rise in popularity in modern drug discovery. Biochemical assays are still being performed for primary screening using huge compound libraries. However, cellular assays are being utilized with more frequency for lead selection and lead profiling, with widespread use of HTS technologies for the functional analysis of drug compounds in live cells.

Cell-based assays provide predictive model systems that allow researchers to observe physiological responses of cells to pharmacological agents and environmental conditions. The term cell-based assay is used to refer to any of a number of different experiments based on the use of live cells. Cell-based *in vitro* assays are emerging as an integral aspect of today's drug discovery process for screening chemical libraries. Technology development has enabled modern primary screening to utilize live cells for HTS. The significant benefit of screening using live cell assays is the generation of more physiologically relevant data and the ability to elucidate compound effect on target biomolecule functions (Cawkill and Eaglestone, 2007). The use of cell-based assays in high-throughput screens is growing in acceptance and popularity. Advantages of cell-based assays include: (1) distinguishing between agonist and antagonist, (2) identification of allosteric modulators, (3) characterization of compound attributes, such as permeability and stability inside of cells, and (4) assessment of cytotoxicity (Kunapuli *et al.*, 2005). Cell-based assays offer a more accurate representation of the real-life model since live cells are used, and also offer the possibility of a dynamic experiment through monitoring the numbers or behavior of the live cells. Cell-based assays can be used to screen molecular libraries for their effects on cell behavior, such as proliferation, toxicity, motility and morphology. In the last few years, cell-based assays using engineered cells and microorganisms have become an increasingly attractive alternative to *in vitro* biochemical assays for HTS in the early phase of the drug discovery process. Cell-based assays predict the effect of the drug not only on a particular target but also on the entire pathway that the target modulates. This gives a more precise interpretation of the drug activity under physiological conditions. Furthermore these assays also provide information on the molecule's toxicity and bioavailability.

Cell-based assays have notable advantages over biochemical assays as they do not require purification of the target protein and therefore eliminate investment of resources to gain the necessary knowledge for obtaining a biochemical active target–this advantage has become particularly important as it would indeed be difficult to set up specific biochemical assays for hundreds of new proteins for which the natural substrates remain largely unknown. The cell-based assays most likely represent the natural physiological state more closely than *in vitro* assays and also cell-based assays can immediately select against compounds that are generally cytotoxic, or that cannot permeate cellular membranes to reach intracellular targets.

Cell-based assays have their own drawbacks, particularly in handling. The cell-based assays are extremely sensitive to alterations in temperature, nutrients, gas flow, contamination, and so on, making them difficult to handle. In addition, the drugs that do not penetrate the cell membrane cannot be studied for efficacy. However, this is considered both as an advantage as it helps in eliminating scores of drug candidates and as a disadvantage as these drug candidates can be modified in order to permeate through the membrane and demonstrate enhanced efficacy.

Cell-based assays should ideally be performed with cells of human origin, which evidently provide the most physiologically relevant model system. However, the effects of redundant processes on the measured output can be difficult to control and to distinguish from the effects that are expected to be specific for the defined target; and genetic manipulation of mammalian cells is generally problematic and time consuming. Moreover, human cells are expensive to culture and sometimes difficult to propagate in automated systems used for HTS.

Animal models, which allow for preliminary predictions of the systemic effects of drugs and have contributed greatly to the advancement of drug testing in the past, often exhibit anatomical and physiological differences between species, which can cause difficulty in data interpretation and also inconsistency in the data. Animal experiments are also costly and time consuming, and have to undergo many regulatory and ethical guidelines. Cell-based assays are easier to use in a high-throughput format than animals, and can uncover important biological issues, such as cellular toxicity or the complex cell biology surrounding the target, that biochemical assays cannot. In this case, cell-based assays are a good compromise between whole organisms and *in vitro* biochemistry systems (Durick and Negulescu, 2001). They have been widely used in drug target validation and the study of drug ADMET (administration, distribution, metabolism, elimination and toxicity).

Cell-based assays usually involve culturing cells as single cells, monolayer cells on a two-dimensional (2D) surface, multilayers or aggregates in a 3-D scaffold or even fresh tissues and organs.

Components of Cell-Based Assays

Cells

The important requirement to develop a cell-based assay is the cells themselves. Cell function assays depend on a reliable source of cells, whether fresh or cryo-preserved, to make accurate and defensible conclusions. Cellular histology platforms also require a systematic and well-defined procedure for collection and preparation to ensure the consistent and reliable source of cells. When the source of cells is patient samples, it is imperative that well-thought-out processes for collection, shipment and storage are implemented to ensure accurate and reliable data.

In some cases, such as proliferation and neutralizing antibody (NAB) assays, a cell line is used as the source of the assay readout. Without a secure source of this cell line, which can be expected to provide a consistent assay reagent, the entire development and validation process is compromised. A description of the cell line is essential and should include how it was developed, media and growth conditions, storage and recovery. References are useful if available. A full description of the cell-banking process is helpful. When using cell lines for a cell-based assay, a master bank should be created to preserve the cells. Cell banking is performed to preserve the characteristics of the cell line to be used. It is recommended that the cell-banking program be implemented as early as possible in the life cycle of assay development. Often it is not known how many passages a cell line can withstand before drift occurs. Cell banking also offers insurance that the cell line can be reestablished in the event of a catastrophe such as microbial contamination, cross contamination with other cell lines or loss of desired characteristics.

As soon as a cell line is introduced into the lab, an initial master bank should be frozen. The number of ampoules will be dependent on how quickly the cells multiply but at least three to five ampoules should be frozen within the first week. Initial evaluation of the cells should be as complete as possible, but should at least examine sterility (mycoplasma, fungi, etc.) growing conditions, viability and the ability to be frozen and recovered from liquid nitrogen. Once convinced of the cell line's integrity, the main master bank should be prepared by thawing an ampoule from the initial bank. Since it is preferable to expand these cells to a high concentration with as few passages as possible, while maintaining high viability, it may be advisable to thaw several of the ampoules, if the inventory of the initial master bank allows it. The number of vials contained in the master bank is dependent on the life expectancy of the assay. It is always prudent to bank more than the expected requirement, even if the master bank must consist of several different and increasing passage numbers due to the slow growth of cells. Once established, the master bank is used as supply for the working stock. Early in the process while the working stock is in culture, the number of passages should be monitored closely and tested at intervals to determine that its integrity is being maintained. Well before the master bank is depleted a sequential master bank should be prepared, if necessary.

Tests critical to the determination of the continued integrity of the cell lines' required characteristics should be conducted throughout the cells' expansion to assess the optimum permissible passage number. If the cells once thawed lose viability, some rescue methods may be employed. Dead cells can be removed by centrifugation or another method. Cells can be nursed to higher viability by expanding in smaller culture volumes/culture plates. Higher concentrations of sera, if used, or other growth supplements, may encourage growth. Such rescue methods could encourage the growth of a variant cell line and further re-characterization would have to be performed.

Assay format

The type of assay to be used will define the development process and validation needed. The data generated by the assay may be quantitative and consist of a continuous numerical value, such as data reported from a regression of a standard curve. Proliferation assays frequently are reported based on this format. Other qualitative formats allow for a discrete or descriptive, numeric-reporting format, where the data are spaced across the axis, or used a descriptive, non-numeric term (e.g., high or low; yes or no). Intrinsic to the assay format is the sensitivity requirement. This must be determined at the initiation of development, based on the intended use to confirm that the platform selected and data reporting will afford the sensitivity to meet the needs of the study.

Critical reagents

It is important to identify which reagents are critical to the assay method so that their qualification, sourcing and lot-to-lot acceptance criteria can be established upfront. Additional assessments conducted during this phase include readout signal (color intensity, MTT, etc.) incubation times, reagent concentrations, and so on.

Effect of Environmental Variables in Cell-Based Assays

Control of environmental conditions in cell-based assays is extremely important. A large number of variables such as cell health, number, metabolic state and phenotype can all have influence on the results of a cell-based assay. The variations in terms of temperature and humidity within the incubator directly affect the results of cell-based assay. Consistent temperature and high humidity contribute to reduction in CVs and control over CO_2 levels helps control pH, an important factor in providing an appropriate environment for cell growth. Even while utilizing buffered media, ionic concentrations have a substantial influence on cell health and metabolic activities. Balanced ionic conditions are very important, when performing assays on ion channels and other metabolic events, including ligand-based cellular activation events. Other environmental factors that can cause variance in the results of cell-based assays are humidity and position of well plates. In order to minimize the variations, various microplate chambers have been developed and used in cell-based assays. Automation is another way of preventing any variance in the assay results.

CO_2 control

Controlling CO_2 levels in an environmental chamber aids in maintaining a proper pH in mammalian cell-based assays. These assays may include ligand-binding assays, signal transduction assays and a variety of G protein-coupled receptor (GPCR) assays.

Proper CO_2 levels, and hence proper pH, is also required when culturing cells for subsequent assays, such as the long-term culture (7–21 days) of Caco-2 cells prior to performing the permeability assay. CO_2 concentrations of 5–7% are sufficient for most applications.

Temperature control

Temperature is the most important factor, which can cause variance in the results if not properly maintained. It can affect the results either directly or indirectly where the cells and/or cellular products or processes are involved in the assays.

Direct effect

The health of all cells is critical in assays that use either the cells or the products of cells and cellular processes. Most mammalian cell cultures represent the *in vivo* conditions best, when cultured at 37ºC. As approximation of *in vivo* conditions will provide the best results that lead to therapeutic drug 'hits' in screening programs, control of the metabolic milieu will yield the most reliable results; for that, temperature is very important.

In addition to mammalian cells, many screening programs related to antibacterial or antifungal drug discovery may also utilize whole and live cell assays. It is important to have precise control over culture temperature in order to eliminate or include the effect of temperature on the results of *in vitro* efficacy studies (such as MIC). The control of overgrowth of some bacterial or fungal species is also a consideration in such programs, as is the same control when developing assays for food or beverage quality.

Culture and assay temperature can have effects on a variety of cellular processes, including phosporylation and glycosylation of proteins. Also, cell growth and other metabolic process kinetics can be affected by temperature. These processes include other posttranslational modifications and 2D and 3D presentation of proteins.

Indirect effects

The indirect effects of temperature control can have significant impact on assay results. Uneven temperature across microplates, slides or other assay formats (petri dishes, microchips) can skew results because of hyperactivation, hypoactivation or inactivation of enzymes or other proteins used in assays. Assay variance due to inappropriate activation of temperature-dependent moieties can also be avoided if the culture temperature is controlled correctly.

Humidity control

Maintenance of optimal humidity is very important in the cell-based assays, as this will be critical for the cell health and assay consistency. Although humidity plays a minor role in variance in results for assays when compared to temperature, it may affect the repeatability in assays by causing change in the well volumes due to evaporation.

Well position

The plate position in the chamber may also influence the results if the gradient across the chamber is greater than 2%.

Contamination

The cells must be protected from contamination by external agents such as bacteria. In some cases, it is necessary to protect laboratory personnel from contamination by the cells (i.e. viral cell lines). If high-sensitivity fluorescence detection is being used, then dust particle contamination must be kept to a minimum, as dust causes false positive readings for these kinds of detection systems.

Receptors

Receptors are proteins that bind a specific ligand, which leads to the activation of a cascade of reactions. These receptors fall under three major categories: (1) peripheral membrane receptors, (2) transmembrane receptors (metabotropic [GPCRs] and ionotropic [ligand-gated ion channels]), and (3) intracellular receptors for steroid and hormones. Due to their pathway-modulating nature, they have been implicated in many disease conditions. Thus it may be a prudent idea to design a drug that inhibits the deleterious effects or enhances its therapeutic effects. The ligand can be peptides or chemicals and those drugs that compete with them can also fall under these two categories. The drugs that bind and modulate the receptors are classified as:

- The mandn fjksdl fsdfjsdfjklsd
- Agonist–which binds to the receptor and alters its function;
- Antagonist–which binds to the receptor's active or allosteric site and alters the agonist's effects; and
- Inverse agonist–which binds to the receptor's active site and induces an effect opposite to that of an agonist.

Ionic Channels

Ionic channels are important drug targets as they have now been recognized for their role in many pathophysiologic conditions. Some of the main conditions caused are chronic pain and many neurologic and cardiac arrythmias. It is mainly the sodium and potassium channels that have been implicated (Kaczorowski *et al.*, 2008).

Mammalian Cell-Based Assays

The assays are basically divided into binding assays and functional assays.

Binding assays

Binding assays generally depict the direct binding of the unlabeled drug and radiolabeled/flourolabeled physiological ligand to the target receptor. This is otherwise called competitive ligand binding as there is a competition between the radiolabeled/flourolabeled ligand and drug for the receptor. Typically the concentration of the radiolabeled/flourolabeled ligand is kept constant while the concentration of the unlabeled drug is varied. If the drug has affinity for the receptor it will compete with the radiolabeled/flourolabeled ligand for the target and displace it. The drug's receptor binding affinity (RBA) can be determined by measuring the amount of radiolabeled/flourolabeled ligand bound to the receptor, thereby arriving at the IC50 (concentration of drug that displaces 50% of radiolabeld ligand) of the drug. The RBA is calculated ideally by dividing the IC50 of the drug by the IC50 of a standard or the radiolabeled/flourolabeled ligand. The detection method could be radiometric (heterogeneous) or flourimetric (homogeneous) (Smith and O'Donnell).

Mepyramine binding assay

A typical example for this is the screening of H1 receptor antagonists for allergic conditions. Under normal circumstances the drug for screening must be checked for its ability to displace the physiological ligand/agonist. But due to the unstable nature of the physiological ligand under laboratory conditions, the drug for screening is first checked for its ability to displace a well-studied standard H1 antagonist mepyramine, which shares close structural similarity to the physiological ligand and is radiolabeled. This can also be used to check the efficacy of the test drug over currently available medication. But the drug's ability to displace mepyramine alone would not provide an idea of the drug's antihistaminic activity. This aspect can be demonstrated only through functional assays, which will establish the drug's efficacy in blocking the signal transduction process, thereby altering the synthesis of metabolites.

As a first step, one has to establish the binding and displacement efficacy of the test drug and for this purpose a binding assay needs to be conducted. The binding assay again is divided into two parts:

1. Saturation binding and
2. Competitive binding.

Saturation binding is done to arrive at the number of receptor sites and the effective concentration of radiolabeled standard histamine antagonist (^{3}H-mepyramine) at which all the receptor sites are occupied by it. However, the standard can also bind nonspecifically to sites other than the receptor on the membrane which leads to ambiguity in calculation. Hence simultaneously the standard drug's nonspecific binding value also needs to be established for that specific concentration at which all the sites are occupied, which has to be deducted from the total binding value. This concentration will later on be carried over to the competitive binding assay, where, as mentioned previously, the concentration is kept constant while the test ligand concentration is varied.

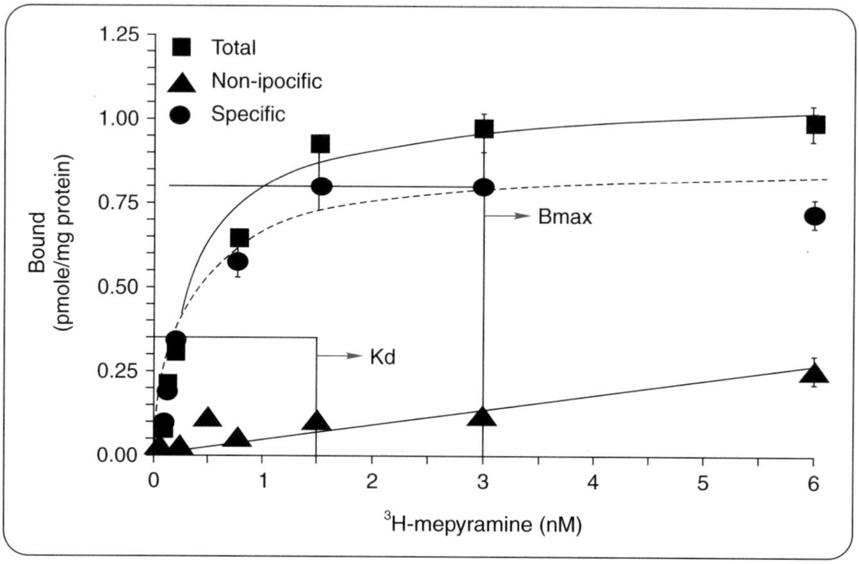

Fig. 3.10

In this case increasing concentrations of radiolabeled ligand are taken and incubated with CHOgpH1 (Chinese hamster ovary cells cloned with guinea pig H1 receptor) cells (Fitzsimons *et al.*, 2004). The total binding is calculated and simultaneously nonspecific binding is also calculated (Fig. 3.10). From this the specific binding values at each concentration of ^{3}H-mepyramine are calculated by the following formula:

Specific binding = (Total binding – Nonspecific binding)

The standard graph is plotted with the specific binding values and Bmax (binding maximum) is plotted, from which Kd (dissociation constant) is determined as

Kd = ½(Bmax).

This is expressed in picomoles/mg protein.

The nonspecific binding can be calculated by blocking all the receptor sites with another antihistamine-like triprolidine or ^{3}H-mepyramine itself. In the former case, the other antihistamine is incubated first with the cells, followed by ^{3}H-mepyramine. This will give an idea of the nonspecific binding of ^{3}H-mepyramine. The graph obtained is always linear as shown in Fig. 3.10, as increasing concentrations of ^{3}H-mepyramine increase nonspecific binding also.

The competitive binding assay is done so as to establish the unlabeled test ligand's ability to displace the standard. The standard concentration as obtained from the saturation binding assay is kept constant over varying concentrations of test ligand in the increasing order. After a specific incubation time the assay mixture is filtered and the filtrate is analyzed in a scintillation counter for each concentration. The displacement efficacy of the test ligand can be obtained from the count of the radiolabeled standard still occupying the receptor sites. If the count remains the same or only a slight decrease is observed then it can be concluded that the test ligand is not efficacious. However, if the count decreases dramatically, then we can ascertain that the test ligand is very efficacious and this can proceed for the functional assays.

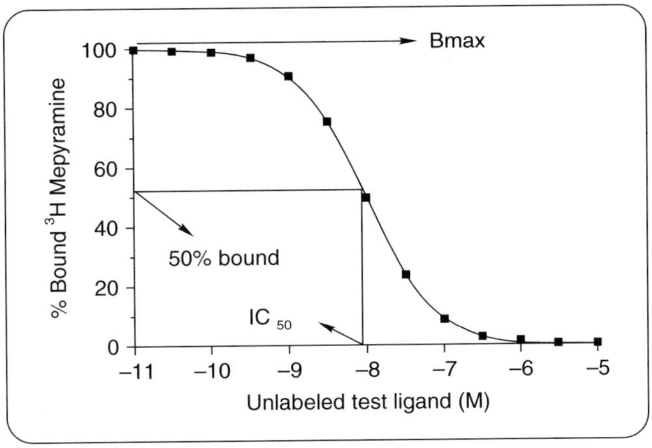

Fig. 3.11

A graph is then plotted with the results obtained and IC50 is also determined from the graph (Fig. 3.11). IC50 is that concentration of the unlabeled test ligand that is required to inhibit or displace 50% of the radiolabeled ligand. If 50% of the radiolabeled ligand is bound, then we can infer that the rest of 50% has been displaced by the unlabeled test ligand. It is usually calculated by the formula given below (www.unmc.edu/.../competition/IC50.htm):

log IC50 = concentration of unlabeled test ligand showing 50% inhibition of control
= 10^{-8} M or
= 10 nM

Functional Assays

Now that we have established the binding efficiency of the test ligand to the receptor, we know that the test drug is more efficacious in blocking the receptor than the standard drug available. But now the question arises as to whether this test drug has the ability to block even the receptor-mediated pathways and thereby block formation of metabolites. This can be established only through certain functional assays. Now taking the present example of histamine and its H1 receptor, the efficacy of the test drug in blocking the H1 receptor-mediated pathway can be demonstrated by a couple of simple functional assays, which are as follows:

1. Formation of [^{3}H]IP (inositol phosphate)
2. Formation of cAMP

Formation of inositol phosphate

Formation of [^{3}H]IP (inositol phosphate) can predict the efficacy of the drug in a concentration-dependent manner up to some extent. It is a well-reported fact that histamine stimulates the production of inositol phosphate through activation of phospholipase C by the histamine–receptor complex. In this case a known amount of [^{3}H]*myo*-inositol (precursor of phophatidylinositol) is incubated with CHO-H1 cells for a particular amount of time. Following this, the cells are stimulated with varying concentrations of histamine in the presence/absence of varying concentrations of test ligands. The reaction is stopped after a particular period of incubation and the radioactive fraction is separated through chromatography and centrifugation and then the [^{3}H]IP formed is measured in a scintillation counter. The drug's efficacy can be determined by analyzing [^{3}H]IP formation as it will be altered according to the increasing concentration of test ligand, since the signal transduction pathway is blocked which in turn blocks production of PLC and thereby blocks formation of [^{3}H]IP. A typical graph representing the [^{3}H]IP production in response to varying concentrations of test ligand is given in Fig. 3.12 (Fitzsimons *et al.*, 2004).

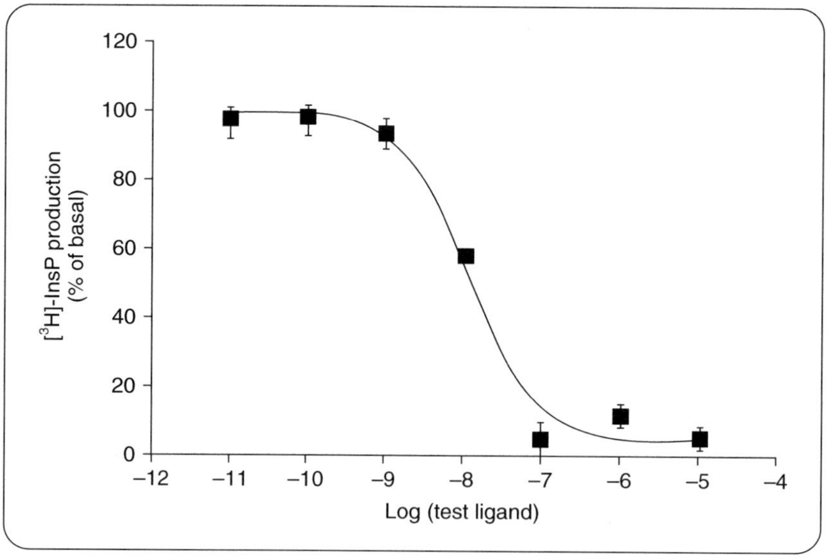

Fig. 3.12

Reporter gene assays

One of the most commonly used functional assays for drug screening would be the reporter gene assays in which a reporter gene is attached downstream to the promoter region of the gene of interest such that when the gene of interest gets expressed so does the reporter gene, whose phenotypic expression is measurable like fluorescence or luminescence. Some of the commonly used reporter genes are Lac Z, GFP and luciferase. In the case of drug screening the expression of a particular gene of interest, which can be assayed through the expression of the reporter construct, is a direct evidence of the efficacy of the test compound in regulating the gene's expression.

For example, when screening antihistaminc molecules, the target is usually the H1 receptor as mentioned previously. But there are three other known histamine receptors (H2, H3 and H4) having varied functions. One of these receptors that is of equal importance as the H1 is the H2 receptor. This receptor is involved in the secretion of gastric acid and present in the gastric cells; overstimulation of this receptor leads to the generation of acidity and subsequent ulcerative conditions. The physiological ligand of H2 receptor is histamine, which modulates the signal transduction pathway in the gastric parietal cells causing the production of gastric acid and cAMP and Ca2+ mobilization (Oda *et al.*, 2000). Thus many anti-H2 molecules are developed, the most popular of which is ranitidine. In order to screen histamine antagonists, the H2 receptor is stimulated with an agonist (histamine), which stimulates the production of intracellular cAMP. This cAMP activates protein kinase A, which in turn activates CREB (cAMP response element binding protein), a transcription factor which binds to cAMP response element (CRE) and mediates gene transcription. The changes in the production of cAMP can be measured by assaying the transcription of CRE-attached luciferase reporter gene in the cell, where once the luciferase gene is expressed it luminesces upon addition of the substrate (which can be measured by a luminometer).

For example, when screening for a novel anti-H2 compound, cell lines expressing the H2 receptors with the luciferase gene cloned onto the CRE gene are taken and treated with varying doses of histamine and the cAMP level in response to histamine treatment is measured through the expression of CRE-attached luciferase reporter using the luminometer that records the luminescence by luciferase. A standard graph is generated from this (Fig. 3.13), following which the cell lines are treated with anti-H2 compounds and the response is recorded using a luminometer. The efficacy of the compound is evaluated by whether it blocks the H2 receptor, thereby inhibiting cAMP production, which is established by the nonexpression of CRE-luciferase gene.

Human Cell-Based Assays

The use of human cells, which retain organ-specific properties, represents important experimental systems for early toxicity screening. Human cell lines are important to mimic the organ- or cell-specific properties, which is extremely important to screen the drug efficiency against specific diseased state. Acute myeloid leukemia (AML) cell lines are one of such commonly used human cell lines to study the drug action against cancer of the myeloid cells leading to abnormal production of white blood cells and hence affecting the production of normal blood cells. In the drug discovery process it is equally important to screen the mechanism action apart from screening the potency of drug compound.

The promising primary human cell culture systems include the following (Li, 2005):

1. Hepatocytes for liver toxicity
2. Renal proximal tubule epithelial cells for nephrotoxicity
3. Vascular endothelial cells for vascular toxicity

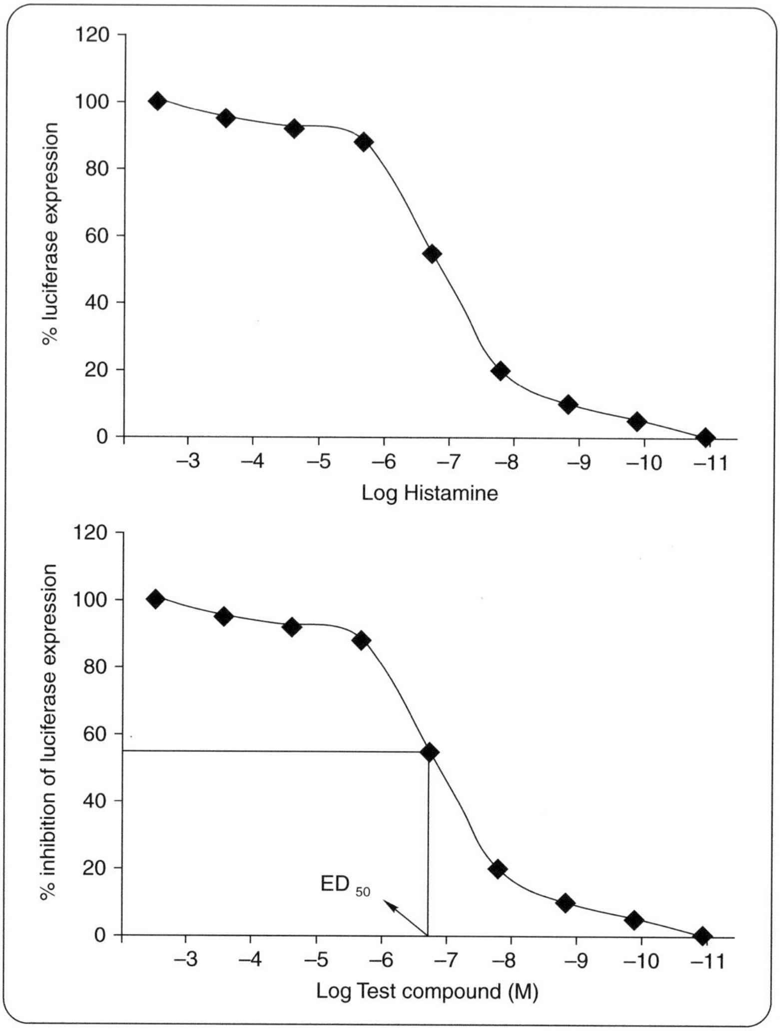

Fig. 3.13

4. Neuronal and glial cells for neurotoxicity
5. Cardiomyocytes for cardiotoxicity
6. Skeletal myocytes for rhadomyolysis

Microbial Cell-Based

Microorganisms such as yeast present a convenient alternative for measuring the activity of defined human proteins in a heterologous, yet cellular (eukaryotic) environment. In yeast cells, the function of human proteins can often be constituted and aspects of some human physiological processes can be produced because of the high degree of conservation of basic molecular and cellular mechanisms between yeast and human cells. The fact that many human proteins function in yeast indicates that the required conformation, stability, protein–protein interaction, and so on are taking place in this eukaryotic organism. This is a fundamental notion for the application of yeast cells in HTS with human target proteins (Hughes, 2002).

Rescue-type assays

Rescue type assays generally involve the rescuing of microbial cells from their inactive state to the proliferation state by compounds that block the growth inactivation factors in these cells. These growth-inactivating factors are proteins that inhibit certain other proteins which are important for the growth and proliferation of these microbial cells (Osawa 2006).

Hence, based on the above principle, an assay can be designed where mutant strains of microbes, such as either *Escherichia coli/Saccharomyces* carrying a point mutation of a certain protein (pA), which is necessary for the growth of the cells in the given media containing a particular nutrient (N1), can be generated. This mutation renders the cells incapable of uptake of N1, thereby inhibiting its growth in the media containing N1. The compound's (C1, C2, C3) to be screened must possess the activity to reverse the mutation such that it rescue's the cell's inability for N1 uptake and aids in the proliferation of growth. A disk diffusion assay can be done where paper disks soaked with the test compounds are placed on the agar plates inoculated with the mutant strains of the microbe. Efficacious compound(s) will reverse the mutation such that the activity of pA is restored, thereby observing growth of cells around the disk alone. The efficacy of the test compounds can be assessed by measuring the zone of growth around the disk. This is only a qualitative assay and is mostly used as a primary screening tool.

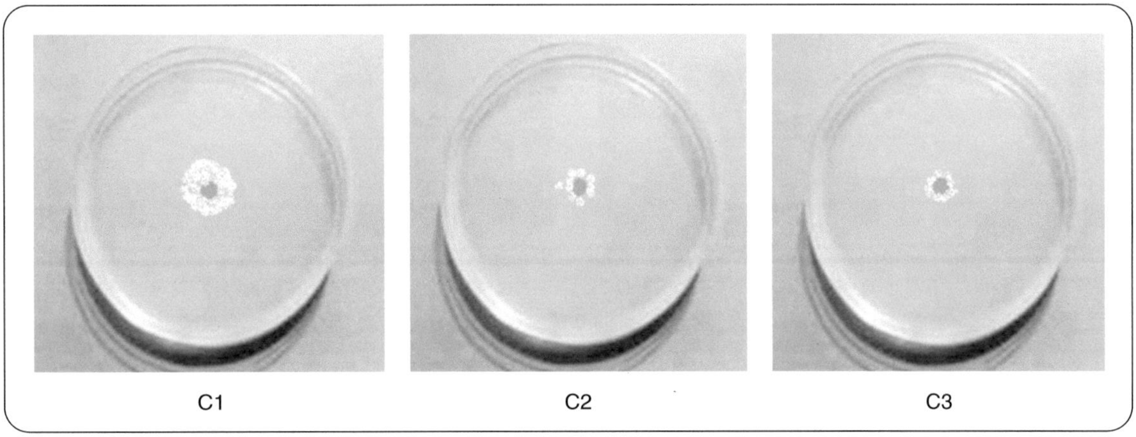

Fig. 3.14

The efficacy of the three compounds is determined through the halo of growth of microbe around the drug-soaked disk, which has rescued the inhibition of growth of the microbe by reversing the mutation of pA, rendering it capable of proliferating in media containing N1. From Fig. 3.14 it can be observed that the halo growth is around the disk (till where the drug has diffused) and measured by the diameter of growth around the disc (mm). C1 seems to be the most efficacious of the three, since the diameter of growth is more compared to that of C2 and C3.

Growth inhibition assays

Growth inhibition assays are typically used for antimicrobial drug screening. The ability of the test compound to inhibit the growth of the organisms will prove the compounds' efficacy. In this assay the agar plates are inoculated with the microbes and the disks soaked with the test compound(s) are placed at the center of the plate and incubated for a predetermined time at optimum temperature and humidity. If the compound(s) is efficacious there will be a clear zone around the disc where the growth of the microbes has been inhibited by the test compound. The diameter of the zone of clearance is measured and compared against the control. This is also a qualitative assay and can be used as a primary screening tool.

Well diffusions can also be performed where on a plate with full growth wells are made and different concentrations of the drug are incubated and the zone of clearance is measured as shown in Fig. 3.15.

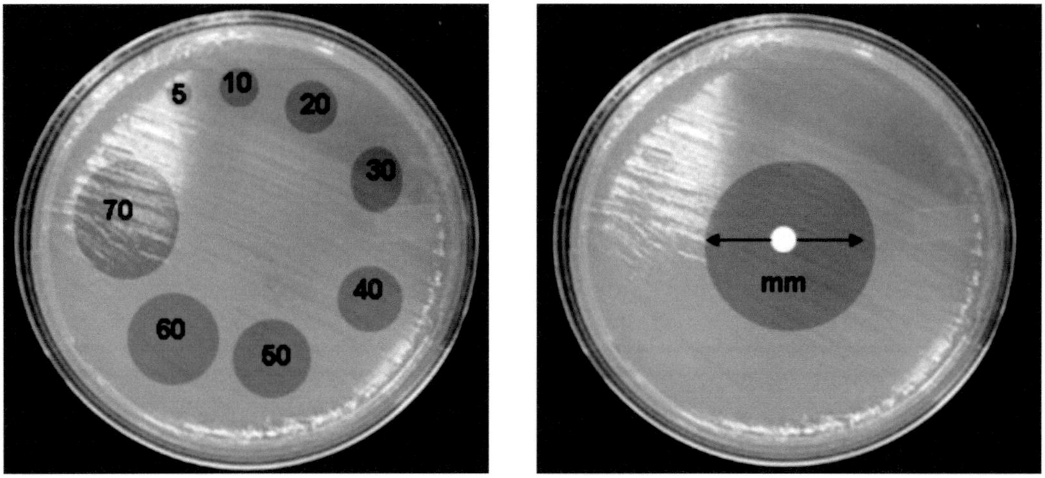

Well Diffusion Assay

Disc Diffusion Assay

(Concentrations (ug/ml)

Fig. 3.15

In case of both the assays the efficacy of the compound can be ascertained and the concentration at which it is efficacious can be determined by measuring the zone of clearance with regard to concentration. From this the IC50 value can be obtained.

Yeast Two-Hybrid Screening Assay

The yeast two-hybrid (Y2H) system, though a very useful tool to screen drugs inhibiting protein–protein interactions, is exploited rarely as a screening tool. The system works basically with two domains of a transcription factor being separated but present in close proximity to each other. These domains are fused to individual proteins. One is called the bait protein, which is usually fused to the binding domain, and the other is called the prey protein, fused to the activation domain. When the two proteins interact they bring the activation and binding domain close to each other, which leads to the transcription factor being activated and thereby promotes transcription of a reporter gene.

A study conducted by researchers (Kato-Stankiewicz *et al*., 2002) illustrated the use of Y2H as a screening tool, where they screened small that inhibits interaction of Ras and Raf proteins, which otherwise leads to the growth of cancer cells.

Cytotoxicity Screening Assays

Cytotoxicity screening of novel compounds with a defined set of standard cell lines (THP-1, COS, Hep G-2, CHO, A549, H 292, PLB 985, COR-L23, COR-L23R, COR-5010, HL-60, MIA-Pa–Ca-2, HeLa) enables to detect the basic possible cytotoxicity effect of novel substances.46 The principle of testing is exposing the cells in growth phase to a drug. The cells are allowed to proliferate in order to distinguish between cells that remain viable and are capable of proliferation and those that remain viable but cannot proliferate. Measuring the succinate dehydrogenase mitochondrial activity of living cells by the specific reagent MTT, the quantity of viable cells can be detected. The enzyme turns the MTT into a brown color by cutting the tetrazolium ring. The amount of produced MTT formazan can be determined spectrophotometrically at 490 nm (Verbanac *et al*., 2005).

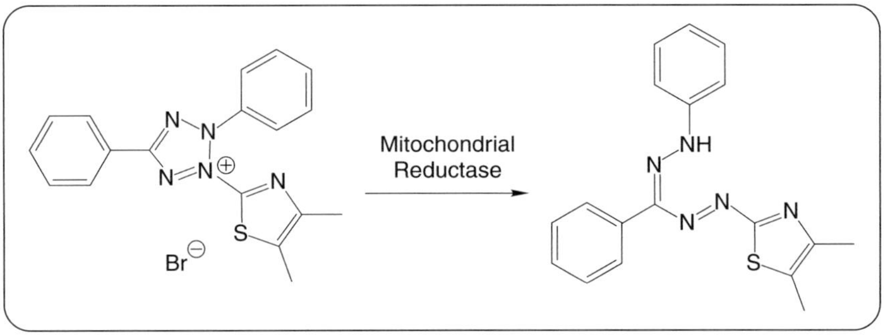

Fig. 3.16 *Principle of MTT Antiproliferative HTS Cytotoxicity Assay*

(3-(4,5-Dimethylthiazol-2-yl)-5-(3-carboxymethoxyphenyl)-2-(4-sulfophenyl)-2*H*-tetrazolium) (MTS) is a more recent alternative to MTT. MTS, in the presence of phenazine methosulfate (PMS), produces a water-soluble formazan product that has an absorbance maximum at 490–500 nm in phosphate-buffered saline. It is advantageous over MTT in that: (1) the reagents MTS + PMS are reduced more efficiently than MTT, and (2) the product is water soluble, decreasing toxicity to cells seen with an insoluble product (Cory *et al*., 1991).

One more approach is followed in order to establish the antiproliferation assays of human or animal blood cells and other primary cell lines based on the adenosine triphosphate (ATP) levels–bioluminescent ATP cytotoxicity screening. This type of screening is intended for the rapid and safe detection of proliferation and cytotoxicity of mammalian cells and cell lines in culture by determination of their ATP levels. ATP can be used to assess the functional integrity of living cells since all cells require ATP to remain alive and carry out their specialized functions. The bioluminescent method utilizes an enzyme, luciferase, which catalyses the formation of light from ATP and luciferin according to the following reaction.

$$\text{ATP} + \text{Luciferin} + \text{O2} \xrightarrow{\text{Luciferase}} \text{Oxyluciferin} + \text{AMP} + \text{PPi} + \text{CO2} + \text{Light}$$

The emitted light intensity is linearly related to the ATP concentration and is measured 565 nm using a luminometer or beta counter. The assay is conducted at ambient temperature[24].

IN VIVO MODELS FOR DRUG SCREENING

In vitro models for screening of drugs can provide one with data on the efficacy of the drug candidate under simulated physiological conditions. But they cannot give precise data on the fate of the drug candidate once it enters a physiological system, as the drug candidate has to face tremendous barriers in order to reach its target. Thus the drug candidate's efficacy inside a physiological system needs to be proved, which can be demonstrated through some *in vivo* experiments. However, a drug candidate cannot be directly evaluated for its efficacy in humans; hence we should look at the next best alternative available, which happens to be nonhuman living organisms such as rodents, rabbits, guinea pigs, pigs, dogs, and so on.

Rats

These rats are a special breed of *Rattus norvegicus*, which were bred by Clark University in 1895 for experimental purposes. Thus this special breed was termed 'the laboratory rat'. These rats are white, calmer and have smaller internal organs compared to their wild counterparts. These rats can selectively breed for specific type of experiments to be performed. Accordingly following are the types of rats developed till now:

- Sprague Dawley rats
- Wistar rats
- Zucker rats
- Long–Evans rats
- Fischer 344 rats
- Lister black-hooded rats
- Holtzman albino strain rats

The laboratory rats have been used to study various disease conditions such as diabetes, inflammation and hypertension.

Mice

Laboratory mouse or *Mus musculus* is the largely used laboratory animal due to its ease of handling and maintenance and for economical reasons. They are generally inbred/outbred/transgenic for various experimental designs. They are frequently used to screen for drugs, as most diseases affecting humans can be expressed effectively in mice due to the high degree of genetic homology. Thus various transgenetic mice such as oncomice, where a foreign gene to induce a cancer has been inserted, or knockout mice, where a specific gene has been knocked out like the fat mice or normally bred mice with immunodeficiency or nonobese diabetic mice that develop type 1 diabetes mellitus, have been developed till date. Also, mice are excellent candidates to study behavioral patterns in humans. Hence, they are being developed to screen drugs that can affect the central nervous system (CNS).

Guinea Pigs

Guniea pigs are probably the most popular animal models to have been developed. Because of their docile nature and ease of handling, they were the primary experimental organisms in the past. Guinea pigs are both outbred and inbred. However, the outbred ones, such as the Dunken–Hartley breed, are the ones most widely used in research. Their main use in scientific experiments is mainly in the field of allergy and respiratory diseases, e.g. anaphylaxis, histamine-induced bronchospasm and other respiratory conditions. Thus, they can be good screening models for drugs like antihistamines. They have been also used to study reproductive disorders.

Other Mammals

Besides the mammals discussed above and the rabbits, the others used are primates, but these are rarely used nowadays and so are hamsters as rodent models.

Rabbits

Rabbits have been used extensively for research purposes as non-rodent species. The commonly used breed for experimental purposes are albino New Zealand white rabbits.

Carrageenan-Induced Paw Edema in Rats

A typical example that can be given is the *in vivo* screening of an anti-inflammatory drug that has been short-listed from *in vitro* screening models. The most commonly used model is carrageenan-induced paw edema in rats for inflammation due to the non-complex nature and reproducibility of the model when compared to others (Buadonpri *et al.*, 2009).

Zebra Fish as a Model for Drug Screening

Zebra fish is a small freshwater teleost and model organism for drug screening. Zebra fish have many advantages to be used as model organism, such as being easy to maintain and breed, a large number of them being possible to be housed in a small space and a relatively short generation time. Zebra fish embryogenesis is rapid and body plant established by 24 h postfertilization. Most of the internal organs are fully developed by 96 h postfertilization. Zebra fish embryo is transparent and external, enabling easy observation of drug effect on the internal organs such as kidney, liver, and so on, in the live organism. This is a great advantage over mammalian model organism, where the embryo development takes place *in utero*. Zebra fish are small and require small amounts of drug compound for assay, and this small size also enables one to use 96-well microplate formats. Drug administration into zebra fish is very simple: a small-molecule drug can be dissolved in water and diffused into the organism. Large-scale farword genetic screenings have been carried out in zebra fish, and many mutants obtained from the genetic screens display phenotypes resembling human diseases, which are also available for the study (Ma *et al.*).

Zebra fish–based assays are being used for studying drug toxicity, including acute toxicity, organ toxicity and developmental toxicity. The transparent nature of zebra fish embryo enables a thorough assessment of drug-induced morphological changes and color changes in the internal organs without the complicated surgery. Zebra fish also develop similar responses to xenobiotic chemicals as mammals do, including generation of oxidative stress and induction of xenobiotic specific enzyme. Zebra fish and mammalian hearts have been shown to exhibit similar characteristics. Many of the small molecules were studied in zebra fish embryonic heart rate and found to cause cardiac QT prolaongation (Ma *et al.*).

Zebra fish can be used as a model for angiogenesis screening and apoptosis screening. Angiogenesis is a sprouting of new blood vessels from the existing ones. Zebra fish have a simple blood circulation system and the angiogenesis in zebra fish is similar to that in many other vertebrates. Several important genes such as VEGF, Fli-1, Flt-1, Tie-1 and Tie-2 have been cloned in zebra fish, which are shown to express in similar pattern to that in mammals. Angiogenic vessels' formation can be monitored by endogenous alkaline phosphatase activity, which is present primarily in vessels during early development. Blood vessels can also be monitored by microangiography, which is obtained by injecting fluorescent microbeads in the circulatory system. HTS assay formats have been developed using 96-well plates to quantify endogenous alkaline phosphatase activity in the embryo (Ma *et al.*).

Apoptosis or programmed cell death is important for homeostasis, and any abnormalities will lead to diseases such as cancer and neurodegenerative diseases. The apoptotic process in zebra fish is similar to mammals and zebra fish homologues of most of the mammalian apoptosis-related genes have been identified, including the Bcl-2 family members, caspases, Ced-4-like molecules, death receptors and ligands and apotosis-related kinases. There is a stereotypic pattern of normal apoptotosis during zebra fish embryo development and any alteration in the normal apotosis events can serve as an assay for apoptosis modulator. Apoptosis in zebra fish can be easily detected using fluorescent labeling techniques such as acridine orange and fluorescent conjugated caspase substrate. Quantitative assays have also been developed in the 96-well microplate format; e.g. acridine orange can be extracted from the whole embryo into individual wells and quantified using fluorescence microplate reader. In addition to the assays described above, zebra fish models are available and are being developed for many other diseases such as neurological, immunological, hematopoietic and metabolic diseases. Many complementary techniques such as transgenesis and gene knockdown are also available for zebra fish, enhancing the power of this model in drug discovery (Ma *et al.*).

EX VIVO MODELS FOR DRUG SCREENING

Ex vivo by definition means outside the living body. It usually involves excision of a particular tissue or organ out of the living system and maintaining it under strict physiological conditions in an apparatus exceeding not more than 24 h. As described previously, *in vitro* screening forms the initial phase of screening. In the advent of obtaining a positive hit, the lead molecule has to be further screened in order to answer questions such as how does the molecule behave in a living system? Is the molecule efficacious in the living system? Does it have site-specific toxicity (tissue it has been targeted to)?

In such cases, the tissue or the organ can be excised from the living organism and studied for its effect on that particular tissue. But this type of screening is rarely performed due to the tedious nature of the experiments. A typical example that could be given would be screening for antihistamines using isolated guinea pig ileum contraction assay.

In this method the guinea pig ileum is excised and immediately connected to a force transducer and transferred into a tissue bath apparatus supplemented with Kreb's-Hansleit buffer, which is continuously gassed with 95% O_2 and 5% CO_2 at 37°C. The equilibration time is of 30–45 min and the buffer is changed every 10 min. A standard graph is drawn for the agonist (histamine) concentration in an increasing dose-dependent manner, with the percentage of ileum contraction as the parameter upon introducing it into the organ bath. The contractile responses are recorded at a resting tension of 0.4–0.5 g isometrically by the force transducer. After obtaining the standard values, the efficacy study is performed where the histamine antagonists/screening agents are introduced into the bath and incubated for a given time followed by the measurement of contractile responses of the ileum to the antagonist. Ideally a potent antagonist will displace histamine from the site leading to relaxation of the ileum.

REFERENCES

Bourguet, N., Torréton, J.-P., Galy, O., Arondel, V., Goutx, M. (2003). Application of a specific and sensitive radiometric assay for microbial lipase activities in marine water samples from the lagoon of Nouméa. *Applied and Environmental Microbiology* **69(12)**:7395–7400.

Buadonpri, W., Wichitnithad, W., Rojsitthisak, P., Towiwat, P. (2009). Synthetic curcumin inhibits carrageenan-induced paw edema in rats. *Journal of Health Research* **23(1)**:11–16.

Cawkill, D., Eaglestone, S.S. (2007). Evolution of cell-based reagent provision. *Drug Discovery Today* **12(19/20)**.

Cory, A.H., Owen, T.C., Barltrop, J.A., Cory, J.G. (1991). Use of an aqueous soluble tetrazolium/formazan assay for cell growth assays in culture. *Cancer Communications* **3(7)**:207–212.

Durick K., Negulescu P. (2001). Cellular biosensors for drug discovery. *Biosensors and Bioelectronics* **16(7–8)**:587–592.

Fan, F., Wood, K.V. (2007). Bioluminescent assays for high-throughput screening. *Assay and Drug Development Technologies* **5(1)**.

Fitzsimons, C.P., Monczor, F., Fernández, N., Shayo, C., Davio, C. (2004). Mepyramine, a histamine H1 receptor inverse agonist, binds preferentially to a G protein-coupled form of the receptor and sequesters G protein. *Journal of Biological Chemistry* **279(33)**:34431–34439.

Hertzberg, R.P., Pope, A.J. (2000). High-throughput screening: New technology for the 21st century. *Current Opinion in Chemical Biology* **4**:445–451.

Hughes, T.R. (2002). Yeast and drug discovery. *Functional and Integrative Genomics* **2**:199–211.

Kaczorowski, G.J., McManus, O.B., Priest, B.T., Garcia, M.L. (2008). Ion channels as drug targets: The next GPCRs. *Journal of General Physiology* **131(5)**:399–405.

Kalanur, S.S., Seetharamappa, J., Mamatha, G.P., Hadagali, M.D., Kandagal, P.B. (2008). Electrochemical behavior of an anti-cancer drug at glassy carbon electrode and its determination in pharmaceutical formulations. *International Journal of Electrochemical Science* **3**:756–767.

Kato-Stankiewicz, J., Hakimi, I., Zhi, G., Zhang, J., Serebriiskii, I., Guo, L., Edamatsu, H., Koide, H., Menon, S., Eckl, R., Sakamuri, S., Lu, Y., Chen, Q.-Z., Agarwal, S., Baumbach, W.R., Golemis, E.A., Tamanoi, F., Khazak, V. (2002). Inhibitors of Ras–Raf-1 interaction identified by two-hybrid screening revert Ras-dependent transformation phenotypes in human cancer cells. *Proceedings of the National Academy of Sciences* USA **99(22)**:14398–14403.

Komatsu, M., Tajima, Y., Ito, T., Yamashiro, Y., Hiramatsu, K. (2009). Use of a sensitive chemiluminescence-based assay to evaluate the metabolic suppression activity of linezolid on methicillin-resistant *Staphylococcus aureus* showing reduced susceptibility to vancomycin. *Journal of Microbiology and Biotechnology* **19(7)**:734–741.

Kunapuli, P., *et al.* (2005). *Assay and Drug Development Technologies* **3(1)**.

Li, A.P. (2005). Preclinical *in vitro* screening assays for drug-like properties. *Drug Discovery Today: Technologies*.

Ma, C., parng, c., Seng, W.L., Zhang, C., Willett, C., McGrath, P. Zebrafish–An *in vivo* model for drug screening. *Drug Discovery* (IPTOnline article).

Ma, H., Horiuchi, K.Y. (2006). Chemical microarray: A new tool for drug screening and discovery. *Drug Discovery Today* **11(13/14)**.

Oda, T., Morikawa, N., Saito, Y., Masuho, Y., Matsumoto, S.-i. (2000). Molecular cloning and characterization of a novel type of histamine receptor preferentially expressed in leukocytes. *Journal of Biological Chemistry* **275(47)**:36781–36786.

Osawa, H., Stacey G., Gassmann W. (2006). ScOPT1 and AtOPT4 function as proton-coupled oligopeptide transporters with broad but distinct substrate specificities. *Biochemical Journal* **393**:267–275.

Ouellet, M., Riendeau, D., Percival, M.D. (2001). A high level of cyclooxygenase-2 inhibitor selectivity is associated with a reduced interference of platelet cyclooxygenase-1 inactivation by aspirin. *Proceedings of the National Academy of Sciences USA* **98(25)**:14583–14588.

Puzanowska-Tarasiewicz, H., Misiuk, W., Mielech-Lukasiewicz, K., Kuzmicka, L. (2009). Spectroscopic and electrochemical analysis of psychotropic drugs. *Indian Journal of Pharmaceutical Sciences* **71(1)**:8–18.

Roda, A., Guardigli, M., Pasini, P., Mirasoli, M. (2003). Bioluminescence and chemiluminescence in drug screening. *Journal of Analytical and Bioanalytical Chemistry* **377(5)**.

Smith, G.C., O'Donnell, J.T. *Process of New Drug discovery and Development*, 2nd edn.

Tijssen, P. (1985). *Practice and Theory of Enzyme Immunoassay*. New York: Elsevier.

Verbanac, D., Jelic, D., Stepanic, V., Tatic, I., Ziher, D., Kostrun, S. (2005). Combined *in silico* and *in vitro* approach to drug screening. *Croatica Chemica Acta* **78(2)**:133–139.

Zheng, W., Spencer, R.H., Kiss, L. (2004). High throughput assay technologies for ion channel drug discovery. *Assay and Drug Development Technologies* **2(5)**.

Zhou, N., Chen, Z., Zhang, D., Li, G. (2008). Electrochemical assay of human islet amyloid polypeptide and its aggregation. *Sensors* **8**:5987–5995.

Ziegler, C. (2000). Cell-based biosensors. *Fresenius' Journal of Analytical Chemistry* **366(6–7)**:552–559.

4

In Vitro/In Vivo Assessment of Human Hepatic Drug Metabolism

Anuj Kapoor and C.N. Ramchand* [1, 2]

[1]*Laila Pharmaceuticals Pvt. Ltd., Chennai, India*

[2]*Visiting faculty, Swinburne University Technology Mebourne, Australia*

After entering the body, drugs are eliminated through either excretion or metabolism in one or more inactive or active metabolites. The stability of the new chemical entity has a significant role *in vivo*, which can affect the safety and efficacy of the new chemical entity.

New chemical entities, which have shorter half-lives, require multiple doses to sustain the plasma levels while the compounds with longer half-lives require a different dosing regimen. Moreover, USFDA guidance documents state that adequate assessment of the safety and effectiveness of a drug should include a description of its metabolism and the contribution of metabolism to overall elimination.

The major site for the metabolism of the drugs or the new chemical entity in development is the liver, where the drug undergoes different phases of metabolism by biotransformation reactions mainly catalyzed by the cytochrome P450 (CYP) family of enzymes located in the endoplasmic reticulum and/or by non-CYP enzyme systems, such as sulfo- and glucuronosyltransferases. Therefore, the most relevant information for new chemical entity metabolic clearance *in vivo* is frequently derived from *in vitro* studies using *in vitro* cellular/subcellular fraction methods.

Determination of the absorption and plasma-bound fraction of the new chemical entity can provide a better suggestion of the *in vivo* hepatic intrinsic clearance. Generally, prediction of the metabolic stability for a new chemical entity involves either measuring metabolite formation from parent entity or disappearance of the parent entity in microsomes or hepatocytes. For example, measurement of

ramchand@lailapharma.com

the disappearance of a new chemical entity can provide an estimate of the metabolic half-life, which can then be used to derive the *in vitro* intrinsic clearance.

In vitro metabolic studies serve as a screening mechanism to rule out the importance of a particular metabolic pathway and drug–drug interactions for unnecessary *in vivo* testing and provide a verdict on certain metabolic pathways, which are important via *in vitro* studies for the further development of a new chemical entity or to prevent further clinical investigations. In addition, *in vitro* metabolic data from multiple species assist in the evaluation of animal species for use in toxicological and pharmacokinetic studies.

To characterize the hepatic metabolic profile of the new chemical entity, liver microsomes and hepatocytes are used for the screening of new chemical entities. Liver microsomes represent a model system which contains a significant portion of Phase I enzymes. A significant disappearance of new chemical entity in the presence of liver microsomes would indicate likely contributions from CYP enzymes and prediction of metabolic stability *in vivo*.

INTRODUCTION

Drug development is a costly and lengthy process involving multiple disciplines. During the preclinical phase of development, drug metabolism experiments are usually conducted in at least two species of animals (a rodent and a non-rodent species) to investigate the pharmacokinetics (PK) and absorption, distribution, metabolism and excretion (ADME) of the new chemical entity (NCE). The primary objectives of these experiments are to understand how the NCE is handled by animals and to derive information that can lead to the understanding of efficacy and potential toxicity in humans. In most drug metabolism laboratories, metabolism studies also are carried out at this stage to collect as much as possible information pertaining to the potential interaction of the NCE of interest with model *in vitro* systems derived from humans, as well as preclinical species. Taken together, these experiments can be costly, time consuming and labor intensive. The emphasis of preclinical metabolism studies should aim for understanding the NCEs with respect to their pharmacodynamics (PD), toxicity and potential adverse effects in humans instead of completing a comprehensive checklist of experiments.

In vitro metabolism systems can be extremely useful in understanding the nature and extent of interactions between NCEs and animal/humans. In many instances, *in vitro* metabolism systems have been shown to reflect the biotransformation pathways of NCEs observed *in vivo* and their effects on drug-metabolizing enzymes (e.g. inhibition and induction). In recent years, the availability of human tissues (liver microsomes, liver slices and hepatocytes) and recombinant cytochrome P450 (CYP) isoforms has provided model systems in which valuable human metabolism information can be obtained for NCEs on metabolite structures, metabolic rates and the enzymes (cytochrome P450 isoforms) responsible for their metabolism. Studies conducted in these biological matrixes of reduced complexity compared to *in vivo* models allow the evaluation of intrinsic metabolic potential or drug—drug interaction mechanisms with respect to specific reactions. In addition, *in vitro* systems derived from various animal species offer the possibility of comparing metabolic pathways among species, including humans, before a compound is tested clinically, and can contribute to the understanding of toxicity and efficacy observed in animals and humans. Two areas of particular interest for the use of *in vitro* studies in the understanding of a new drug are:

1. the relationship of metabolic pathways and PK/PD and
2. the prediction of drug interaction potential in humans.

The early knowledge about the metabolism of an NCE and its affinity to certain drug-metabolizing enzymes helps in the drug development process by providing important information for the selection of a lead compound from among a number of substances pharmacologically equally effective in their therapeutic response. *In vitro* metabolic studies give information about the metabolic stability and possible interactions between compounds that have affinity for the same drug-metabolizing enzymes. *In vitro* metabolic studies and affinity screenings have a role in determining the reasonable dose ranges *in vivo* studies of test species and human volunteers.

Testing the effects of an NCE on CYP-specific model activities and the effects of CYP-specific reference inhibitors on the metabolism of an NCE in human liver microsomes *in vitro* gives information about the affinity of an NCE for CYP enzymes and permits *in vivo* predictions about the behavior of the NCE in man (metabolic pathways, intrinsic clearance, and so on), which helps to design *in vivo* studies for revealing possible interactions.

IN VIVO PROFILING OF A NEW CHEMICAL ENTITY

In this section, profiling of new chemical entity *in vivo* has been explained in order to have an overview of the *in vivo* pharmacokinetic properties of potential new medicines in laboratory animals (rats, mice and guinea pigs). Pharmacokinetic studies are performed to test how much of an NCE is absorbed from the site of administration (e.g. from the gastrointestinal tract, or from a subcutaneous injection), and to see how long they remain in the circulation. These factors are important as they will determine if the potential NCE is suitable for progression into pharmacodynamic models (e.g. animal models of human diseases), and will provide essential dosing information for these studies. Demonstration of efficacy (i.e. the desired drug effect) in animal models is required before a potential NCE can be tested in human volunteers or patients.

Pharmacokinetic testing in animals takes place at the end of an extensive *in vitro* drug discovery cascade, which weeds out the compounds that are not potent enough or not specific enough, have an undesirable metabolic profile or are unsuitable for other reasons such as solubility or problems with chemical synthesis. Example of this would be an *in vitro* cell-based assay to determine the potency of a novel drug, where the cells have been manipulated to express a human receptor, and metabolic profiling studies, which are performed using recombinant human and animal liver enzymes. These stages ensure that only carefully selected small subsets of a potential NCE are progressed into animal models. Although use is made of computer-based simulations to assist us in identifying the most appropriate compounds to progress into further testing, there is still no better way to determine the pharmacokinetic properties of new compounds than by performing studies in animals. As these compounds will need to be tested for efficacy in animal models before they can be administered to humans, it is appropriate that PK is determined in these same species. Compounds which do not meet the desired pharmacokinetic properties will not be used in pharmacodynamic studies, and this prevents unnecessary animal experiments being performed. In addition, the pharmacokinetic data obtained can itself be used to guide the selection of compounds for further development.

For most NCEs, oral bioavailability is a key requirement as this will allow the formulation of the medicine as a tablet, although as stated earlier there are some for which parenteral (i.e. intravenous) administration or subcutaneous dosing is more appropriate. In some instances the demonstration of efficacy in animal models requires the injection of the compound directly into the abdominal cavity; hence, to provide information on the likely plasma exposure and duration of action, this route will occasionally be used. Rats, mice and guinea pigs are the key experimental species that are used in pharmacodynamic efficacy and safety studies, and that is why we will use these animals for our pharmacokinetic experiments. These species are among the lowest in terms of evolutionary development but having a well-defined and comparable physiology to man. The most common sort of pharmacokinetic study requires the dosing of one group of animals with a test compound intravenously and another group to receive the dose via the oral route. This enables us to calculate the oral bioavailability and thereby rank compounds on the basis of their ability to absorb following oral dosing. These studies are generally performed in rats, although some studies using mice and guinea pigs may be required. The sampling of blood from rats and guinea pigs can be achieved by surgical cannulation of blood vessels. Rats can also be sampled by taking blood directly from the tail tip and mice will generally be sampled only under terminal anesthesia. An additional set of animals may undergo long-term pharmacokinetic studies following a single dose of compound, where blood samples will be taken from the tail tip very frequently over a period of up to 2 months. In all the studies performed, the amount of blood taken and the duration of the study are limited, and at the end of all procedures animals are humanely sacrificed.

The next stage of pharmacokinetic testing is the identification of drug metabolites and the routes by which these are cleared from the body. This provides very important information regarding the enzymatic pathways and organs involved in excretion. The most simple experiment is to dose the animals with test compound and collect blood urine and feces, which may contain the compound or its metabolites. Collection of urine and feces is achieved by using specially designed cages having a gridded floor, which allows urine and fecal pellets to fall through. For some compounds it may be more appropriate to look for metabolites in the bile fluid, and this is achieved by surgical cannulation of the bile duct under a general anesthetic. Once the animals have recovered from surgery the compound is dosed and the bile fluid collected from the conscious animal using the cannula. These studies give detailed information on their metabolism and excretion prior to selection of development candidates, and in total including the urine/feces studies.

Recently there have been concerns that coadministration of some drugs in humans can have serious consequences in terms of side effects due to them acting on liver enzymes. This can occur if one drug inhibits an enzyme that is key to the metabolism of another and thereby changes the pharmacokinetic properties of that compound. *In vitro* studies using isolated or recombinant liver enzymes can provide us with much information regarding the likelihood of such a significant interaction, but it may be necessary to provide *in vivo* evidence that these phenomena can occur under real physiological conditions. These studies are only intended to identify changes in pharmacokinetic parameters and toxicity is not expected.

Progression of potential new chemical entity into animal models of disease is a key step in advancing a new compound towards becoming a drug for use in humans. Animal disease models often require repeated dosing of compounds over several days to demonstrate efficacy, and in these circumstances it may sometimes be useful to know how much compound is present in plasma after multiple doses. After multiple doses of drug the compound can start to accumulate and give rise to higher plasma concentrations than can be seen after a single dose.

Taken as a whole, the pharmacokinetic studies will provide us with essential information with which we can advance a potential NCE for further development from *in vitro* experiments to preclinical animal models of disease and ill health. Detailed pharmacokinetic profiling will avoid using inappropriate compounds in pharmacodynamic studies, which are unlikely to be successful in man, at an early stage.

CYTOCHROME P450 ENZYMES INVOLVED IN XENOBIOTIC METABOLISM

The CYPs belong to a superfamily of enzymes consisting of microsomal hemoproteins that catalyze the oxidative, peroxidative and reductive metabolism of a wide variety of endogenous and exogenous compounds. This superfamily is divided into families and subfamilies based on the homology of amino acid sequences (Nelson *et al.*, 1996). Members of the same family exhibit about 40% amino acid sequence identity, and the members of the same subfamily possess greater than 55% identity. Most biotransformation of xenobiotics is done by enzymes from the families CYP1, CYP2 and CYP3, accounting for about 70% of human hepatic microsome CYPs (with CYP3 accounting for approximately 30%). The human CYP1 family contains several members that include CYP1A1, -1A2 and -1B1. CYP1A2 represents about 13% CYP enzymes in human liver as determined by immunoblots, and has been identified to be involved in the metabolism of a number of marketed drugs, such as acetaminophen, clomipramine and imipramine. The CYP2 family contains several subfamilies including CYP2A, CYP2B, CYP2C, CYP2D and CYP2E. The role of subfamilies CYP2A, CYP2B and CYP2E in drug metabolism has been shown to be insignificant. The CYP2C subfamily is complex and contains at least seven members. CYP2C8 and CYP2C9 are the two major isoforms in the CYP2C family and account for 35% and 60% of the total subfamily, respectively. Although CYP2C19 is a minor isoform that accounts for only about 1% of the CYP2 family, this enzyme, along with CYP2C8 and -2C9, plays a very important role in drug metabolism. CYP2C9 is responsible for the metabolism of ibuprofen, tolbutamide and torsemide. Drugs metabolized by CYP2C8 include taxol and retinoids. CYP2C19 is the major isozyme metabolizing diazepam, omeprazole and clomipramine. Another very important isozyme in the CYP2 family is CYP2D6. Although CYP2D6 constitutes approximately 2% of the total hepatic CYPs, it metabolizes a wide variety of drugs including cardiovascular drugs, antidepressants and antipsychotics. So far, CYP2D6 is perhaps the second most important CYP enzyme in drug metabolism and has been shown to be responsible for metabolizing over 30% of the drugs on the market. In the CYP3 family, three isoforms have been identified in human liver. Expression of CYP3A5 appears to be polymorphic and is found in about 20% of the population. CYP3A7 is only detected in fetus liver. Both CYP3A5 and 3A7 did not play important roles in drug metabolism. Human CYP3A4 is the most abundant isoform in all CYP families, constituting about 29% of total CYP proteins, and it also has been recognized to be the most important isoform in drug metabolism. To date, metabolism catalyzed by CYP3A4 is the major elimination route for nearly 50% of the marketed drugs. Because of their importance in drug metabolism, both CYP3A4 and CYP2D6 are often involved in drug–drug interactions.

Variation of Cytochrome P450s

The expression of CYP enzymes varies between individuals due to genetic and environmental factors and some diseases. These factors produce interindividual variation in the rates and metabolic pathways of xenobiotics. One example of genetic factors influencing the interindividual variation is the polymorphic expression of at least CYP2A6, CYP2C9, CYP2C19 and CYP2D6 among the population. The frequency of poor metabolizers (PMs) varies between races and ethnic groups. Some dietary compounds, cigarette smoking, alcohol and drugs may cause induction or diminution of the expression of certain CYPs (Pelkonen and Breimer, 1994; Pelkonen *et al.*, 1998).

When several drugs are administered simultaneously, there is always a risk of pharmacokinetic interactions. One drug can modulate the CYP-mediated metabolism of another if the drugs are metabolized by the same enzyme. On the other hand, one drug can inhibit the metabolism of another drug by binding to the same enzyme without being itself metabolized. These interactions can be studied by *in vitro* methods using cultured hepatocytes or subcellular organelles derived from the human liver (Boobis, 1995; Pelkonen *et al.*, 1998). Table 4.1 summarizes the xenobiotic-metabolizing human hepatic CYPs.

Table 4.1 *Summary of Xenobiotic-Metabolizing Human Hepatic CYPs*

CYP	*Preferred Substrate and Reaction*	*Inhibitor*
1A2	Phenacetin (O-deethylation)	Furafylline, fluvoxamine
	7-Ethoxyresorufin (O-deethylation)	Fluvoxamine
2A6	Coumarin (7-hydroxylation)	Methoxsalen, pilocarpine
2B6	7-Ethoxy-4-trifluoromethylcoumarin	
2C8	Taxol (hydroxylation)	Quercetin
2C9	Tolbutamide (methyl hydroxylation)	Sulfaphenazole
	Diclofenac (hydroxylation)	
	S-Warfarin (7-hydroxylation)	
2C19	*S*-Mephenytoin (4-hydroxylation)	Teniposide, fluconazole
	Omeprazole (oxidation)	Fluconazole
2D6	Debrisoquine (4-hydroxylation)	Quinidine
	Dextromethorphan (O-deethylation)	
	Bufuralol (1′-hydroxylation)	
	Chlorzoxazone (6-hydroxylation)	Diethyldithiocarbamate
	Aniline (4-hydroxylation)	
3A4	Testosterone (6β-hydroxylation)	Troleandomycin, ketoconazole, gestodene
	Midazolam (1-hydroxylation)	
	Nifedipine (dehydrogenation)	

CYP1A Subfamily

The human CYP1A subfamily consists of two members: CYP1A1 and CYP1A2. CYP1A2 is mainly expressed in the liver, while CYP1A1 is primarily expressed in extrahepatic tissues. CYP1A1 is induced by cigarette smoking and polycyclic aromatic hydrocarbon (PAH)-type inducers in extrahepatic tissues, mainly the lung and placenta. In the liver, CYP1A1 is expressed at a very low level (Guengerich, 1991; McKinnon *et al.*, 1991; Pasanen and Pelkonen, 1994; Raunio *et al.*, 1995; Pelkonen *et al.*, 1998). CYP1A1 has activity toward some PAHs (Guengerich, 1991).

The constitutively expressed CYP1A2 in human liver is inducible by, for example, environmental compounds, such as constituents of cooked meat, cruciferous vegetables, cigarette smoke, PAHs and polychlorinated biphenyls (Adams *et al.*, 1997). The metabolic activation of some arylamines, such as 4-aminobiphenyl, 2-aminoanthracene and 2-naphthylamine, is done by CYP1A2 (Guengerich, 1991).

CYP1A2 represents about 15% of the total CYP enzymes in human liver (Pelkonen and Breimer, 1994; Shimada *et al.*, 1994). There is some variability between individuals in the CYP1A2 enzyme levels in the human liver (Shimada *et al.*, 1994). Because of the large interindividual variation in CYP1A2 activities, the *in vivo* testing of this enzyme has been quite difficult to evaluate (Kunze and Trager, 1993). CYP1A2 substrates among the currently used drugs include theophylline, caffeine, olanzapine, ondansentron, paracetamol, phenacetin and propranolol. Caffeine and theophylline have been considered as *in vivo* diagnostic probes. The usually employed *in vitro* substrate is ethoxyresorufin, which seems to be quite specific to CYP1A2 (Burke *et al.*, 1985). The substrates and their enzyme kinetic parameters have been reviewed by Pelkonen *et al.* (1998).

Furafylline and fluvoxamine have been the most widely used *in vitro* diagnostic inhibitors. Furafylline is a potent and selective mechanism-based inactivator of CYP1A2 (Sesardic *et al.*, 1990), but it has no function as an *in vivo* inhibitor because of its interactions with caffeine (Tarrus *et al.*, 1987).

Fluvoxamine is also used as an *in vivo* diagnostic inhibitor for CYP1A2 (Brosen *et al.*, 1993; Rasmussen *et al.*, 1995). Fluvoxamine is known to inhibit moderately CYP2D6 and CYP2C19, though at a higher concentration range than CYP1A2 (Jeppesen *et al.*, 1996), but not CYP1A1, CYP2A6, CYP2E1 or CYP3A4 *in vitro*. Venkatakrishnan and co-workers have shown that fluvoxamine inhibits CYP2C19 equally potently as CYP1A2 in lymphoblast-expressed human CYPs and, to a slightly lesser extent, CYP2C9 and CYP3A4 (Von Moltke *et al.*, 1995; 1996; Venkatakrishnan *et al.*, 1999).

CYP2A Subfamily

In humans, there are three genes in the CYP2A subfamily: *CYP2A6* codes the enzyme catalyzing coumarin 7-hydroxylation (about 10% of total P450), while the product of *CYP2A7* is inactive and *CYP2A13* is not expressed in the liver (Pelkonen *et al.*, 2000). In the olfactory mucosa, CYP2A13 is highly expressed as a catalytically active protein (Gu *et al.*, 2000). Recently, CYP2A6 has been reported to be polymorphically expressed in the human liver (Oscarson *et al.*, 1998). No endogenous substrate for CYP2A6 has been found.

It has been recently shown that CYP2A6 participates in the metabolism of nicotine (Cashman *et al.*, 1992; Nakajima *et al.*, 1996b) and its metabolite cotinine (Nakajima *et al.*, 1996a).

This enzyme also catalyzes the metabolic activation of several procarcinogens and promutagens, such as aflatoxin B_1 (Yun *et al.*, 1991; Salonpää *et al.*, 1993) and several nitrosamines (Yamazaki *et al.*, 1992; Tiano *et al.*, 1994). Some drugs and chemicals, including halothane and coumarin, which is widely used as a probe substance for CYP2A6 both *in vitro* and *in vivo*, are also metabolized by this enzyme (Rendic and Di Carlo, 1997; Pelkonen *et al.*, 1998).

Draper and co-workers (1997) have extensively studied the commonly employed P450 substrates and inhibitors with regard to their effect on CYP2A6-catalyzed coumarin 7-hydroxylation. They also screened the effects of some commonly used solvents on the same reaction. They found that many of the studied chemicals were inhibitors of CYP2A6, although earlier presumed to be selective for some other CYPs. For example, ketoconazole is used as a CYP3A4-specific inhibitor, but it was also found to inhibit CYP2A6 quite potently. Also, many commonly used organic solvents inhibit coumarin 7-hydroxylation at substrate concentrations near K_m.

More substrates and inhibitors currently known to be metabolized by or to interact with CYP2A6 *in vitro* and *in vivo* have been summarized by Pelkonen *et al.* (2000).

CYP2B Subfamily

CYP2B6 is the only active member of the CYP2B subfamily in human, although the *CYP2B7* gene has also been found in the genome (Czerwinski *et al.*, 1994). For a long time, it was thought that CYP2B6 would not be expressed in every human liver. For example, Mimura *et al.* (1993) assessed 50 human liver samples by immunoblotting analysis with antimonkey P4502B antibody for CYP2B6 and found only about of the livers to contain the protein (see also Yamano *et al.*, 1989, and Shimada *et al.*, 1994). The highest level of CYP2B6 found by Mimura and co-workers was <2% of the total P450. Today, several groups have shown that this enzyme is expressed in every human liver, but the levels of expression differ between individuals (Ekins *et al.*, 1997; Stresser & Kupfer, 1999). The amount of CYP2B6 protein seems to be below 1% of the total P450 present in the human liver, and the reason for the earlier reports about non-expressing individuals is probably the weak sensitivity of either the antibodies used or the detection methods. Today, there are very sensitive and specific anti-peptide antibodies available for quantitative immunological studies (Stresser and Kupfer, 1999). Similarly to the other studies on CYP2B6, they showed the expression of this enzyme to be highly variable.

CYP2B6 has been postulated to be co-regulated with CYP3A4 or at least to be inducible by the same inducers, such as rifampicin and dexamethasone, as well as by phenobarbital in cultured human hepatocytes (Strom *et al.*, 1996).

The catalytic activity of CYP2B6 has recently been under efficient research by many groups. Ekins and co-workers (1997, 1998) have especially evaluated several chemicals and drugs as specific substrates for this enzyme. Among the suggested CYP2B6-catalyzed reactions are O-deethylation of 7-ethoxy-4-trifluoromethylcoumarin (7-EFC), N-demethylation of *S*-mephenytoin, stereoselective hydroxylation of RP 73401 [3-cyclopentyloxy-*N*-(3,5-dichloro-4-pyridyl)-4-methoxybenzamide], to RPR 113406 (Stevens *et al.*, 1997) and bupropion hydroxylation (Faucette *et al.*, 2000). The availability of the other selective substrates presented above, RP 73401 and its CYP2B6-formed metabolite RPR 113406 prepared by Rhône-Poulenc Rorer Co., is unknown. Recently, Kobayashi *et al.* (1999) evaluated the role of CYP2B6 in the N-demethylation of *S*-mephobarbital by using 10 cDNA-expressed human CYPs. They found that only CYP2B6 catalyzed the reaction. Also, the activity correlated strongly with the immunodetectable CYP2B6 levels in microsomes from 10 individual human livers. This activity is probably quite usable if the substrate, *S*-mephobarbital, could be easily separated from its *R*-enantiomer. The metabolite, phenobarbital, is commonly used as a P450-inducing agent (Pelkonen *et al.*, 1998).

Orphenadrine has been widely used as an inhibitor of CYP2B6, though its selectivity toward this isoform is questionable (Murray and Reidy, 1990; Chang *et al.*, 1993; Ekins *et al.*, 1997; Guo *et al.*, 1997). Although actively searched, no selective inhibitor for CYP2B6 has been found yet.

CYP2C Subfamily

The CYP2C subfamily is the second most abundant CYP protein in the human liver, representing about 20% of the total P450 (Shimada *et al.*, 1994). This subfamily consists of three active members in the human liver, namely CYP2C8, CYP2C9 and CYP2C19. Of these, CYP2C9 and CYP2C19 have been characterized to be polymorphically expressed (Goldstein and De Morais, 1994; Gill *et al.*, 1999).

CYP2C8 has been assumed to play an unimportant important role in drug metabolism since it is expressed at very low levels in the human liver. Still, the new, very potent anticancer drug, taxol, for example, is partly metabolized by CYP2C8 (Harris *et al.*, 1994; Sonnichsen *et al.*, 1995). CYP2C8 also participates in the metabolism of the endogenic agents retinol and retinoic acid (Leo *et al.*, 1989). The involvement of this member of the CYP2C subfamily in the metabolism of NCEs has been difficult to study because there is no good, specific substrate and inhibitor for this isoform. In many cases, CYP2C8 also participates, to a small extent, in the metabolism of the CYP2C9 substrates (Wrighton *et al.*, 1993b).

CYP2C9 is the major CYP2C isoform in the human liver (Goldstein and De Morais, 1994), and it has been shown to be genetically polymorphic with at least three different alleles that produce differently active protein. The functional consequences of these polymorphisms are not yet clear, although CYP2C9 has a major role in the metabolism of many clinically important, weakly acidic drugs, such as *S*-warfarin (Rettie *et al.*, 1992), tolbutamide, phenytoin (Doecke *et al.*, 1991), sulfamethoxazole (Cribb *et al.*, 1995) and many of the nonsteroidal anti-inflammatory compounds (Leeman *et al.*, 1993) as well as the new drug in this class, a cyclooxygenase-II selective inhibitor, celecoxib (Tang *et al.*, 2000). The frequencies of the two variant alleles, *CYP2C9*2* and *CYP2C9*3*, have been reported to range from 7% to 19% in Caucasian populations (Furuya *et al.*, 1995; Sullivan-Klose *et al.*, 1996; Stubbins *et al.*, 1996).

With CYP2C19, the genetic polymorphism leads to the PM phenotypes exhibiting less active or completely inactive *S*-mephenytoin 4′-hydroxylase. This PM phenotype is produced by at least two major and several minor variant alleles of CYP2C19 (Goldstein and De Morais, 1994), and, consequently, CYP2C19 substrates are not metabolized as expected (Pelkonen *et al.*, 1998). This may lead to accumulation of the drug and to *in vivo* concentrations exceeding the therapeutic level and producing unexpected toxic effects. The search for CYP2C19-selective inhibitor both *in vitro* and *in vivo* is under way, since omeprazole, which is usually employed, also inhibits other CYPs (Funck-Brentano *et al.*, 1997). The deficiency of the 4′-hydroxylation pathway of *S*-mephenytoin occurs in 2–5% of the Caucasian population (Relling *et al.*, 1990).

CYP2D Subfamily

The human genome includes only one functional gene in the CYP2D subfamily, namely *CYP2D6* (Nelson *et al.*, 1996). There also exist two *CYP2D7* pseudogenes and two pseudogenes of *CYP2D8* (Heim and Meyer, 1992; Nelson *et al.*, 1996). More than 60 allelic variants have been reported for *CYP2D6*. Of these, most affect the activity of the expressed protein. CYP2D6 represents 1–5% of the total P450 (Pelkonen and Breimer, 1994; Shimada *et al.*, 1994; Pelkonen *et al.*, 1998), and 7–8% of the Caucasian population are PMs for this enzyme (Heim and Meyer, 1992).

The search for endogenous substrates for CYP2D6 has recently become more interesting because it has been shown that CYP2D6 is associated with Parkinson's disease (Barbeau *et al.*, 1985; Armstrong *et al.*, 1992; Smith *et al.*, 1992; Agúndez *et al.*, 1995) and with susceptibility to develop liver and lung cancer (Idle, 1981; Ayesh *et al.*, 1984; Agúndez *et al.*, 1994; Caporaso *et al.*, 1995; Bouchardy *et al.*, 1996). Martínez *et al.* (1997) suggested a neurotransmitter, tryptamine, as an endogenous substrate for CYP2D6. The metabolism of tryptamine into tryptophol was catalyzed in an NADPH-dependent manner and inhibited by a specific CYP2D6 inhibitor, quinidine.

One common feature of CYP2D6 substrates is that they contain at least one basic nitrogen atom at a distance of 5 or 7 Å from the oxidation site. Second, there is a planar hydrophobic area near the oxidation site; third, the substrates exhibit a negative molecular electrostatic potential above the planar part of the molecule (Koymans *et al.*, 1992; Strobl *et al.*, 1993; de Groot *et al.*, 1997). The drugs known to be substrates for this enzyme include antiarrhythmic and other cardiovascular drugs, β-adrenergic blocking agents, tricyclic antidepressants, neuroleptics and many other commonly used therapeutical agents (Cholerton *et al.*, 1992). The mostly used *in vitro* model reactions are dextromethorphan O-demethylation, debrisoquine 4-hydroxylation and bufuralol 1′-hydroxylation. Of these substrates, debrisoquine is also employed in *in vivo* studies as a CYP2D6 model substance, although its use is becoming more difficult because it is not marketed any more (Pelkonen *et al.*, 1998, and references therein).

As a reference inhibitor for CYP2D6, quinidine is widely used in drug metabolism studies. It is a specific and potent inhibitor with a K_i value of 0.06 μM for CYP2D6, and the CYP next in sensitivity, CYP3A4, has a K_i value around 10 μM (Broly *et al.*, 1989; Bourrie *et al.*, 1996).

Due to the fact that numerous drugs on the market are metabolized by CYP2D6 and the polymorphic nature of the expression of this protein, it is strongly suggested that the affinities of the NCEs on this CYP form should be characterized to predict and to possibly avoid drug–drug interactions.

CYP2E Subfamily

The coding region of *CYP2E1* is highly conserved in different ethnic groups and species. There are significant inter-ethnic differences in polymorphisms, but there is no clear evidence of any of the reported polymorphisms to be related to altered *in vivo* activities. All the reported polymorphisms are found in the noncoding regions of the gene, suggesting an important role in the biotransformation of endogenous substances (Ronis *et al.*, 1996; Yin *et al.*, 1997).

The CYP2E1 expression is regulated by many factors. For example, fasting elevates the level of the protein by increasing the transcription of the gene (Johansson *et al.*, 1990) and diabetes by stabilizing the mRNA (Song *et al.*, 1987), while isoniazid increases the translation efficiency (Park *et al.*, 1993) and affects the enzyme stabilization similarly to ethanol and imidazole (Eliasson *et al.*, 1990).

The CYP2E1 substrates include very few clinically important drugs. Actually, only paracetamol (Patten *et al.*, 1989), caffeine (Gu *et al.*, 1992), chlorzoxazone (Peter *et al.*, 1990) and enflurane (Thummel *et al.*, 1993) are worth mentioning here. Most organic solvents and anesthetics, short-chain alcohols and many nitrosamine and azo carcinogens (Hong and Yang, 1985; Yang *et al.*, 1985; Sohn *et al.*, 1991; Koop, 1992) are also xenobiotic substrates of this enzyme. CYP2E1 participates in the metabolism of many endogenous substances, such as lipid peroxidation products (Terelius and Ingelman-Sundberg, 1986), ketones (Koop and Cassazza, 1985) and fatty acids, such as linoleic and arachidonic acids (Laethem *et al.*, 1993). A number of other small-molecular CYP2E1 substrates are listed in the review article by Ronis *et al.* (1996).

Pyridine is a specific *in vitro* inhibitor and inhibits CYP2E1 at relatively low concentrations (Hargreaves *et al.*, 1994; Taavitsainen *et al.*, unpublished results). The metabolite of disulfiram, diethyldithiocarbamate, has also been used as an *in vitro* inhibitor (Guengerich *et al.*, 1991; Brady *et al.*, 1991), though its selectivity is questionable (Yamazaki *et al.*, 1992).

CYP3A Subfamily

The CYP3A subfamily represents about 30% of the total P450 content in the human liver (Pelkonen and Breimer, 1994; Shimada *et al.*, 1994), although the levels of the protein may vary 40-fold among individuals (Guengerich, 1995a). This subfamily consists of three members (Nelson *et al.*, 1996): CYP3A4 is the most abundant CYP enzyme in the human liver and it is expressed in several tissues, but the expression in the liver and small intestine is of major interest in view of the metabolism of drugs and other xenobiotic chemicals (Guengerich, 1999). CYP3A5 is a minor, polymorphic CYP3A enzyme, which is expressed in the lungs (Kivistö *et al.*, 1996; Anttila *et al.*, 1997) and the colon (Gervot *et al.*, 1996). About 20% of individual adults express CYP3A5 at a high level in the liver (Guengerich, 1999). CYP3A7 is expressed in fetal liver and the adult endometrium and placenta (Schuetz *et al.*, 1993; Hakkola *et al.*, 1994).

The members of the CYP3A subfamily have overlapping catalytic specificities, but some selectivity exists. CYP3A4 participates in the metabolism of about half of the drugs in use today (Bertz and Granneman, 1997). For example, testosterone 6β-hydroxylation, midazolam 1′- and 4-hydroxylation, nifedipine oxidation and erythromycin N-demethylation are catalyzed by this enzyme. The known substrates of CYP3A4 vary in size, from small molecules such as acetaminophen (M_r 151), to cyclosporin A (M_r 1201) (Guengerich, 1999). In addition to the substrates listed above, we could further mention the physiologically important progesterone and andostenedione (Waxman *et al.*, 1991), cortisol, quinidine, diltiazem, lidocaine, lovastatin, troleandomycin, warfarin and triazolam (Guengerich and Shimada, 1991; Wrighton and Stevens, 1992).

CYP3A is inducible by many drugs, e.g. rifampicin, dexamethasone, carbamazepine and phenobarbital-type inducers (Pelkonen *et al.*, 1998). The induction of CYP3A has an effect on the interindividual variation and affects both bioavailability and drug–drug interactions (Guengerich, 1999).

The inhibitors of CYP3A have a wide variety of chemical structures. For example, azole-type fungicides, ketoconazole and itraconazole, are potent inhibitors. Ketoconazole also inhibits other CYPs than CYP3A4, but at a concentration of 1 μM it is relatively selective for CYP3A4 (Newton *et al.*, 1994; Baldwin *et al.*, 1995). Gestodene, a progesterone analog with a steroid structure, has been long known as a mechanism-based CYP3A inhibitor (Pelkonen *et al.*, 1998). Gestodene is also a substrate for CYP3A4.

The substrate specificity and catalytic features of CYP3A4 have recently been a target of active research. It has been shown by many groups that the properties of CYP3A4 have not yet been thoroughly elucidated (Ueng *et al.*, 1997; Korzekwa *et al.*, 1998; Wang *et al.*, 2000). For example, the role of cytochrome b_5, divalent cations and rate-limiting steps in the catalysis are still under study (Guengerich, 1999). Wang *et al.* (2000) studied the *in vitro* drug–drug interaction patterns with four commonly used CYP3A4 substrates. The results indicated that CYP3A4 is a very complex enzyme and that its interaction patterns are substrate dependent.

Thanks to the unique properties of CYP3A4, the enzymatic processes catalyzed by CYP3A4 do not always follow the typical competitive inhibition kinetics. A substrate can either inhibit or stimulate the *in vitro* metabolism of another substrate, or activate its own metabolism (Shou *et al.*, 1994). The kinetics can be either cooperative or allosteric, depending on the binding sites of the two substrate/inhibitor molecules, one molecule of two substrates each or one molecule of the substrate and an effector (Shou *et al.*, 1994; Ueng *et al.*, 1997; Korzekwa *et al.*, 1998; Guengerich *et al.*, 1999; Wang *et al.*, 2000).

Although the cooperativity in CYP3A4-catalyzed reactions has been known for a long time, there has not been any major progress in this field. A great majority of studies suggest that there are at least two distinct binding sites for the substrate and the effector. The location of the effector binding site–whether at the active site or at a separate allosteric site–is not yet known (Ueng *et al.*, 1997). Harlow and Halpert (1998) presented a model for cooperativity, which suggests that the substrate and effector molecules bind at adjacent sites and are both part of a large binding cavity. This model agrees with the one presented by Shou *et al.* (1994), with the exception that they suggested two catalytic sites, both of them with access to the reactive oxygen.

Based on these results, it is concluded that the active site of CYP3A4 is very large and flexible, which postulation is supported by the wide substrate selectivity. Shou and co-workers (1994) also suggested that the activator, when binding to the active site, excludes water molecules from the substrate cavity and prevents the hydrogen peroxide release. These models combined could together explain the atypical CYP3A4 kinetics, including activation, autoactivation, mutual inhibition, partial inhibition, substrate inhibition, biphasic saturation curves and alteration of regiospecificity.

Still, although much effort has been invested in CYP3A4 research, there may still be many properties of this enzyme that need to be studied. One should bear in mind the likelihood that because CYP3A4 plays such an important role in xenobiotic metabolism, its catalysis may not be very simple in nature. The conclusions drawn on the basis of only one substrate or inhibitor should be regarded as tentative.

METHODS FOR STUDYING *IN VITRO* METABOLISM OF NCEs

Overview of Preclinical Studies

Preclinical studies consist of animal studies (on the PK and PD of the compound, toxicological studies) and animal and human tissue–derived *in vitro* studies. Because of the problems in extrapolating the results of animal studies to humans, various *in vitro* methods have been developed by employing human tissue–derived systems (Wrighton *et al.*, 1993). Also, the regulatory authorities have begun to increasingly demand that the issues concerning metabolism and toxicity in test species compared to humans should be actively clarified in early preclinical tests. This is done by utilizing liver preparations from humans and trying to find the test species that most closely resemble human metabolism and the production of toxic intermediates (Yuan *et al.*, 1999).

It is important to elucidate the *in vitro* metabolism and the putative interactions at the time of planning other preclinical and early clinical studies. In the next few sections, human tissue–derived preclinical *in vitro* systems will be briefly discussed.

Human-Derived *In Vitro* Systems in Preclinical Drug Metabolism Research

There are several approaches to preclinical metabolism studies. The enzyme sources in these studies are human-derived systems currently under rapid development and evaluation. These systems consist of liver microsomes, hepatocytes and cell lines heterologously expressing drug-metabolizing enzymes, liver slices and individually cDNA-expressed enzymes in host cell microsomes. Each of these will be discussed briefly here. Table 4.2 shows a comparison of different human-derived *in vitro* methods.

Human Liver Microsomes

Human liver microsomes are fractionated from subcellular organelles by differential ultracentrifugation. Microsomes are formed from smooth endoplasmic reticulum (ER) during tissue homogenization (Boobis, 1995). A microsomal fraction from human liver contains a full complement of P450 enzymes, which makes it a suitable tool for studying inhibitory interactions and CYP-catalyzed metabolite formation (Kremers, 1999). By employing relevant cofactors and other reaction components, one can readily investigate and distinguish between P450s, flavin-containing monooxygenases (FMOs) and glucuronosyltransferases. Microsomes are relatively easy to prepare, and enzymatic activities are stable during prolonged storage (Beaune *et al.*, 1986; Yamazaki *et al.*, 1997), if the original tissue is correctly handled and frozen immediately after excision (Kremers, 1999). The validation and harmonization of assay procedures between different laboratories in this respect, too, would lead to less inter-laboratory variation in the same assays (Boobis *et al.*, 1998; Kremers, 1999).

Human Hepatocytes

Hepatocytes contain the full compartment of Phase I and Phase II enzymes, and the whole metabolite pattern can therefore be detected in incubations with hepatocytes. Other effects of an NCE, such as the induction of drug-metabolizing enzymes and possible toxic effects, can also be elucidated (Morel *et al.*, 1990; Maurel, 1996; Ferrini *et al.*, 1997; Li *et al.*, 1997).

The utilization of human primary hepatocytes is restricted, because sufficient liver samples are quite difficult to obtain and hepatocytes are difficult to preserve for later use. Some successful attempts to cryopreserve primary hepatocytes have been described (Guillouzo *et al.*, 1995). A prolonged culture method has also been published, in which hepatocytes are maintained for over 30 days (Kono *et al.*, 1997), preserving some of their drug-metabolizing activities and inducibility instead of the standard for up to 1 week. Hepatocytes can be subjected to several test and washout periods during their lifetime. This method, together with the cryopreservation method, enables more efficient use of a single hepatocyte batch than before.

Table 4.2 *Comparison of* In Vitro *Enzyme Sources Used in Preclinical Research*

Enzyme Sources	*Availability*	*Advantages*	*Disadvantages*
Microsomes	Relatively good, from transplantations or commercial sources	Easy to obtain. Also commercially available. Relatively inexpensive technique.	Contain only Phase I DMEs and UDP-glucuronosyltransferases. Require strictly specific substrates and inhibitors or antibodies for individual DMEs.
cDNA-expressed individual CYPs	Good, commercially available	Can be utilized with high-throughput screening (HTS) substrates. The role of individual CYPs in the metabolism of an NCE can be easily studied.	The effect of only one enzyme at a time can be evaluated
Immortalized cell lines	Available at request; not many adequately characterized cell lines exist	Non-limited source of enzymes	The expression of most DMEs is poor or absent if characterized at all
Primary hepatocytes	Relatively difficult to obtain, relatively healthy fresh tissue needed. Commercially available. Cryopreservation possible.	Contain the whole complement of DMEs. The induction effect of an NCE can be studied.	Require specific techniques and well-established procedures. The levels of many DMEs decrease rapidly during cultivation.
Liver slices	Relatively difficult to obtain, fresh tissue needed. Cryopreservation possible.	Contain the whole complement of DMEs and cell–cell connections. The induction effect of an NCE can be studied.	Require specific techniques and well-established procedures

Data partially adapted from Wrighton *et al.* (1993) and Skett *et al.* (1995).

Permanent Cell Lines

Immortalized cell lines that express one or more drug-metabolizing enzymes could be valuable tools in preclinical studies, but for most CYPs this approach has failed (Daujat *et al.*, 1996; Gonzalez and Korzekwa, 1995). When whole-cell systems are used, one must know which P450s are really expressed as functional proteins and which are liable to fade out during cultivation. Many of the cell lines used lack the complement of enzymes present in hepatocytes *in vivo*. On the other hand, when studying direct interactions with the enzyme, whole-cell systems could be too complex (Boobis, 1995).

Liver Slices

Of the systems presented here, precision-cut liver slices resemble most closely the *in vivo* situation, which contain not only the enzymes of the whole liver but also the connections between individual cells. The technique of maintaining liver slices is demanding. The thickness of a slice has to be minimal within the limits of the optimal number of cell layers and oxygen and nutrient transportation (Vickers *et al.*, 1995). Recently, methods for cryopreservation of tissue slices have been developed (e.g., Fisher *et al.*, 1993; Ekins *et al.*, 1996; de Kanter *et al.*, 1998; Glöckner *et al.*, 1998; de Graaf *et al.*, 2000). These methods allow for a more flexible use of slices, because viability and CYP activities seem to be preserved quite well (de Graaf *et al.*, 2000; Renwick *et al.*, 2000).

cDNA-Expressed Enzymes

Drug-metabolizing enzymes are available commercially as heterologously expressed enzyme systems. In these preparations, an individual enzyme is produced in the ER of a eukaryote host cell. The expression of human liver CYPs in different artificial systems has become easier due to the rapid development of recombinant DNA techniques (Gonzalez *et al.*, 1991). The systems employed for the production of cDNA-expressed CYPs include bacteria (Fisher *et al.*, 1992; Gillam *et al.*, 1993), yeast (Guengerich *et al.*, 1991a; Peyronneau *et al.*, 1992), mammalian cell lines (Guengerich, 1995b) and baculovirus systems (Asseffa *et al.*, 1989). cDNA-expressed enzymes are a valuable tool in the search for the enzymes participating in the metabolism of an NCE. Because the enzymes are studied in isolation from other hepatic enzymes and because they lack the whole complement of hepatic enzymes, the *in vivo* predictive value of the data obtained from heterologously expressed enzyme systems has been debated (Rodriguez, 1999).

If the inhibition of the metabolism of an unknown compound is studied in a single enzyme system, one should take into account that *in vivo* there are different amounts of individual enzymes in the human liver. The cofactor supply may also affect the relative contribution of certain CYPs. As it was pointed out above, the contribution of one enzyme to the specific metabolic route may not be so significant as it seems on the basis of cDNA-expressed enzymes (Rodriguez, 1999).

As an affinity-screening tool, cDNA-expressed enzymes are valuable. It is also the most useful system allowing a high-throughput screening (HTS) technology for P450 studies today, because of the difficulties and high costs in the detection of multiple substrates and metabolites produced in the HTS applications of other techniques, such as human liver microsomes (White, 2000). The detection of these multiple metabolites requires novel, highly sensitive mass spectrometry tools, whereas cDNA-expressed systems can utilize the conventional measurement of fluorescence metabolite production for multiple enzymes (see, for example, www.gentest.com).

Measures of Metabolism in *In Vitro* Systems

Metabolic Stability of a New Chemical Entity

The metabolic stability of an NCE determines, to a great extent, its future as a drug candidate (see, for example, Kuhnz and Gieschen, 1998). If an NCE is rapidly metabolized in human liver preparations, its bioavailability *in vivo* is most probably too low for it to be a drug candidate. This naturally depends on the administration route of the drug. By determining the time and concentration dependence of metabolite formation from an NCE on the disappearance of the NCE *in vitro* in an appropriate system, its metabolic fate and half-life *in vivo* can be predicted. Similar studies performed in human and test species give valuable information for the selection of test species for pharmacokinetic and toxicological *in vivo* studies.

Identification of Metabolites and Metabolic Routes

Today, there are effective methods for metabolite identification and subsequent construction of metabolic routes. Metabolite identification can be developed from incubations with human liver preparations, homogenates or microsomes (Kremers, 1999). For example, mass spectrometric (MS) methods employing high-performance liquid chromatography (HPLC) as a separative tool have evolved into extremely sensitive and accurate techniques. Through these methods, it is possible to determine with high accuracy the exact molecular masses and metabolite structures. As analytical methods, these techniques are at their best in skillful and highly experienced hands.

Sample preparation for MS studies is a critical step, since the available chemical information of an NCE is often limited. The incubation conditions and the reaction-terminating reagent have to be chosen so as not to alter the parent compound or the metabolites chemically and to keep the recovery of the substrate and the metabolites close to 100%. Otherwise, it is impossible to predict the pathways for biotransformation.

Identification of CYPs Metabolizing a New Chemical Entity

After characterizing the metabolic stability and metabolic routes of an NCE, the *in vivo* prediction requires clarification of the drug-metabolizing enzymes that participate in the *in vitro* biotransformation of the NCE. The methods usually employed for this purpose are presented below.

After determining the initial velocity conditions and enzyme kinetic parameters, the CYPs involved in the metabolism of an NCE can be characterized by chemical and antibody inhibitors selective or specific for respective CYPs. It is important to select the substrate concentration correctly: near or preferably below the determined K_m values, if the analytical method for metabolite detection allows it. In case the *in vivo* concentrations are known, it is recommendable to use substrate concentrations close to the therapeutic level, if at all feasible.

Utilization of CYP-Selective Chemical Inhibitors

Numerous compounds have been characterized for their inhibitory potency against different CYPs. Many of them are selective for only the desired enzyme at relatively low concentrations, e.g. furafylline for CYP1A2 (Sesardic *et al.*, 1990; Clarke *et al.*, 1994; Bourrie *et al.*, 1996; Racha *et al.*, 1998); CYP2C9 is selectively inhibited by sulfaphenazole (Bourrie *et al.*, 1996); quinidine is potent inhibitor for CYP2D6 though metabolised via CYP3A4 (Bourrie *et al.*, 1996); pyridine seems to be quite selective for CYP2E1 (Hargreaves *et al.*, 1994; own unpublished results), and there are many selective inhibitors for CYP3A4, of which ketoconazole is the most widely used, although it also affects other CYPs (Schmider *et al.*, 1995; Bourrie *et al.*, 1996). For CYP2A6 and CYP2C19, the search for selective chemical inhibitors is still under way (Draper *et al.*, 1997; III).

Utilization of CYP-Specific Antibodies

Today, there are several commercial sources for CYP-specific inhibitory antibodies. The products usually are well characterized and not very expensive. Inhibitory antibodies usually are targeted toward a sequence at or near the substrate-binding site. The antigen can be selected in such a way that the resulting antibody only inhibits the target CYP. Inhibitory antibodies raised specifically against a certain CYP form are a good tool in distinguishing between CYPs established as equally possible NCE-metabolizing CYPs by other methods. Antibodies can also be used if there are no sufficiently specific chemical inhibitors available for a certain enzyme (e.g., CYP2B6; Stresser and Kupfer, 1999).

cDNA-Expressed CYPs

Similarly to CYP-specific inhibitory antibodies, cDNA-expressed enzymes are convenient tools when a specific activity or a selective chemical inhibitor cannot be used in metabolic studies. With the expressed enzymes, the relative roles of individual CYPs cannot be quantitatively estimated, mainly due to the interindividual variation in the levels of individual active CYPs in the liver (Guengerich, 1995b). cDNA-expressed CYPs can also be used in the HTS methodology when the goal is to screen large numbers of compounds (White, 2000).

Recombinant enzymes can be used to ascertain the role of a certain CYP in the metabolism of an NCE. Still, the biotransformation of an NCE by a single CYP does not necessarily mean its participation in the reaction *in vivo* (IV). When taking into account the proportion of a certain CYP in the human liver, the activity obtained for the whole liver can be extrapolated to the prediction of the participation of this enzyme (Rodrigues, 1999).

Correlation Analysis

For correlation analysis, a well-characterized bank of human liver samples is needed. The number of individual livers should be at least 10 (preferably more) to demonstrate the interindividual variation in the battery of activities. In correlation analysis, the measured CYP-specific activities are correlated against the rate of the metabolic pathway of an NCE in every individual liver sample. Another approach is to correlate the levels of an individual CYP determined by Western blot analysis against the NCE activity (Beaune *et al.*, 1986; Guengerich and Shimada, 1991; Guengerich, 1995b). When correlating the levels of each CYP protein to the activity of an NCE, one should take into account that any inactive protein could also contribute to the estimation of protein levels in each liver. This could lead to an erroneous correlation, because the inactive CYP proteins do not participate in the metabolism of the NCE (Guengerich, 1995b). If there is a sufficient number of individual samples, statistical significance can also be considered. Still, a correlation plot would give all the information needed for the evaluation of the participating CYPs. The higher the correlation between the activities, the larger the likelihood that the respective CYP enzyme is responsible for the metabolism of the NCE. For correlation analysis, the initial velocity conditions and the substrate concentrations near K_m, or preferably the concentrations found *in vivo* should be used to avoid nonspecific metabolism of substrates (Guengerich, 1995b).

Particularly with CYP3A4, the correlation analysis is somewhat complicated because of the peculiar nature of the CYP3A4 catalytic mechanism (Harlow and Halpert, 1998; Guengerich, 1999).

Measures of the Affinities of a New Chemical Entity for CYPs

Inhibition of CYP-Catalyzed Model Reactions by a New Chemical Entity

From the therapeutic point of view, it is also important to know which drug-metabolizing enzymes the substance under development has affinity to. For example, a compound inhibiting CYP3A4 could affect the *in vivo* concentrations of numerous drugs and other xenobiotics metabolized via this CYP, since over 50% of the drugs on the market are biotransformed by CYP3A4 (Pelkonen and Breimer, 1994; Bertz and Granneman, 1997). In recent years, severe adverse reactions due to interactions with CYP3A4 have led to the withdrawal of some drugs from the market. For example, terfenadine coadministrated with azole antimycotics caused potentially lethal ventricular arrhythmias (Monahan *et al.*, 1990). Another example is mibefradil, the plasma concentrations of which were highly elevated by CYP3A4 inhibitors, leading to serious side effects (Kleinbloesem *et al.*, 1995; Siepmann *et al.*, 1995). Such economically consequential decisions could have been avoided if the affinity of the new compounds to CYPs had been recognized and correctly interpreted at the early phases of the drug development process (Siepmann and Kirch, 2000).

The effect of an NCE on CYP-specific activities is studied by co-incubating a series of dilutions of the study substance with a reaction mixture and a specific substrate. The effect of an NCE is described as the concentration of the studied compound causing 50% inhibition of the CYP-specific activities (Boobis, 1995). If there is affinity toward some CYP-enzyme, the apparent K_i can be determined. By comparing the effects of an NCE on the CYP-specific activities to the respective effects of diagnostic inhibitors, a tentative prediction of the *in vivo* situation can be made.

Spectral Interaction Studies

Spectral interaction studies have been used from the early years of P450 research to recognize P450 ligands. Compounds that have affinity to a CYP-active site coordinate toward the heme iron of the protein, causing a change in the spin equilibrium of heme iron. The binding can produce several types of spectral changes that can be monitored by spectrophotometric scanning according to the procedure presented by, for example, Jefcoate (1978).

In Vitro–In Vivo Scaling of an NCE

General

The very first attempts to predict *in vivo* pharmacokinetic parameters from *in vitro* experiments were presented by Rane *et al.* (1977). In general, *in vitro–in vivo* scaling consists of two approaches: prediction of the intrinsic clearance (Cl_{int}) of an NCE and prediction of drug–drug interactions. In the literature, methods for both purposes are extensively presented (Obach *et al.*, 1997; Ito *et al.*, 1998a, 1998b). Some of the methods will be reviewed briefly in the following sections.

Other pharmacokinetic parameters, such as plasma half-life, volume of distribution and oral bioavailability, have also been considered for the estimation of *in vivo* kinetics on the basis of *in vitro* studies (Obach *et al.*, 1997; Ito *et al.*, 1998a, 1998b). Many *in vivo* factors affect the results of extrapolation. One of these is the binding to plasma and tissue proteins and, ultimately, the volume of distribution of drug. The effect of binding with numerous different compounds has been studied, and the general conclusion seems to be that, with highly lipophilic drugs, protein binding does not play a very important role in prediction accuracy (Kurz and Fichtl, 1983; Pacifici and Viani, 1992; Obach *et al.*, 1997; von Moltke *et al.*, 1998).

Considerations regarding Assay Conditions for New Chemical Entity Studies

Initial velocity conditions

When the metabolic routes of an NCE are recognized either in liver microsomes or in liver homogenate from the human or the test species, a method for the separation and, if a reference substance is available, quantification of metabolites is required. Determination of the initial velocity conditions is important for an accurate determination of the enzyme kinetic parameters of metabolite formation reactions. The determination of the IC_{50} values for CYP-selective diagnostic inhibitors is best performed if the substrate concentration used is selected from within the linear part of the time and protein dependence curve for the metabolite formation from an NCE. When possible, the substrate concentration should be close to the achieved concentrations *in vivo* or at least close to the K_m value (Guengerich, 1995b; Yuan *et al.*, 1999).

Apparent enzyme kinetic parameters K_m and V_{max}

The determination of apparent enzyme kinetic parameters in human liver preparations with different substrates has been presented in various publications and is also available as teaching material (e.g. Boobis, 1995), and it will not be considered in detail here. Basically, there are two approaches available for this purpose: (1) the use of graphical presentations and derivations for Michaelis–Menten kinetics and (2) the use of an iterative software for calculating the parameters from untransformed data using the Michaelis–Menten equation. The latter approach is nowadays most widely used, since it gives somewhat more accurate and more reproducible values than the graphical method. Still, the graphical method is also in use and, if properly handled, gives results accurate enough for practical purposes.

Prediction of the intrinsic clearance (Cl_{int})

For the prediction of intrinsic clearance, one should be familiar with specific information about the enzymes participating in the metabolism of an NCE. This includes the identity of the enzymes and the enzyme kinetic parameters for the NCE with metabolizing enzymes. Without this information, it is still possible to derive K_m and V_{max} by following substrate consumption. This approach does not reveal the parameters for individual metabolic routes, but allows the prediction of overall intrinsic clearance (Cl_{int}) and produces information about the bioavailability of the drug under study.

For example, Ito *et al.* (1998a, 1998b) have studied extensively the quantitative prediction of *in vivo* drug clearance and drug interactions from *in vitro* studies. Both publications would be worth an introduction, but are too extensive to be reviewed here.

Basically, the *in vitro* metabolism can be converted into its *in vivo* counterpart. From the Michaelis–Menten equation for the velocity (v) of metabolite formation,

$$v = \frac{V_{max} * [S]}{K_m + [S]}$$

When $K_m >> [S]$, the reductions of the equation lead to the general expression that the intrinsic clearance (Cl_{int}) is

$$Cl_{int} = V_{max}/K_m, \text{ where}$$

V_{max}/K_m is presented as volume/time. This constant can be compared to the respective *in vivo* value obtained from pharmacokinetic studies. Obach *et al.* (1997) presented an extensive survey, where they compared values obtained from *in vitro* studies of 50 compounds to the respective *in vivo* results. In that study, 12 different methods for clearance predictions were used, of which four were employed to predict values for *in vitro* half-life (t) and, consequently, to predict clearance, four utilized *in vitro* enzyme kinetic data and four were allometric methods, in which the respective human prediction was derived from animal studies. Obach *et al.* (1997) concluded that there is no single method to exactly predict human *in vivo* pharmacokinetic parameters from *in vitro* data, but many of the tested methods yielded a satisfactory level of accuracy to warrant decision making in the drug discovery process. Generally, for the compounds that were highly protein bound, the predicted clearance was underestimated, if the degree of binding was taken into account. Especially for the prediction of the volume of distribution, the plasma protein-binding factor must be included in the calculations. It should be noted that if an NCE binds extensively to plasma protein, it is most probable that it also binds to microsomal proteins. On the whole, the presented methods for estimating *in vivo* pharmacokinetic values from *in vitro* data provide a certain window of accuracy. For example, the estimation of t from *in vitro* enzyme kinetic data gives results accurate enough for the purpose of finding out the dosage regimens for an NCE.

Extrapolation of Cl_{int} to in vivo *clearance in the whole organism*

When extrapolation of Cl_{int} to the *in vivo* clearance in the whole organism is done, some preliminary information or assumptions are needed. These are presented in, for example, reviews by Ito *et al.* (1998a, 1998b) and Obach (1997). If the studied compound is metabolized via more than one pathway, the intrinsic clearances of these pathways need to be summed up to achieve a total Cl_{int} for the study system (microsomes, whole-cell systems, liver slices):

$$Cl_{int\,1} + Cl_{int\,2} + Cl_{int\,3} \ldots + Cl_{int\,n} = Cl_{int\,tot}, \text{ where}$$

1, 2, 3, ..., *n* represent the different metabolic pathways. The assumptions needed for scaling to the clearance of the whole organism are the amount of microsomal protein per gram of liver wet weight, the wet weight of the whole liver of the organism, the liver blood flow and the weight of the organism. Information of distribution volume is also needed. If some organ other than the liver, such as the kidneys or the intestine, will participate significantly in the elimination of the studied compound, their Cl_{organ} has to be taken into account when scaling to the clearance of the whole organism.

Apparent K_i and type of inhibition

It is important to determine the apparent inhibition constant K_i for a compound that inhibits the metabolism of an NCE, for it is used in *in vivo* interaction predictions (Ito *et al.*, 1998a). The use of initial velocity conditions in this series of assays is extremely important because conditions that do not fulfill the linear velocity demand would lead to an underestimation of the inhibitory potency of an NCE (Yuan *et al.*, 1999).

The determination of the apparent K_i value is done either by fitting lines by linear regression analysis into the Dixon plot or any secondary plot, or by an iterative nonlinear curve fitting and calculations based on the known Michaelis–Menten kinetics for the type of inhibition (Boobis, 1995).

Prediction of drug–drug interactions

Drug–drug interactions that may alter pharmacokinetics could occur at several sites, including gastrointestinal absorption, plasma and/or tissue protein binding, transporter proteins and metabolism (Ito *et al.*, 1998b). The prediction of hepatic clearance is an important prerequisite for the prediction of drug–drug interactions, and the accuracy of the prediction method is dependent on the accuracy of the clearance prediction. The interaction prediction is complicated if there are multiple CYPs participating in the biotransformation of the NCE. In that case, the relative contribution of each enzyme has to be taken into account (Obach *et al.*, 1997).

Also, the type of inhibition (competitive, noncompetitive or uncompetitive) of the NCE is a valuable item of information. Independently of the inhibition type–except in the case of uncompetitive inhibition–when the substrate concentration is much lower than K_m, the degree of inhibition (R) is expressed as follows:

$$R = \frac{v(\text{with inhibitor})}{v(\text{without inhibitor})} = \frac{1}{1 + [I]/K_i}$$

This is usually the case in therapeutic use (Ito *et al.*, 1998b).

The determination of the inhibitor concentration *in vivo* is very difficult (or impossible), and the unbound concentration of an inhibitor is therefore usually utilized when calculating the degree of inhibition. However, as discussed above, the total concentration may be more appropriate to use in these calculations (Obach *et al.*, 1997). The interindividual variation should also be considered, though it is problematic to take into account when extrapolating *in vivo* from *in vitro* studies (Ito *et al.*, 1998a, 1998b).

When the inhibition of a CYP enzyme causes interactions, it has to be examined both from the point of view how the NCE affects other drugs administered simultaneously and how the other drugs affect the metabolism or therapeutic effect of the NCE. Clinically, if the half-lives of simultaneously administered drugs were equal or nearly equal, it would be possible to schedule the dosing regimens in such a way that the drugs do not interfere with each other's effects (Obach *et al.*, 1997). If an NCE inhibits the activity of some CYP enzymes, the *in vivo* concentrations of the drugs metabolized by these CYPs might increase dangerously. This was the case with mibefradil, which is a potent inhibitor of both the drug-transporting P-glycoprotein and CYP3A *in vitro* (Siepmann *et al.*, 1995; Krahenbuhl *et al.*, 1998; Mullins *et al.*, 1998; Spoendlin *et al.*, 1998; Prueksaritanont *et al.*, 1999; Wandel *et al.*, 2000). When the CYP enzymes catalyzing the oxidative reactions of an NCE are identified, there would already exist some candidates for inhibiting the reactions. For example, if an NCE is metabolized predominantly by CYP3A4, it is most probable that classical CYP3A4 inhibitors such as azole antimycotics (e.g. Varhe *et al.*, 1994; von Moltke *et al.*, 1996) or grapefruit juice (e.g. Proppe *et al.*, 1995; Armeer and Weintraub, 1997; Kivistö *et al.*, 1999) could cause an elevation in the *in vivo* concentrations of the NCE.

CONCLUSIONS

Pharmaceutical research is an extremely complicated endeavor that encompasses several diverse disciplines, which are united by the common goal of discovering and developing new, safe and effective therapeutics. Drug metabolism and pharmacokinetics is an important determinant of the action of a compound *in vivo*, and therefore plays a significant role in modern drug discovery. New tools and approaches have been developed, including *in vitro* HTS, rapid bioanalytical methodologies and *in silico* methodologies to predict passive absorption and metabolic clearance, and to minimize drug–drug interaction potential. Understanding of the way in which physicochemical properties determine DMPK (particularly drug absorption, clearance, protein binding and distribution) is increasing. However, some fundamental processes remain to be fully elucidated, including the *in vivo* impact of nonspecific binding in *in vitro* screens, and the functional significance of intestinal and hepatobiliary transporter proteins. The use of transgenic animals is beginning to contribute to an understanding of the contribution of transporter proteins to drug bioavailability (intestinal and hepatic drug uptake/efflux) and drug interactions, and to play a role in validating projections for humans. Future studies are likely to focus on the evaluation of the various *in vitro* human CYP induction screens available, with particular emphasis on their predictive value regarding what will happen when the compounds are administered to humans. The science of DMPK has evolved in response to changes in drug discovery to the point where it now makes a much greater contribution to lead selection and optimization than it did in the past. This trend is likely to continue as DMPK further increases the efficiency and effectiveness of the discovery and development of new medicines.

REFERENCES

Alavijeh, M.S., Palmer, A.M. (2004). The pivotal role of drug metabolism and pharmacokinetics in the discovery and development of new medicines. *IDrugs* **7(8)**:755–763.

Benet, L.Z., Cummins, C.L., Wu, C.Y. (2003). Transporter–enzyme interactions: Implications for predicting drug–drug interactions from *in vitro* data. *Current Drug Metabolism* **4(5)**:393–398.

Blakey, G.E., Lockton, J.A., Perrett, J., Norwood, P., Russell, M., Aherne, Z., Plume, J. (2004). Pharmacokinetic and pharmacodynamic assessment of a five-probe metabolic cocktail for CYPs 1A2, 3A4, 2C9, 2D6 and 2E1. *British Journal of Clinical Pharmacology* **57(2)**:162–169.

Eddershaw, P.J., Beresford, A.P., Bayliss, M.K. (2000). ADME/PK as part of a rational approach to drug discovery. *Drug Discovery Today* **5(9)**:409–414.

Houston, J.B., *et al.* (1997). Prediction of hepatic clearance from microsomes, hepatocytes and liver slices. *Drug Metabolism Reviews* **29**:891.

Jones, H., Housto, J.B. (2004). Use of the substrate depletion approach for determining *in vitro* metabolic clearance: Time dependencies in hepatocyte and microsomal incubations. *Drug Metabolism and Disposition*.

Lin, J., Sahakian, D.C., de Morais, S.M., Xu, J.J., Polzer, R.J., Winter, S.M. (2003). The role of absorption, distribution, metabolism, excretion and toxicity in drug discovery. *Current Topics in Medicinal Chemistry* **3(10)**:1125–1154.

Obach, R.S. (1999). Prediction of human clearance of twenty-nine drugs from hepatic microsomal intrinsic clearance data: An examination of *in vitro* half-life approach and nonspecific binding to microsomes. *Drug Metabolism and Disposition* **27(11)**:1350–1359.

Philpot, R.M. (1991). Characterization of cytochrome P450 in extrahepatic tissues. *Methods in Enzymology* **206**:623–631.

Riley, R.J., Martin, I.J., Cooper, A.E. (2002). The influence of DMPK as an integrated partner in modern drug discovery. *Current Drug Metabolism* **3(5)**:527–550.

Roberts, S.A. (2003). Drug metabolism and pharmacokinetics in drug discovery. *Current Opinion in Drug Discovery and Development* **6(1)**:66–80.

Selick, H.E., Beresford, A.P., Tarbit, M.H. (2002). The emerging importance of predictive ADME simulation in drug discovery. *Drug Discovery Today* **7(2)**:109–116.

USFDA (2006). Draft Guidance for Industry: Drug Interaction Studies—Study Design, Data Analysis, and Implications for Dosing and Labeling. US Food and Drug Administration.

Wheeler, C.W., Guenthner, T.M. (1990). Spectroscopic quantitation of cytochrome P-450 in human lung microsomes. *Journal of Biochemical Toxicology* **5(4)**:269–272.

Yan, Z., Caldwell, G.W. Evaluation of cytochrome P450 inhibition in human liver microsomes. In: *Optimization in Drug Discovery: In Vitro Methods*.

5

Drug Targets in *Mycobacterium Tuberculosis*

Vanaja Kumar[x]

Tuberculosis Research Centre, Chennai, India

INTRODUCTION

Five decades of tuberculosis (TB) control program using potentially efficacious drugs and the availability of bacillus Calmette-Guérin (BCG) vaccine have failed to reduce the prevalence of tuberculosis infection in most parts of the world. It has been reported that more than 3 billion people have been vaccinated with BCG, but still TB kills more than 50,000 people every week and approximately one-third of the world population is asymptomatically infected by *Mycobacterium tuberculosis* (Dye *et al*., 2002).

Current chemotherapy for TB relies on drugs that inhibit bacterial metabolism (Zhang, 2005). According to their mode of action, TB drugs can be grouped as cell wall inhibitors (isoniazid [INH], ethambutol, ethionamide, cycloserine), nucleic acid synthesis inhibitors (rifampicin [RIF], quinolones), protein synthesis inhibitor (streptomycin, kanamycin) and inhibitors of membrane energy metabolism (pyrazinamide, PZA).

The existing TB drugs are therefore only able to target actively growing bacteria and not the slow-growing bacteria or slowly metabolizing bacteria that persist after the growing bacteria have been killed by bactericidal drugs (Mitchison *et al*., 1980). Sterilizing activity describes the ability to eliminate latent or "dormant" bacteria that survive inside the host macrophages. Although RIF and PZA are partially sterilizing drugs and play an important role in shortening the therapy from 12–18 months to 6 months, persistent bacilli are not eradicated completely by currently available

---

[x] *vanaja_kumar@hotmail.com*

drugs (Chopra *et al.*, 2003). Thus, although achieving a clinical cure, the current TB chemotherapy does not achieve a bacteriological cure since the therapy cannot completely eradicate all bacilli in the lesions (McCune and Tompsett, 1956).

Drug Resistance as a Major Problem

Drug resistance in tuberculosis is a matter of great concern for TB control program since there is no cure for some resistant strains of *M. tuberculosis*. New drugs for treatment, new diagnostic methods and an effective vaccine are the need of the hour for the reason that these strains could spread around the world killing thousands of people.

Even after shortening DOTS (Directly Observed Treatment, Short-Course) to 6 months, an important practical issue in the treatment is patient compliance. Treatment for 6 months is still a lengthy drug administration period and noncompliance most often contributes to the development of multidrug-resistant (MDR-TB) strains. Alternative second-line drugs then come into use, but multidrug-resistant strains that also exhibit resistance to these second-line drugs (XDR-TB) are now on the rise.

MDR-TB, defined as resistance to at least RIF and INH, is a compounding factor for the control of the disease, since patients harboring MDR strains of *M. tuberculosis* need to be put on alternative treatment regimens involving second-line drugs that are more costly, more toxic and less effective. Whereas, extensively drug resistant (XDR) strains are defined as having resistance to INH and RIF in addition to three of the six main classes of second-line drugs, viz. aminoglycosides, polypeptides, fluoroquinolones, ethionamide, cycloserine and paraaminosalicylic acid (Centers for Disease Control and Prevention, 2006).

XDR-TB constitutes an emerging threat for the control of the disease and the further spread of drug resistance, especially in HIV-infected patients (Gandhi *et al.*, 2006). As a result, rapid detection of drug resistance to both first- and second-line antituberculous drugs has become a key component of the TB control program.

Existing Drug Targets and the Need for New Ones

Most of the currently used antituberculous drugs were developed in the 1950s and arose from microbiological screens of libraries of natural or chemical compounds, or as a result of serendipitous leads (Cole, 2002). The existing drugs that are targeting cellular process and their molecular target have been enumerated (McKinney, 2000).

Although the existing drugs have an immense value in controlling TB, the emergence of drug-resistant strains and the inability of the existing drugs to act against the latent forms of the bacilli have led to further challenges for the antitubercular drug discovery.

Impact of Complete Genome Sequence of *Mycobacterium Tuberculosis*

Sequencing the whole genome of *M. tuberculosis* is one of the major events that happened in the history of tuberculosis and has revolutionized the tuberculosis research. The genome sequence of

M. tuberculosis has provided new dimensions to tuberculosis researchers around the world. Finding a new drug against tuberculosis is largely dependent on our ability to amalgamate post-genomic information with the newly developed fields of transcriptomics and proteomics.

The availability of the mycobacterial genome sequence has set up a platform to answer the questions that remained unanswered over the years. Though genome sequencing definitely reveals more than 'the tip of an iceberg', it still needs to be supplemented with additional information such as gene function, regulation and interactions. A combination of all of this knowledge holds promise for the development of new intervention regimens against TB (Chakhaiyar and Hasnain, 2004).

With the emergence of bioinformatics and on account of using genomics and proteomics technologies that are highly heterogeneous in nature, a massive amount of data is generated and stored in different databases. The future goal of bioinformatics is to integrate these databases together into a single portal so as to generate knowledge from the available information to acquire a clear picture of the amazing pathogen *M. tuberculosis* and the disease it causes.

DRUG TARGET IDENTIFICATION

Tuberculosis compounded by the problem of drug resistance has triggered the search for newer drugs and hence new drug targets (Hasan *et al.*, 2006). Drug target identification involves acquiring a molecular-level understanding of a specific disease state and includes analysis of gene sequences, protein structures, protein–protein interactions and metabolic pathways (Augen, 2002; Smith, 2004). In the age of genomics, the process of drug target identification needs to incorporate and integrate different sources of data, including genetic, transcriptomic, proteomic and metabolomic data (Jiang and Zhou, 2005).

Genomics

Genomics is the study of entire set of genes in the genome and their functions. The availability of whole genome details of 857 bacteria has generated data that demand advanced technologies, thereby posing a major challenge to exploit the same. Further, this leads to identifying and characterizing new virulent factors and drug targets.

The complete genome sequence of *M. tuberculosis* has opened new vistas in diagnosis, epidemiology and vaccine development (Cole *et al.*, 1998). Automated DNA sequencing allows the direct comparison of specific genes among large populations of isolates. The determination of complete genomic sequence of strains using new technologies such as DNA microarrays and computational biology has provided a whole genome perspective on genomic content, gene regulation and metabolism.

The use of differential expression to monitor whole genome expression is now a powerful approach, which will result in the definition of differentially expressed genes important in pathogenesis. This will provide useful targets for the rational design of new drugs and vaccine candidates for *M. tuberculosis*. These studies are likely to confirm the reality of 'transcriptomics' as a technical deliverable for hypothesis-driven research into mycobacterial pathogenesis, vaccine and drug research (Ahmed and Hasnain, 2004).

Proteomics

Proteomics is defined as the study of the protein products of the genome, and their interactions and functions. Similarly, the proteins expressed at a given time in a given environment constitute a proteome (Dove, 1999). Target identification, one of the key steps in drug discovery process, relies on the timely knowledge of biological cause and effect in the course of disease, which ultimately rests on the knowledge of protein function and regulation (Burbaum and Tobal, 2002).

Identification of drug target has fostered through applied genomics because both high-throughput methods and tools that allow nucleic acid amplification have enabled large-scale profiling of expressed genes (Nuttall, 2001). However, analysis of the information produced by genomics, when measured against comparable information regarding protein expression, has led to the conclusion that message abundance fails to correlate with protein quantity (Pandey and Mann, 2000). As a result, the development of drug discovery technologies has begun to shift from genomics to proteomics. This shift has occurred not only in target discovery but also in many other areas of the process including patient treatment and care (Simpson and Dorow, 2001).

Recent technological advances in separation and identification (mass spectrometry [MS], protein chip technologies and phage display), bioinformatics and technologies that detect protein interactions and activities (activity-based assays and two-hybrid assays) have a vital role to play in all the areas of drug discovery, from target identification to assessment of drug efficacy both in preclinical (target selectivity) and clinical situations (patient response).

Bioinformatics

Bioinformatics plays a key role in the exploitation of genomic, transcriptomic and proteomic data to gain insights into the molecular mechanisms that underlie disease and to search for targets that will lead to new drugs (Searls, 2000; Dahl *et al.*, 2002; Whittaker, 2003).

With the use of bioinformatics tools, the genome of *M. tuberculosis* can be searched for identifying new genes belonging to an existing class of drug targets. One essential requirement for a drug target is to understand its function. Accurate function prediction of gene products using computational tools has become an important issue in the field of bioinformatics (Hennig *et al.*, 2003; Gabaldon and Huynen, 2004). By searching similar protein sequences with known function annotations, one can draw some inferences about the function of the uncharacterized gene. More sophisticated methods of incorporating sequence information such as sorting signals, posttranslational modifications and domains to predict protein function have also been developed (Jiang and Zhou, 2005).

Three-dimensional structures of proteins being highly correlated with their functions help in elucidating their functions. The TB Structural Genomics Consortium (TBsgc) consists of 415 active members and is involved in the determination and analysis of three-dimensional structures of proteins on the genome scale. The goals of the consortium are to discover new folds providing representative structures for all protein families, to discover function from structure and to characterize new drug targets. The structural and functional information present in the TBsgc database will form a basis for understanding *M. tuberculosis* pathogenesis and for structure-based drug design.

Cui *et al.* (2009) have analyzed the protein–protein interaction (PPI) map of *M. tuberculosis* and unraveled the function of hypothetical protein as well as a potential signaling pathway. The PPI network developed in this study, coupled with the findings of potential signal proteins, provides a basis for understanding the potential virulence and infection mechanisms of *M. tuberculosis*.

Raman *et al.* (2008) reported a comprehensive *in silico* target identification pipeline, targetTB, for *M. tuberculosis*. The pipeline incorporates a network analysis of the protein–protein interactome, a flux balance analysis of the reactome, experimentally derived phenotype essentiality data, sequence analyses and a structural assessment of targetability, using novel algorithms. Flux balance and network analysis are used to identify proteins critical for survival of *M. tuberculosis*, followed by comparative genomics with the host, finally incorporating a novel structural analysis of the binding sites to assess the feasibility of a protein as a target. Further analyses include correlation with expression data and non-similarity to gut flora proteins as well as 'anti-targets' in the host, leading to the identification of 451 high-confidence targets. These targets are further explored to identify broad-spectrum antibiotic targets and specific *M. tuberculosis* targets using phylogenetic profiling against 228 pathogen genomes.

Phage-Based Discovery

Over the evolutionary period, phages have mastered the art of killing their host bacteria. Phages arrest critical cellular processes and redirect the host cell for phage reproduction. Phage-mediated bacterial inhibition is exploited for drug target discovery. Phages produce proteins that inhibit host cell machinery. The targets of these phage proteins can act as ideal drug targets. These targets have been evolutionarily and biologically validated. Diversified targets can be identified by this method. Mimicking the growth inhibitory effect of phage protein by a chemical compound offers better solution for drug discovery.

Phage ORFs inhibitory to bacteria are identified and used as baits to identify target proteins in host bacteria. The targets are then validated. Several targets have been identified and validated in *Staphylococcus* using this novel phage-based method (Liu *et al.*, 2004). ORF104 of *Staphylococcus* phage 77 inhibits DNA synthesis. The target was identified as Dna I, helicase loader of *Staphylococcus aureus*. The targets of several other ORFs of *Staphylococcus* phages have also been identified. ORF16 inhibits Dna I (helicase loader), ORF25, ORF168 and ORF240 inhibit Dna N (DNA pol III ß subunit), ORF78 inhibits Dna G (DNA primase), ORF140 inhibits PT R14 and ORF67 inhibits RNA synthesis (Brown *et al.*, 2004).

Small phages such as enterobacteria phage Qß and φx174 have different lytic mechanisms. Single-gene lytic systems are attractive for drug target discovery as they inhibit the cell wall biosynthesis. A2 protein of a phage inhibits the mur A enzyme of cell wall biosynthesis (Bernhardt *et al.*, 2001). Further the single gene is resolved into small peptides. The structures of both target and phage proteins are deciphered to design a new antibiotic. Phage proteins that target different steps in cell wall synthesis may lead to the identification of more targets. Initiatives in this approach with mycobacteriophages hold promises for detection of novel drug targets in *M. tuberculosis*.

NOVEL TARGETS

Existing antibiotics act only on a few targets. Several new targets have been identified and studied. Genes involved in persistence, cell wall synthesis, metabolism, and so on, are essential for survival and virulence and are identified as drug targets. Some of them are validated *in vitro* and *in vivo* as potential targets.

Persistence Targets

Persistence is the hallmark of the disease and around one-third of the world's population is latently infected with TB. Eradication of TB is difficult because of the persistence of *M. tuberculosis* for several decades and recurrence of infection.

M. tuberculosis DNA-equivalent to 10^5 organisms per organ has been measured in treated mice, which were negative for culture. This shows that a small percentage of bacteria persist even after chemotherapy. This is known as the physiological resistance to drugs.

The current regimens are ineffective against persistent populations as they act on a growing population of bacteria. Hence, a long duration of treatment is required, leading to patient noncompliance and development of drug resistance. Drugs targeting persistent bacteria are the need of the hour to eradicate TB. Understanding the metabolic pathways contributing to persistence and resuscitation will aid in identifying potential targets (Murphy and Brown, 2008).

In vitro dormant models have been designed. Certain genes expressed in these *in vitro* dormant models and in *in vivo* animal infection serve as good targets. They are listed below.

Isocitrate Lyase

Metabolism of bacteria grown *in vitro* is different from the natural population of bacteria existing *in vivo* in lungs (Bloch and Segal, 1956). It has been proved that mycobacteria exhibit preference to lipids *in vivo*. Thus fatty acids are a source of carbon and energy during chronic infection.

Glyoxylate cycle is an important lipid metabolic pathway and is absent in humans. Isocitrate lyase (ICL) is an enzyme of glyoxylate cycle that is involved in the utilization of host-derived lipids. ICL is upregulated during infection of macrophages, induced in stationary phase and hypoxic cultures. It is also required for survival in lung during persistent infection in mouse (McKinney *et al*., 2000). It is a validated persistence target.

Rv3133c/DosR

Rv3133c/DosR is a transcription factor, induced by hypoxia. All genes upregulated by hypoxia need Rv3133c/DosR for induction. Rv3133c/DosR is a transcription factor of the two-component response regulator class (Park *et al*., 2003). DosR is required for long-term survival of *Mycobacterium bovis*. This has been explored as a drug target.

Cyclopropane synthetase

Cyclopropane synthetase is required for cording, persistence and virulence. Cyclopropane rings are modifications of membrane lipids that are present in various bacteria. Gene pcaA codes for cyclopropane synthetase and is required for the synthesis of proximal cyclopropane ring of alpha mycolates. The transposon mutant of pcaA replicates *in vivo* but does not persist. They can act as good targets as they are absent in humans. Drugs against these targets may shorten chemotherapy (Glickman *et al.*, 2000).

RelMtb

Persistence of mycobacteria is associated with the shutdown of active metabolism by a broad transcriptional program called the stringent response. RelMtb initiates the stringent response. Deletion of RelMtb affects the long-term viability. The mutant strain is unable to produce chronic infection. It is a potential target for treating latent infection (Dahl *et al.*, 2003).

Targeting Cell Wall Biosynthesis

Mycobacterial cell envelope is a complex structure comprising of mycolic acid, peptidoglycan, arabinogalactan and non-covalently associated collection of polar lipids. This unique structure specific to mycobacteria and related species contribute to both the survival and drug resistance. Thus, the cell wall biosynthesis pathway acts as a good target, as there is no homology in humans. Many of the currently available drugs target cell wall biosynthesis. Several other new potent targets are also present in cell wall.

Peptidoglycan Biosynthesis

Alanine racemase and D-Ala-D-Ala ligases of peptidoglycan synthesis are validated targets. Inactivation of alanine racemase is found to affect the survival of mycobacteria and is inhibited by D-cycloserine.

Arabinogalactan Biosynthesis

Arabinan not only plays a structural role but is also found to be important in sensing mechanisms. EmbA and EmbB are involved in the formation of the terminal hexa-arabinofuranoside portion of arabinogalactan. Ethambutol, one of the first line drugs, inhibits the Emb proteins. This target has been validated by knockout experiments *in vitro* (Wolucka, 2008).

AftA, arabinofuranosyl transferase, catalyzes the addition of the arabinofuranosyl residue to the galactan core. It is essential for cell viability, and disruption of this enzyme is lethal to *M. tuberculosis* (Sassetti *et al.*, 2003; Wolucka, 2008). The essentiality of the gene makes it an attractive target.

Phosphoribosyltransferase, UDP-galactopyranose mutase, galactofuranosyl transferase and dTDP-6-deoxy-L-lyxo-4-hexulose reductase are other enzymes involved in arabinogalactan synthesis. They were found to be essential for survival *in vitro* (Mdluli and Spigelman, 2006). These enzymes are also being explored as drug targets.

Targeting Fatty Acid Synthesis

The FAS II pathway of fatty acid synthesis is unique to bacteria and is absent in humans. Thus, it is an attractive drug target pathway.

Inh A

Inh A is the target of a first-line drug, INH. The elongation step of FAS II pathway is catalyzed by inh A (Banerjee *et al.*, 1994). Crystal structure is available for inh A, FabH, and MabA and they serve as potent targets. Mab A participates in the synthesis of long-chain fatty acids. Mab A of mycobacteria is distinct from other bacteria, making it an attractive target.

Methyltransferases mmA4 participate in the modification of meromycolates and they are an attractive target. The inhibitor of its cofactor, *S*-methyl adenosine, inhibits *M. tuberculosis* (Mdluli and Spigelman, 2006).

pKS3 catalyzes the condensation step in mycolic acid synthesis. Acyl-AMP ligase, FadD32 and AccD4-containing acyl-coenzyme A (CoA) carboxylase are also found to be essential for growth. Deletion of genes in *in vitro* cultures affects the viability.

Mycocerosic pathway is found in the cell wall of pathogenic bacteria. Enzymes in this pathway are essential for growth and are identified as potent drug targets. The acyl coA transferase involved in methyl malonyl coA synthesis is also identified as a potential drug target.

Targets of Amino Acid Biosynthesis

It is an important pathway rich in potent targets. Any drug developed against this pathway is lethal as the organism cannot utilize amino acids from the host. LysA, LeuD, TrpD, Proc, LeuA and dihydropicolinate reductase are validated by the knockout method. Mutant is attenuated in the mouse model.

Arginine Biosynthesis

Biosynthesis of arginine is essential. ArgF mutant is not viable *in vitro* and is found to be attenuated in mouse. These findings denote that *M. tuberculosis* is unable to obtain arginine from the host, qualifying it as a potent target.

Shikimate Pathway

The absence of this pathway in mammals makes it an attractive option as a potent drug target. This pathway is highly essential for *M. tuberculosis*. The enzymes AroA, -B, -C, -E, -G, -K and -Q associated with this pathway have been validated *in vitro*. The product of the pathway is chorismate and is intermediate in the synthesis of aromatic amino acids, folic acid and quinones (Ducati *et al.*, 2007).

Synthesis of Branched-Chain Amino Acid

Acetohydroxy acid synthase catalyzes the synthesis of branched-chain amino acids. It is an important target for antimycobacterial agents. Several inhibitors are available with activity against *M. tuberculosis* (Le *et al.*, 2007). Inhibitors have also been designed by structural modeling.

Peptide Deformylase

Peptide deformylase (PDF) catalyzes an important step in protein synthesis. It removes the N-terminal formyl group from nascent proteins, making it an ideal target for antibacterial drug development. By transposon site hybridization it is found to be essential for growth of *M. tuberculosis*. Deletion of gene is lethal to *M. bovis*. Inhibitors have been designed for PDF and are found to be potent antimycobacterial agents (Teo *et al.*, 2006).

Cofactor Biosynthesis

Biotin Biosynthesis

Diaminopelargonic acid aminotransferase (DAPA AT) is an enzyme of biotin biosynthetic pathway. This enzyme catalyzes the transamination of 8-amino-7-oxononanoic acid. It is involved in the long-term survival of *M. tuberculosis* and is a potential therapeutic target. Amiclenomycin from actinomycetes is found to irreversibly inhibit *M. tuberculosis* and the target was found to be DAPA AT (Mann and Ploux, 2006).

DNA Synthesis

NAD-Dependent DNA Ligase

NAD is an essential cofactor, which is required for redox balance and energy metabolism as well as for the activity of the NAD-dependent DNA ligase in prokaryotes. NAD-dependent DNA ligase catalyzes the joining of nicks between bases in double-stranded DNA. NAD-dependent DNA ligases are validated novel targets not present in humans. Inhibitors are designed that affect only the NAD-dependent ligase but not the ATP-dependent ligase present in humans. The domain in *M. tuberculosis* ligase (MtuLigA) is characterized and potent inhibitors have been studied *in vivo*. Inhibitors specific for each bacteria may be designed in future (Srivastava *et al.*, 2007).

DNA Gyrase

Fluoroquinolones inhibit DNA gyrase. DNA gyrase catalyzes negative supercoiling of DNA. Double-stranded nicks are created by the enzyme. DNA gyrase is required for various processes such as DNA replication, transcription and recombination. Newer fluoroquinolones exhibit high inhibitory activity against active and nonreplicating *M. tuberculosis* (Mdluli and Spigelman, 2006).

NadD and NadE

Recycling of exogenously acquired nicotinamide is an important and functional pathway in *M. tuberculosis*; however, the organism shows considerable flexibility in switching between recycling and *de novo* synthesis of NAD, suggesting that interrupting one of them alone would be non-lethal. Obviously, the two common enzymes shared by both pathways, viz. *nadD* and *nadE*, are the viable drug targets.

Others

NADH Menaquinone Oxidoreductase

NADH menaquinone oxidoreductase is an enzyme of respiratory chain. Several inhibitors such as phenothiazines show potent activity.

Cytochromes P450

The genome sequence of *M. tuberculosis* has revealed a number of cytochrome P450 enzymes, suggesting fundamental physiological roles for these enzymes. Several azole drugs, known inhibitors of cytochromes P450, have been shown to have potent antimycobacterial activity, and the most effective azoles have extremely tight binding constants for one of the Mtb P450s (CYP121). The structure of CYP121 has been determined at atomic resolution, revealing novel features of P450 structure. The structure provides a platform for design of inhibitor molecules as novel antitubercular agents (Munro *et al.*, 2003).

ATP Synthase

ATP synthase is a membrane-bound enzyme that catalyzes the formation of ATP. Though ATP synthase is present in humans, sequence similarity is very less (Cole and Alzari, 2005). Diaryquinolone inhibits ATP synthase, leading to ATP depletion and thus affecting viability (Andries *et al.*, 2005). ATP synthase is found to be essential in *M. tuberculosis* by transposon site mutagenesis. Diaryquinolone can shorten the duration of therapy. It has synergistic activity with PZA and the combination of PZA and diaryquinolone is found to have a high sterilizing effect.

Glutamine Synthetase (Gln A1)

Glutamine synthetase is an important enzyme of nitrogen metabolism. It is found to be essential for growth *in vivo*. It is essential for virulence (Tullius *et al.*, 2003) and is exploited as a drug target.

ideR, Regulatory Protein

ideR, regulatory protein is a metal-dependent regulator and is found to be an essential gene in *M. tuberculosis*. IdeR is required for iron-dependent siderophore production and oxidative stress response (Rodriguez *et al.*, 2002).

Deoxy-D-xylulose-5-phosphate Reductoisomerase

Deoxy-D-xylulose-5-phosphate reductoisomerase (DXR) is a potential target for antitubercular chemotherapy and is absent in mammals. C-methyl-D-erythritol-4-phosphate (MEP) pathway is essential for isoprenoid biosynthesis. This is essential for growth and survival. DXR is an important enzyme of this pathway. It catalyzes the conversion of deoxy-D-xylulose-5-phosphate to methyl-D-erythritol-4-phosphate. Structural model and inhibitors against DXR can be designed (Singh *et al.*, 2007).

Toxin Antitoxin Modules

M. tuberculosis has 38 toxin–antitoxin (TA) modules that are potent targets. Drugs that activate toxin production or inactivate antitoxin expression can be designed. Several *relBE* and nine mazEF loci are found in *M. tuberculosis* (Zhang, 2005).

Virulence Factors

Drugs targeting virulence factors are noted as a paradigm shift in antimicrobial drug discovery. These antiinfectives are not alternative to antibiotics but they can also be used as one more weapon against deadly mycobacteria. Erp mutant grows well in *in vitro* culture but not in mice. Though its function is unknown it serves as a potent target (Berthet *et al.*, 1998). Granuloma-specific genes coding PE/PE-PGRS family of proteins are also found to be important in virulence. They can serve as potent targets. Phthiocerol dimycocerosate (PDIM) is a virulence factor. Mutant growth is impaired only *in vivo* but not *in vitro* and it acts as a potent target. Phenolic glycolipids (PGLs) are small molecular virulence factors. FaD22 is an essential enzyme in PGL biosynthesis and is found to be a drug target. Conventional drug screening will not identify these targets, as they are expressed only *in vivo*.

PRIORITIZING DRUG TARGETS

With the enormous number of drug targets available, it is now important to prioritize the drug target. It is now feasible to have a computational approach to rank and prioritize the targets based on various factors such as metabolic choke points, essentiality of gene and persistence (Hasan *et al.*, 2006). Automated tools have been developed to identify essential genes (Singh and Ghosh, 2006).

CONCLUSION

The availability of the complete genome sequence of *M. tuberculosis* has revolutionized and facilitated a more rational approach for new drug targets and drug discovery. Knowledge regarding essentiality of gene *in vivo* and *in vitro*, functional characterization, high-throughput crystallographic studies and structural elucidation of proteins leading to structure-based drug designing will aid in the discovery of potent drugs against the most potent targets. This will pave a way for the discovery of drugs that are effective against persisters and MDR TB strains, making eradication of tuberculosis a dream come true.

ACKNOWLEDGMENTS

The author acknowledges the help of Suganya Selvaraj, Sameer Hassan and Balaji Subramanyam in the preparation of this chapter.

REFERENCES

Ahmed, N., Hasnain, S.E. (2004). Genomics of *Mycobacterium tuberculosis*: Old threats & new trends. *Indian Journal of Medical Research* **120(4)**:207–212.

Andries, K., Verhasselt, P., Guillemont, J., Gohlmann, H.W., Neefs, J.M., Winkler, H., *et al.* (2005). A diarylquinoline drug active on the ATP synthase of *Mycobacterium tuberculosis*. *Science* **307(5707)**:223–227.

Augen, J. (2002). The evolving role of information technology in the drug discovery process. *Drug Discovery Today* **7(5)**:315–323.

Banerjee, A., Dubnau, E., Quemard, A., Balasubramanian, V., Um, K.S., Wilson, T., *et al.* (1994). inhA, a gene encoding a target for isoniazid and ethionamide in *Mycobacterium tuberculosis*. *Science* **263(5144)**:227–230.

Bernhardt, T.G., Wang, I.N., Struck, D.K., Young, R. (2001). A protein antibiotic in the phage Qbeta virion: Diversity in lysis targets. *Science* **292(5525)**:2326–2329.

Berthet, F.X., Lagranderie, M., Gounon, P., Laurent-Winter, C., Ensergueix, D., Chavarot, P., *et al.* (1998). Attenuation of virulence by disruption of the *Mycobacterium tuberculosis* erp gene. *Science* **282(5389)**:759–762.

Bloch, H., Segal, W. (1956). Biochemical differentiation of *Mycobacterium tuberculosis* grown *in vivo* and *in vitro*. *Journal of Bacteriology* **72(2)**:132–141.

Brown, E.D. (2004). Drugs against superbugs: Private lessons from bacteriophages. *Trends in Biotechnology* **22(9)**:434–436.

Burbaum, J., Tobal, G.M. (2002). Proteomics in drug discovery. *Current Opinion in Chemical Biology* **6(4)**:427–433.

Centers for Disease Control and Prevention. (2006). Emergence of *Mycobacterium tuberculosis* with extensive resistance to second-line drugs—Worldwide, 2000–2004. *MMWR* **55(11)**:301–305.

Chakhaiyar, P., Hasnain, S.E. (2004). Defining the mandate of tuberculosis research in a postgenomic era. *Medical Principles and Practice* **13(4)**:177–184.

Chopra, P., Meena, L.S., Singh, Y. (2003). New drug targets for *Mycobacterium tuberculosis*. *Indian Journal of Medical Research* **117**:1–9.

Cole, S.T., Alzari, P.M. (2005). Microbiology. TB—A new target, a new drug. *Science* **307(5707)**:214–215.

Cole, S.T., Brosch, R., Parkhill, J., Garnier, T., Churcher, C., Harris, D., *et al.* (1998). Deciphering the biology of *Mycobacterium tuberculosis* from the complete genome sequence. *Nature* **393(6685)**:537–544.

Cui, T., Zhang, L., Wang, X., He, Z.G. (2009). Uncovering new signaling proteins and potential drug targets through the interactome analysis of *Mycobacterium tuberculosis*. *BMC Genomics* **10(1)**:118.

Dahl, J.L., Kraus, C.N., Boshoff, H.I., Doan, B., Foley, K., Avarbock, D., *et al.* (2003). The role of RelMtb-mediated adaptation to stationary phase in long-term persistence of *Mycobacterium tuberculosis* in mice. *Proceedings of the National Academy of Sciences USA* **100(17)**:10026–10031.

Dahl, S.G., Kristiansen, K., Sylte, I. (2002). Bioinformatics: From genome to drug targets. *Annals of Medicine* **34(4)**:306–312.

Dove, A. (1999). Proteomics: Translating genomics into products? *Nature Biotechnology* **17(3)**:233–236.

Ducati, R.G., Basso, L.A., Santos, D.S. (2007). Mycobacterial shikimate pathway enzymes as targets for drug design. *Current Drug Targets* **8(3)**:423–435.

Dye, C., Williams, B.G., Espinal, M.A., Raviglione, M.C. (2002). Erasing the world's slow stain: Strategies to beat multidrug-resistant tuberculosis. *Science* **295(5562)**:2042–2046.

Gabaldon, T., Huynen, M.A. (2004). Prediction of protein function and pathways in the genome era. *Cellular and Molecular Life Sciences* **61(7–8)**:930–944.

Gandhi, N.R., Moll, A., Sturm, A.W., Pawinski, R., Govender, T., Lalloo, U., *et al.* (2006). Extensively drug-resistant tuberculosis as a cause of death in patients co-infected with tuberculosis and HIV in a rural area of South Africa. *Lancet* **368(9547)**:1575–1580.

Glickman, M.S., Cox, J.S., Jacobs, W.R., Jr. (2000). A novel mycolic acid cyclopropane synthetase is required for cording, persistence, and virulence of *Mycobacterium tuberculosis*. *Molecular Cell* **5(4)**:717–727.

Hasan, S., Daugelat, S., Rao, P.S., Schreiber, M. (2006). Prioritizing genomic drug targets in pathogens: Application to *Mycobacterium tuberculosis*. *PLoS Computational Biology* **2(6)**:e61.

Hennig, S., Groth, D., Lehrach, H. (2003). Automated Gene Ontology annotation for anonymous sequence data. *Nucleic Acids Research* **31(13)**:3712–3715.

Jiang, Z., Zhou, Y. (2005). Using bioinformatics for drug target identification from the genome. *American Journal of Pharmacogenomics* **5(6)**:387–396.

Le, D.T., Lee, H., Chung, Y., Yoon, M., Choi, J. (2007). Virtual screening of tubercular acetohydroxy acid synthase inhibitors by structural analysis of its models. *Bulletin of the Korean Chemical Society* **28(6)**:947–952.

Liu, J., Dehbi, M., Moeck, G., Arhin, F., Bauda, P., Bergeron, D., *et al.* (2004). Antimicrobial drug discovery through bacteriophage genomics. *Nature Biotechnology* **22(2)**:185–191.

Mann, S., Ploux, O. (2006). 7,8-Diaminoperlargonic acid aminotransferase from *Mycobacterium tuberculosis*, a potential therapeutic target. Characterization and inhibition studies. *FEBS Journal* **273(20)**:4778–4789.

McKinney, J.D. (2000). *In vivo veritas*: The search for TB drug targets goes live. *Nature Medicine* **6**:1330–1333.

McKinney, J.D., Höner zu Bentrup, K., Muñoz-Elías, E.J., Miczak, A., Chen, B., Chan, W.T., *et al.* (2000). Persistence of *Mycobacterium tuberculosis* in macrophages and mice requires the glyoxylate shunt enzyme isocitrate lyase. *Nature* **406(6797)**:735–738.

Mdluli, K., Spigelman, M. (2006). Novel targets for tuberculosis drug discovery. *Current Opinion in Pharmacology* **6(5)**:459–467.

Mitchison, D.A. (1980). Treatment of tuberculosis. The Mitchell lecture 1979. *Journal of the Royal College of Physicians (London)* **14(2)**:91–95, 98–99.

Munro, A.W., McLean, K.J., Marshall, K.R., Warman, A.J., Lewis, G., Roitel, O., *et al.* (2003). Cytochromes P450: Novel drug targets in the war against multidrug-resistant *Mycobacterium tuberculosis*. *Biochemical Society Transactions* **31(Pt. 3)**:625–630.

Murphy, D.J., Brown, J.R. (2007). Identification of gene targets against dormant phase *Mycobacterium tuberculosis* infections. *BMC Infectious Diseases* **7**:84.

Murphy, D.J., Brown J.R. (2008). Novel drug target strategies against *Mycobacterium tuberculosis*. *Current Opinion in Microbiology* **11(5)**:422–427.

Nuttall, M.E. (2001). Drug discovery and target validation. *Cells Tissues Organs* **169(3)**:265–271.

Pandey, A., Mann, M. (2000). Proteomics to study genes and genomes. *Nature* **405(6788)**:837–846.

Park, H.D., Guinn, K.M., Harrell, M.I., Liao, R., Voskuil, M.I., Tompa, M., *et al.* (2003). Rv3133c/dosR is a transcription factor that mediates the hypoxic response of *Mycobacterium tuberculosis*. *Molecular Microbiology* **48(3)**:833–843.

Raman, K., Yeturu, K., Chandra, N. (2008). targetTB: A target identification pipeline for *Mycobacterium tuberculosis* through an interactome, reactome and genome-scale structural analysis. *BMC Systems Biology* **2**:109.

Rodriguez, G.M., Voskuil, M.I., Gold, B., Schoolnik, G.K., Smith, I. (2002). ideR, an essential gene in *Mycobacterium tuberculosis*: Role of IdeR in iron-dependent gene expression, iron metabolism, and oxidative stress response. *Infection and Immunity* **70(7)**:3371–3381.

Sassetti, C.M., Boyd, D.H., Rubin, E.J. (2003). Genes required for mycobacterial growth defined by high density mutagenesis. *Molecular Microbiology* **48(1)**:77–84.

Searls, D.B. (2000). Using bioinformatics in gene and drug discovery. *Drug Discovery Today* **5(4)**:135–143.

Simpson, R.J., Dorow, D.S. (2001). Cancer proteomics: From signaling networks to tumor markers. *Trends in Biotechnology* **19(10)**:S40–48.

Singh, N., Avery, M.A., McCurdy, C.R. (2007). Toward *Mycobacterium tuberculosis* DXR inhibitor design: Homology modeling and molecular dynamics simulations. *Journal of Computer-Aided Molecular Design* **21(9)**:511–522.

Singh, V.K., Ghosh, I. (2006). Kinetic modeling of tricarboxylic acid cycle and glyoxylate bypass in *Mycobacterium tuberculosis*, and its application to assessment of drug targets. *Theoretical Biology and Medical Modelling* **3**:27.

Smith, C. (2004). Drug target identification: A question of biology. *Nature* **428(6979)**:225–231.

Srivastava, S.K., Dube, D., Kukshal, V., Jha, A.K., Hajela, K., Ramachandran, R. (2007). NAD^+-dependent DNA ligase (Rv3014c) from *Mycobacterium tuberculosis*: Novel structure-function relationship and identification of a specific inhibitor. *Proteins* **69(1)**:97–111.

Teo, J.W., Thayalan, P., Beer, D., Yap, A.S., Nanjundappa, M., Ngew, X., *et al.* (2006). Peptide deformylase inhibitors as potent antimycobacterial agents. *Antimicrobial Agents and Chemotherapy* **50(11)**:3665–3673.

Tullius, M.V., Harth, G., Horwitz, M.A. (2003). Glutamine synthetase GlnA1 is essential for growth of *Mycobacterium tuberculosis* in human THP-1 macrophages and guinea pigs. *Infection and Immunity* **71(7)**:3927–3936.

Whittaker, P.A. (2003). What is the relevance of bioinformatics to pharmacology? *Trends in Pharmacological Sciences* **24(8)**:434–439.

Wolucka, B.A. (2008). Biosynthesis of D-arabinose in mycobacteria—A novel bacterial pathway with implications for antimycobacterial therapy. *FEBS Journal* **275(11)**:2691–2711.

Zhang, Y. (2005). The magic bullets and tuberculosis drug targets. *Annual Review of Pharmacology and Toxicology* **45**:529–564.

6
Anti-diabetic Drugs

Madhulika Dixit*

Department of Biotechnology, IIT Madras, Chennai, India

INTRODUCTION

The prevalence of diabetes and its associated risk factors are increasing at an alarming rate worldwide. The primary cause for the same appears to be a change in lifestyle on account of increased urbanization and fast-food culture. Up to 80% of deaths in patients with diabetes are caused due to the associated cardiovascular complications. By and large the anti-diabetic drugs belong to two major categories: oral hypoglycemic agents (OHAs) and insulin. The OHAs include insulin sensitizers such as metformin and thiazolidinediones and insulin secretagogues such as sulfonylureas. Insulin therapy, which is a must for type 1 diabetes and for type 2 diabetes with OHA failure, involves either short-acting or long-acting analogues. This chapter would provide an overview of the commonly used anti-diabetic drugs, their mode of action, pharmacokinetics and their beneficial and/or harmful side effects.

Diabetes is a progressive metabolic disorder characterized by disturbances in insulin action and glucose utilization. As a result, it is clinically defined by hyperglycemia in peripheral circulation. It is estimated that 1 in every 5 patients in the age group of 60–70 years suffers from diabetes and its associated complications (King *et al.*, 1998; Sicree *et al.*, 2003). The revised diagnostic criteria following from the WHO guidelines for diabetes are: fasting plasma glucose (FPG) $\geq$ 126 mg/dl, symptoms of diabetes along with random plasma glucose (RPG) $\geq$ 200mg/dl or a 2-h post 75 g glucose load $\geq$ 200 mg/dl in oral glucose tolerance test (OGTT). Clinically these observations are seen when more than 70% of the β-cells of islets of Langerhans have undergone functional aberration. Alternatively, it is also observed when the response of glucose-metabolizing tissues such as liver,

*mdixit@iitm.ac.in

skeletal muscles or adipose tissue to insulin are compromised, a state more commonly referred to as insulin resistance. Before we deal with types of anti-diabetic drugs available in the market, it is necessary to have an overview of how glucose metabolism is regulated in healthy individuals and what are the various types of diabetes.

MAINTENANCE OF BLOOD GLUCOSE

Upon intake and digestion of food, the released glucose is absorbed in the gastrointestinal (GI) tract, from where it is forwarded to the circulating blood. Through the circulatory system, this monosaccharide reaches peripheral and metabolic tissues to be utilized as the major energy source. Whenever there is an excess of glucose in circulation, the surplus is stored as glycogen in liver and skeletal muscles (via glycogenesis) and as fats in adipose tissue (lipogenesis). In contrast, under fasting states, glucose is obtained from its stored form though glycogenolysis (glycogen breakdown) and gluconeogenesis (synthesis of glucose from noncarbohydrate sources) in liver. Additionally, in adipose tissue, the stored fats undergo lipolysis to release energy. Hence, in a healthy individual, optimum levels of glucose in blood are achieved via feedback mechanisms between circulation and metabolic tissues. Two major counteracting hormones that are instrumental in bringing about this balance are insulin and glucagon.

Insulin Secretion and Action

Insulin is a 51-amino-acid-long polypeptide hormone consisting of two chains (A and B). It is secreted by the β-cells of islets of Langerhans in pancrease in response to increased blood glucose. Due to increased intracellular levels of ATP in these cells, there is closure of ATP-sensitive K^+ channels, thereby causing membrane depolarization, consequent Ca^{2+} influx and fusion of insulin-containing vesicles for insulin secretion (Tengholm and Gylfe, 2008). The classical insulin-responsive tissues are liver, skeletal muscle and fat. In the liver, insulin promotes conversion of glucose to glycogen while inhibiting gluconeogenesis. In skeletal muscle and adipose tissue, it promotes glucose uptake, glycogen synthesis and fat storage. It also prevents oxidation of fatty acids into ketone bodies in the adipose tissue. Hence, by and large, its role is to lower the blood glucose upon release from pancreas. Interestingly, secretion of insulin by pancreas is also promoted by some of the enteric hormones such as glucagon-like peptide-1 (GLP-1) and gastric inhibitory peptide, which are released in response to food intake (Gautier *et al.*, 2008).

Glucagon

Glucagon is a 29-amino-acid-long peptide hormone secreted by the α-cells of the islets of Langerhans of the endocrine pancreas in response to lower blood glucose. It essentially opposes the effects of insulin by enhancing glycogen breakdown and gluconeogenesis in liver. It also promotes the oxidation of fatty acids in adipose tissue to form ketone bodies as alternate energy source (especially in brain during fasting state) (Quesada *et al.*, 2008). For an overview of the maintenance of blood glucose by insulin and glucagons, please refer to Fig. 6.1.

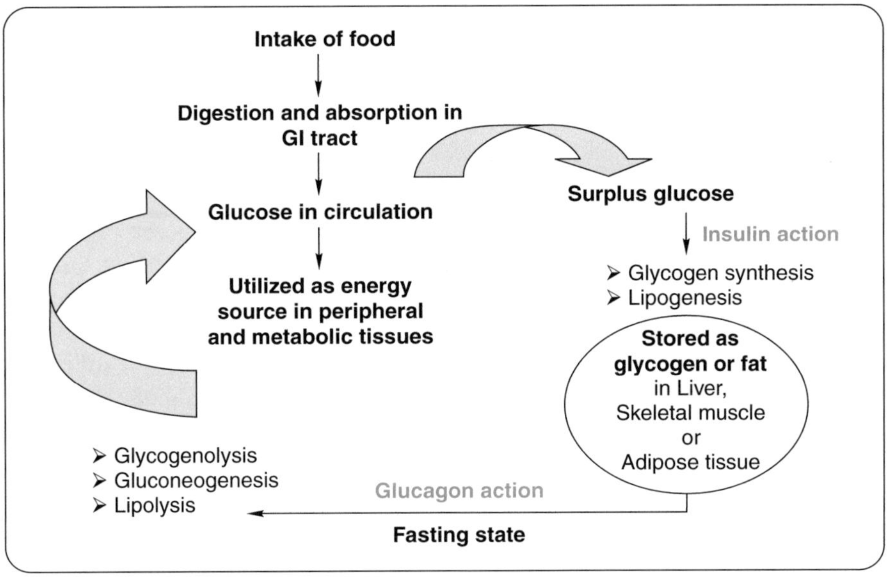

Fig. 6.1 *Schematic Representation of Maintenance of Blood Glucose Level*

TYPES OF DIABETES

Hyperglycemia observed in diabetes can result from one of the following reasons:

1. Decreased secretion of insulin by the β-cells.
2. Compromised response of metabolic tissues to insulin (insulin resistance).
3. Increase in counter-regulatory hormone glucagon, which opposes the insulin action.

Hence any approach toward designing drugs for diabetes treatment has to take into account the various pathways it wishes to target in order to have an ultimate beneficial response with regard to blood glucose regime. Additionally, based on the primary cause of diabetes, it is categorized into three main categories (Guillausseau *et al.*, 1997):

1. Type 1 diabetes: This refers to the autoimmune destruction of pancreatic β-cells causing insulin deficiency. These patients have an absolute requirement of insulin injections.
2. Type 2 diabetes: This is caused due to either insulin resistance of target tissues or decrease in overall insulin secretion. The initial stages of this type of diabetes can be regulated by diet management and lifestyle modification in the form of regular exercises to enhance endogenous insulin secretion. Later stages require medical intervention in the form of insulin secretagogues (e.g. sulfonylureas) or insulin sensitizers (e.g. metformin). It is in the terminal stages, when the β-cells have lost the capacity to produce and secrete insulin, that the patient is administered external insulin.
3. Gestational diabetes: This form of diabetes is associated with pregnancy. It is usually observed during the second half of gestation and is usually caused due to anti-insulin effects

of chorionic somatomammotropin, prolactin or cortisol. Recommended treatment is insulin injections.

ANTI-DIABETIC DRUGS

Based upon the inherent nature of diabetes, different classes of anti-diabetic drugs are now available in the market. These drugs would decrease the circulating levels of glucose either by stimulating production and secretion of endogenous insulin from pancreas or by enhancing the responsiveness of target tissues toward insulin. The class of drugs which bring about these changes are broadly classified as oral hypoglycemic agents (OHAs). However, in patients suffering from type 1 diabetes or gestational diabetes, the only mode of treatment is either natural insulin preparations or insulin analogues (Ajjan and Grant, 2006; Kitabchi *et al.*, 2001. It should also be noted that based upon the severity of the disease and its associated complications, these drugs are either given as monotherapy or in combination with other drugs to achieve maximal effects (Massi-Beneditti and Orsini-Federici., 2008). For an overview of various classes of anti-diabetic drugs available, please refer to Fig. 6.2.

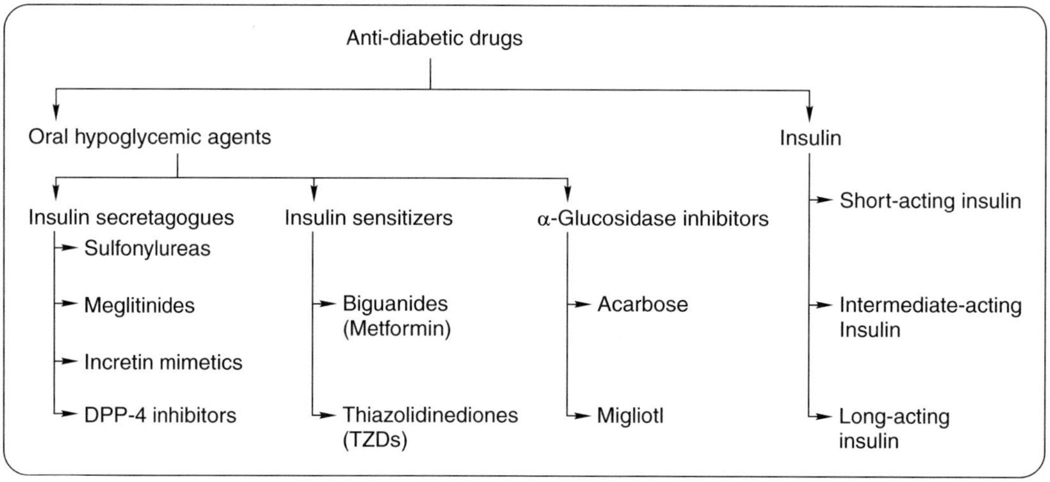

Fig. 6.2 *Summary of Types of Anti-diabetic Drugs*

Oral Hypoglycemic Agents

OHAs, as the name suggests, are administered orally to achieve normoglycemia in diabetics (Leyetan, 2007). They achieve it through any of the following modes:

1. Increase the secretion of insulin by the pancreas (insulin secretagogues).
2. Improve the sensitivity of liver, skeletal muscle and adipose tissue toward glucose-lowering effects of insulin (insulin sensitizers).

3. Decrease the absorption of glucose from the GI tract.

Hence the target organs for these agents can be pancreas, liver, adipose tissue, muscles or the GI tract.

Insulin Secretagogues

Sulfonylureas

These agents, discovered by Marcel Janbon and colleagues, stimulate the release of insulin from pancreatic β-cells by inhibiting the ATP-sensitive potassium channels. Upon binding to their cognate receptor complex (SUR1), which also houses the ATP-sensitive K^+ channel, they induce membrane depolarization and opening of Ca^{2+} channels. This is followed by an increased release of insulin from the intracellular storage vesicles (Proks *et al.*, 2002). They are also reported to increase the number of insulin receptors on insulin-responsive tissues to augment glucose uptake via the GLUT4 translocation. Structurally all the members of this family contain a central *S*-phenylsulfonyl urea structure. Coming to the pharmacokinetics, these drugs are readily absorbed in the GI tract, metabolized in liver via the cytochrome P450 system prior to excretion through urine. Both short- and long-acting sulfonylureas are available in market, and their choice of use depends upon the propensity of the patient to develop hyperglycemia. Due to fewer side effects, the second-generation drugs such as glimepiride and glibenclamide are commonly in use (Massi-Beneditti, 2003; Rendell, 2004). These agents are taken 30 min prior to meal and their effect can last up to 24 h. Among the two, glimepiride has a rapid onset and prolonged effect due to its faster reversible association with the receptor. The biggest drawback of these drugs is that their use is contingent upon the presence of residual β-cell function. Major side effects are episodes of hypoglycemia and weight gain due to edema. Occasionally a patient may exhibit GI discomfort in the form of vomiting and nausea.

Meglitinides

Commonly referred to as 'short-acting secretagogues', they function in a fashion similar to sulfonylureas. However, they have a distinct binding site on the SU receptor as compared to the sulfonylureas. These drugs potentiate glucose-mediated insulin release. Compared to sulfonylureas they are absorbed in the intestine faster, with their levels peaking within an hour. Two common members of this class are repaglinide from Novo Nordisk and Starlix (Dornhorst, 2001). Since the activity of these drugs is partly glucose dependent, the effectiveness of the drug is compromised in the presence of relatively less glucose. Compared to sulfonylureas, they exhibit a lower risk of hypoglycemia but are far more expensive. The side effect is weight gain.

Peptide analogues

This class of drugs includes incretin mimetics and dipeptidyl peptidase 4 (DPP-4) inhibitors. Incretins are a class of hormones secreted by the GI tract that are released in response to food intake. Two main members as previously mentioned are GLP-1 and gastric inhibitory peptide, both of which promote insulin release from the islets of Langerhans (Gautier *et al.*, 2008). However, they both get inactivated via the catalytic cleavage mediated by DPP-4. Available incretin mimetics such as exenatide essentially bind to the GLP receptors on the β-cells of the pancrease to cause insulin release. Exenatide is a 39-amino-acid-long synthetic molecule exhibiting 53% homology with GLP1. It is also resistant to cleavage by DPP-4 (Briones and Bajaj., 2006; Cyetkovic and Plosker, 2007; Davidson *et al*., 2008). The acute insulinotrophic effects include glucose-dependent insulin release, improved β-cell mass and delayed gastric emptying, thereby delaying the onset of postprandial hyperglycemia. Interestingly, it also impairs glucagon's secretion, thereby decreasing liver-mediated glucose output. The major side effects of exenatide are headache, nausea, diarrhea and dyspepsia. Another example of GLP-1 analogue is liraglutide (Feinglos *et al*., 2005).

The common inhibitors of DPP-4 are vildagliptin and sitagliptin (Crepaldi *et al*., 2007). Both of them report lesser episodes of hypoglycemia and both are reported to favor β-cell regeneration and differentiation. Recent studies have shown that DPP-4 inhibitors are successful in maintaining reduced levels of HbA_{1c} up to a year. Measurement of glycosylated of hemoglobin (HbA_{1c}) is considered to be a fair mode of evaluating a patient's glycemic status for the preceding 3 months.

Insulin Sensitizers

Biguanides

These dimethyl guanidine derivatives were first discovered in extracts of *Galega*, commonly known as French lilac. Currently, the only available viable treatment option from this family is metformin (Stack, 2008). Other members (phenformin and buformin) were withdrawn from market due to associated fatal lactic acidosis. The exact mode of their action is still unclear; however, they decrease hepatic gluconeogenesis while activating glucose uptake by peripheral tissues such as skeletal muscles. They also decrease the intestinal absorption of glucose. Interestingly, recent reports demonstrate the beneficial cardiovascular effects of metformin, because of its ability to improve the lipid profiles. It does so by facilitating conversion of low-density lipoprotein (LDL) to high-density lipoprotein (HDL) and by inhibiting triglyceride formation in liver (Raskin *et al*., 2008). Metformin is absorbed via the small intestine and is excreted in urine without alteration. It is usually the first line of treatment for diabetics. Advantages of metformin include reduced risk of hypoglycemia, favorable effect on lipid profile and weight loss. The disadvantages are, however, nausea, abdominal discomfort and, in rare cases for metformin, lactic acidosis.

Thiazolidinediones

Glitazones, as thiazolidinediones (TZDs) are commonly called, are drugs that bind to a class of nuclear receptors called peroxisome proliferator-activated receptor-gamma (PPARγ). Upon binding to these receptors through PPARγ responsive elements (PREs), they activate the transcription of numerous insulin-responsive genes such as lipoprotein lipase (LPL) and GLUT4. They hence improve the insulin sensitivity by increasing glycogen synthesis in liver and lipogenesis in adipose tissue. They also enhance intracellular signaling by increasing the tyrosine kinase activity of the insulin receptor. Beneficial effects of these drugs on lipid profile are also reported as they decrease the triglyceride levels. They are absorbed in the gut and are metabolized by the hepatic cytochrome P450 system. The major members in this class are rosiglitazone, pioglitazone and troglitazone (Bradley, 2002; Alarcón de la Lastra *et al*., 2004). The major side effect of these compounds is water retention leading to edema and occasionally liver damage or hepatitis as seen with troglitazone. On one hand, ADOPT study, PROactive 5 and DREAM trials have shown the beneficial effects of TZDs on management of diabetes and its associated cardiac complications; on the other hand, a retrospective meta-analysis on rosiglitazone has suggested a higher risk of coronary artery disease (Kretz and Friedmann, 2006; Erdman *et al.*, 2007; Mannucci *et al.*, 2008).

α-Glucosidase Inhibitors

These oral anti-diabetic drugs are neither insulin secretagogues nor are they insulin sensitizers. Instead, they delay the breakdown of complex sugars such as starch into glucose, thereby directly affecting the onset of postprandial hyperglycemia. They are essentially competitive inhibitors of *α*-glucoside enzymes present in the brush border cells of the small intestine. These membrane-bound enzymes hydrolyze oligosaccharides to monosaccharide moieties such as glucose. The most widely used members of this family are acarbose and miglitol (Godbout and Chiasson, 2007; Hansfeld and Schaper, 2008). While acarbose is a pseudo-tetrasaccharide, miglitol resembles a monosaccharide sugar. Less than 2% of acarbose is absorbed through gut while miglitol has a better absorption. Hence, acarbose is directly excreted though the fecal route, while miglitol is excreted through urine. In addition to inhibiting *α*-glucosidase, acarbose also inhibits pancreatic *α*-amylase (the enzyme responsible for hydrolyzing starch). Some of the disadvantages of these drugs are flatulence and diarrhoea. Their use is usually recommended for treating prediabetic patients exhibiting impaired glucose tolerance (IGT).

Insulin Preparations and Insulin Analogues

Insulin therapy is must for a type 1 diabetic patient and has to be initiated in type 2 diabetics when the OHAs fail. It is also recommended for pregnant women suffering from gestational diabetes. Based on the duration of action, various types of insulin preparations and insulin analogues are available (Mayfield and White, 2004). They are mainly classified into three categories: short-acting insulin, intermediate-acting insulin and long-acting insulin. Additionally they are classified based on the source of insulin, which can be human, bovine or porcine. It would be needless to say that human insulin preparation is the least immunogenic. Among the animal sources of insulin, porcine insulin is less antigenic and it differs from human insulin at a single amino acid, to be precise the 30th amino acid in B chain of insulin, which is replaced by an alanine as opposed to a threonine residue at the same position in humans (Watkins PJ, 1982). In order to enhance the duration of insulin action, these are made available as zinc or protamine suspensions. Insulin analogues on the other hand are genetically engineered versions of human insulin. Through mutagenesis strategies, one or more amino acids are specifically replaced by more suitable residues to enhance the potency.

Short-Acting Insulin

They are rapid-acting insulin with the onset of action within half an hour of administration. Their effects last up to 8 h. Currently available preparations in this category are Actrapid, Humulin and a highly purified beef insulin called Hypurin Bovine Lente. Among the analogues the members are lispro and aspart.

Intermediate-Acting Insulin

These are usually available as isophane insulin suspensions, e.g. neutral protamine Hagedorn or as zinc suspension (e.g. lente). Their effects start within an hour of injection and lasts for up to 24 h.

Long-Acting Insulin

These are essentially insulin analogues with prolonged half-life and their duration of action lasts for up to 34–40 h. The available ones in the market are Lantus (glargine) and Levemir (detemir). In glargine, the aspartate residue at Position 21 of A chain is replaced by glycine to improve its bioavailability. Glargine has no peak of action as such; instead, it is released into circulation at a constant rate. Similarly, detemir has a prolonged action due to its ability to bind tightly to serum albumin the main carrier protein in bloodstream. Among the two, determir is associated with lesser episodes of weight gain as opposed to glargine (Barnett, A., *et al.*, 2008).

In addition to these, mixed preparations of insulin with varying combinations of regular and intermediate insulin are available in the market to achieve optimum glycemic responses based on the patient's requirement and state of disease. They are usually available as mixtures of 30% rapid-acting and 70% of intermediate-acting insulin. Since these insulin preparations exhibit biphasic responses with regard to insulin effects, they score advantage over multiple insulin injections. However, there is no hard and fast rule as to which insulin preparation is better than the other, as the need of insulin regime varies from patient to patient. Readers are recommended to the excellent articles by Watkins (Watkins, PJ, 1982), MacPerson *et al.* (1990) and Barnett, A. *et al.* for suggested insulin regimes to be followed based on patient requirements. Major complications arising due to insulin therapy are episodes of hypoglycemia, weight gain and edema, and, in rare cases, insulin allergy.

CONCLUSIONS

Diabetes, being a metabolic disorder of glucose imbalance, essentially requires treatment addressing the issues of hyperglycemia. Based on the extent of disease, the therapy is usually initiated with the use of OHAs unless it is a type 1 patient. These agents are essentially sulfonylureas, metformin or TZDs. Incretin mimetics and DPP-4 are newer-generation OHAs that are being considered for treatment. An alternative approach, which is mainly used in impaired glucose tolerant patients, is the use of α-glucoside inhibitors such as acarbose and miglitol. Insulin therapy on the other hand is a must for type I diabetics or in type 2 patients where OHAs have failed to deliver desirable effects.

REFERENCES

Ajjan, R.A., Grant, P.J. (2006). Cardiovascular disease prevention in patients with type 2 diabetes: The role of oral anti-diabetic agents. *Diabetes and Vascular Disease Research* **3(3)**:147–158.

Alarcón de la Lastra, C., Sanchez-Fidalgo, S., Villegas, I., Motilva, V. (2004). New pharmacological perspectives and therapeutics potential of PPAR-gamma agonists. *Current Pharmaceutical Design* **10(28)**:3505–3524.

Barnett, A., Begg, A., Feher, D.M., Hamilton, S., and Munro, N. (2008). Insulin for type 2 diabetes: choosing a second line regimen. *International Journal of Clinical Practice* **62(1)**:1647–1653.

Bradley, C. (2002). The glitazones: A new treatment for type 2 diabetes mellitus. *Intensive and Critical Care Nursing* **18(3)**:189–191.

Briones, M., Bajaj, M. (2006). Exenatide: A GLP-1 receptor agonist as novel therapy for type 2 diabetes mellitus. *Expert Opinion in Pharmacotherapy* **7(8)**:1055–1064.

Crepaldi, G., Carruba, M., Comaschi, M., Del Prato, S., Frasjese, G., Paolisso, G. (2007). Dipeptidyl peptidase 4 (DPP-4) inhibitors and their role in type 2 diabetes management. *Journal of Endocrinological Investigation* **30(7)**:610–614.

Cvetkovic, R.S., Plosker, G.L. (2007). Exenatide: A review of its use in patients with type 2 diabetes mellitus (as an adjunct to metformin and/or a sulphonylurea). *Drugs* **67(6)**:935–954.

Davidson, J.A., Parente, E.B., Gross, J.L. (2008). Incretin mimetics and dipeptidyl peptidase-4 inhibitors: Innovative treatment therapies for type 2 diabetes. *Arquivos brasileiros de endocrinologia e metabologia* **52(6)**:1039–1049.

Dornhorst, A. (2001). Insulinotropic meglitinide analogues. *Lancet* **358**:1709–1716.

Erdman, E., Dormandy, J.A., Charbonnel, B., Massi-Benedetti, M., Moules, I.K., Skene, A.M. (2007). The effect of pioglitazone on recurrent myocardial infarction in 2445 patients with type 2 diabetes and previous myocardial infarction. Results from PROactive (PROactive05). *Journal of American College of Cardiology* **49(17)**:1772–1780.

Feinglos, M.N., Saad, M.F., Pi-Sunyer, F.X., An, B., Santiago, O. (Liraglutide Dose-Response Study Group) (2005). Effects of liraglutide (NN2211), a long acting GLP-1 analogue, on glycaemic control and body weight in subjects with type 2 diabetes. *Diabetic Medicine* **22(8)**:1016–1023.

Gautier, J.F., Choukem, S.P., Girard, J. (2008). Physiology of incretins (GIP and GLP-1) and abnormalities in type 2 diabetes. *Diabetes and Metabolism* **Suppl. 2**:S65–72.

Godbout, A., Chiasson, J.L. (2007). Who should benefit from the use of alpha-glucosidase inhibitors? *Current Diabetes Reports* **7(5)**:333–339.

Guillausseau, P.J., Tielmans, D., Virally-Monod, M., Assayag, M. (1997). Diabetes: From phenotypes to genotypes. *Diabetes and Metabolism* **Suppl. 2**:14–21.

Hanefeld, M., Schaper, F. (2008). Acarbose: Oral anti-diabetes drug with additional cardiovascular benefits. *Expert Review of Cardiovascular Therapy* **6(2)**:153–163.

King, H., Aubert, R.E., Herman, W.H. (1998). Global burden of diabetes 1995-2025; Prevalence, numerical estimates and projection. *Diabetes Care* **21**:1414–1431.

Krentz, A.J., Friedmann, P.S. (2006). Type 2 diabetes, psoriasis and thiazolidinediones. *International Journal of Clinical Practice* **60(3)**:362–363.

Levetan, C. (2007). Oral anti-diabetic agents in type 2 diabetes. *Current Medical Research and Opinion* **23(4)**:945–952.

MacPherson, J.N., and Feely, J. (1990). Insulin. *British Medical Journal.* **300**:731–736.

Mannucci, E., Monami, M., Lamanna, C., Gensini, G.F., Marchionni, N. (2008). Pioglitazone and cardiovascular risk. A comprehensive meta-analysis of randomized clinical trials. *Diabetes, Obesity and Metabolism* [doi: 10.1111/j.1463–1326 2008.00892.x.PMID 18505403].

Massi-Beneditti, M. (2003). Glimepiride in type 2 diabetes mellitus: A review of the worldwide therapeutic experience. *Clinical Theapeutics* **25(3)**:799–816.

Massi-Beneditti, M., Orsini-Federici, M. (2008). Treatment of type 2 diabetes with combined therapy: What are the pros and cons? *Diabetes Care* **31(2)**:S131–135.

Mayfield, J.A., White, R.D. (2004). Insulin therapy for type 2 diabetes: Rescue, augmentation, and replacement of β-cell function. *American Family Physician* **7(3)**:489–500.

Proks, P., Reimann, F., Green, N., Gribble, F., Ashcroft, F. (2002). Sulfonylurea stimulation of insulin secretion. *Diabetes* **51(3)**:S368–376.

Quesada, I., Tuduri, E., Ripoll, C., Nadal, A. (2008). Physiology of the pancreatic alpha-cell and glucagons secretion: Role in glucose homeostatis and diabetes. *Journal of Endocrinology* **199(1)**:5–19.

Raskin, R. (2008). Why insulin sensitizers but not secretagogues should be retained when initiating insulin in type 2 diabetes. *Diabetes/Metabolism Research and Reviews* **24(1)**:3–13.

Rendell, M. (2004). The role of sulphonylureas in the management of type 2 diabetes mellitus. *Drugs* **64(12)**:1339–1358.

Sicree, R., Shaw, J., Zimmet, P. (2003). The global burden of diabetes. In: Gan, D. (ed.), *Diabetes Atlas*, 2nd ed, 15–71. Brussels, Belgium: International Diabetes Federation.

Stack, T. (2008). Metformin: A review. *Drugs of Today (Barcelona, Spain: 1998)* **44(4)**:303–314.

Tengholm, A., Gylfe, E. (2008). Oscillatory control of insulin secretion. *Molecular and Cellular Endocrinology* doi: 10.1016/j.mce.2008.07.009.

UK Prospective Diabetes Study (UKPDS) Group (1998). Intensive blood glucose control with sulphonylureas or insulin compared with conventional treatment and risk of complications in patients with type 2 diabetes (UKPDS 33). *Lancet* **352**:837–853.

Watkins, P.J. (1982). ABC of Diabetes. *British Medical Journal.* **284**:1929–1932.

7

'GPCROMICS': Exploring and Exploiting GPCROMES for Drug Discovery

Lavanya Madhuri Balivada and Gopala Krishna Aradhyam*

Department of Biotechnology, Indian Institute of Technology Madras, Chennai 600 036, India

INTRODUCTION

G protein-coupled receptors (GPCRs) form the largest superfamily of proteins in the human body (Gether, 2000). About 3–4% of the vertebrate genome codes for these extensive and diverse membrane receptors, which are involved in several kinds of signal transduction pathways (Vázquez-Prado *et al.*, 2003). Of the >2000 genes coding for GPCRs, about two-thirds code for odorant receptors, ~215 for ligand receptors and ~160 for orphan receptors (Schöneberg *et al.*, 2004). These receptors are responsible for metabolic, physiological and neurological maintenance of most biological systems, from nematodes like *Caenorhabditis elegans* to humans (Prossnitz, 2004). However, the number of GPCRs increases with increasing complexity of the organism (Fredriksson *et al.*, 2005). GPCRs were named so since they transduce signals intracellularly with the help of G proteins (guanine-nucleotide binding proteins). Though all known GPCRs share a common characteristic structure of having seven transmembrane domain (7TM domain), functionally they are fairly diverse. This functional diversity is fulfilled by a wide array of ligands and downstream effector molecules in the signal transduction pathway.

Membrane protein dynamics has found re-invigorated interest probably because most of the drugs in the market are targeted to receptors, especially GPCRs. Drugs targeting members of this protein

---

* *agk@iitm.ac.in*

superfamily represent the core of modern medicine. GPCRs are the most aggressively investigated drug targets in the pharmaceutical industry. Today >60% of the drugs target GPCRs because of their extracellular domains that impart ability to transduce signals into intracellular responses. GPCRs present a wide range of opportunities as therapeutic targets for diseases such as cancer, diabetes, obesity and many others because these receptors are expressed and are active in every organ of the body. Due to their extensive, exclusive and unique role in various signaling pathways, GPCR-defective diseases play an important role in drug discovery and development. Functional characterization of a disease causing mutant GPCR is extremely essential to correlate receptor mutation with the observed phenotype. Studying ligand-induced structural changes in receptors also proves immensely helpful in drug discovery. Though receptor agonists or antagonists do not affect its functionality, they cause different structural changes in the receptor in response to the ligand (Kenakin, 2003). Much of recent attention is toward studying constitutively active receptor systems in order to learn more about the receptor–drug interaction and thus its screening for potential candidate molecules (Chen *et al.*, 1999). Such constitutively active receptors are more advantageous as such systems are highly sensitive to agonists and exhibit increased capability to detect ligands.

GRAFS CLASSIFICATION OF GPCRs

Initially, GPCRs were classified into different families based on their sequence homology, activating ligands, effector molecules involved and the pathway of signal transduction (Table 7.1) (Gether, 2000). This system of classification included three major families of GPCRs based on their structural homology (families A, B and C). While yeast pheromone receptors form two unrelated families (families D and E), four receptors from *Dictyostelium discoideum* form the last family (family F). The main drawback of this system was that some of the families were restricted to receptors from a single species. Moreover, with the sequencing of the human genome, many of the mammalian receptors could not be assigned to any of the six existing classes of GPCRs. Hence, Fredriksson *et al.* (2003) suggested a new system of classification based on chromosomal positions of genes and fingerprint motifs (Fig. 7.1). According to this new system of classification, represented as 'GRAFS' (each letter standing for the name of the family of receptors; Glutamine, Rhodopsin, Adhesin, Frizzled and Secretin), all GPCRs share a common ancestor and are believed to have evolved by exon shuffling and gene duplication (Perez, 2003). Fredriksson *et al.* (2005) expanded the GRAFS system to identify and classify GPCRs from different eukaryotic genomes using hidden Markov models (HMMs). They observed that many classes of GPCRs, though absent in vertebrates, are present in other taxa. Moreover, the five classes of GPCRs found in mammals are present in organisms known to exist much before the divergence of nematodes in the natural history of evolution (Fredriksson *et al.*, 2005). The largest family of GPCRs, the rhodopsin family, has been subdivided into 19 sub-families when compared to 6 families in the earlier classification. Some of the GPCRs, which could not be assigned to any of the five families, were grouped into 'other 7TM' family. The GRAFS system of classification overcomes the drawbacks of the 'A to F family' system of classification of GPCRs. For example, this system differentiates the adhesion and secretin family of receptors, which were otherwise classified into a single Family B in the A to F classification system (Fredriksson *et al.*, 2003).

Table 7.1 *Three of the Most Important Classes of GPCR Superfamily*

Family	*Representative Receptors*	*Characteristic Features*	*Ligands*	*Expression*	*References*
A	Rhodopsin, Adrenergic, Dopamine, Chemokine	• The largest and the most studied with >90% of known GPCRs • Low homology, few conserved residues; characteristic '*DRY*' motif in the second cytoplasmic loop • Palmitoylated cysteine at the C-terminus gives the appearance of a fourth cytoplasmic loop	Light, epinephrine, peptides, lipids, lipoproteins, monoamines nucleotides	Retina, cardiac muscle, brain	Gether, 2000 Wess, 1998
B	Glucagon, Calcitonin	• Characteristic disulfide bridge connecting ECL2 and ECL3 • Long hormone binding N-terminus (100–150 amino acid residues) with several cysteines, thus contains many disulfide bonds • Peptide ligand binding site involves various contact points from N-terminus and the three extracellular loops	Peptides	Islets of Langerhans, thyroid	Gether, 2000 Schöneberg *et al.*, 2004 Kristiansen, 2004
C	GABA, Taste, Pheromone	• Extensively long N-terminus (500–600 amino residues long) • Very and short and highly conserved intracellular loop 3	Na^{+2} ions, H^{+} ions, sugars, amino acids, plant alkaloids	CNS, taste buds of tongue	Gether, 2000

Note: In addition to the above-mentioned families, there also occur families D, E and F, which code for yeast pheromone receptors and few cAMP receptors from the slime mold *Dictyostelium discoides* (Gether, 2000; Wess, 1998.).

STRUCTURE

GPCRs are also called as '7TM' or 'hepta-helical receptors' due to their common structural characteristics (Pierce *et al.*, 2002). All of them have 20–30 hydrophobic amino acid residue, long seven tandemly arranged transmembrane (TM) helices with an extracellular N-terminus (7–3000 residues), an intracellular C-terminus (12–400 residues), three cytoplasmic loops and three extracellular loops (5–250 residues) (Fig. 7.2) (Morris and Malbon, 1999). Though the TMs are highly conserved among closely related GPCRs, the loops are comparatively variable while the N- and C-termini are the most diverse elements, adding to their ability to recognize diverse extracellular ligands and different cytoplasmic G proteins (Fredriksson *et al.*, 2005).

Though the number of GPCRs and data concerning them are increasing exponentially, little success has been met in the field of crystal structures of GPCRs. The difficulty in mimicking the membrane environment *in vitro* makes crystallization of the receptors a tedious and time-consuming process. Overexpression of the mammalian receptors in bacterial or insect cell lines has its own limitations (Beeley and Sage, 2003). The unavailability of posttranslational modification machinery

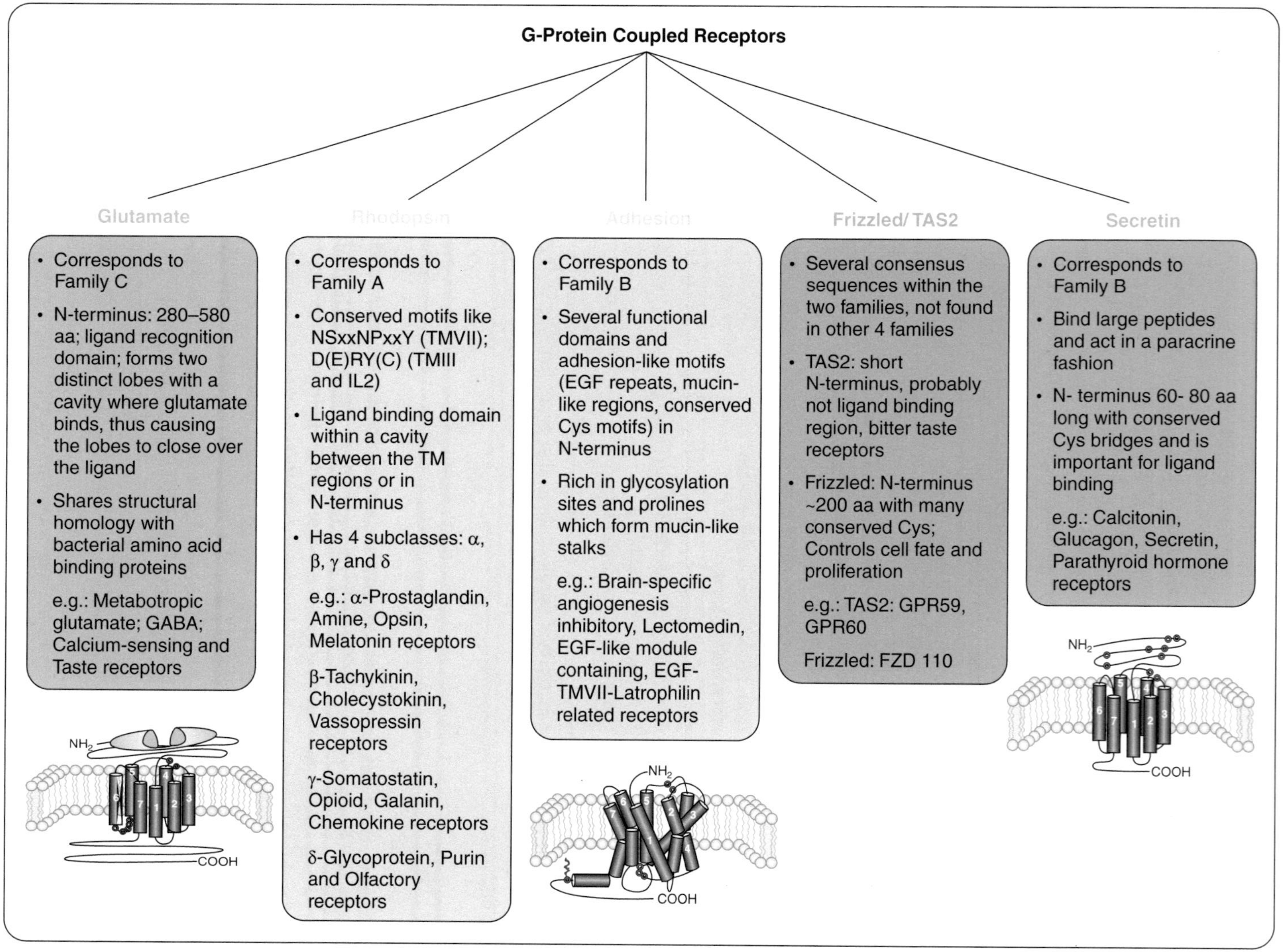

Fig. 7.1 *'GRAFS' System of Classification of G Protein-Coupled Receptors (Fredriksson et al., 2003)*

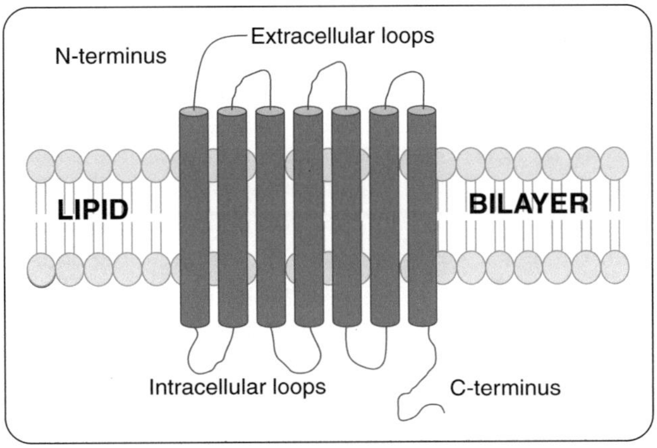

Fig. 7.2 *Cartoon Representation of a Typical GPCR, Showing the Seven Transmembrane Regions, Extracellular N-Terminus, Intracellular C-terminus, Three Extracellular Loops and Three Intracellular Loops. Almost all the GPCRs are Targeted to the Plasma Membrane and Therefore their Extracellular Loop Regions are Very Good Targets for Drugs to Act On.*

in bacteria and the difference in the cell wall composition of bacteria and mammals make it difficult to stabilize the GPCR in one conformational state long enough to crystallize it (Beeley and Sage, 2003). Even if the receptor is overexpressed, it is difficult to stabilize it to a level sufficient for crystallization trials. It is also difficult to keep the receptor functional after solubilization and purification. Moreover, high-resolution structural analysis of GPCRs has been hindered by their low natural abundance and difficulty in producing and purifying significant quantities of the recombinant protein homogeneously and modified post-translationally. X-ray structures of bovine rhodopsin, with and without retinal and β_2-adrenergic receptor, are the only crystal structures of GPCRs available (Palczewski *et al.*, 2000; Salom *et al.*, 2006; Rasmussen *et al.*, 2007). The crystal structure of rhodopsin reveals that Helix VII is involved in interaction with the chromophore ligand. To aid this, the extracellular region of the receptor forms stacks of β-sheets, which shield the chromophore from the extracellular matrix (Okada and Palczewski, 2001). The availability of high-resolution structure of rhodopsin and adrenergic receptors makes it possible to predict and model the structure and functional sites of interaction of the agonist molecules in other GPCRs. For example, bovine rhodopsin and human dopamine D_2 receptor are ~20% identical, ~25% in just the TM regions. This allows us to mimic the structure of rhodopsin on dopamine, especially in the TM regions (Ballesteros *et al.*, 2001). Based on sequence alignment and homology modeling, most of the residues involved in intracellular ligand binding for β-adrenergic receptors were shown to be present toward the interior of the TM helices (Gether and Kobilka, 1998). However, with the recently solved crystal structure of β_2-adrenergic receptor, it is clear that this receptor differs from rhodopsin in the 'DRY' region. The cytoplasmic interactions involving cytoplasmic loop 2, which contains the DRY region, TM3 and TM6, are found to be weaker than in rhodopsin and this has been attributed to the increased basal-level activity of the receptor (Rasmussen *et al.*, 2007).

BIOGENESIS

GPCR export from the endoplasmic reticulum (ER) and trafficking to the plasma membrane is a highly regulated process. Any mutation leading to improper folding of the receptor and, hence, retention of the receptor in ER, leading to its aggregation, causes an abrogation of signal transduction. This may result in activation of death signals of the cell (Duvernay *et al.*, 2005). Most of the signature motifs for export from ER are present in the membrane-proximal C-terminus of the receptor (Table 7.2) (Duvernay *et al.*, 2005). GPCR-laden vesicles from ER migrate to the endoplasmic reticulum–Golgi intermediate compartment (ERGIC) to Golgi apparatus, and finally to the *trans*-Golgi network (TGN). During the process of export, GPCRs also undergo posttranslational modifications in the form of glycosylation or lipid modification. Mature receptors are then transported to their final functional destination, the plasma membrane (Duvernay *et al.*, 2005). Receptor dimerization has also been shown to be responsible for their proper folding, trafficking to the plasma membrane and their activity. Studies have proved that some receptors are transported from the ER only after their successful self-dimerization (Duvernay *et al.*, 2005).

Table 7.2 *Various Motifs Found in the Membrane Proximal C-Terminus of GPCRs Which Play a Role in Receptor Export and Trafficking from ER to the Plasma Membrane*

Receptor	*Motif*	*Function*	*References*
β-Adrenergic Vasopressin V2	$-^{410}DSLL^{413}-$ $-^{335}E(X)_3LL^{340}-$	• Sorting signal for TGN • Mediator of endocytosis at the plasma membrane • Recycling of the internalized receptor to the plasma membrane • Regulation of receptor targeting to lysosomes	Gether and Kobilka, 1998 Morello and Bichet, 2001
Dopamine	$-^{333}F(X)_3F(X)_3F^{341}-$	• Cell surface expression • Promotes receptor interaction with chaperones	Gage *et al.*, 2001 Bermack *et al.*, 2001
Vasopressin V3	$-^{341}FN(X)_2LL(X)^{3L350}-$	• Receptor export from ER • Trafficking to the membrane	Robert *et al.*, 2005
α-Adrenergic Angiotensin II type 1	$-^{433}F(X)_6IL^{441}-$ $-^{309}F(X)6LL^{317}-$	• Highly conserved motif in GPCRs • Export from ER • Expression at cell surface • Agonist-induced activation of receptor	Zhou *et al.*, 2006 Dong *et al.*, 2007

The export mechanism of GPCRs also involves the efficient coordination of many different ER-resident chaperones, receptor activity modifying proteins (RAMPs) and other accessory proteins (Fig. 7.3). RAMPs also exhibit chaperone activity by aiding receptors in folding and trafficking from intracellular compartment to the plasma membrane. This was first shown for calcitonin gene–related peptide receptor (Duvernay *et al.*, 2005). RAMPs are also known to affect the receptor glycosylation and their functional structure, as is evident from the fact that they are transported to the plasma

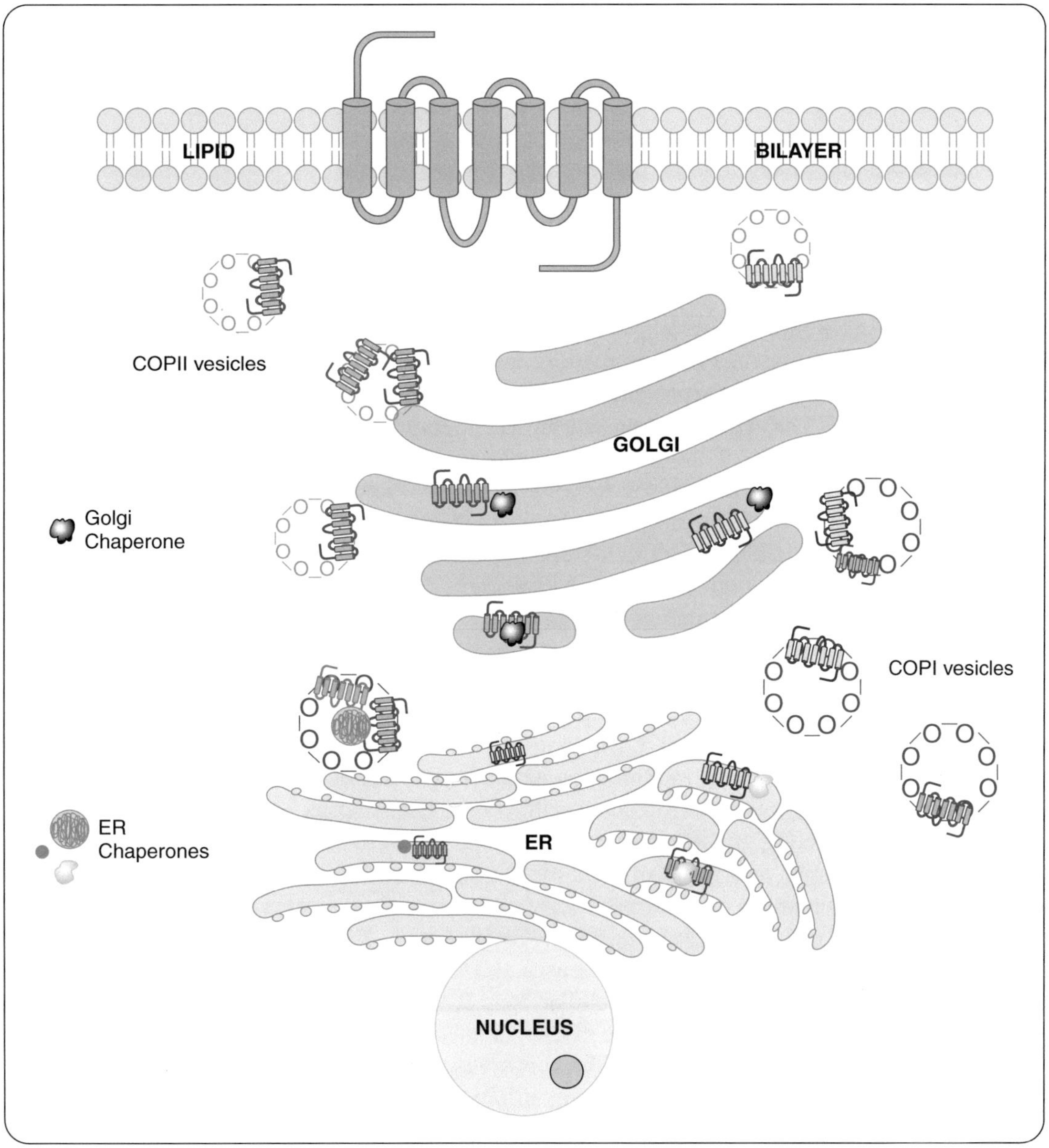

Fig. 7.3 *Biogenesis of GPCR from ER to Plasma Membrane through Golgi with the Help of Various Chaperones, RAMPs and Clathrin-Coated Pits Proteins involved in the Trafficking are also Potential Drug Targets. (For color figure please see Plate 6)*

membrane along with the receptor (Duvernay *et al.*, 2005). Poyner and group (Conner *et al.*, 2004) have shown that RAMPs specifically interact with a section of Class B GPCRs, like the calcitonin (CT) receptor, calcitonin receptor-like (CL) receptor, adrenomedullin (AM) receptor and amylin

(AMY) receptor. Due to heterodimerization among these receptors and also heterodimerization among RAMP-1, -2 and -3, these receptors exhibit significant cross-reactivity to RAMPs. RAMPs also aid the receptor in interacting with its ligand, as shown for CL receptor, which in the absence of RAMPs does not bind to any ligand (Conner *et al.*, 2004). Moreover, it has been shown that CL receptor and RAMPs associate with each other in the Golgi, to form a stable complex that is transported to the plasma membrane and finally internalized as such (Kuwasako *et al.*, 2000; Leuthäuser *et al.*, 2000; Hilairet *et al.*, 2001).

GPCRs having N-linked oligosaccharides are also assisted by chaperones such as calnexin and calreticulin for proper folding, prevention of exit of incompletely or mis-folded and oligomerized proteins from the ER and their premature degradation (Hammond and Helenius, 1995). Glucose-related protein 98 (Grp98) and binding immunoglobulin protein (BiP) prevent the aggregation of newly synthesized proteins, thus helping them to fold correctly. BiP, a 78 kDa glucose-related heat shock protein, and Grp98, a 98 kDa protein, use ATP/ADP to regulate proper protein folding by protein disulfide isomerases (PDIs) (Li and Lee, 2006). Members of the PDI family and Erp57 catalyze rate-limiting steps in folding of the newly synthesized receptor (Hammond and Helenius, 1995). Thus, chaperone-mediated folding of the receptor helps the 'export quality receptors' to bypass the scrutiny of ER quality control system (Chapple *et al.*, 2001). *ninaA (neither inactivation nor after-potential A)*, RanBP2 and ODR-4 (odorant-response abnormal receptor 4) are some chaperone-like proteins that also help in the regulation of GPCR export (Duvernay *et al.*, 2005). These proteins act by stabilizing the receptor conformation and promoting receptor delivery to the membrane (Chapple *et al.*, 2001; Duvernay *et al.*, 2005). Apart from interactions with these proteins, ER export of the receptors also depends on the kind of motif (conserved amino acid sequence) they carry.

The status of posttranslational modification in the form of N-linked glycosylation of the receptor also determines the fate of receptor trafficking to membranes. It is considered to be the most common form of posttranslational modification, with almost 95% of the GPCRs being glycosylated. Glycosylation plays an important role in many cellular processes such as lectin-based sorting along the secretory pathway, targeting to a lysozome as a consequence of mannose-6-phosphate modification, ER-associated degradation as a result of mannose trimming, quality control through calnexin cycle, folding through the alteration of hydrophobicity, protection from protease-mediated degradation, immune evasion, cell–cell interaction, and so on (Lanctot *et al.*, 2005).

Glycosylation usually occurs at the consensus *'NXS/T'* motif (where X is any amino acid other than proline), usually localized in extracellular loop 2 of the receptor. Studies with human AT_1 receptor have shown that positioning of the glycosylation site within the receptor also plays a crucial role (Lanctot *et al.*, 2005). Introduction of the conserved glycosylation motif in extracellular loop 1 of this receptor leads to a significant decrease in affinity and transportation of the receptor to the cell surface, while localization of this lipid moiety within extracellular loop 3 of the same receptor leads to cell surface localization-deficient mutants which exhibited normal affinity to the ligand. However, shifting the glycosylation site by two residues in the extracellular loop 2 led to a mis-folded receptor, which did not exhibit any trafficking deficiencies (Lanctot *et al.*, 2005).

Studies with follicle-stimulating hormone (FSH), β_2-adrenergic and histamine receptors have shown that such a modification plays a very important role in cell surface expression of the receptors (Duvernay *et al.*, 2005). For example, the interaction of R^{337} mutant of the arginine vasopressin-receptor2 (AVPR2) with calnexin leads to the absence of this mutant receptor on the cell surface leading to nephrogenic diabetes insipidus (NDI) (Morello *et al.*, 2001). Furthermore, the lutenizing hormone (LH) receptor requires this lipid moiety only for its proper folding, and once properly folded and trafficked to the membrane, glycosylation has no role to play in ligand binding or receptor activation (Wheatley and Hawtin, 1999). Mutating the glycosylatable asparagine residues in AT_1 receptor showed that this modification is necessary for cell surface targeting of the receptor. A large fraction of the unglycosylated receptor was trapped in the ER (Lanctot *et al.*, 2005). Glycosylation of prostaglandin D_2, $F_{2\alpha}$, E_2, PGI_2 and A_2 thromboxane was required for normal sorting of the receptor to plasma membrane and efficient ligand binding (Coleman *et al.*, 1994). Naturally occurring mutations in retinal rhodopsin's two highly conserved N-linked glycosylation sites lead to the autosomal disorder of retinitis pigmentosa (Sung *et al.*, 1991).

It has been shown that for receptors such as somatostatin, rhodopsin, β_2-adrenergic, thyroid-stimulating hormone (TSH) and gastrin-releasing peptide, glycosylation is extremely important for increased affinity to ligand binding and/or G protein coupling (Spiro, 2002). Human prostacyclin receptor has two consensus glycosylation sites, viz. its N-terminus and extracellular loop 1. Glycosylation of this receptor is important for membrane targeting of the receptor and subsequent ligand binding and effective downstream signaling (Zhang *et al.*, 2001). Similar studies with CL receptor have shown that of the three glycosylation sites it carries in its extracellular loops and N-terminus, glycosylation of the asparagine in its N-terminus (Asn^{123}) is necessary for ligand binding and signal transduction, rather than cell surface expression (Kamitani and Sakata, 2001). However, mutating asparagines in the other two glycosylation sites did not bring about any change in receptor targeting or function compared to the wild-type receptor. Moreover, Asn^{123} glycosylation of the CL receptor is necessary for its interaction with RAMPs and its proper folding. Studies with neurokinin 1 (NK1) receptor, which has two glycosylation sites, showed that mutating any one of these sites resulted in a receptor that was no different from the wild type. However, double mutants of the NK1 receptor for these two glycosylation sites led to partial functioning of the receptor (Tansky *et al.*, 2007). This double mutant was also rapidly internalized, implying that glycosylation of this receptor mainly plays a role in receptor stabilization at the plasma membrane.

Another important post-translational modification is phosphorylation of the receptor. Phosphorylation/dephosphorylation states are one of the most important regulatory events controlling whether the receptors are switched on or off. Though there is no conserved motif for phosphorylation, serine, tyrosine, histidine and threonine are the most commonly phosphorylated residues. Phosphorylation plays an important role in the life cycle of a GPCR, mainly by desensitizing the receptor after agonist binding. For example, phosphorylation of somatostatin receptor is necessary for proper internalization and desensitization after binding of somatostatin (Liu and Schonbrunn, 2001). Similarly, phosphorylation of rhodopsin by rhodopsin kinase or of β-adrenergic receptor by cAMP-dependent protein kinase A leads to uncoupling of the receptor–G protein complex (McDowell and Kuehn, 1977; Sibley *et al.*, 1985). Phosphorylation of β-adrenergic receptor by β-adrenergic receptor kinase leads to rapid desensitization of the ligand-bound receptor (Sibley *et al.*, 1985).

Sulfation of GPCRs is another late post-translational modification occurring in the Golgi. Sulfation occurs on tyrosines in the conserved '*Y-D/E-Y*' motif (Costagliola *et al.*, 2002). It has been shown that sulfation of an N-terminal tyrosine in the chemokine C–C motif 5 receptor (CCR_5) is necessary for its binding to HIV-1 gp120 protein (Farzan *et al.*, 1999). Moreover, it has been observed that sulfation of the receptors TSH, LH and FSH is necessary for increased affinity of ligand binding, resulting in efficient receptor activation. Furthermore, unsulfated TSH has been implicated in Grave's disease, which is responsible for stimulating autoantibodies in these patients (Bonomi *et al.*, 2006). Studies with the lysosphingolipid mediator sphingosine 1-phosphate (S1-P) receptor showed that sulfation of this receptor is essential for regulation and migration of T cell functions (Fieger *et al.*, 2005). Recently, Sakmar and group have shown by NMR spectroscopy that three cysteines in the N-terminal region of $CXCR_4$ receptor are necessary for high-affinity binding of the receptor to stroma-cell derived factor 1 (SDF-1) (Seibert *et al.*, 2008; Veldkamp *et al.*, 2008). This interaction is essential for normal embryonic development and abrogation of this interaction has been implicated in many types of cancers.

Other post-translational modifications of GPCRs include palmitoylation, prenylation and/or myristoylation (Bouvier *et al.*, 1995). Rhodopsin, α_{2A}-adrenergic, β_2-adrenergic, D_1 dopamine and LH receptors have palmitoylated cysteines (Cys) in the C-terminal domain (Kristiansen, 2004). The conserved position of Cys in this domain suggests the important role of palmitoylation in regulating the accessibility of this domain to various kinases and other interacting molecules. Though fatty acid modification of receptors has been proved experimentally only for rhodopsin, it has been extended to other GPCRs also (Moench *et al.*, 1994). Palmitoylated cysteines have been shown to be absolutely necessary for processing of LH, canine H_2 histamine, CCR_5 chemokine receptors and also bovine rhodopsin (Qanbar and Bouvier, 2003). Increased radiolabeled palmitate incorporation was observed in activated M_2 muscarinic and 5-hydroxytryptamine 4A (5-HT_{4A}) receptors. Moreover, activation of β_2-adrenergic receptor increased the turnover rate of receptor-bound palmitate (Kristiansen, 2004). A cysteine-to-glycine (C341G) palmitoylation-deficient mutant of β_2-adrenergic receptor was unable to couple to $G_{\alpha s}$ and was found to be hyperphosphorylated. Depalmitoylation leads to receptor phosphorylation with subsequent uncoupling of the GPCR–G protein complex and endocytosis. Palmitoylation-deficient mutants of human somatostatin 5 (sst5), mouse thyrotropin-releasing hormone (TRH) and human AVPR2 though had no effects on agonist-stimulated signal transduction, these mutant receptors still exhibited decreased rates of agonist-promoted internalization (Qanbar and Bouvier, 2003). However, palmitoylation-deficient mutants of LH receptor were found to be internalized twice faster than the wild-type receptors (Kawate and Menon, 1994).

LIFE CYCLE OF GPCRs

Receptor Activation

GPCRs in the plasma membrane are activated by a large variety of ligands, such as amines, glycoproteins, peptides, amino acids, photons, nucleosides, nucleotides, prostanoids, fatty acids, phospholipids, Ca^{2+} ions, odorants, tastants and pheromones, which bind to their extracellular surface. About 70–80% of known hormones and neurotransmitters are known to transduce cellular signals by activating GPCRs (Kristiansen, 2004).

Activation results in rearrangement of the cytoplasmic loops of the receptor, due to the rigid body movement of the TM helices (Fig. 7.4). In rhodopsin, Helices III and VI, and to a certain extent Helix II, exhibit up to 8 Å movements, resulting in rearrangement of the cytoplasmic loops of the receptor (Palczewski *et al.*, 2000; Stenkamp *et al.*, 2002). Helix movements of rhodopsin are the effect of

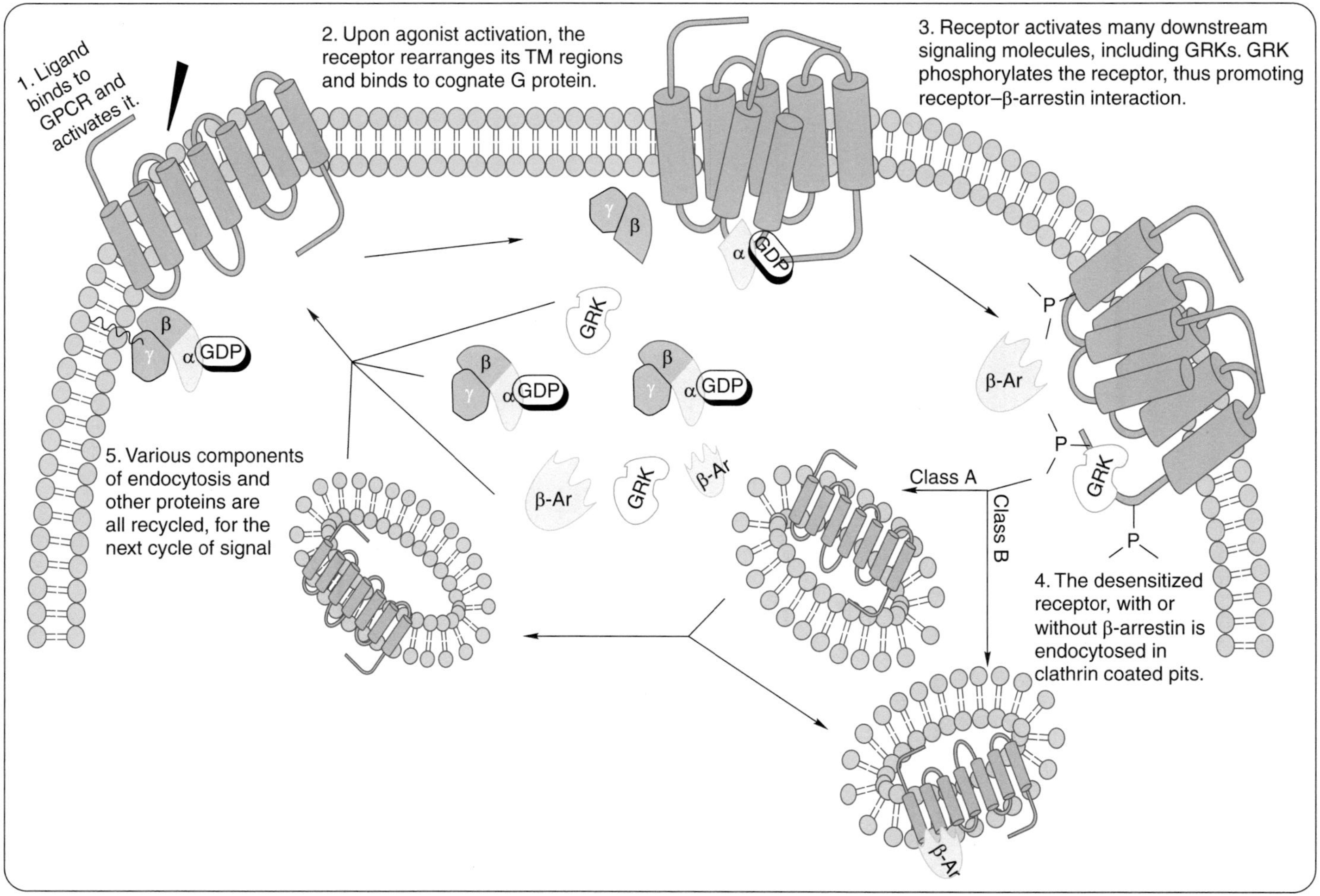

Fig. 7.4 *Life Cycle of a GPCR*

(Upon activation due to agonist binding, the transmembrane helices of the receptor rearrange themselves. The activated receptor activates many downstream effector molecules such as G proteins and many enzymes, finally translating the external signal into an internal stimulus. The activated receptor is phosphorylated by protein kinases, thus promoting arrestin binding to the receptor. The desensitized receptor along with arrestin is endocytosed and internalized, to be recycled to the plasma membrane.)

changes in its chromophore structure, upon absorption of light (Palczewski *et al.*, 2000). This, in turn, leads to changes in intramolecular constraints on the *'DRY'* motif found in the second cytoplasmic loop of this receptor (Palczewski *et al.*, 2000). Arginine in this motif is extensively conserved among GPCRs and plays a major role in the activation of G proteins and, hence, subsequent downstream signaling (Palczewski *et al.*, 2000). Mutations of this arginine lead to constitutive activation of many GPCRs like the cannabinoid receptor and the histamine H_2 receptor (Hager *et al.*, 1995; Rana *et al.*, 2001). However, there may be more than one interaction site between the receptor and its cognate G protein (Hargrave *et al.*, 1993).

Mutations in the ligand-binding sites of receptors have varied effects. For example, a lysine-to-glycine (K296G) mutation, in TM7, in the chromophore attachment site of rhodopsin, leads to its constitutive activation, which in turn leads to constitutively activated transducin (i.e. in the absence of light and 11-*cis*-retinal) (Robinson *et al.*, 1994). This has been implicated in RP, where degeneration of rods occurs due to the reduced usage of rhodopsin-inactivating machinery such as rhodopsin kinases (Sibley *et al.*, 1985). A specific aspartate (D^{100}) in TM3 of human 5-HT_{4a} receptor is necessary for ionic interaction between the receptor and the ligand. Mutating this residue to asparagine leads to inability of the receptor to bind 5-hydroxytryptamine (5-HT), thus stimulating cAMP production (van Rhee and Jacobson, 1996). A particular serine (S^{153}) in the extracellular loop 2 is highly conserved in the rhodopsin family of GPCRs. In human 5-HT_{4a}, this residue is replaced with a proline, which develops a kink in the TM helix of the receptor. Though this mutation has no effect on serotonin-induced cAMP production, it is necessary for ligand selectivity of this receptor (Mialet *et al.*, 2000). Serotonin receptor also has a hydrophobic ligand-binding pocket with conserved phenylalanine and asparagine residues in cytoplasmic loop 3 (F^{275}, F^{276} and N^{279}). F275A, F276A and N279L mutations of this receptor lead to decreased serotonin affinity of the GPCR. Moreover, double mutants of this receptor, just like the Y302A in cytoplasmic loop 3 and S197A in TM5 mutants, decrease both ligand binding and serotonin-induced adenylyl cyclase activity (Mialet *et al.*, 2000). Similar studies with prostacyclin receptor, whose activation is important for relaxation of vascular smooth muscle and prevention of blood coagulation, showed that mutation of a highly conserved arginine in TM7 (R279A) to alanine led to protein expression being one-third as less as what it was, and also its ligand binding efficiency, while a Y75A mutation in TM2 further reduced the affinity of this receptor toward the ligand, to be one-fiftieth of what it was (Stitham *et al.*, 2003).

Nicotinic acid receptor is implicated in mediating the anti-lipolytic activities of nicotinic acid (niacin). In addition to a tryptophan in the extracellular loop2 and /phenylalanine/tyrosine (W^{91}/F^{276}/Y^{284}) in TM7, in the ligand-binding pocket of this receptor, a specific arginine in TM3 (R^{111}) also plays an important role by acting as an anchor for the carboxylate ligands. A mutation of tyrosine at position 91, in extracellular loop 2, to serine (Y91S) showed that though this residue has no role in receptor activation, it remarkably decreases the ability of the receptor to respond to nicotinic acid. An R111A mutation in TM3 of the nicotinic acid receptor results in inability of the receptor to bind nicotinic acid even though the receptor is normally expressed and localized to cell surface. These residues are therefore crucial for ligand-dependant receptor activation. Moreover, C100A and C177A in TM3 and extracellular loop 2 mutations of this receptor lead to its decreased stability, meaning that these residues are important for receptor stabilization. They aid in formation of disulfide bonds between extracellular loop 2 and N-terminal tail of the receptor (Tunaru *et al.*, 2005).

Apart from mutations in the ligand binding pockets, there also occur mutations that disrupt the interhelical interactions of GPCRs, which affect receptor activation. Helix–helix interactions of rhodopsin have a highly conserved signature, with >80% amino acid identity across this family of GPCRs (Eilers *et al.*, 2002). For example, a serine-to-tyrosine mutation (S140Y) in 'DRS' motif present in the extracellular loop 2 of the somatostatin receptor leads to almost 100% increase in ligand binding efficiency, with ~60% increase in receptor internalization. However, a leucine-to-alanine (L140A) mutation exhibits no difference in affinity to the ligand, decreases the receptor internalization by ~50% and impairs G protein coupling to the receptor (Arora *et al.*, 1995).

Receptor Desensitization

Desensitization refers to the attenuation of receptor activity after ligand-mediated stimulus. This involves phosphorylation, uncoupling of the receptor from its cognate heterotrimeric G protein, internalization to vesicles from the cell surface and downregulation of receptor synthesis (Ferguson, 2001). Active state GPCRs are phosphorylated by second-messenger dependent protein kinases leading to rapid uncoupling of the GPCR–G protein complex (Gurevich and Gurevich, 2006). Phosphorylation of the receptor leads to arrestin binding, which in turn is responsible for the uncoupling reaction (Fig. 7.4). Arrestins also aid in endocytosis of the receptor into clathrin-coated pits (CCPs) by acting as adapter molecules. They link the phosphorylated receptor to the clathrin lattice through protein–protein interactions (von Zastrow, 2003). Many mutations in GPCRs have been shown to affect receptor downregulation and desensitization. A G22S mutation in 5-HT_{1A} leads to the attenuation of agonist-promoted downregulation and functional desensitization of the receptor. However, this does not have any effect on ligand binding (Ferguson, 2001). R16G, Q27E, T164I and C341G mutations lead to enhanced agonist-promoted downregulation of the β_2-adrenergic receptor. These mutations have been implicated in asthma, hypertension and heart failure (Sadee *et al.*, 2001). A specific arginine-to-histidine (R137H) mutation of the vasopressin receptor leads to constitutive desensitization by arrestin, implying that the phosphorylated receptor is engulfed by intracellular vesicles even in the absence of agonist (Barak *et al.*, 2003). This is implicated in nephrogenic diabetes insipidus (Barak *et al.*, 2001). It has also been shown that two non-conserved serine residues,viz. S^{188} and S^{421}, respectively, in the cytoplasmic loop 2 and C-terminus of 5-HT_{2A} receptor are extremely important for agonist-mediated desensitization (Gray *et al.*, 2003). Mutating these residues renders the receptor resistant to desensitization.

Receptor Endocytosis and Internalization

In the process of recycling GPCRs from the plasma membrane, GTPases (a class of enzymes that hydrolyze guanine triphosphates) such as Rab and Sar1 play an important role in trafficking of receptors. Many Rab GTPases have been identified that regulate ER–Golgi transport, endocytosis and trafficking of GPCRs between early, late and recycling endosomes and lysosomes (Table 7.3). While most of these Rab GTPases regulate internalization of the receptor from endosomes to plasma membrane or vice versa, some of them interact directly with the receptor. For example, Rab5 interaction with angiotensin II receptor type 1 (AT_1) receptor has been shown to be very important for fusion of endocytic vesicles (Duvernay *et al.*, 2005). Rab1 regulates export of cystic fibrosis transmembrane conductance regulator (CFTR) receptor by aiding in transport of the receptor from ER to cell surface in a cell-specific manner (Duvernay *et al.*, 2005). Similar to Rab GTPases, Sar1 GTPase is also essential for GPCR regulation and trafficking. Sar1 GTPase forms a complex with the structural coat complexes Sec23/Sec24 and Sec13/Sec31 heterodimers that help in deformation and budding of the COPI vesicle containing the receptor (Bickford *et al.*, 2004; Gürkan *et al.*, 2006). Sar1 GTPase is also important for the formation and budding of COPII vesicles in the ER membrane and, hence, assists in GPCR export from the ER. Moreover, it has been shown that the β_2-adrenergic receptor complexes $G_{\beta\gamma}$ and adenylyl cyclase II in the ER (Dupré *et al.*, 2006, 2007). Sar1 has specifically been shown to be necessary for ER export, membrane targeting and signal regulation of α_{2B}-adrenergic, β_2-adrenergic and AT_1 receptors (Dong *et al.*, 2008).

Table 7.3 *Different Rab GTPases Involved in GPCR Export and Trafficking to the Membrane (Gether and Kobilka, 1998)*

Rab	*GPCR*	*Function*
1	Angiotensin II type 1 β_2-Adrenergic	Transport from ER to the Golgi
4	β_2-Adrenergic	Recycling of internalized receptor from endosome to plasma membrane
5	Chemokine 2	Recycling of internalized receptor from plasma membrane to endosome
7	Opioid	Targeting to lysosomes for degradation
11	Muscarinic	Transport from endosome to plasma membrane

Endocytosis is the process by which the agonist-activated and -desensitized receptor is removed from the cell surface. Endocytosis of the desensitized receptor is important as it regulates the cell surface expression of the receptor and processes them for recycling so that there is continued signaling (Ferguson, 2001). Endocytosis leads to downregulation of the receptor for long-term desensitization (Tsao *et al.*, 2001). Though the most common mechanism of receptor endocytosis is arrestin dependent and/or dynamin/clathrin dependent, it can also be arrestin independent and dynamin/clathrin dependent, or arrestin–dynamin/clathrin independent (Santini *et al.*, 2002). Arrestin–dynamin/clathrin-dependent endocytosis involves the distribution of the receptor–arrestin complex into preexisting clathrin-coated pits. These invaginations then pinch off from the membrane with the help of dynamin (Sever, 2002).

Intracellular trafficking of receptors and their internalization are highly dynamic and regulated processes, which not only help in receptor desensitization but also help in dephosphorylation and resensitization of the receptor (Fig. 7.4) (Oakley *et al.*, 1999). The intracellular trafficking pathway of GPCRs is determined by many factors. Specific sequences in the intracellular domains of these receptors determine the course of the receptor pathway. A tyrosine-specific sequence has been identified to regulate GPCR endocytosis. The common $NP(X)_3Y$ motif found in the third intracellular loop of many GPCRs shows similarity with *NPXY* internalization signal (Pippig *et al.*, 1995; von Zastrow, 2003). Mutating this motif in β_2-adrenergic receptors leads to its decreased internalization; surprisingly though the same mutation in gastrin-releasing peptide hormone (GRPH) receptor has no effect (von Zastrow, 2003). It has been shown that phosphorylation of residues in the third intracellular loop of dopamine D_2 receptor by protein kinase C is necessary for both receptor desensitization and internalization (Namkung and Sibley, 2004). Similarly, in the case of M_1 muscarinic acetylcholine (mACh) receptor also, the receptor internalization signal is present within the serine/threonine-rich region in the third intracellular loop. This region is probably the site for phosphorylation and hence promotes receptor endocytosis (Moro *et al.*, 1993). Strengthening this view have been observations showing that binding properties of the receptors for arrestins lead to different patterns of internalization (Futter *et al.*, 1996; Shenoy and Lefkowitz, 2003). GPCRs have been divided into two classes based on their affinity for arrestin and subsequent trafficking patterns (Shenoy and Lefkowitz, 2003). β-arrestin directs Class A receptors, such as β_2-adrenergic receptors, to CCPs but does not internalize with them. On the other hand, β-arrestin is also internalized along with Class B receptors, such as the V_2 vasopressin receptor (Palczewski *et al.*, 1991) (discussed in the next subsection). This fate of β-arrestins is determined by self-ubiquitination–deubiquitination patterns (Shenoy and Lefkowitz, 2003). Arrestin ubiquitination and deubiquitination also play a very important role in determining the intracellular trafficking pathway of GPCRs.

Post-endocytic Pathway of the Receptor

Once a receptor has been internalized, it can either be downregulated or be resensitized. Downregulation is the process where the receptor is targeted to the lysosomes and degraded within them (Ferguson, 2001). Endocytosis promotes proteolysis of the receptor and their subsequent trafficking to lysosomes. Though accessory proteasomes or cellular endoproteases are involved in receptor downregulation, the exact machinery involved and the mechanism is still unclear (Tsao *et al.*, 2001). Ligand-induced conformational changes in the receptor and/or activation of downstream effectors control and regulate the lysosomal degradation of the epidermal growth factor (EGF) and β_2-adrenergic receptors (Pippig *et al.*, 1995; Futter *et al.*, 1996).

Receptor desensitization and resensitization are two very important mechanisms in the lifetime of a receptor. Decrease in receptor responsiveness to agonist with time acts as a feedback mechanism preventing receptor overstimulation. Receptor desensitization involves interaction of the receptor with various proteins like second messenger dependent protein kinases, G protein receptor kinases (GRKs) and arrestins (Ferguson, 2001). A receptor endocytosed to intracellular compartments or downregulated is also said to be desensitized (Doss *et al.*, 1981; Trejo and Coughlin, 1999). Receptor resensitization involves recycling of a functionally active receptor back to the membrane (Prossnitz, 2004). Like downregulation, resensitization is also regulated by endocytosis. The endocytosed receptor is brought in contact with phosphatases, which dephosphorylate the receptor, thus resensitizing it. These resensitized receptors are recycled back to the plasma membrane in a functional state (Pippig *et al.*, 1995 Pitcher *et al.*, 1995). Arrestin-free form of the receptor is recycled to the membrane with the help of various phosphatases and adapter proteins (Prossnitz, 2004).

The importance of arrestin in receptor internalization and resensitization is evident from the fact that in the absence of arrestin, receptor fails to recycle even though it is internalized. However, introducing arrestin into the cell reverses this defect. In the absence of arrestin, majority of the internalized receptors are found in the perinuclear-recycling compartment. But in the presence of arrestin, very little receptor population is found in the perinuclear recycling compartment, indicating effective entry and exit of the receptor from this compartment (Prossnitz, 2004). Interaction of β-arrestins with receptors can be in two different ways. In Class A receptors, for example, the β_2-adrenergic receptor, upon ligand stimulation, the activated receptor binds to arrestin. However, this interaction is stable till the receptor–arrestin complex comes in contact with CCPs and the receptor is internalized by the pit. Since the receptor binds to arrestin with low affinity, arrestin dissociates from the receptor just before CCP internalizes the receptor for degradation (Pippig *et al.*, 1995). On the other hand, in Class B receptors, such as the angiotensin II receptor type 1a, the agonist-activated receptor binds to arrestin with high affinity and this complex is as such internalized by the CCPs (Tohgo *et al.*, 2002). In addition to agonist-activated receptors, arrestins also bind to GRK-phosphorylated GPCRs with high affinity (Lohse *et al.*, 1992). Thus, arrestins must have the ability to recognize and bind many GPCRs in many different conformations. In β_2-adrenergic receptor, GRK phosphorylation increases the affinity of the receptor for arrestin. However, a tyrosine-to-alanine (Y236A) mutant of β_2-adrenergic receptor, which lacks phosphorylation by GRKs, is still able to bind to arrestins. In this case, arrestin ameliorates the internalization of the receptor by CCPs (Ferguson *et al.*, 1996). Moreover, it has been shown that rat thyrotropin-releasing hormone receptor loses its β-arrestin-dependent internalization property when threonine and serine casein kinase II sites in the C-terminus of the receptor are mutated as T365A, T371A and S383A (Hanyaloglu *et al.*, 2001).

OLIGOMERIZATION OF GPCRs

GPCRs were considered to be acting as monomers at the membrane surface. However, several reports have confirmed the presence of oligomeric nature of GPCRs at the membrane. It is now a well-known fact that most of the GPCRs belonging to the glutamate family under GRAFS classification exist in dimerized or oligomerized states (Jones *et al.*, 1998; Kaupmann *et al.*, 1998; White *et al.*, 1998). Oligomerization of GPCRs, however, can have varied implications; for example, the efficacy, affinity and potency of the ligand or agonist may vary for the monomeric and oligomeric receptors. Moreover, homo- or hetero-oligomerization of the receptor adds up to the functional activity and stability of the receptor variability, which might also affect its subcellular localization and desensitization. Finally, development of multivalent drugs with high affinity for the receptor that target specific oligomeric receptors and hence increase the selectivity of drug action may also be possible. For example, a thiadiazole derivative that is a potent multivalent drug which binds to m3 muscarinic receptor has 100 times higher affinity for the receptor than the conventional monomeric drug carbachol (Rajeswaran *et al.*, 2001). These oligomerized receptors can be held together either by covalent bonds like disulfide bonds or non-covalent bonds like hydrophobic bonds, or both (Nikbin *et al.*, 2003). The regions of interactions in the two receptors that come closer for dimerization are the coiled-coil domains present in the C-terminus or the TM helices. A coiled-coil domain present in the C-terminus of $GABA_B$ R_1 and R_2 receptors is largely responsible for heterodimerization of these receptors (Nikbin *et al.*, 2003). A motif present toward the cytoplasmic face of the sixth TM helix of β_2-adrenergic receptor is responsible for the homodimerization of β_2-adrenergic receptor. This has also been confirmed by competitive peptide binding assays (Hebert *et al.*, 1996).

The most common form of oligomerization occurs as homo- or heterodimerization, as opposed to oligomerization of the receptors (Milligan *et al.*, 2004). Dimerization affects ligand selection, as has been shown for dopamine receptors 1 and 2 (Maggio *et al.*, 1999). When these two receptors are co-expressed in cells, they readily dimerize. This leads to increased agonist binding sites on the dimer when compared to the monomeric receptor (Maggio *et al.*, 1999). This suggests that dimerization of the receptor affects affinity of the ligand for the dimeric receptor. However, on the other hand, ligand binding may also promote or inhibit receptor dimerization (Terillon and Bouvier, 2004). Studies with leukotriene B1 receptor and most of the glutamate family of GPCRs have shown that even though the receptors exist as dimers or oligomers, a single receptor within this complex is sufficient for activating its cognate G protein and subsequent downstream signaling (Hlavackova *et al.*, 2005; Pin *et al.*, 2005; Damian *et al.*, 2006). Homodimerization involves interaction of the receptors mostly via their C- or N-termini, but rarely involves the TM regions (Milligan *et al.*, 2004). On the other hand, heterodimerization involves interaction of TM regions of the participating receptors. Heterodimerization has been observed to be more common in receptors that are closely related than in distantly related ones (Milligan *et al.*, 2004).

Dimerized receptors can come in contact with each other via their TM regions in two different ways (Fig. 7.5). *Contact dimerization* occurs when two different TM bundles are packed due to

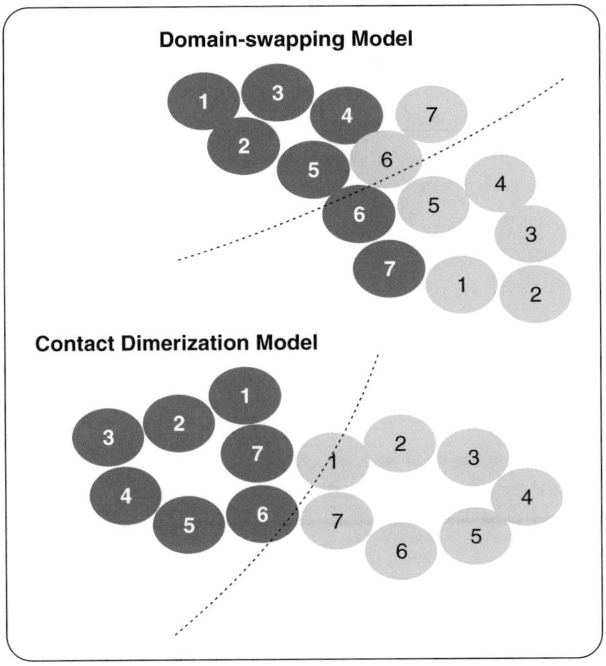

Fig. 7.5 ***Dimerization Models of GPCRs***

(Though dimeric models of GPCRs is becoming a widely accepted theory, two main models of dimeric GPCR activity have been proposed. Domain swapping occurs when TM bundles of the two receptors interpenetrate and the interacting TMs of both the receptors act as one receptor. For example, in this Figure, TM1–5 of one receptor (blue) interlace with TM6 and TM7 of the other receptor (pink) and act as one single receptor molecule. Contact dimerization occurs when the TM bundles of the two receptors come together that would otherwise face the lipid membrane, but each one has its own separate binding site.)

interactions in different binding sites at the interface that would otherwise face the lipid environment (Schulz *et al.*, 2000). It was first observed in rhodopsin, based on a two-dimensional (2D) electron diffraction map. The contact interface of the two tightly packed 7TM domains of the two receptors is located between the lipid-oriented TM receptor regions (Schulz *et al.*, 2000). The second kind of interaction is the *domain-swapped dimerization*, where polypeptides from two different receptors appear as interlaced units due to the interpenetration of their TM bundles (Gouldson *et al.*, 1998). In this kind of dimeric interaction, the two receptors exchange their N- and C-terminal domains and fold around the hydrophilic interface formed due to this exchange (Schulz *et al.*, 2000). Chimeras between muscarinic receptor and α_{2C}-adrenergic receptor support the domain-swapping model (Maggio *et al.*, 1993).

However, radio-ligand binding assays, site-directed mutagenesis, computational analyses, molecular modeling and receptor co-expression studies have localized the regions of GPCRs that are involved in cross-linking with each other, to TM1, TM4-6 and the cytoplasmic loops 1 and 2 (Paul *et al.*, 2004). Radio-ligand binding studies showed that dopamine D_2 and LH receptors exist as dimers (Ng *et al.*, 1996; Nikbin *et al.*, 2003). Immunoblot analysis of dopamine D_2 receptors expressed in insect cell lines exhibited two major bands, one 44 kDa and the other 90 kDA. Further, competitive peptide binding studies confirmed the existence of this receptor as dimer (Ng *et al.*, 1996). Presence of bradykinin B_2 receptor dimers was proved by cross-linking experiments. Endogenously expressed bradykinin receptors were cross-linked using maleimidobenzoyl-*N*-hydroxysuccinimide ester and later detected by anti-bradykinin antibodies. The agonist bradykinin was found to promote dimerization of the receptor (AbdAlla *et al.*, 1999). $GABA_B$ R_1 and R_2 receptors are inactive when expressed individually, although $GABA_B$ R_2 manages to fold properly and traffic correctly to the membrane. When co-expressed, these two receptors form functionally active dimers. It was suggested that on heterodimerization with $GABA_B$ R_1, $GABA_B$ R_2 masks the ER retention signal and in the process aids in proper folding of $GABA_B$ R_1, thus functioning like a chaperone (Nikbin *et al.*, 2003). Dimerization may also control activity of the receptor. β_2-adrenergic receptor dimerizes upon increased concentrations of the agonist as a means to decrease affinity of the receptor for the ligand by masking the second ligand-binding site (Limbird *et al.*, 1975). Another evidence for the role of receptor dimerization in activation of downstream signaling molecules comes from rhodopsin–transducin interactions. The cytoplasmic surface of rhodopsin is about half the size of heterotrimeric transducin. This suggests that each monomer of rhodopsin might interact with a different domain of the heterotrimeric G protein; for example, one monomer might interact with the G_α and the other with the $G_{\beta\gamma}$ subunit. This may serve as a basis for dissociation of the heterotrimer into G_α and $G_{\beta\gamma}$ subunits with subsequent release of GDP (Overton and Blumer, 2000).

Further, heterologous expression systems and a combination of different methodologies like co-immunoprecipitation, chemical cross-linking, bioluminescence resonance energy transfer (BRET) and Förster resonance energy transfer (FRET) have poured some insight into the biochemical nature of GPCR oligomerization. It has been shown that chemokine receptors CCR_2, CCR_5, $CXCR_1$, $CXCR_2$ and $CXCR_4$ exist as homodimers. CCR_2 is also known to heterodimerize with $CXCR_4$ and $CXCR_5$. $CXCR_1$ and $CXCR_2$ are also reported to heterodimerize with each other. These dimerizations are ligand independent. Hernanz-Falcon and co-workers (2004) have shown that TM1 and TM4 of CCR_5 are involved in dimerization by domain swapping. Mutating residues in these TM regions do not promote homodimerization and coupling to the cognate G protein and other downstream effector molecules. Similarly, in cells that express both CCR_5 and CCR_2 receptors, it has been shown that stimulating these receptors with ligands specific for both the receptors induces signaling that is 100-fold lesser than activation of the monomeric receptors. Moreover, homodimerization of CCR_5 and heterodimerization of CCR_2 with CCR_5 receptors have been shown to prevent entry of the human immunodeficiency virus (HIV) into the cell. This can be used to regulate and modify anti-HIV therapy.

The subcellular compartment where receptor dimerization or oligomerization occurs is yet to be established. Several studies report that oligomerization of the receptors occurs in the ER and that the oligomer is transported to the cell membrane (Overton and Blumer, 2000; Terillon and Bouvier, 2004). Disruption of the dimerization motif of β_2-adrenergic and α-factor receptor hinders cell surface expression of the receptors (Salahpour *et al.*, 2004). Oligomerization of the receptors masks specific signals or hydrophobic patches, which would otherwise lead to retention of the receptors in the ER (Nikbin *et al.*, 2003). Oligomerization of some other receptors has been shown to be ligand mediated. While some receptors maintain their oligomeric status throughout the signaling process, some others cycle between the monomeric and oligomeric states (Milligan *et al.*, 2004; Terillon and Bouvier, 2004). Moreover, some receptors, such as the α_{2C}- and α_{1D}-adrenergic receptors, use another GPCR, a β_2-adrenergic receptor in this case, to get a 'free-ride' to the plasma membrane (Uberti *et al.*, 2005; Prinster *et al.*, 2006). Similar studies with a truncated, ER-retained form of rhodopsin showed that in presence of wild-type rhodopsin, cell surface expression of the truncated receptor increased (Concepcion *et al.*, 2002).

As the picture about the monomeric nature of GPCRs changes to dimeric and oligomeric forms, drug-designing mechanisms also need to change to accommodate this new idea about GPCRs. Drugs have to be modified to act on sites other than the conventional monomeric sites on the receptors. Newer strategies that allow interaction of the drug only with the heterodimeric GPCR have to be developed. One such mechanism proposed by George *et al.* (2002) uses dimeric ligands. The monovalent ligands are covalently linked such that their interaction with the GPCR is stabilized. Such a divalent ligand, 6′-guanindinonaltrindole (6′-GNTI), has been developed that selectively recognizes the δ- and κ-opioid heterodimers and not the homodimeric receptors (Waldhoer *et al.*, 2005).

GPCRs IN SPECIALIZED MEMBRANE DOMAINS: LIPID RAFTS AND CAVEOLAE

Lipid rafts are planar domains present in the outer lipid bilayer of the cell membrane, which are enriched in specific lipids like glycosphingolipids and cholesterol. This makes the membrane more organized and rigid compared to the surrounding, less organized phospholipid bilayer (Brown and London, 1998). On the other hand, caveolae are 50–100-nm-diameter flask-shaped invaginations in the plasma membrane of certain cells. The characteristic shape of caveolae is due to the presence of caveolae-specific proteins caveolin-1, -2 and -3 (Chini and Parenti, 2004). Numerous GPCRs and their accessory proteins, such as G proteins, receptor tyrosine kinases (RTKs) and phosphatases, are found in these caveolae (Chini and Parenti, 2004). Some GPCRs are almost exclusively located in the detergent-resistant membranes (DRMs) under basal conditions (Chini and Parenti, 2004).

The molecular mechanisms underlying the avidity and subsequent trafficking of the GPCRs to these rafts/caveolae are not clear yet. Extracellular regions of GPCRs mediate signals for these mechanisms, as interaction of these regions with the lipids and/or proteins in the bilayer is feasible. Studies with EGF receptor have shown that interaction of the extracellular region of this receptor with gangliosides acts as a targeting signal for the localization of these receptors to DRMs (Chini and Parenti, 2004). Interaction of the TM regions of a receptor with lipids and proteins in DRMs dictates domain localization for agonist binding. Toward this direction molecular docking studies have shown cholesterol-binding sites on the α-helices of GPCRs (Politowska *et al.*, 2001). A caveolin-scaffolding domain has been implicated in the identification of caveolin-binding domains in GPCRs (Couet *et al.*, 1997). Caveolins also act as molecular chaperones and help in routing the receptor to the plasma membrane (Wyse *et al.*, 2003). Caveolin-1 is responsible for regulating the activity of many serotonergic and purinergic receptors that use $G_{q\alpha}$ for downstream signaling. Caveolin-1 also modulates the activity and is required for membrane targeting of 5-HT_{2A} receptors (Bhatnagar *et al.*, 2001). It has been shown that caveolin-1 promotes association of 5-HT_{2A} receptors with $G_{q\alpha}$ (Bhatnagar *et al.*, 2004). Caveolin-1 also interacts with EGF receptor although it seems to inhibit its activity, leading to internalization of the receptor (Couet *et al.*, 1997).

Lipid rafts have also been shown to render stability and to decide the fate of GPCRs (Kifor *et al.*, 2003). First, a GPCR can be localized to the rafts/caveolae upon agonist binding and then be internalized via rafts (Chini and Parenti, 2004). Second, the receptor might move into rafts after agonist stimulation, activate specific signaling events, move out of the rafts and eventually get internalized by CCPs (Wyse *et al.*, 2003). Third, the receptor may be localized to the rafts by default (Chun *et al.*, 1994). Finally, a receptor may be localized to lipid rafts by default but leaves the rafts after agonist binding, for internalization by CCPs (Chini and Parenti, 2004).

Cholesterol also plays an important role in the functioning and organization of GPCRs (Ostrom and Insel, 2004). This is evident from cholesterol depletion studies using different cholesterol binding agents. These compounds bind cholesterol and thus disrupt the architecture of the lipid rafts by depleting cholesterol in these rafts. Depletion of cholesterol from rafts rich in endothelin A receptor leads to diminished co-localization of Trp-1 receptor and decreased endothelin response (Ostrom and Insel, 2004). The cyclic nucleotide–gated ion channels show abolished response to stimulation by agonists in the absence of cholesterol from rafts (Brady *et al.*, 2004). Phosphosphingolipids and polyunsaturated fatty acids like docosahexaenoic acid (DHA) help in the efficient signaling of rhodopsin (Mitchell *et al.*, 2003). DHA also reduces rhodopsin activation and hence, the receptor's coupling efficiency with G proteins (Niu *et al.*, 2004; Barnett-Norris *et al.*, 2005). Loss of DHA in rafts of central nervous system and retina leads to defective learning, memory, olfactory discrimination, and so on.

CONSTITUTIVE ACTIVITY OF RECEPTORS

According to recent reports, about 40% of known GPCRs, such as the β-adrenergic receptors, H_3 histamine receptors and TSH receptors, exhibit a constitutive basal level of activity (Schöneberg *et al.*, 2004). This basal level of activity of the wild-type receptor is necessary for normal physiological functions. Any abnormality in basal-level activity indicates a shift in the ratio of basal level activated receptor and ground state receptor from the wild type. Such abnormally active GPCRs may lose specificity in signaling due to gain of functional sites, which may interact with more than one G protein family (Schöneberg *et al.*, 2004). To get an in-depth view of the diseases caused due to malfunctioning of GPCRs, an *a priori* knowledge about the receptor structure, activation, desensitization, oligomerization, signaling pathway, and so on, is essential (Morris and Malbon, 1999). GPCRs are activated by a wide range of ligands binding to different sites on the receptor. The binding sites for ligands may be within the pocket formed by the 7TM embedded within the membrane, as for biogenic amines, or pockets formed by the extracellular loops of the receptor, as for peptides, or in the N-terminus, as for glutamate, bradykinin, Ca^{+2}, glycoprotein hormones, and so on (Sadee *et al.*, 2001). Any mutations in these active sites of interaction may lead to altered ligand or cellular trafficking of the receptor (Sadee *et al.*, 2001).

For example, narcotic tolerance and dependence are regulated due to the constitutive activity of μ-opioid receptor (Burford *et al.*, 2000). The upregulation of constitutive activation of the receptor after treatment of a patient with opiates also accounts for this (Wang *et al.*, 1994). An opioid receptor can be activated by at least two ligands binding to different sites on the receptor. Peptide endorphins bind to the extracellular loops while opioid alkaloids bind to the 7TM core of the receptor (Befort *et al.*, 1996). Thus, ligand binding and structural integrity of the receptor for proper functioning and efficient signal transduction depend on the sequence variation of the receptor.

Many missense mutations cause constitutive activation of GPCRs (Ren *et al.*, 1993). A tyrosine-to-any amino acid (T373X) mutation in the α_2-adrenergic receptor leads to increased constitutive activation of the receptor, thus resulting in agonist-independent inhibition of adenylyl cyclase. This is due to activation of G_i protein by the agonist-independent activated receptor (Coughlin, 1994). Constitutive activation of GPCRs has also been implicated in many diseased states. A lysine-to-glutamine (K296Q) mutation in the TM7 of rhodopsin causes its constitutive activation, leading to RP (Keen *et al.*, 1991). An alanine-to-lysine (A357K) mutation causing constitutive activation of H_3 histamine receptor leads to accumulation of high levels of cAMP in the cell (Takahashi *et al.*, 2003).

Certain human diseases such as familial male precocious puberty, hyperfunctioning thyroid adenoma and hypocalcemia are caused due to certain mutations leading to constitutive activation of GPCRs such as the LH, thyrotropin and Ca^{+2}-sensing receptors, respectively (Han *et al.*, 1998). Constitutively active rhodopsin mutants have been implicated in retinal diseases. A glycine-to-aspartate (G90D) or an alanine-to-glutamate (A292E) mutation in rhodopsin is responsible for congenital night blindness, while a lysine-to-glutamate/methionine (K296E and K296M) mutation causes autosomal dominant RP (Hargrave *et al.*, 1993). However, the activated receptor need not always effectively transduce downstream signaling. For example, the K296E mutation-carrying mice are constitutively phosphorylated, bind β-arrestin and thus prevent activation of the cognate G protein, transducin (Li *et al.*, 1995). The R16G and Q27E mutations in a β_2-adrenergic receptor cause enhanced agonist-promoted downregulation of the receptor (Green *et al.*, 1994). These mutations cause altered agonist-mediated regulation, leading to nocturnal-type asthma (Han *et al.*, 1998). A lysine-to-asparagine (K47D) mutation-containing variant of the Ca^{+2}-sensing receptor has been implicated in the autosomal dominant form of hypocalcemia. This codon is essential for Ca^{+2} sensing (Okazaki *et al.*, 1999). Jansen's metaphyseal chondrodysplasia is caused due to gain-of-function mutations in the parathyroid hormone (PTH) receptor. The histidine-to-arginine (H223R) and threonine-to-proline (T410P) variants of the PTH receptor are constitutively active in an agonist-independent fashion

(Schipani *et al.*, 1997). Loss-of-function mutations like the glycine-to-serine (G40S) mutation of the glucagon receptor leads to decreased affinity of the receptor for glucagons and has been implicated in type II diabetes mellitus (Rhee *et al.*, 2000).

DISEASES CAUSED DUE TO MALFUNCTIONING OF GPCRs

GPCRs control a variety of physiological functions in the human body. Many mutations have been reported in GPCRs, which lead to improper folding of the receptors and their subsequent retention and aggregation in the ER. This means that any mutation in the genes coding for these proteins can cause acquired or inherited diseases (Table 7.4). Till date >600 loss-of-function mutations and >100 gain-of-function mutations have been found in GPCRs. Loss-of-function mutations prevent the receptor from reaching its destination or impair its action, if at all it manages to reach its site of action. On the other hand, gain-of-function mutations cause constitutive activation of the receptor or activation of the receptor in the absence of a proper ligand. Diseases due to the former are normally acquired and cannot be transmitted, probably due to reproductive inability and/or limited lifespan, while diseases due to the latter are usually inherited. Some of the diseases arising from gain-of-function mutations of GPCRs include hyperthyroidism, congenital stationary night blindness and dominant and sporadic hypo-parathyroidism, caused due to activating mutations of TSHR, rhodopsin and Ca^{+2}-sensing receptor, respectively (Schöneberg *et al.*, 2004). However, loss-of-function mutations are apparent only when both the alleles of the receptor gene are affected. Many loss-of-function mutations are responsible for diseased conditions like congenital nephrogenic diabetes insipidus, color blindness, dwarfism, and so on. However, certain diseased states are implicated due to the rare dominant negative effects of a loss-of-function mutant receptor (allele), as in rhodopsin. In the autosomal dominant form of RP, misfolding and improper trafficking of the receptor leads to the death of rod cells (Coughlin, 1994; Schöneberg *et al.*, 2004).

About 4% of defective receptor synthesis is due to problems in posttranslational modifications and splicing mechanisms (D'Souza-Li *et al.*, 2001). Large or complex insertions/deletions may lead to loss of signal sequences, which affect transportation of the receptor to its site of action. Such receptors are retained in the ER (Schöneberg *et al.*, 2004). However, when these receptors were transported to the membranes, they behaved properly. Many Rhodopsin and Secretin family (GRAFS system) receptors are believed to be involved in diseased states due to loss of disulfide bonds in their extracellular loops (Savarese *et al.*, 1992). Mutations in any other potential site may hinder posttranslational modifications of the receptor. Defective Rab GTPase trafficking of the receptors also leads to disease states (Gether and Kobilka, 1998). About 13% of the disease-causing mutations of GPCRs have been shown to induce agonist-independent activation of the receptor. These mutations are believed to be responsible for as many as 30 different monogenetic human diseases (Schöneberg *et al.*, 2004).

Mutations, Deletions and Polymorphisms

Many mutations (missense, nonsense, complex deletions or insertions), which may or may not affect the reading frame, may affect efficient transcript formation, thus influencing other downstream

Table 7.4 *Mutations in Various Regions of GPCRs, Implicated in Many Major Diseases, Classified based on Their Occurrence in the GPCR (Russo et al., 1995; Schöneberg et al., 2004)*

Region	*Mutant Receptor: Disease State*	*Mutations/ Polymorphisms*	*Functional Consequence*	*Features*
N-terminus	Rhodopsin: Retinitis pigmentosa	Thr4Lys Asn15Ser Thr17Met Pro23His Pro23Leu Gln28His	Affects N-glycosylation	• 36–154 residues • Motifs for N-glycosylation • Residues for intracellular trafficking (Arg) • Residues for proper folding (Cys) • Residues for ligand binding, activation, down regulation
	β_2-Adrenergic receptor: Nocturnal-type asthma	Arg16Gly	Increased agonist-promoted downregulation of the receptor	
	h5-HT_1A: Psychiatric disorders	Gly22Ser	Attenuated receptor downregulation and desensitization	
	M3 muscarinic receptor	Pro242Ala Pro505Ala Pro540Ala	Lower receptor cell surface expression	
Transmembranes	V2 receptor: Nephrogenic diabetes insipidus	Lys44Pro Trp164Ser Ser167Thr Ser167Lys Arg113Trp ΔVal278/279	Retention of the protein in pre-Golgi compartment, altered ligand binding	• 7α-Helices • Helix–helix interactions contribute to functional tertiary structure of the receptor • Receptor folding, stability, ligand binding, ligand-induced conformational changes for G protein coupling
	Endothelin B receptor: Hirschsprung's disease	Cys109Arg Trp276Cys	Defective receptor processing, transport, cell surface expression and G protein binding	
	Calcium-sensing receptor: Familial hypoparathyroidism and sporadic hypoparathyroidism	Phe788Cys Leu77Arg	Truncated receptor and hence no functional dimerization of the receptor	
	Dopamine 2 receptor: Schizophrenia	Pro310Ser Ser311Cys	Reduced ligand binding affinity	

(Contd)

(Table 7.4 Contd)

Region	***Mutant Receptor: Disease State***	***Mutations/ Polymorphisms***	***Functional Consequence***	***Features***
Intracellular loops	Class A GPCRs with E/DRY/H motif	Arg137His	Constitutive activation of the receptor, its interaction with regulatory proteins, impair receptor-mediated signal transduction	• Structural stability • Receptor interactions with signaling and regulatory proteins • Consensus sites for posttranslational modifications • Receptor desensitization and internalization
	V2 receptor: X-linked nephrogenic diabetes insipidus	Arg135Gly Arg135Leu Arg135Pro Arg135Trp	Unable to couple to Gs	
	Rhodopsin: Retinitis pigmentosa	Ala623Ile Ala623Ser Ala623Val	No release of GDP from the G protein even after binding to the receptor	
	Thyroid-stimulating hormone: Thyroidism	Gly185Cys Arg202Cys	Constitutively active receptor	
Extracellular loops	V2 receptor: X-linked nephrogenic diabetes insipidus	Arg334Cys	Impaired binding of ligand, reduced downstream signaling	• Disulfide bridges formed by the two conserved Cys residues of EL1 and EL2 • Residues responsible for proper receptor folding • Formation of ligand binding pocket
	$P2Y_2$ receptor: Cystic fibrosis and Chronic bronchitis		Altered generation of second messengers affecting calcium channels	
C-terminus	α_{1a}-adrenergic receptor: Benign prostatic hypertrophy	Cys492 variants	Varied palmitoylation sites	• Ser/Thr serve as sites for G protein receptor kinase phosphorylation and receptor desensitization • Cysteine residues are palmitoylated • G protein binding domain
	Endothelin B receptor: Hirschsprung's disease		Reduced ligand-induced intracellular calcium levels and inhibition of adenylyl cyclase activity	

processes of the receptor. Defects due to alterations at various stages of GPCR synthesis, processing and transportation are mainly classified into four classes, as shown in Fig. 7.6.

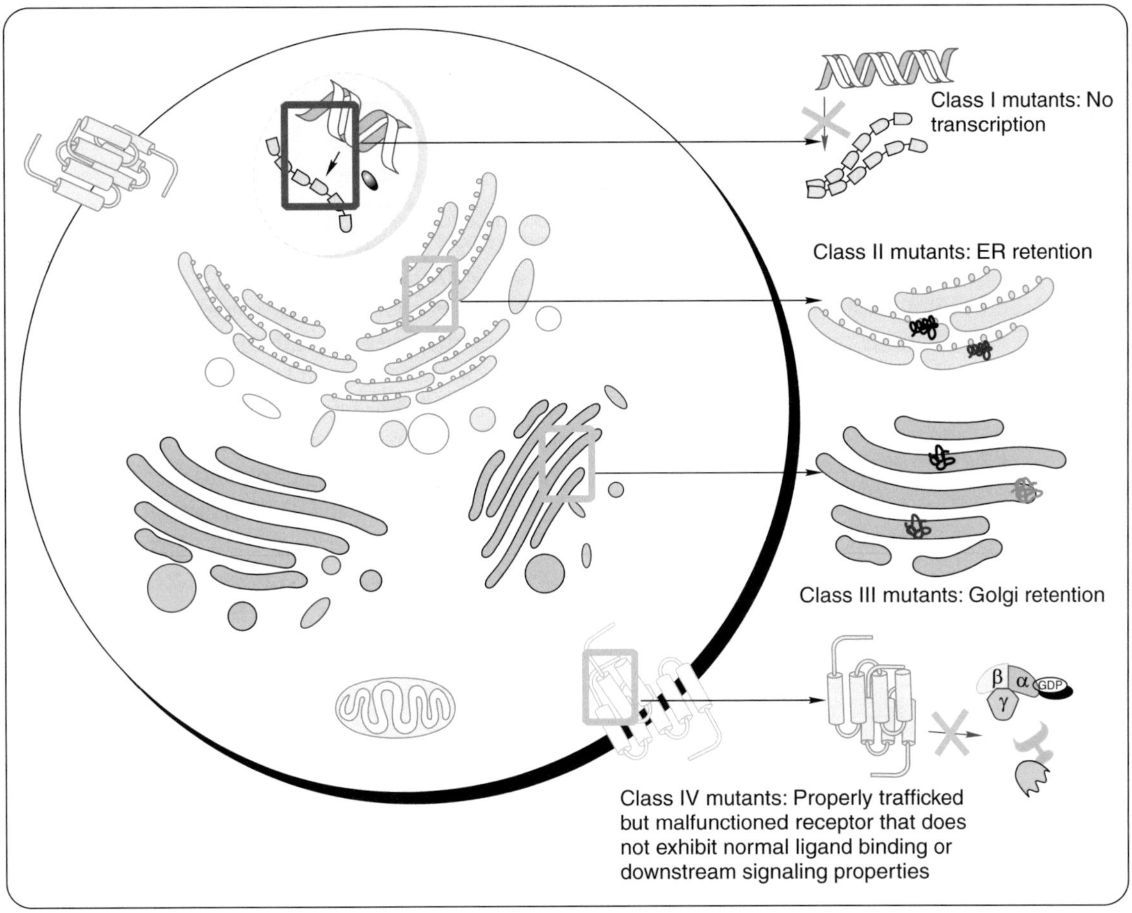

Fig. 7.6 ***Defects in GPCR Functioning Can Be because of Many Mutations in GPCR-Encoding Gene. Various Classes of Defects in GPCRs, which Lead to Their Dysfunction, have been Elucidated. (For color figure please see Plate 7)***

Diseases caused due to dysfunction of GPCRs are based on alterations at the genomic level or receptor biogenesis and trafficking. *Class I defect* of receptors implies either complete or partial deletion of the gene encoding the receptor or mutations in the promoter region of the same gene (Schöneberg *et al.*, 2004). The '*18q-syndrome*' is caused due to large deletions in chromosome 18 in humans, which harbors the melanocortin type 4 (MC_4) receptor and galanin type 1 receptor (Savarese *et al.*, 1992). *Class II* mutations affect stability and translation of mRNA, posttranslational modifications leading to accumulation and retention of the receptor in ER. A dominant negative mutant of MC_4 receptor is improperly folded and forms complexes within the ER leading to its retention in ER. A C271R mutation of the MC_4 receptor, implicated in severe early-onset obesity, causes misfolding of the receptor, as a new disulfide bridge is formed within the extracellular loop 3 of the receptor (Cody *et al.*, 1999). *Class III* mutations are those that affect the structure of the receptor, leading to inefficient receptor trafficking to the membrane and their retention in the Golgi. These mutations promote degradation of the receptor by trafficking them to endosomes or lysosomes. The K44P and Y128S mutations occurring in vasopressin V_2 receptor lead to retention of the receptor either in the pre-Golgi or the Golgi compartments, thus reducing its cell surface expression (Oksche and Rosenthal, 1998). Finally, *class IV* mutations affect receptor signaling by altering ligand binding and G protein coupling of the receptor. Mutations in the endothelin receptor, implicated in Hirschsprung's disease, though traffic the receptor properly to the membrane and also allow receptor–ligand interactions as in wild-type receptors, but still exhibit impaired coupling to G proteins. Such conditions are very rare (Inamura *et al.*, 2000).

Mutant receptors that escape the quality control check of the ER might end up showing inefficient binding to their ligands or may not get activated at all to transduce signals (Chapple *et al.*, 2001; Schöneberg *et al.*, 2004). Studies with mACh receptors and G_q/G_i coupled receptors proved that normal GPCRs could turn tumorigenic in the presence of excess ligands. Mutations causing agonist-independent receptor/G protein coupling were identified as a cause of many malignant tumors and carcinomas (Schöneberg *et al.*, 2004). The first clues of cellular transformation and GPCR signaling were obtained from '*mas*' oncogene, whose protein product has a typical GPCR structure (Whitehead *et al.*, 2001). Natural activating mutations of GPCRs cause hyperplasic growth of receptor cells. According to literature, about 80% of thyroid adenomas are due to gain-of-function TSH receptor mutations. Similarly, mutations in TSH and LH receptors have been shown to be responsible for thyroid insular carcinoma and testicular carcinoma, respectively (Schöneberg *et al.*, 2004).

Rhodopsin and Retinitis Pigmentosa

Rhodopsin is a prototypical GPCR, whose crystal structure was the first to be solved (Palczewski *et al.*, 2000). It is present in the membranes of photoreceptor cells and uses a photon of light to activate itself. Mutations in this receptor have been linked to many retinopathies, like RP and X-linked congenital stationary night blindness (Mendes *et al.*, 2005).

The gene coding for this 348-residue-long receptor has been mapped to 3q21-q24 (Bunge *et al.*, 1993). Just like any other protein, rhodopsin is also synthesized in the ER and transported to Golgi for posttranslational modifications. The post-Golgi rhodopsin vesicles are then transported to the outer segment of a specialized ciliary compartment where phototransduction occurs. Rhodopsin consists of an opsin apoprotein and a retinylidene chromophore linked to a conserved Lys in the TM region of the receptor via a Schiff's base (Menon *et al.*, 2001).

Rhodopsin is the first GPCR whose crystal structure was solved (Palczewski *et al.*, 2000). Crystal structure data show that rhodopsin has two mannose glycosylation sites in the N-terminal region. While helix III is the longest of the seven helices of this receptor, the cationic helix VIII (H8) is the shortest. H8 is formed by the region comprising of Asn^{310} to Cys^{323} (White *et al.*, 2001). This H8 is involved in interaction of the receptor with phospholipids in the membrane and also coupling of the receptor to its G-protein, transducin (Ernst *et al.*, 2000; Isele *et al.*, 2000; Marin *et al.*, 2000; Hessel *et al.*, 2001). Analysis of the crystal structure also shows the presence of a β-strand (Ser^{186}–Ile^{189})

in the extracellular loop 2, which is necessary for binding the chromophore via Glu^{181} and Tyr^{191}. Moreover, this β-strand is stabilized by disulfide bonding and forms a lid that traps the chromophore in its pocket. The chromophore 11-*cis*-retinal is covalently attached to Lys^{296} in helix VII of the receptor. The chromophore is completely buried within the TM regions, more toward the extracellular side, and is shielded from the external aqueous environment by the β-strands and extracellular loops of rhodopsin. Moreover, cytoplasmic loops 2 and 3 are also involved in the interaction of transducin with the receptor (Marin *et al.*, 2001).

Upon photochemical isomerization, due to activation of rhodopsin by light, a series of spectroscopically well-defined intermediates are produced, which also results in the conversion of retinal to all-*trans*-retinal. Metarhodopsin (R*) is one such intermediate that transmits signal of the absorbed light by rhodopsin to its cognate G protein, transducin. This interaction between metarhodopsin and transducin leads to an exchange of GDP for GTP on the G protein. This now active G protein–GTP complex activates downstream effector molecules such as phosphodiesterase which hydrolyze cGMP resulting in hyperpolarization of the rod membrane.

Mutations in rhodopsin gene and the receptor are so many that they have been divided into different classes. Class I mutations generally occur in the cytoplasmic C-terminus and resemble wild-type rhodopsin in trafficking to the membrane and binding to the chromophore. Class II mutations are more infrequent than Class I mutations in occurrence and lead to defective receptors that are not properly folded and are unstable. Mutations of rhodopsin implicated in RP have been tabulated (Table 7.4). More than 45 mutations, ~39 of which are amino acid substitutions, have been observed in the mutant receptor causing this disease. Although the mutations are scattered throughout the receptor, they are concentrated around the disulfide bonds linking extracellular loops 1 and 2, the chromophore binding pocket and the C-terminus (Tao, 2006).

Many mutations in the gene coding for rhodopsin have been shown to form the molecular basis of RP. RP is probably the best studied among diseases caused by defective GPCRs. It is a slowly progressive bilateral degeneration of the retina and the pigmented epithelium of the choroid. It is a group of photoreceptor dystrophies in which the rod and cone cells degenerate. RP is a form of retinal degeneration, wherein abnormalities of the photoreceptors or the retinal pigment epithelium (RPE) lead to a progressive loss of vision. Patients suffer from retinal dystrophy and night blindness, subsequently leading to complete loss of vision. RP can be autosomal dominant (20–25%), autosomal recessive (15–20%) or X-linked dominant/recessive (45–50%). One of the main proteins implicated in RP is rhodopsin, which is responsible for about 25% of autosomal dominant forms of RP (Berson *et al.*, 1991). Most of the RP mutations are missense, dominantly inherited and lead to a misfolded protein. Literature shows that retinal cells become apoptotic during RP, probably due to lack of proper multimeric complex formation in disk membranes (Abdulaev, 2003). Currently there is no treatment for RP. However, progression of the disease can be delayed by administering vitamin A intake (Berson *et al.*, 1993).

Thyroid-Stimulating Hormone Receptors and Thyroid Disorders

Mutations of the TSH receptor have been implicated in many diseases such as congenital hypothyroidism, hyperthyroidism, thyroid tumors and even the autoimmune Grave's disease (Paschke *et al.*, 1996; Nebel *et al.*, 1999). The constitutive gain-of-function mutations of the TSH receptor stimulate growth and differentiation of thyrocytes, leading to overproduction of the thyroid hormone (Russo *et al.*, 1995). This may lead to congenital hyperthyroidism due to transfer of thyroid-stimulating antibodies from mother to fetus. Activating mutations of the TSH receptor cause toxic adenoma and sporadic non-autoimmune hyperthyroidism, while inactivating mutations lead to hypothyroidism and resistance to TSH (Tao, 2006). Recently, a case of euthyroid hyperthyrotropinemia was discovered, wherein a mutation (Arg310Cys) in the TSH receptor leading to its constitutive activation was reported but the patient was resistant to TSH (Russo *et al.*, 2000).

TSH and its cognate receptor, TSH receptor, are the key regulators and modulators of thyroid function in the body. It was only about 40 years after the discovery of TSH was it found that this hormone exerts its functions through a protein in the plasma membrane (Uhlenhuth, 1927; Pastan *et al.*, 1966). Forty years since the discovery of the TSH receptor, though the crystal structure of the receptor is not yet available, we now know for sure that this receptor is at the center of many human disorders of the thyroid gland, including its role as an autoantigen in Grave's disease (Pastan *et al.*, 1966). Moreover, mice carrying natural inactivating mutations in the TSH receptor show impaired gastrointestinal immunity (Stein *et al.*, 1994; Wang *et al.*, 1997).

The TSH receptor belongs to the rhodopsin family with a large extracellular domain, which accounts for about half of the entire molecular size of the receptor (Kohn *et al.*, 1989 1995; Rees *et al.*, 1988; Singh and Curtiss, III, 1994). The gene for human TSH receptor has been mapped to 14q31 (Rousseau-Merck *et al.*, 1990). In addition to the thyroid tissue, this gene is also expressed in lymphocytes, adipocytes, retro-ocular fibroblasts, neuronal cells and astrocytes, though the possible function of this extrapituitary secretion is not understood (Mengistu *et al.*, 1994; Paschke and Geenen, 1995; Graves and Davies, 2000; Crisanti *et al.*, 2001). This gene codes for the 764-amino-acid-long TSH receptor with a molecular weight (m.w.) of 86.5 kDa.

The receptor consists of a long hydrophilic domain (1–418), in addition to seven hydrophobic TM regions with extracellular and intracellular loops (419–682) and a short C-terminus (683–764). The receptor also has leucine-rich repeats, characteristic of glycoprotein hormones (Kajava *et al.*, 1995; Bhowmick *et al.*, 1996). Homology modeling of the extracellular domain of the TSH receptor with porcine ribonuclease inhibitor, the first protein in which the leucine-rich repeats were discovered, showed that the extracellular domain of TSH receptor has six to nine leucine-rich repeats. These repeats, each of which is a β-sheet, is oriented toward the interior circumference of a horseshoe-like tertiary structure to which the hormone binds. However, TSH receptor differs from these glycoprotein hormone receptors as it undergoes many more activating gain-of-function mutations than any other glycoprotein hormone receptor (van Sande *et al.*, 1995; Vassart *et al.*, 1995). Moreover, the extracellular domains of some of the mature TSH receptors also get cleaved into two subunits, subunit A and subunit B. Also, a proteolytic degradation or cleavage of a small portion of the extracellular domain of this receptor is necessary for a functionally active receptor (Rees *et al.*, 1988; Zhang *et al.*, 1995; van Sande *et al.*, 1996; Rapoport *et al.*, 1998). However, the significance of this cleavage into two subunits is not yet clear (Rapoport *et al.*, 1998; Graves and Davies, 2000). Also, unlike other glycoprotein hormone receptors, TSH receptor is considered to be quite noisy since it transduces signal via adenylyl cyclase even in the absence of its ligand (Cetani *et al.*, 1996). There also occur two unique insertions in the TSH receptor, an 8-amino-acid insert (38–45) in the N-terminal region and a 50-amino-acid insert (317–366) in the C-terminal region (Wadsworth *et al.*, 1990; Rapoport *et al.*, 1998). While the former insert is important for TSH and stimulating antibody binding, the function of the larger insert is yet to be determined. The four cysteines in the extracellular domain, $Cys^{24, 29, 31, 41}$, form the conformational epitope for binding of stimulating antibodies to the TSH receptor (Chen *et al.*, 2001). TSH receptor is posttranslationally glycosylated at $Asn^{77, 99, 113, 177, 198, 302}$, of which mutation of Asn^{77} and Asn^{113} leads to a significant change in the localization and functional activity of the TSH receptor (Russo *et al.*, 1991). Moreover, deletion of the signal peptide of TSH receptor prevents the *in situ* processing of the receptor as well as its glycosylation (Akamizu *et al.*, 1990; Ban *et al.*, 1992). Other posttranslational modifications of the TSH receptor include amidation and tyrosine sulfation. Sulfation of tyrosines in the extracellular domain of TSH receptor has been shown to contribute to the interaction of the receptor with positively charged residues in TSH and also help in binding to autoantibodies (Costagliola and Vassart, 2000; Haugen *et al.*, 1999).

Upon binding of TSH to its receptor in thyroid cells, the activated receptor stimulates the downstream effector molecules, which ultimately lead to release of secondary messengers like cAMP, inositol 1,4,5-triphosphate (IP_3) and diacylglycerol (DAG) (Vassart and Dumont, 1992; Szkudlinski *et al.*, 2002). This results in the regulation of thyroidal gene expression. The TSH receptor exerts its downstream signaling effect via a range of G proteins. Immunoblotting studies with subtype specific antibodies raised against different G protein alpha subunits showed the interaction of the receptor with G_i protein (Laugwitz *et al.*, 1996). Studies where membranes of thyroid gland were photolabeled with [α^{32}P]GTP showed the interaction of the receptor with G_s, G_o, G_{i1}, G_{i2}, G_{i3}, G_q, G_{11}, and G_{13} subtypes of G protein. Moreover, the TSH receptor stimulating antibodies increased the incorporation of [α^{32}P]GTP while the TSH receptor blocking antibodies completely abolished photolabeling. This means that G protein activation is mainly due to receptor activation and not a direct effect of TSH on the G protein (Allegeier *et al.*, 1994). However, TSH receptor mediates its downstream signaling mainly via G_s and G_q proteins, leading to activation of adenylyl cyclase and phospholipase C (Allegeier *et al.*, 1994). However, activation of phospholipase C requires much higher concentrations of TSH than does activation of adenylyl cyclase.

Many site-directed mutagenesis studies, molecular modeling, studies with synthetic peptides and various enzymatic and immunological approaches have helped identify the importance of the extracellular domain of TSH receptor for ligand binding and signal transduction. Studies, where about 98% of the extracellular domain of TSH receptor has been deleted, show that this leads to a constitutively active receptor (Zhang *et al.*, 2000). This means that the extracellular domain of this receptor inhibits constitutive activation of the TM regions. Moreover, such mutations in the extracellular domain and the extracellular loops of this receptor are the strongest activating mutations reported so far for TSH receptor (Duprez *et al.*, 1997). However, it is also important to note that these two regions play a very important role in ligand binding to the receptor and subsequent downstream signaling by the receptor. Deleting just the amino acids 339–367 in the extracellular domain of TSH receptor also led to a constitutively active receptor (Zhang *et al.*, 1995). Such constitutively activating mutations of the receptor help it to eliminate certain intra-receptor interactions, very similar to those occurring on binding of the ligand to the receptor. These mutations also vary the basal and TSH-induced activation rates of the receptor (Tonacchera *et al.*, 1997; Fremont *et al.*, 2001). However, deleting the entire extracellular domain led the receptor being trapped in ER and not trafficked to the plasma membrane. At least 10 amino acids in the extracellular domain are necessary for proper trafficking of the receptor to the plasma membrane. Numerous TSH antibodies binding to different parts of the extracellular domain of TSH receptor lead to its activation or inhibition (Rapoport *et al.*, 1998; Oda *et al.*, 2000). Parallelism between receptor binding and activation for various TSH mutants and no significant shift in $GTP_{\gamma}S$ on binding to TSH receptor implies that there occurs no distinction between the recognition and activation sites of the receptor (Akamizu *et al.*, 1994; Kosugi *et al.*, 1996; Szkudlinski *et al.*, 1996; Grossmann *et al.*, 1997).

TSH receptor stimulating antibodies or antagonists disrupt the interaction between the extracellular domain and the extracellular loops of the receptor, whereas TSH receptor blocking antibodies, also known as TSH analogs or agonists, promote the interaction between these two regions of the receptor and hence help in agonist binding to the receptor. These antibodies are central to the autoimmune Grave's disease. Studies also show that a peptide generated from amino acids 352–366 of TSH receptor which is used to produce specific antibodies against the receptor is reactive to most Grave's sera. This peptide forms the most hydrophilic region of TSH receptor and is also the most immunogenic region of the receptor. The C-terminus of the extracellular domain of TSH receptor that binds TSH and stimulating antibodies with high affinity is, however, not necessary for agonist response. Mutation or deletion of specific residues in the extracellular domain, Tyr^{385}, Cys^{301} and Cys^{390}, affects the affinity of TSH and blocking antibodies for the receptor but has no effect on stimulating antibody binding to the receptor (Kosugi *et al.*, 1991; Kohler *et al.*, 1996). Also, substitution mutation of $Cys3^{01}$ with Ser exhibits a 50-fold decrease in the K_d (affinity) value of TSH and 20-fold decrease in the EC_{50} value of TSH-induced cAMP release. Mutating the same Cys to Glu, though, almost completely abolishes TSH binding to the receptor, and does not show any change in TSH-induced cAMP release. Site-directed mutagenesis and peptide and chimeric studies have shown that Thr^{40} and Cys^{41} along with Leu^{57}, Ser^{69}, Ala^{71}, Phe^{72}, Ser^{74}, Leu^{75}, Pro^{76} and other specific residues (30–61) form the epitope for the stimulating antibody binding. Mutations of any of these residues in the TSH receptor do not bind any TSH nor induce any release of cAMP, even though the receptor is expressed normally on the cell surface (Kosugi *et al.*, 1993). Similarly, peptide studies have shown that TSH binding site on the receptor is between residues 303 and 382. The conserved Cys in extracellular loop of glycoprotein hormone receptors, Cys^{494} and Cys^{569} in case of TSH receptor, has been shown to be important for TSH binding and autoantibody interaction. These mutations are mainly localized in the intracellular loop 3 and TM3, though some of them have been found in other regions of the receptor (Russo *et al.*, 1995).

Grave's disease (first described by Dr Robert Graves in 1835), also known as Basedow's disease or Graves–Basedow disease, is the condition of goiter with exophthalmus (bulging or protuberance of one or both the eyes) (von Basedow, 1840/1945; Graves, 1835/1940). This is the most common form of hyperthyroidism in the world. It is a polygenic multifactorial disease without the Mendelian pattern of inheritance. This disease is more common in women than in men, though a clear-cut genetic factor has not been found yet. Grave's disease is an autosomal dominant non-autoimmune hereditary form of hyperthyroidism caused due to constitutive activation of the TSH receptor (Schöneberg *et al.*, 2004). Antibodies are produced against TSH receptor, and, in some cases, also against T3 and T4 thyroid hormones (Tomer and Davies, 1993). These anti-TSH receptor antibodies bind to the receptor and cause its constitutive activation. This stimulated TSH receptor causes overproduction of the T3 and T4 hormones in follicular cells of the thyroid gland. Excess production of these hormones leads to enlargement of the thyroid gland, a condition termed as *goiter*. Constitutive activation of the receptor leads to increased cAMP levels within the cell (Tomer and Davies, 1993). Expression of TSH receptor in retro-orbital and connective tissue is responsible for extrathyroidal manifestations of this disease, as in ophthalmopathy and pretibial myxedema. This disease can be treated with the help of antithyroid drugs (such as carbimazole, methimazole and propylthiouracil) or by thyroidectomy (removal of the thyroid gland). TSH receptor antagonists or stimulating antibodies that block the actions of the receptor can also help in treating the disease.

T cells and B cells that are reactive to thyroid antigens, including the TSH receptor, infiltrate the thyroid gland, leading to the production of antibodies against the receptor. This results in hyperthyroidism with thyroiditis, associated with thyroglobulin and thyroid peroxidase. Owing to these factors, Grave's disease is categorized as autoimmune thyroiditis type 3. Grave's thyroid gland is enlarged due to hypertrophy and hyperplasia of thyroid follicles. Antibodies to thyroglobulin and thyroid peroxidase are also observed in Grave's patients. There also occurs spontaneous hypothyroidism in about 25% of Grave's patients. This disease occurs in about 1% of women and 0.1% of men. However, there is a 30–50% concordance in monozygotic twins and about 7% incidence in HLA-identical siblings (Tomlinson *et al.*, 2008).

Currently, there are three types of antibodies against TSH receptors: thyroid stimulating immunoglobulins that act as long-acting thyroid stimulants, thyroid growth immunoglobulins and thyrotropin-binding inhibiting immunoglobulins. Thyroid stimulating immunoglobulins are usually the IgG class of antibodies which stimulate the cells much slower and longer than the TSH receptor, thus leading to excess hormonal production. Thyroid growth immunoglobulins bind to the TSH receptor directly and cause growth of the follicular cells in the thyroid gland. Thyrotropin-binding inhibiting immunoglobulins, as the name indicates, inhibit binding of TSH to its receptor. Moreover, these antibodies mimic TSH binding to the receptor, thus causing thyroid hormone production.

Hashimoto's thyroiditis is the first autoimmune disease to be discovered. This autoimmune disease was first described by Hashimoto Hakara in 1912 when he came across four cases of goiter and termed this condition as struma lymphomatosa or lymphomatous goiter. However, the autoimmune nature of this disease was established only when Roitt *et al.* (1956) discovered autoantibodies against thyroglobulin in patients with Hashimoto's thyroiditis. An year later, autoantibodies to thyroid; peroxidase were also discovered in these patients. This disease, which represents itself as hypothyroidism or goiter or both, commonly affects middle-aged women and is the primary cause of sporadic goiter in children. Hashimoto's thyroiditis is associated with HLA-D3 and HLA-D5. Though this disease is known to have a high familial predisposition, it has also been found to be associated with Down's syndrome, familial Alzheimer's and Turner's syndrome. Moreover, Hashimoto's has also been found to coexist with other autoimmune diseases such as pernicious anemia, diabetes mellitus, chronic hepatitis, Sjögren's syndrome, adrenal insufficiency and also Grave's disease.

Though it is a common form of hypothyroidism, in some cases it can lead to transient hyperthyroid thyrotoxicosis, termed as *hashitoxicosis* (Kidd *et al.*, 1980). Autoantibodies are produced against thyroid peroxidase, thyroglobulin and the TSH receptors, which leads to destruction of the thyroid hormone–producing follicles in the thyroid gland (Volpe, 1979; Tomer and Davies, 1993). Etiology of this disease is unknown; however, genetic and environmental factors are believed to be involved. Like Grave's disease, viral or bacterial infection, especially *Yersinia enterocolitica*, is also assumed to be involved (Valtonen *et al.*, 1986; Wenzel *et al.*, 1991; Toivanen and Toivanen, 1994). Moreover, T cells in patients with this disease show restrictive antigenic response, indicating that specific antigenic stimulus, like an infection, is involved (Katzin *et al.*, 1989). Hypothyroid Hashimoto's disease is treated by taking thyroid hormone pills, which help in recovering normal thyroid levels.

Both humoral and T cell–mediated immune responses which activate CD_4 or helper T cells (T_H) are believed to play a major role in the pathology of this disease. Apart from bacterial and viral infections in the body which can elicit this activation of T cells, studies have shown that thyrocytes expressing HLA-DR antigen become antigen-presenting cells and hence expose thyroid proteins to the CD_4 T_H cells, thus eliciting autoimmune response. Upon activation, these T cells stimulate B cells to produce antibodies against thyroid proteins like thyroglobulin, thyroid peroxidase and TSH receptor. Recently, another pathway describing production of these thyroid antibodies has been proposed wherein the intra-thyroid cells having cytotoxic T cells (T_C) with suppressor activity are involved. However, another study shows that follicular cells in Hashimoto's thyroiditis exhibit deep staining for the death receptor Fas and its cognate ligand FasL. The apoptotic inhibitory protein Bcl-2 shows decreased expression in the thyroid follicles of Hashimoto's patients. The thyroid follicular cells in Hashimoto's also seem to have an antibody-independent thyroid cell injury which involves inducing apoptosis in these cells by upregulating Fas and FasL and downregulating Bcl-2 activities.

Many mutations in the TSH receptor also cause *hyperfunctioning thyroid adenomas*. Somatic mutations Asp619Gly and Ala623Ile in the TSH receptor have been implicated in these adenomas (Parma *et al.*, 1993). Specific missense mutations in the gene coding for TSH receptor that translate to F631C, T632I and D633E have also been identified in thyroid adenomas. These mutations have been observed only in DNA of thyroid cells and not in any other cell in the body (Porcellini *et al.*, 1994). Though currently there are no drugs that act on TSH receptor directly to treat hyperthyroidism, the first line of treatment includes drug therapy with propylthiouracil and methimazole, both of which act on the enzymes in thyroid gland. In cases where drug therapy fails, radio-iodine therapy is used, wherein the patient is administered radioactive iodinated water. This radioactive iodine is quickly absorbed by the hyperactive thyroid cells, which are destroyed rapidly due to radiation. In some severe cases, where both drug and radioactive iodine therapy fail, thyroidectomy is performed. TSH receptor antagonists are still in developmental stages. Hoermann *et al.* (1992) developed a peptide TSH receptor antagonist. This peptide is derived from human choriogonadotropin hormone and acts by blocking the TSH receptor completely. It also prevents binding of the blocking antibodies to the receptor and thus prevents cAMP production. Hence, this peptide can be a potential drug, especially for treatment of Grave's hyperthyroidism.

While TSH receptor antagonists can be used to treat hyperthyroidism and thyroid cancers, TSH receptor agonists can be used to treat hypothyroidism and in diagnosing thyroid cancers. Recently, Moore *et al.* (2006) developed a small molecule, thieno[2,3-*d*]pyrimidine **3** (Org 41841), that only acts as a partial agonist for the luteinizing hormone/choriogonadotropin receptor (LHCGR), but a complete agonist for the TSH receptor. Initial docking studies showed that this molecule formed hydrogen bonds specifically with TM3 of TSH receptor. The effect of this agonist was detected by measuring the amount of cAMP released. The mutation of a specific glutamate in the TM3 to alanine (E506A) disrupted the interaction between the agonist and the receptor. Moreover, docking studies showed that this small agonist bound to a cleft formed by TM3–6 of the TSH receptor. Further studies and clinical trials are yet to confirm the future of this chemical compound as a potential drug for at least a few, if not all, thyroid disorders. Recently, Neumann *et al.* (2008) developed another low molecular weight TSH receptor antagonist, NIDDK/CEB-52. Org 41841 was chemically modified by molecular modeling to produce this new antagonist that inhibits the activation of TSH receptors by TSH or the stimulating antibodies and will be useful to treat diseases involved in hyperthyroidism.

Melanocortin-4 Receptors and Obesity

The melanocortin receptors are unique in the sense that they are able to recognize different kinds of peptide agonists, encoded by the pro-opiomelanocortin (POMC) gene and two inverse agonists or antagonists, agouti and agouti-related protein (AGRP) (Smith and Funder, 1988; Dinulescu and Cone, 2000). The POMC gene is expressed in the pituitary, brain and some peripheral tissues like the skin, and codes for adrenocorticotrophin (ACTH), the melanocyte-stimulating hormones (MSH), α-MSH, β-MSH and γ-MSH, as well as the opioid peptide β-endorphin. While the agouti gene is exclusively expressed in epithelial follicular cells, the AGRP gene is expressed in the hypothalamus and adrenal gland. The five receptor subtypes are each coded by a separate gene. MC_1 receptor is expressed in melanocytes and is responsible for regulation of pigment production (Chhajlani and Wikberg, 1992; Mountjoy *et al.*, 1992). MC_2 receptor is a typical adrenocorticotrophin receptor and is expressed in adrenal cortex, where it regulates the synthesis of glucocorticoid hormones (Mountjoy *et al.*, 1992). Defects in MC_4 receptor cause dominant severe early obesity (Farooqi *et al.*, 2003). MC_3 and MC_5 receptors, though expressed in neuronal cells and cells of the exocrine gland, respectively, have not yet been characterized. Apart from the above, this set of receptors also play a role in adrenal steroidogenesis, energy homeostasis, exocrine gland secretion, inflammation and cardiovascular function. Table 7.5 sheds more light on these receptors.

Table 7.5 ***Melanocortin Receptor Subtypes, Their Genomic Location, Ligand Binding Affinities and Role in Human Diseases***

Subtype	*Chromosomal Location*	*Length*	*α-MSH Binding Affinity*	*Disease Implicated*	*References*
MC_1	16q24.3	317	8.4	Skin cancer Melanomas	MacNeil *et al.*, 2002 Mountjoy *et al.*, 1992
MC_2	18p11.21	297	9.8 for ACTH (does not bind α-MSH)	Pituitary adenomas Primary adrenal insufficiency disorders	MacNeil *et al.*, 2002 Kapas *et al.*, 1996
MC_3	20q13.2	360	8.0–8.4	Obesity Myocardial infarction	Gantz *et al.*, 1993b Schioth *et al.*, 1996 Oosterom *et al.*, 1999 Adan *et al.*, 1999
MC_4	18q21.3	332	7.4–8.0	Obesity Hyperphagia	Gantz *et al.*, 1993a Mountjoy *et al.*, 1994 Adan *et al.*, 1999 Yang *et al.*, 2000
MC_5	18p11.2	325	6.9	–	MacNeil *et al.*, 2002 Chhajlani *et al.*, 1993

The single exon gene coding for MC_4 receptor has been mapped to chromosome 18q22 (Gantz *et al.*, 1993a; Sundaramurthy *et al.*, 1998). The 332-amino-acid-long MC_4 receptor belongs to the rhodopsin family of GPCRs. Upon ligand binding (α-MSH), the MC_4 receptor activates the downstream G_s protein, which in turn transduces the signal by stimulating adenylyl cyclase, ultimately leading to the release of cAMP (Gantz *et al.*, 1993a, 1993b; Mountjoy *et al.*, 1994). This also forms the basis for assaying the functionality of the receptor by measuring cAMP and Ca^{2+}, in cells *in vitro* (Gantz *et al.*, 1993a, 1993b; Mountjoy *et al.*, 2001).

The MC_4 receptor binds to α-MSH and ACTH with equal and highest affinity (pK_i of 7.4–8.0), followed by β-MSH and with the least to γ-MSH (Adan *et al.*, 1999; Yang *et al.*, 2000; MacNeil *et al.*, 2002). However, the receptor also binds the native antagonists with almost equal or higher potency that it binds the agonist. Affinity of the receptor for its inverse agonist AGRP is 9.3 pIC_{50} (Fong *et al.*, 1997). Mouse MC_4 receptor binds to its antagonist agouti with a pK_d value of 7.3 (Kiefer *et al.*, 1998). The recombinant MC_4 receptor expressed in bacterial cells has been shown to have a pIC_{50} value of 7.06 (Rosenfeld *et al.*, 1998).

The stimulation of MC_4 receptor by α-MSH in the hypothalamus leads to a series of anorexigenic signals. These signals ultimately cause a feeling of satiety and hence reduce food intake (Farooqi *et al.*, 2003). Many inactivating mutations of the MC_4 receptor produce a dysfunctional protein, thus leading to a condition called *dominant early onset* or *severe obesity* (Biebermann *et al.*, 2003; Lubrano-Berthelier *et al.*, 2003). The first frameshift mutation in MC_4 receptor was discovered in 1998 and related to severe early-onset obesity. Till date about 80 mutations of the MC_4 receptor that may be nonsense, missense or frameshift have been linked to this disease. These mutations fail to stimulate downstream signaling of the MC_4 receptor, even when α-MSH is bound to the receptor. Hence, the downstream signals are not initiated and the person is left with a feeling of insatiety. Moreover, these mutations lead to a dysfunctional receptor, which is retained in the ER and hence exhibits poor cell surface expression (Nijenhuis *et al.*, 2003; Yeo *et al.*, 2003). The knockout mice for MC_4 receptor have been shown to become obese, hyperphagic, hyperinsulinemic and hyperglycemic (Huszar *et al.*, 1997).

These various mutations of the MC_4 receptor lead to abrogation of the receptor functions, either partially or completely. There can be null mutations (W16X, Y35X, Q43X and L64X, the first two in the N-terminal region and the last two in TM1) in the receptor, which lead to defective protein synthesis or accelerated degradation of the receptor resulting in a complete loss of the receptor pool from the cell. In addition to the various substitution mutations (TM1: S58C, N62S; intracellular loop 1: P78L; TM2: N97D, G98R, I102S; extracellular loop 1: L106P; TM3: I125K; TM4: R165Q/W; intracellular loop 3: N240S; TM6: L250Q; extracellular loop 3: C271R/Y and TM7: Y287X) that bring about a frameshift, there also occur deletion (CTCT at codon 148 in intracellular loop 2) and insertion (TGAT at codon 244 in TM7) mutations that lead to the defective receptor being retained in the ER. The N97D, L106P, I125K, I137T (TM3) and I316S (C-terminus) mutation-carrying receptors, though, are folded and trafficked properly to the plasma membrane, and have an impaired ligand binding efficiency, either due to decreased affinity or decreased ligand binding capacity. Defective receptors carrying D90N (TM2), I137T and A175T (TM4) mutations though effectively bind the ligand at the membrane, are not able to transduce the signal intracellularly. The mutation in MC_4 receptor gene translating into a D90N mutation in the receptor has been reported to be exerting a dominant negative effect. Just about a decade ago it was discovered that the MC_4 receptor deficiency leads to a co-dominantly inherited obesity syndrome.

Obesity refers to increase in the mass of adipose tissue and is determined by body mass index (BMI). Obesity is majorly associated with many other diseased conditions such as osteoarthritis, diabetes, cancer, cardiovascular diseases, blood pressure, blood cholesterol and the like. Like many other diseases, many genetic and environmental factors are involved in causing obesity. Various genetic disorders such as the Prader–Willi syndrome, Bardet–Biedl syndrome, diseases caused due to mutations in leptin and melanocortin receptors and leptin deficiency syndrome have been implicated with obesity. *Dominant severe early-onset obesity* first occurs in children under 10 years of age. Adults and children alike exhibit an increased resistance to insulin, leading to a condition called *hyperinsulinemia*. About 30% of these patients experience pancreatic β-cell failure and type 2 diabetes. In addition to hyperinsulinemia, these patients also exhibit *hyperphagia*, increased bone mineral density and early onset of puberty. This disease is inherited in an autosomal dominant manner, wherein heterozygotes exhibit obesity phenotypes, while the homozygotes exhibit much severe obesity (Hinney *et al.*, 2003). The obesity phenotypes in heterozygotes have been attributed to haplo-insufficiency because the MC_4 receptor molecules expressed by the normal gene copy are not sufficient to bring out effective functioning of the receptor in controlling food intake (Vaisse *et al.*, 2000). Farooqi *et al.* 2003 have shown that MC_4 receptor deficiency is also associated with hypertension and lowers blood pressure significantly. This suggests that MC_4 receptor also modulates blood pressure by exerting its activity on the sympathetic nervous system.

Many mutations of the MC_4 receptor have been implicated in dominant severe early-onset obesity. In a study by Vaisse *et al.* (2000), eight rare mutations were found in obese patients. A 47-48G insertion in the N-terminal region of the MC_4 receptor leads to the synthesis of an aberrant peptide that contains the first 16 amino acids as the wild-type MC_4 receptor, but also an additional 12 amino acids due to frameshift. An L250Q mutation in the intracellular loop 3 of the receptor leads to a constitutively active receptor that has increased basal activity and a 10-fold higher affinity for its ligand, α-MSH. T150I, I170V, R165W and I301T mutations lead to a receptor with decreased activation rates. Further studies have shown that these receptors have about 80% less affinity for α-MSH and hence the conclusion that receptors carrying these mutations either are not trafficked properly to the cell surface or have reduced affinity for the ligand. These various mutations of the MC_4 receptor lead to abrogation of the receptor functions, either partially or completely. There can be null mutations (T11S, W16X, R18C, Y35X, Q43X and L64X, the first four in the N-terminal region and the last two in TM1) in the receptor, which lead to defective protein synthesis or accelerated degradation of the receptor resulting in a complete loss of the receptor pool from the cell. In addition to the various substitution mutations (TM1: S58C, N62S; intracellular loop 1: P78L; TM2: N97D, G98R, I102S; extracellular loop 1: L106P; TM3: I125K; TM4: R165Q/W; intracellular loop 3: N240S; TM6: L250Q; extracellular loop 3: C271R/Y; TM7: Y287X) that bring about a frameshift, there also occur deletion (CTCT at codon 148 in intracellular loop 2) and insertion (TGAT at codon 244 in TM7) mutations that lead to the defective receptor being retained in the ER (Yeo *et al.*, 2003). The N97D, L106P, I125K, I137T (TM3) and I316S (C-terminus) mutation-carrying receptors, though, are folded and trafficked properly to the plasma membrane, and have impaired ligand binding efficiency, due to either decreased affinity or decreased ligand binding capacity. Defective receptors carrying D90N

(TM2), I137T and A175T (TM4) mutations though effectively bind the ligand at the membrane and are not able to transduce the signal intracellularly. The mutation in MC_4 receptor gene translating into a D90N mutation in the receptor has been reported to be exerting a dominant negative effect. Though treatment of severe early-onset obesity is through monitoring diet and physical activity, drugs which can effectively treat this disease are still not available. These drugs are being developed based on studies which show that presence of the mutated MC_4 receptor in the cell does not hinder the functional activity of the wild-type MC_4 receptor. Thus, drugs are being developed which can stimulate production of these wild-type MC_4 receptors in cells (Ho and MacKenzie, 1999; Yeo *et al.*, 2003).

Chemokine Receptors and HIV Infection

Chemokines are *chemo*tactic cyto*kines* that are produced by virtually all cells in the body. These chemokines have varied functions ranging from antimicrobial activity to leukocyte trafficking to apoptotic activity to regulating gene expression. They exert their activity by binding to specific membrane receptors, the chemokine receptors. Chemokine receptors have been implicated in many diseases like Chagas disease, lung diseases, inflammation, autoimmune diseases, cancer and even infection by the HIV (Table 7.6). Chemokine receptors are a class of GPCRs sharing similarity with the rhodopsin superfamily of receptors. There are about 18 subtypes of chemokine receptors in the human body that recognize about 50 different ligands (Table 7.7) (Yoshida *et al.*, 1998; Zaballos *et al.*, 1999; Homey *et al.*, 2000; Schweickart *et al.*, 2000; Yoshie and Zlotnik, 2000). These receptors are further classified, and hence named, based on the number and spacing of conserved cysteines, as CC, CXC, CX_3C and C classes. Of these, CC and CXC types are more common. In addition to these chemokine receptors, there also exist three other 7TM receptors that bind chemokines, namely Duffy receptor, D_6 receptor and CCX-CKR receptor (Nibbs *et al.*, 2003). However, the functional importance of these three receptors is yet to be established.

Table 7.6 *Chemokine Receptor Subtypes, Their Cellular Localization and Role in Human Diseases*

Subtype	*Chromosomal Location*	*Length*	*Receptor Cell Type*	*Disease Implicated*	*References*
CCR_1	3p21	355	T-cells, monocytes, eosinophils, basophils	Rheumatoid arthritis Multiple sclerosis	Su *et al.*, 1996 Samson and Labhe *et al.*, 1996 Amat *et al.*, 2006 Saeki and Naya, 2003
CCR_2	3p21	374	Monocytes, immature dendritic cells, memory T-cells	Artherosclerosis Rheumatoid arthritis Multiple sclerosis type 2 Diabetes mellitus	Charo *et al.*, 1994 Samson *et al.*, 1996b

(Contd)

(Table 7.6 Contd)

Subtype	Chromosomal Location	Length	Receptor Cell Type	Disease Implicated	References
CCR_3	3p21.3	355	Eosinophils, basophils, mast cells, T-helper cells, platelets	Allergic asthma Rhinitis	Samson and Soularue *et al.*, 1996
CCR_4	3p24	360	T-helper cells, mature dendritic cells, basophils	Graft rejection Parasitic infection	Samson and Soularue *et al.*, 1996
CCR_5	3p21	352	T-cells, monocytes	HIV-1 co-receptor Transplant rejection	Samson and Libert *et al.*, 1996
CCR_6	6q27	374	Regulatory T-cells, memory T-cells, B-cells, dendritic cells	Allergic asthma	Liao *et al.*, 1997 Baba *et al.*, 1997
CCR_7	17q12–q21.2	378	T-cells, mature dendritic cells	–	Schweickart *et al.*, 1994
CCR_8	3p22	355	Helper T-cells, monocytes, dendritic cells	–	Zaballos *et al.*, 1996
CCR_9	3p21.3	357	T-cells, IgA-positive plasma cells	Inflammatory bowel disease	Zaballos *et al.*, 1999
CCR_{10}	17q21.1–q21.3	362	T-cells	–	Marchese *et al.*, 1994
$CXCR_1$	2q35	350	Neutrophils, monocytes	Inflammatory lung disease	Lee *et al.*, 1992 Holmes *et al.*, 1991
$CXCR_2$	2q35	360	Neutrophils, monocytes	COPD Angiogenic tumors	Lee *et al.*, 1992 Murphy and Tiffany, 1991
$CXCR_3$	Xq13	368	Helper T-cells, mast cells, mesangial cells, microvascular endothelial cells, neoplastic cells	Inflammatory skin disease Multiple sclerosis Transplant rejection Angiostatic tumor growth	Loetscher *et al.*, 1998a
$CXCR_4$	2q21	352	Almost ubiquitous expression	HIV-1 co-receptor Tumor metastases Haematopoiesis	Loetscher *et al.*, 1994, 1998b Feng *et al.*, 1996
$CXCR_5$	11q23.3	372	B-cells, follicular helper T-cells	–	Dobner *et al.*, 1992
$CXCR_6$	3p21	342	Natural killer cells, memory T-cells, helper T-cells	Inflammatory liver disease Artherosclerosis	Loetscher *et al.*, 1997
CX_3CR_1	3p21.3	355	Macrophages, endothelial cells, smooth muscle cells	Artherosclerosis	Combadiere *et al.*, 1998
XCR_1	3p21.3–p21.1	333	T-cells, natural killer cells	Rheumatoid arthritis Nephropathy	Yoshida *et al.*, 1998

Table 7.7 *The Numerous Ligands for the Chemokine Receptors and Their Affinities*

Subtype	*Ligands*	*Ligand Binding Affinity*	*References*
CCR_1	CCL3 (MIP-1α) CCL5 (RANTES) CCL7 (MCP-3) CCL14 (HCC1)	7.8–10.2 6.8–8.2 8.1 7.4	Hesselgesser *et al.*, 1998 Combadiere *et al.*, 1995 Chou *et al.*, 2002
CCR_2	CCL2 (MCP-1) CCL8 (MCP-2) CCL7 (MCP-3) CCL13 (MCP-4)	9.3–10.2 8.6 8.4–8.7 8.6–8.7	Mirzadegan *et al.*, 2000 Lüttichau *et al.*, 2003 Uguccioni *et al.*, 1997
CCR_3	CCL13 (Eotaxin-2) CCL7 (MCP-3) CCL5 (RANTES)	8.7–10.3 8.6–9.2 8.5–9.3	Uguccioni *et al.*, 1997 Daugherty *et al.*, 1996
CCR_4	CCL17 CCL22 (MDC)	8.7 9.2	Imai *et al.*, 1998
CCR_5	CCL3 (MIP-1α) CCL5 (RANTES) CCL3 (MIP-1β) CCL14 (HCC1) CCL11 (Eotaxin)	7.7 9.2–9.7 8.0–8.9 7.2 7.7	Zoffmann *et al.*, 2001 Napier *et al.*, 2005 Ruffing *et al.*, 1998 Blanpain *et al.*, 1999
CCR_6	CCL20 (MIP-3β)	7.9–8.5	Power *et al.*, 1997 Baba *et al.*, 1997
CCR_7	CCL19 CCL2	7.7–9.0 9.3	Yoshida *et al.*, 1997 Yoshida *et al.*, 1998
CCR_8	CCL1	8.5–9.8	Dairaghi *et al.*, 1999
CCR_9	CCL25	–	–
CCR_{10}	CCL27 CCL28		
$CXCR_1$	CXCL8 CXCL6	8.8–9.5 7.0	Lee *et al.*, 1992 Wuyts *et al.*, 1998
$CXCR_2$	CXCL1 CXCL2 CXCL3 CXCL8 CXCL5 CXCL6	8.4–9.7 7.0–9.1 7.8–9.2 8.8–9.5 6.9–9.0 7.0	Lee *et al.*, 1992 Ahuja and Murphy, 1996 Wuyts *et al.*, 1998
$CXCR_3$	CXCL9 CXCL10 CXCL11	7.3–8.3 7.8–9.8 10.4–10.5	Weng *et al.*, 1998 Heise *et al.*, 2005
$CXCR_4$	CXCL12	7.7–8.2	Loetscher *et al.*, 1998b Hesselgesser *et al.*, 1998

(Contd)

(Table 7.7 Contd)

Subtype	*Ligands*	*Ligand Binding Affinity*	*References*
$CXCR_5$	CXCL13	–	Legler *et al.*, 1998
$CXCR_6$	CXCL16	1.0	Wilbanks *et al.*, 2001
CX_3CR_1	CXCL1	8.9	Garin *et al.*, 2003
XCR_1	XCL1 XCL2	8.0	Yoshida *et al.*, 1998

Though chemokine receptors share common structural features with the rhodopsin family of GPCRs, there also exist some unique features. Chemokine receptors have prolines in their TM regions, which are not found in TMs of other GPCRs. Upon ligand binding, the '*DRY*' motif in intracellular loop 2 and the '*NPXXY*' motif in TM7 play a major role in chemokine receptor activation (Aramori *et al.*, 1997; Gosling *et al.*, 1997; Ballesteros *et al.*, 2001; Lagane *et al.*, 2005). Typically, the charged Asp-Arg residues in the '*DRY*' motif form ionic bonds with residues in the TM6, which form an ionic lock. However, upon activation, these bonds are broken, leading to rearrangement of TM regions. This results in opening up the receptor for G protein access (Gether *et al.*, 1997; Ballesteros *et al.*, 2001; Ghanouni *et al.*, 2001). But owing to the large molecular size of chemokines, the rearrangement of TM regions of the chemokine receptor needs to follow a different mechanism, which is assumed to be provided by the occurrence of prolines in its TM regions. These prolines produce a kink in the TM helices of the receptor and thus also affect the orientation of the loop regions in the receptor. Studies have shown that a '*TXP*' motif in TM2 of CCR_5 and CCR_2 produces a kink in TM2 helix such that its extracellular end is brought close to the TM3 helix. This opens up the chemokine receptor for ligand binding and signaling (Govaerts *et al.*, 2001; Arias *et al.*, 2003).

Upon activation by a ligand, the chemokine receptor, owing to structural changes, couples to the G_i or G_o family of G proteins to transduce downstream signaling by inhibiting adenylyl cyclase activity and activating calcium channels, ultimately leading to the inhibition of cAMP accumulation and Ca^{2+} influx, respectively (Aramori *et al.*, 1997; Oh *et al.*, 2002). In addition, ligand-induced changes also lead to phosphorylation of certain residues in the C-terminus of the receptor. The phosphorylated receptor then binds to β-arrestin and directs the receptor toward internalization, desensitization and subsequent resensitization (Aramori *et al.*, 1997; Barlic *et al.*, 1999, 2000; Orsini *et al.*, 1999; Sun *et al.*, 2002; Richardson *et al.*, 2003; Galliera *et al.*, 2004; Oppermann, 2004; Lagane *et al.*, 2005). In receptors like $CXCR_4$, activation of the receptor results in binding of the ubiquitin protein to the receptor, thus directing the receptor for degradation to lysosomes (Marchese and Benovic, 2001; Marchese *et al.*, 2003).

The chemokine receptors have very high affinity for their ligands, ranging from pK_i 7.7 to pK_i 10.3 (Table 7.7) (Ruffing *et al.*, 1998; Baba *et al.*, 1999; Blanpain *et al.*, 1999; Zoffmann *et al.*, 2001). Ligand selectivity and binding by the chemokine receptor is a very complicated topic, mainly due to the fact that each ligand can recognize multiple receptors. The conserved cysteines in the N-terminal region and the extracellular loops of the receptor play a major role in ligand binding. Each of the receptors has four conserved cysteines, one in the N-terminus and one each in the extracellular loops. Cysteines in extracellular loops 1 and 2 form a disulfide bond, which is necessary for proper trafficking of the receptor to the plasma membrane and also for signal transduction (Blanpain *et al.*,

1999; Ai and Liao, 2002). Moreover, these receptors also have cysteine clusters in their C-terminus that are sites of palmitoylation and help in membrane anchorage, forming a fourth cytoplasmic loop. Mutating these cysteines produces palmitoylation-deficient receptors that are retained in the ER. However, these mutant receptors possess ligand binding activity similar to the wild-type receptor, but have reduced ligand-induced downstream signaling, as has been shown for the CCR_5 receptor (Damaj *et al.*, 1996; Percherancier *et al.*, 2001). Exceptions to palmitoylation are CCR_1, CCR_3, CCR_{11} and D_6 as they do not have any C-terminal cysteines. In addition to palmitoylation, sulfation of tyrosines also plays a major role in ligand binding by the chemokine receptors. Many chemokine receptors have N-terminal tyrosine clusters that are sulfated in the Golgi apparatus. It has been shown for CCR_5 receptor that sulfation of these tyrosines is essential for ligand binding and HIV entry into the cell. Moreover, peptide studies have shown that peptides derived from the N-terminal of CCR_5 containing sulfated tyrosines are able to interact with gp120 coat protein of HIV, while the unsulfated peptide does not bind to the viral coat protein (Farzan *et al.*, 1999; Cormier *et al.*, 2000; Seibert *et al.*, 2002). Like many rhodopsin family GPCRs, chemokine receptors also possess the typically conserved '*DRY*' motif in intracellular loop 2, which helps in G protein coupling and also probably in β-arrestin binding and ligand-induced internalization of the receptor. Moreover, mutating this *DRY* motif leads to a constitutively active receptor, as has been shown for $CXCR_2$ (*VRY*) (Burger *et al.*, 1999).

Owing to the functional diversity of chemokine receptors, many different assay methods have been developed to detect a functionally expressed receptor in *in vitro* conditions. The most commonly used assays are based on the measurement of amount of cAMP (a measure of cAMP accumulation as a result of G_i activation) and Ca^{2+} (due to Ca^{2+} influx as a result of activation of calcium channels) levels in cells, transfected with receptor and its subsequent activation (Zhao *et al.*, 1998; Baba *et al.*, 1999). Other methods for assaying the functional receptor include detection of apoptosis in neuroblastoma cells due to activation of caspase-3 (Cartier *et al.*, 2003). Oh *et al.* (2002) developed a novel assay method that uses Ba^{2+} as the charge carrier to measure Ca^{2+} currents in human embryonic kidney (HEK) cells that stably express N-type calcium channels and CCR_5 receptor. Detecting HIV fusion and infection in human HeLa cells expressing both CD_4 (cluster of differentiation) molecules and CCR_5 receptor also forms a reliable assay (Choe *et al.*, 1996).

HIV (discovered by Luc Montagnier in 1983) is responsible for acquired immunodeficiency syndrome (AIDS). HIV infection requires interaction of the viral coat protein gp120 with the CD_4 molecules on the target cell surface (Basmaciogullari *et al.*, 2006). In addition to T cells, it also infects mononuclear phagocytes and mucosal dendritic cells (Geijtenbeek *et al.*, 2001). Once infected, HIV affects the patient lifelong, more so due to the asymptomatic nature of the disease for as long as 8–10 years post-infection. Many key factors such as cytokines, immune system and other factors that favor or inhibit replication of HIV play a major role in controlling and balancing the diseased and healthy lifestyle of an individual. Recent reports indicate the involvement of a "co-receptor" also. Many co-receptors belonging to the chemokine receptor family (CCR_2, CCR_3, CCR_5 and CCR_8) have been implicated in HIV-1 infection (Gallo and Lusso, 1997; Berger *et al.*, 1999; Murdoch and Finn, 2000). The first report came in 1995 when Cocchi and colleagues (Cocchi *et al.*, 1995) discovered that three chemokines, RANTES, macrophage inflammatory protein (MIP)-1α and MIP-1β, were able to inhibit infection by HIV-1, HIV-2 and simian immunodeficiency virus (SIV). Later in 1996, Feng and co-workers identified a receptor-like cofactor involved in HIV infection and entry into the cell (Feng *et al.*, 1996). Coincidentally, in early 1996, the receptor for the above three chemokines was discovered and designated as CCR_5 (Combadiere *et al.*, 1996; Samson, Labbe *et al.*, 1996). Consequently, the role of $CXCR_4$ receptor was also elucidated in HIV infection (Berger *et al.*, 1999). Though *in vitro* co-receptor studies showed the probable role played by other chemokine receptors such as CCR_{2b}, CCR_3, CCR_8, CX_3CR_1 and others in HIV infection, they are still yet to be confirmed (Berger *et al.*, 1999). It was again in 1996 when studies showed that a 32 bp homozygous deletion in the coding sequence of CCR_5 gene conferred almost complete resistance to HIV infection (Liu *et al.*, 1996; Samson, Libert *et al.*, 1996). All this also led to a new system of classification for the HIV. For example, the β-chemokine receptor CCR_5 is required for infection by macrophage tropic strains of HIV-1 while the α-chemokine receptor $CXCR_4$ is essential for T-cell tropic strains of HIV-1 for effective infection (Lee *et al.*, 1998). Viruses that use only CCR_5 for infection are termed R_5, while HIV that use only $CXCR_4$ for infection are called X_4. However, dual-tropic strains of HIV that use both CCR_5 and $CXCR_4$ for infection are termed X_4R_5 (Wyatt and Sodroski, 1998).

HIV can be transmitted from infected patients to normal individuals by blood transfusions, mother-to-fetus transmission or sexual intercourse (the most common mode). Both X_4 and R_5 virions are present in the semen, but R_5 pathway is more common. This is due to the fact that spermatozoa express CCR_3 and CCR_5 receptors exclusively but not $CXCR_4$ receptors (Muciaccia *et al.*, 2005). HIV can enter the cell by combined interaction effects of the envelope protein gp160, CD_4 and CCR_5/$CXCR_4$ receptors. On binding to CD_4, gp160 undergoes a conformational change which leads to the exposure of its chemokine binding domain. This then interacts with the chemokine receptors to form a stable complex that aids in cell penetration (Chan and Kim, 1998). The chemokine receptor has very low affinity for gp120 as such, but this increases drastically when CD_4 molecule is bound to gp120 (Chan and Kim, 1998). The crystal structure of the trimolecular complex consisting of CD_4, gp120 and a single-chain human antibody is now solved (Chan and Kim, 1998).

The N-terminal domains of CCR_5 and $CXCR_4$, which are posttranslationally sulfated, are mainly involved in interaction with HIV-1 (Doranz *et al.*, 1997). Apart from this domain, the second extracellular loop of the receptor is also known to be involved in the interaction process (Brelot *et al.*, 1997). Many inactivating mutations, in the form of deletions, missense and nonsense mutations in the receptors, render incomplete, yet strong resistance to HIV-1 after exposure (Tao, 2006). Some mutations in the extracellular domain of the receptors impair, either completely or partially, ligand binding by the receptor, while others lead to intracellular trapping and poor cell surface expression of the receptor (Tao, 2006). A 32 bp deletion in the coding region of CCR_5 gene confers resistance to the cell against HIV-1 infection (Tang and Kaslow, 2003; Lusso, 2006). Due to this deletion, a receptor with only four TM regions is produced, which is retained primarily in the ER (Rana *et al.*, 2001). A recent report also confirms the involvement of this deletion in schizophrenia (Rasmussen *et al.*, 2006). Another polymorphism linked to CCR_5 and HIV is the m303 polymorphism. This mutation introduces a premature stop codon in the receptor. However, this has been observed to confer protection against HIV infection only in heterozygotes CCR_5-Δ32/m303. No homozygotes have been reported so far (Quillent *et al.*, 1998).

Current treatment for HIV is known as highly active antiretroviral therapy (HAART). Antiretroviral medications approved by the Food and Drug Administration (FDA) fall into six categories: non-nucleoside reverse transcriptase inhibitors (NNRTIs) such as delavirdine, efavirenz, etravirine and nevirapine; nucleoside reverse transcriptase inhibitors (NRTIs) such as abacavir, lamivudine, zidovudine and didanosine; protease inhibitors (PIs) such as saquinavir, atazanavir and ritonavir; fusion inhibitors such as maraviroc; entry inhibitors such as enfuvirtide and integrase inhibitors such as raltegravir. Chemokine receptor antagonists such as RANTES-derived peptides and specific derivatives of piperazine and spiro diketopiperazine that inhibit activity of CCR_5 receptors and SDF-1-derived synthetic peptides, 1-deoxynojirimicin and the like that target $CXCR_4$ receptors are in the pipeline (Nagasawa *et al.*, 1996; Schols *et al.*, 1997; Ma *et al.*, 1998; Baba *et al.*, 1999; Delgado *et al.*, 2001; Nardese *et al.*, 2001; Strizki *et al.*, 2001).

Dopamine Receptors, Schizophrenia and Parkinson's Disease

Dopamine is an important neurotransmitter in the brain that exerts its action via the dopamine receptors (Carlsson *et al.*, 1957, 1958). These receptors are key modulators of neuroendocrine signaling and hence control factors like motivation, learning and fine motor movement. It has also been implicated in several neuropsychiatric disorders such as social phobia, Tourette's syndrome, attention-deficit hyperactivity disorder, neuroleptic malignant syndrome, drug and alcohol dependence, schizophrenia and Parkinson's disease (Schneier *et al.*, 2000; Hummel and Unterwald, 2002; Mihara *et al.*, 2003; Faraone and Khan, 2006; Fuxe *et al.*, 2006; Kienast and Heinz, 2006).

It is almost three decades since the discovery of the first two dopamine receptors, D_1 and D_2, by Kebabian and Calne. It took another 10 years for the discovery of three more dopamine receptor subtypes, D_{3-5}. While dopamine D_1 receptor, found in striatal and retinal membranes, acts by activating adenylyl cyclase, dopamine D_2 receptor acts by inhibiting adenylyl cyclase or prolactin release or by inhibiting release of dopamine from dopaminergic fibres (Kebabian *et al.*, 1972; Brown and Makman, 1973; Seeman *et al.*, 1975; Creese *et al.*, 1976; Onali and Schwartz, 1983). An alternative splicing mechanism produces two subtypes of D_2 receptor, D_{2L} (long) and D_{2S} (short), which differ by 29 amino acids in the intracellular loop 3 (Dal Toso *et al.*, 1989; Giros *et al.*, 1989; Monsma *et al.*, 1989). Dopamine D_3 receptor, which is specifically localized in the ventral striatum, bears significant homology to its predecessor, D_2 receptor (Sokoloff *et al.*, 1990). Similar to the D_2 receptor, two different isoforms of D_3 receptor were also discovered, which differed in about 21 amino acid residues in the intracellular loop 3 (Fishburn *et al.*, 1993). Like D_3 receptor, D_4 receptor is also homologous to D_2 receptor and is expressed in extrastriatal brain regions (Van Tol *et al.*, 1992). D_4 receptor also has allelic variants, which differ by about a 48 bp imperfect repeats (Van Tol *et al.*, 1992). The D_5 receptor is highly homologous to D_1 receptor in function and signaling, and hence is also referred to as D_{1B} receptor. It is exclusively expressed in certain limbic areas of the brain (Sunahara *et al.*, 1991; Tiberi *et al.*, 1991). Hence, these five receptors can be divided into D_1-like and D_2-like. Upon activation by its ligand, dopamine, D_1-like receptors activate G_s proteins which then activate adenylyl cyclase, thus leading to accumulation of intracellular cAMP, while D_2-like receptors act by inhibiting adenylyl cyclase via G_i protein. Moreover, genes coding for D_1-like receptors do not contain any introns in their coding sequences, while the genes coding for D_2-like receptors carry introns, located in similar positions on the gene, in their coding sequences.

Schizophrenia is an archetypal major psychotic disorder. It starts in late adolescence. It can exhibit positive or negative symptoms. Positive symptoms include delusions and hallucinations, while negative symptoms include restricted affect, anhedonia and apathy. It is characterized by psychosis (loss of contact with reality), hallucinations (false perceptions), delusions (false beliefs), disorganized speech and behavior, flattened effect (restricted range of emotions), cognitive deficits (impaired reasoning and problem solving) and occupational and social dysfunction along with marked decrease in psychosocial functioning. About 10% of patients with Schizophrenia commit suicide. It occurs in about 1% of the population with 8 times higher prevalence rate in lower and higher socioeconomic classes. Of schizophrenics, 70% become ill between the ages of 15 and 35, with peaks between 15 and 24 in men and 25 and 35 in women. It affects men and women equally.

Excessive activity of the brain neurotransmitter, dopamine, has been implicated in this disease. It has been shown that drugs that block dopamine receptors, *phenothiazines*, somehow seem to reduce schizophrenic progression, while drugs that stimulate dopamine receptors, *amphetamines*, promote schizophrenia (Brown, 1994). Cell surface expression of D_1 receptors is highly reduced in schizophrenic patients, and, hence, there occurs reduced dopamine binding. However, D_2 class receptors (especially D_4 receptors) are expressed at a very high rate, leading to increased dopamine binding (Seeman *et al.*, 1993; Sedvall and Farde, 1995). In addition to dopamine, glutamate, another neurotransmitter in the brain, and its receptor have also been implicated in schizophrenia (Konradi and Heckers, 2003). Decreased levels of the metabotropic glutamate receptors (mGlu2/3) have been found in schizophrenic patients. Glutamate is also known to affect dopamine functioning in the brain (Coyle *et al.*, 2003). Based on these receptor systems, the 'dopamine hypothesis of schizophrenia' and the 'glutamate hypothesis of schizophrenia' have been proposed, which suggest pathologic involvement of the dopamine and glutamate receptors, respectively, in Schizophrenia (Seeman *et al.*, 2005; Lisman *et al.*, 2008).

Drugs that treat schizophrenia are called *neuroleptics*. Dopamine receptor antagonists form a major class of these drugs. These drugs act by binding to the dopamine receptor, thus preventing dopamine binding to the receptor, as a result of which there is no effective downstream signaling. Moreover, glutamate-blocking drugs such as ketamines mimic the symptoms of schizophrenia (Lahti *et al.*, 2001). Based on drug-related studies, serotonin 2C receptors are also believed to be involved in schizophrenia (Castensson *et al.*, 2003).

Parkinson's disease refers to a group of degenerative disorders of the central nervous system that lead to impairment of motor skills and speech, ultimately resulting in tremors, postural instability and loss of physical movement in advanced conditions. Many factors are responsible for causing these motor skill deficiences, such as genetics, toxins, head trauma, cerebral anoxia and, sometimes, even drugs (Jankovic, 2008). It is an idiopathic, slowly progressing degenerative central nervous system disorder. It is characterized by slow and decreased movements (bradykinesia and hypokinesia, respectively); at a later stage even they may become difficult to initiate (akinesia). These kinetic inabilities are caused due to muscular rigidity, restal tremors and postural instability. It normally affects people above 50 years of age, but very rarely is also seen in children (termed as *juvenile parkinsonism*). Statistically, it affects about 1 in every 250 above 40 years of age and 1 in every 100 above 60 years of age. Though, genetic factors are believed to play a major role in the occurrence of this disease, in very rare cases it is a late complication arising out of viral encephalitis (a very rare flu-like infection that causes inflammation of the brain). Many PARK genes have been identified that seem to play a role in Parkinson's. All these symptoms may lead to dementia and depression. Patients may also have orthostatic hypotension, constipation and urinary hesitancy. Clinical diagnosis is by identifying the patient's medical history and neuroimaging. It can be confirmed by other characteristic features such as resting tremors, decreased movements and/or rigidity. Infrequent blinking, loss of facial expressions, impaired postural reflexes and characteristic gait abnormalities also add up to efficiently diagnosing the disease.

Tremendous loss of the brain neurotransmitter, dopamine, has been attributed to be one of the main causes of this disease. It has been observed that about 80% of dopamine-synthesizing cells are lost from the brain. D_2 dopamine receptor has also been believed to be involved in this disease, since decreased levels of the receptor have been found in patients suffering from Parkinson's (Pizzolato *et al.*, 1993). Treatment includes administering dopamine or D_2 dopamine receptor agonists (Ferrari-Toninelli *et al.*, 2008). Typically, when the brain initiates an action, nerve cells in the basal ganglia help smooth muscles to coordinate postural changes by transmitting signals to the thalamus. The thalamus then transmits these signals back to the cerebral cortex. All these signals are transmitted by the chemical neurotransmitter dopamine. This disease occurs due to the depigmentation and loss (about 60%) of some very important nerves like the substantia nigra and locus coeruleus, which leads to depletion (about 70%) of dopamine in the brain. Moreover, loss of brain stem dopaminergic cell groups is also observed. Characteristic Lewy bodies are also observed in Parkinson's disease. Secondary parkinsonism occurs due to loss of or interference with dopamine activity in the basal ganglia subsequent to other genetic disorders, drugs or exogenous toxins. For instance, the antipsychotic drugs that are used to treat paranoia and schizophrenia block the action of dopamine on nerve cells. Parkinson's can be treated by a number of drugs such as levodopa, dopamine agonists, anticholinergics, antihistamines, antidepressants, propanolol and amantadine. Though none of these drugs can cure the disease completely, they make movement easier, thus adding up to the functional lifetime of the patient. A recent research suggests the implantation of dopamine-producing brain cells from human fetal tissue into the brain of person affected with Parkinson's. However, it is still in its experimental stages.

Glutamate Receptors and Alzheimer's Disease

Glutamate is the major excitatory neurotransmitter involved in exciting most of the neuronal synapses via ion channels and the ionotropic channels such as the N-methyl-d-aspartate (NMDA) receptor. The NMDA receptors bind glutamate as their ligand to fine-tune the amplification or inhibition of presynaptic, postsynaptic and glial mechanisms (Nakanishi, 1992; Schoepp and Conn, 1993; Pin and Duvoisin, 1995). For it to bind glutamate, the receptor must be open and the membrane must be depolarized. Depolarization of the membrane occurs due to a Mg^{2+}-dependent blockade of the receptor at membrane resting potential. Once activated, there occurs an influx of Ca^{2+}, which alters the properties of the neuron by stimulating many cellular processes. However, excess Ca^{2+} is also toxic to the cell and forms the basis of many neurodegenerative disorders like Alzheimer's. Though these receptors are responsible for learning, memory and development, they can also cause extensive neuronal damage and brain injury.

Some of the important features of NMDA receptors have been tabulated (Table 7.8). The NMDA receptors use two ligands—glutamate and glycine—for activation, and pass calcium ions to mediate synaptic transmission and neuronal plasticity (Liu and Zhang, 2000). About seven genes code for different subunits of the NMDA receptors, represented by a glycine-binding subunit-NR1, glutamate-binding subunit-NR2A-D and another glycine-binding subunit-NR3A-B (Cull-Candy *et al.*, 2001). The NR1 subunit has eight splice variants. Each subunit has an N-terminal region, a ligand-binding domain, a transmembrane region and a C-terminal region. These subunits form homodimers via disulfide bonding, as in Cys^{79} for $NR1_{1A}$ subunit (Schorge and Colquhoun, 2003; Papadakis *et al.*, 2004). The homodimers of NR1 and NR2 come together, face back to back and form the tetrameric NMDA receptor, forming an ion channel between the two dimers (Stephenson, 2006; Paoletti and Neyton, 2007). The varied functional diversity of the receptor is a result of different combinations of the subunits assembling to form a functional receptor (Chatterton *et al.*, 2002). Any mutations leading to misfolding of the region involved in formation of the disulfide bonds produces a receptor that is retained in the ER (Schorge and Colquhoun, 2003). Upon binding the dual agonists (glutamate and glycine), under proper membrane voltage, the receptor opens up, resulting in Ca^{2+} influx, which acts as a second messenger and modulates synaptic transmission and neuronal plasticity.

Table 7.8 *NMDA Receptor Subtypes, Their Ligand Binding Efficiencies and Their Role in Human Diseases*

Subtype	*Chromosomal Location*	*Length*	*Ligand Binding Affinity*	*Disease Implicated*	*References*
$mGlu_1$	6q24	1194	6.4–6.5	Parkinson's	Desai *et al.*, 1995 Stephan *et al.*, 1996 Dunah *et al.*, 2004
$mGlu_2$	3q21.31	872	4.9	Parkinson's	Flor *et al.*, 1995 Martí *et al.*, 2002 Johnson *et al.*, 1999 Tsai and Coyle, 2002
$mGlu_3$	7q21.1–q21.2	877	7.4	Dyskinesias	Schoepp *et al.*, 1999 Emile *et al.*, 1996 Johnson *et al.*, 1999
$mGlu_4$	6p21.3	912	4.9–5.5	–	Flor *et al.*, 1995 Thomsen *et al.*, 1997
$mGlu_5$	11q14.2	1212	6.1	–	Minakami *et al.*, 1993 Minakami *et al.*, 1994 Mutel *et al.*, 2000
$mGlu_6$	5q35	877	5.2	–	Laurie *et al.*, 1997 Hashimoto *et al.*, 1997
$mGlu_7$	3p26.1–p25.1	915	3.1	–	Wu *et al.*, 1998 Makoff *et al.*, 1996 Wright *et al.*, 2000
$mGlu_8$	7q31.3–q32	908	5.0–5.7	–	Wu *et al.*, 1998 Scherer *et al.*, 1997

The NMDA receptors contain various domains that help them interact with other proteins, such as the PDZ-domain containing proteins (PSD-95 and SAP-102), and direct them to ER and Golgi and ultimately to the cell membrane. NR2A has an ER export sequence, His-Leu-Phe-Tyr, in the C-terminus that directs it out of the ER, once assembled into a functional NMDA receptor (Hawkins *et al.*, 2004). PSD-95 and other members of this family, such as PSD-93, SAP-102, and SAP-97, modulate and regulate NMDA clustering and control its phosphorylation and dephosphorylation mechanisms. Moreover, this association also protects the NMDA receptor from calpain cleavage and also helps in cell surface trafficking and subsequent endocytosis of the receptor (Stephenson, 2006).

Once translated, NMDA receptors are variously posttranslationally modified. Some of the functions of the subunits and the receptor as a whole are mediated by these posttranslational modifications. Phosphorylation of serine and tyrosine residues in the C-terminus is the major form of posttranslational modification. The extracellular N-terminus is a major target for glycosylation. NR1 needs to be in glycosylated form for efficient dimerization with NR2 (Huggins and Grant, 2005). Moreover, cysteines in the subunits can also be nitrosylated. NMDA receptor activation produces nitric oxide in some synapses. This nitric oxide is responsible for S-nitrosylation of specific cysteine residues, as in the NR2A subunit. This also results in downregulation of ion channel activity. Many NMDA receptors are also subject to calpain cleavage. Susceptibility to this Ca^{2+}-dependent calpain cleavage depends on the maturity of the synapse and, in some cases, also on the state of the receptor. NR2 subunits are cleaved by calpain in their C-terminus. The receptors are also ubiquitinated, as a part of their degradation and internalization process.

Glutamate receptors have been widely implicated in Alzheimer's disease. Overstimulation of the NMDA receptors, which bind excess glutamate in brain, leads to cell death, and this condition is called *excitotoxicity*. Alzheimer's (first discovered by Alois Alzheimer in 1901) is the most common form of dementia which affects the memory, thinking and reasoning abilities of the affected individual. It usually occurs in people aged over 60 years (Brookmeyer *et al.*, 1998). Patients affected by Alzheimer's exhibit loss of neuronal and synaptic activity in cerebral cortex and certain subcortical regions of the brain. It is a progressive cognitive deterioration and is characterized by senile plaques, β-amyloid deposits and neurofibrillary tangles in cerebral cortex and subcortical gray matter. Loss of neurons due to extracellular amyloid deposition and neurofibrillary tangles leads to cerebrocortical atrophy, resulting in reduced glucose utilization. It accounts for about 65% of dementia cases in the old-aged and is the most common cause of dementia. Due to longer life expectancy in women, it is twice as much common in women than in men. It affects about 4% of people aged 65–74 years and about 30% of those above 85 years of age. Genetic and environmental factors have been implicated in this disease.

The first reports of the involvement of the NMDA receptors in Alzheimer's came in 1985, when Greenamyer and co-workers found that there was a 57% decrease in glutamate uptake in brains of patients suffering from Alzheimer's (Greenamyer *et al.*, 1985). Several studies later confirmed a decrease in the number of NMDA receptors in the hippocampal region of Alzheimer's brains (Geddes *et al.*, 1986; Greenamyer *et al.*, 1987; Represa *et al.*, 1989 Jansen *et al.*, 1990). Moreover, D'Aniello *et al.* (1998) have shown that Alzheimer's brains had reduced levels of D-aspartate, explaining the low functionality of NMDA receptors and hence decreased memory in these hippocampal regions. Several immunocytochemical studies supported the above data. Immunolabeling studies for NMDA receptor in the hippocampus of Alzheimer's patients exhibited a huge drop, owing to loss of hippocampal cells (Aronica *et al.*, 1998). However, the intensity of immunolabel was found to be almost the same, and in some cases much higher than control, in the remaining surviving cells of the hippocampus (Aronica *et al.*, 1998; Ikonomovic *et al.*, 1997). *In situ* hybridization studies later showed that there was very little or almost no NMDA mRNA expressed in certain parts of the hippocampus of Alzheimer's brains (Ulas and Cotman, 1997).

Treatment for Alzheimer's is by employing acetylcholinesterase inhibitors such as donepezil, rivastigmine and galantamine that improve daily activities and cognitive and neuropsychiatric symptoms. Recently, an NMDA receptor antagonist, mementine, has been approved for Alzheimer's, which slows the progression of the disease. It acts by blocking the NMDA receptors and, hence, preventing their overstimulation by glutamate (Lipton, 2006).

Alzheimer's is mainly believed to be caused due to accumulation and formation of tangles and plaques by the abnormally folded A-beta (also known as Aβ or β-amyloid precursor protein (β-APP)) or the tau (τ) proteins in the brain (Hashimoto *et al.*, 2003). APP, under normal conditions, is responsible for neuronal growth and survival, and repair of the wounded neurons (Turner *et al.*, 2003). However, due to unknown reasons, there occurs proteolysis of APP into a 39–43-amino-acid-long peptide, the β-APP, which aggregates to form senile plaques (Ohnishi and Takano, 2004). In addition, the τ protein, which is involved in microtubular stability, undergoes chemical changes, leading to its hyperphosphorylation and subsequent aggregation (Hernández and Avila, 2007). This leads to impaired Ca^{2+} homeostasis in the cell, thus inducing apoptosis (Yankner *et al.*, 1990). Clinical manifestations of Alzheimer's include early memory loss and visuospatial disturbances. As the disease progresses, patients may have hallucinations, get paranoid and also experience sleep–wake cycle abnormalities.

Serotonin Receptors and Depression

Like dopamine and NMDA, serotonin is also a major neurotransmitter in the body. A study suggested that there occurred reduced or no RNA editing of these serotonin receptors in schizophrenic patients (Sodhi *et al.*, 2001). Since these receptors are almost ubiquitously present in the body, from the gastrointestinal tract to the cardiovascular and central nervous systems, they have been implicated in a wide range of diseases, such as irritable bowel syndrome, psychiatric illnesses (like schizophrenia and mood disorders), Alzheimer's, behavioral problems and also some cardiopulmonary diseases.

Serotonin receptors belong to Class A rhodopsin family of GPCRs. The transmembrane regions bind the ligand serotonin or 5-HT, hence these receptors are also called 5-HT receptors (Kroeze *et al.*, 2002). There are six classes of 5-HT receptors in mammals: 5-HT_1 (5-HT_{1A}, 5-HT_{1B}, 5-HT_{1D}, 5-HT_{1E}, 5-HT_{1F}), 5-HT_2 (5-HT_{2A}, 5-HT_{2B}, 5-HT_{2C}), 5-HT_4, 5-HT_5 (5-HT_{5A}, 5-HT_{5B}), 5-HT_6 and 5-HT_7. This diversity is a result of alternative splicing and RNA editing. Indeed, RNA editing of the mRNA coding for these serotonin receptors plays a very important role in determining the functional diversity and activity of the receptor. RNA editing with adenosine deaminase has been shown to control the constitutive activation of the receptor, thus regulating the maximum constitutive activation exhibited by the unedited receptor. This editing leads to a variant of the receptor in intracellular loop 2, which in turn also affects the receptor–G-protein coupling (Burns *et al.*, 1997; Fitzgerald *et al.*, 1999; Niswender *et al.*, 1999; Wang *et al.*, 2000). In some cases, RNA editing has been shown to affect the interaction of the receptor with arrestins and G protein receptor kinases (GRKs), thus affecting the desensitization and internalization of the receptor (Flomen *et al.*, 2004). Important characteristic features of the genomic organization and ligand-binding efficiencies of the serotonin receptor subtypes have been tabulated (Table 7.9).

Table 7.9 ***Serotonin Receptor Subtypes and Their Dual Ligand Binding Constants and the Human Diseases Implicated***

Subtype	*Chromosomal Location*	*Length*	*Ligand Binding Affinity*		*Disease Implicated*	*References*
			5-HT	*5-CT*		
5-HT_{1A}	5q11.2–q13	422	9.1–9.7	9.4–10.3	Schizophrenia Substance abuse disorder	Fargin *et al.*, 1989 Stam *et al.*, 1992 Newman-Tancredi *et al.*, 1992 Newman-Tancredi *et al.*, 1998
5-HT_{1B}	6q13	390	7.4–9.0	7.7–8.8	Lung cancer Pulmonary hypertension	Parker *et al.*, 1993 Mochizuki *et al.*, 1992 Weinshank *et al.*, 1992 Takai *et al.*, 2001 Kaumann and Levy, 2006
5-HT_{1D}	1p36.3–p34.3	377	8.0–9.0	8.6–9.2	Migraine Neurogenic inflammation	Weinshank *et al.*, 1992 Leysen *et al.*, 1996 Hamblin and Metcalf, 1991 Hamel *et al.*, 1993 Petty *et al.*, 1997
5-HT_{1E}	6q14–q15	365	8.0–8.2	5.1–5.5	Neuroblastomas	Zgombick *et al.*, 1992 Levy *et al.*, 1994 Adham *et al.*, 1993 McAllister *et al.*, 1992 Pranzatelli, 1992
5-HT_{1F}	3p12	366	7.7–8.0	6.1	Migraine headaches	Adham *et al.*, 1993 Adham *et al.*, 1997 VanDenBrink *et al.*, 1998
5-HT_{2A}	13q14–q21	471	6.0–8.4	6.5	Schizophrenia Depression Alzheimer's	Stam *et al.*, 1992 Knight *et al.*, 2004
5-HT_{2B}	2q36.3–q37.1	481	7.9–8.4	6.7–6.9	Pulmonary hypertension	Schmuck *et al.*, 1994 Kursar *et al.*, 1994 Kaumann and Levy, 2006
5-HT_{2C}	Xq24	458	6.8–8.6	5.2–6.7	Obesity	Stam *et al.*, 1994 Knight *et al.*, 2004 McCarthy *et al.*, 2005
5-HT_{4}	5q31–q33	387	5.9–7.0	–	Stress-induced anorexia Hypersensitivity	Blondel *et al.*, 1998 Mialet *et al.*, 2000 Compan *et al.*, 2004

(Contd)

(Table 7.9 Contd)

Subtype	*Chromosomal Location*	*Length*	*Ligand Binding Affinity*		*Disease Implicated*	*References*
			5-HT	*5-CT*		
5-HT_{5A}	7q36.1	357	6.7–6.9	7.6–7.7	Schizophrenia	Rees *et al.*, 1994 Grailhe *et al.*, 2001 Birkett *et al.*, 2000
5-HT_6	1p36–p35	440	6.8–7.5	6.1	Parkinson's	Kohen *et al.*, 1996 Boess *et al.*, 1997
5-HT_7	10q21–q24	479	–	9.0–10.0	Migraine	Stam *et al.*, 1997 Krobert *et al.*, 2001 Thomas *et al.*, 1998

Of all the 5-HT receptors, 5-HT_1 and 5-HT_2 classes are the best studied. Upon ligand binding, the 5-HT_1 and 5-HT_5 receptors are activated and transduce the signal intracellularly by activating the G_i or G_o class of G-proteins. However, some reports suggest the accumulation of cAMP by these serotonin receptors via G_{i2} and adenylyl cyclase II activation (Nichols and Nichols, 2008). Moreover, these receptors also act by opening up K^+ channels, leading to neuronal hyperpolarization. 5-HT_2 receptors mediate their action by promoting hydrolysis of inositol phosphates to increase intracellular Ca^{2+} levels, via G_q and G_{11} proteins (Loric *et al.*, 1995; Launay *et al.*, 1996). These receptors also stimulate the phosphoinositide-specific enzyme phospholipase C for their efficient signal transduction mechanism (Fargin *et al.*, 1989; Albert *et al.*, 1999; Lin *et al.*, 2002). 5-HT_3 receptors are ligand-gated ion channels that are responsible for depolarizing the plasma membrane. 5-HT_4, 5-HT_6 and 5-HT_7 are G_s-coupled receptors that mediate their actions by stimulating adenylyl cyclase to accumulate cAMP intracellularly (Nichols and Nichols, 2008).

Not many mutational studies have been reported so far for serotonin receptors. Two polymorphisms of 5-HT_{1A} occuring in the N-terminus of the receptor, Gly22Ser (G225) and Ile28Val (I28V), do not seem to have any effect on receptor functionality (Nakhai *et al.*, 1995). An Arg219Leu polymorphism of the 5-HT_{1A} receptor has been implicated in Tourette's syndrome (Lam I., 1996). Another mutation, Ala50Val (A50V), occuring in the TM1 of 5-HT_{1A} receptor, makes the receptor unresponsive to its ligand, 5-HT (Del Tredici *et al.*, 2004). The single nucleotide polymorphism Gly861Cys (G861C) occurring in the gene coding for 5-HT_{1B} has been reported in cases of attention-deficit hyperactivity disorder, substance and alcohol abuse and major depression (Hasegawa *et al.*, 2002; Hawi *et al.*, 2002; Huang *et al.*, 2003; Quist *et al.*, 2003). Similarly, three SNPs in the gene coding for 5-HT_{1D} have been related to anorexia (Thr1123Gly (T123G), Thr628Cys (T628C) and Ala2190Gly (A190G)) (Bergen *et al.*, 2003). Knockout mice for 5-HT_{2A} receptor fail to contract smooth muscles of the intestine on stimulation by 5-HT (Fiorica-Howells *et al.*, 2002). 5-HT_{2B} knockout mice develop serious heart defects. Studies have also shown that overexpression of 5-HT_{2B} receptor leads to ventricular hypertrophy caused due to mitochondrial proliferation (Nebigil *et al.*, 2000, 2001, 2003).

Depression refers to severe or even chronic levels of sadness, helplessness and disinterest arising out of excess anger, grief, guilt, anxiety, fear and despair. Depression can be major depression, dysthymia, depression due to a general or physical condition and substance-induced depressive disorder. Depression can occur at any age, but typically develops during mid-teens to thirties. Heredity, changes in neurotransmitter concentrations, altered neuroendocrine functions and psychosocial factors play a major role in causing depression. Neurotransmitter levels including abnormal regulation of cholinergic, catecholaminergic (noradrenergic and dopaminergic) and serotonergic (5-HT) neurotransmission are the genetic factors responsible for depression. Depression causes psychomotor, cognitive and other kinds of dysfunctions such as poor concentration and fatigue, in addition to the discouraged and low mood. Sometimes, anxiety and panic attacks take over during depression. Occurrence of suicidal tendencies is common in cases of severe depression. Diagnosis is based on identification of the symptoms. Severity is assigned by the duration of symptoms, degree of disability and pain. However, additional laboratory tests help distinguish depression from other disorders such as hypothyroidism and Parkinson's.

Many genetic and environmental factors play a major role in causing depression (Post, 1992). Genetically, depression has been related to an imbalance in the serotonin receptor system. Depression and suicidal tendencies occur when the stress hormone, adrenal glucocorticoid, from the adrenal gland interacts with serotonin receptors in the brain during stress and anxiety, along with the limbic–hypothalamic–pituitary–adrenal axis (Chalmers *et al.*, 1993). However, the mineralocorticoid and glucocorticoid receptors in the hippocampus control and downregulate the release of stress hormone and avoid the state of depression (de Kloet *et al.*, 1998).

The exact receptor subtypes involved and the changes occurring in these receptors in a depressed individual are still not very clear. Studies have shown that while the serotonin 5-HT_{1A} and 5-HT_{2A} receptors increase tremendously in cases of stress, depression and suicide, the number of glucocorticoid and mineralocorticoid receptors decreases rapidly (de Kloet *et al.*, 1988; Berendsen, 1995). Studying the changes occurring in brains of animal models when antidepressants are administered might shed some light on the changes occurring in serotonin receptors. However, studies have shown that antidepressants result in hypersensitive postsynaptic and hyposensitive presynaptic receptors.

Treatment includes medication with antidepressants such as desipramine and imipramine or steroid suppressants such as ketoconazole (Murphy *et al.*, 1991; Lopez *et al.*, 1998). While mild cases of depression can be treated by counseling and psychotherapy, severe cases or cases where there is recurrence of depression more than once need medical help also. There exist many classes of antidepressants that can be used to treat depression, such as selective serotonin reuptake inhibitors (SSRIs), serotonin modulators or 5-HT_2 blockers, serotonin-norepinephrine reuptake inhibitors, dopamine-norepinephrine reuptake inhibitors and heterocyclic antidepressants.

Adrenergic Receptors and Asthma

Adrenergic receptors are involved in mediating functions of the sympathetic nervous system. These receptors activate themselves upon binding a neurotransmitter and a neurohormone (norepinephrine and epinephrine, respectively). While the former is released from the sympathetic nerve endings, the latter is released by the adrenal medulla. These receptors modulate circulatory, metabolic, respiratory and central nervous system homeostasis. The importance of these receptors is evident from the role they play in a number of diseases, such as hypertension, angina pectoris, congestive heart failure, asthma, depression, prostatic hypertrophy and glaucoma.

It was in 1948 that these adrenoceptors were classified as α- and β-adrenoceptors (Ahlquist, 1948). Now, the major classes of adrenoceptors include α_1, α_2 and β, each of which has specific subtypes

(Table 7.10) (Bylund *et al.*, 1994). The α_1-receptors are G_q-coupled receptors while α_2-receptors are G_i coupled. Upon activation by a ligand, the α_1-receptors rearrange themselves and couple to G_q proteins. This then activates phospholipase C, leading to release of inositol triphosphate and increase in intracellular Ca^{2+} levels (Michelotti *et al.*, 2000; Hague *et al.*, 2003). In some cases, these receptors have shown to stimulate phospholipase D and activate protein kinase C and mitogen-activated

Table 7.10 *Adrenoceptor Subtypes, Their Dual Ligand Binding Constants and Role in Human Diseases*

Subtype	*Chromosomal Location*	*Length*	*Ligand Binding Affinity*		*Disease Implicated*	*References*
			Epinephrine	*NorEpinephrine*		
α_{1A}	8p21–p11.2	466	6.3	5.8–6.0	Benign prostatic hyperplasia Hypertension	Shibata *et al.*, 1995 Forray *et al.*, 1994 Gu *et al.*, 2006 Bruno *et al.*, 1991
α_{1B}	5q23–q32	519	6.5	6.2	Gastric cancer Intestinal metaplasia	Ramarao *et al.*, 1992 Noda *et al.*, 2007
α_{1D}	20p13	572	7.2	7.4	Hypertension	Yang-Feng *et al.*, 1990 Yang-Feng *et al.*, 1994 Hu and Hoffman, 1993
α_{2A}	10q24–q26	450	5.6–8.3	5.6–8.4	Hypertension Attention-deficit/ hyperactivity syndrome	Kobilka *et al.*, 1987 Li *et al.*, 2006
α_{2B}	2p13–q13	450	5.2–6.2	5.6–9.0	–	Weinshank *et al.*, 1990 Jasper *et al.*, 1998
α_{2C}	4p16	462	5.8–6.2	5.9–8.7	Cardiac hypertrophy	Regan *et al.*, 1988 Jasper *et al.*, 1998
β_1	10q24–q26	477	6.0	6.0	Obesity Cardiomyo-pathy	Frielle *et al.*, 1987 Dionne *et al.*, 2002 Kurland *et al.*, 2002
β_2	5q31-q32	413	6.2	5.4	Hypertension Myocardial infarction	Kobilka *et al.*, 1987 January *et al.*, 1997 Liapakis *et al.*, 2004 Herrmann *et al.*, 2002
β_3	8p12–p11.2	408	3.9–4.7	4.7–6.3	Insulin resistance Gestational diabetes mellitus Breast cancer	Lelias *et al.*, 1993 Emorine *et al.*, 1989 Popp *et al.*, 2004 Strosberg., 1997 Huang *et al.*, 2001

protein kinases (Michelotti *et al.*, 2000; Hague *et al.*, 2003). Activated α_2-receptors activate the G_i protein, which leads to a decrease in intracellular cAMP by inhibiting adenylyl cyclase activity (Bylund and Ray-Prenger, 1989). Some studies have shown the involvement of G_s protein in the life cycle of α_2-receptors (Eason *et al.*, 1992). β-receptors, on the other hand, use G_s to transduce signal intracellularly. The activated receptor couples to G_s protein, which stimulates adenylyl cyclase, thus leading to an increase in cAMP accumulation (Stiles *et al.*, 1984; Wenzel-Seifert *et al.*, 2002).

Recently, the crystal structure of β_2-adrenergic receptor was solved by Rasmussen *et al.* (2007). While it was evident that the β_2-adrenergic receptor shared structural characteristics similar to that of rhodopsin (both belong to the same family), the presence of extensive and frequent kinks in the TM regions, especially TM7, of this receptor differentiate it from rhodopsin. Moreover, the ligand binding site of β_2-adrenoceptor corresponds to the retinal binding site of rhodopsin. As described in earlier mutational studies, Asp^{113}, Val^{114}, Phe^{289}, Phe^{290} and Asn^{312} seem to be involved in efficient interaction between the adrenergic receptor and the ligand (Strader *et al.*, 1989; Chelikani *et al.*, 2007; Rasmussen *et al.*, 2007). The crystal structure also draws attention to the highly conserved '*DRY*' motif in the intracellular loop 2 of the adrenergic receptor, as in rhodopsin. This motif acts as an ionic switch, maintaining the receptor in an inactive conformation.

Various mutagenesis and biochemical studies with β-adrenoceptors have shown that the 7TM regions of the receptor bundle together and form a cleft for the ligand, about 11° below the extracellular surface. Interactions between epinephrine and its β-adrenergic receptor have been well studied. There occurs an ionic bonding between the amino group of the catechol ring in epinephrine and carboxylate side chain of Asp in TM3. There also occurs hydrogen bonding between hydroxyl groups of catechol and serine residues in TM5. The aromatic–aromatic interactions between the phenyl ring of epinephrine and Phe in TM6 are prominent. Moreover, the hydrogen bonding between the chiral benzylic β-hydroxyl group of epinephrine and Asn in TM6 is responsible for the stereoselectivity of epinephrine for its receptor.

Assaying for the α_{1A}-adrenoceptors involves isolated strips of vas deferens and prostate tissue containing glandular and smooth muscle cells, in rats and humans, respectively (Ohmura *et al.*, 1992; Ford *et al.*, 1997). While α_{1B}-adrenoceptors use rat spleen, α_{1D}-adrenoceptors use rat aortic ring and skeletal muscle arteriole to check the functionality of the expressed receptor (Hieble and Ruffolo, Jr., 1996; Leech and Faber, 1996; Stam *et al.*, 1998). However, all these receptors are assayed for their ability to contract these respective tissues. The human α_{2A}-adrenoceptors can be assayed for by overexpressing them in HT29 cells and measuring the inhibition of cAMP via adenylyl cyclase activity using intact cells. This makes use of the radioactive ^{3}H-adenine pre-labeling technique (Bylund and Ray-Prenger, 1989). Assays for α_{2B}- and α_{2C}-adrenoceptors also involve measuring of the cAMP inhibited, similar to α_{2A}-adrenoceptors, but use NG108 cells as host (Bylund and Ray-Prenger, 1989). The functionality of β-adrenoceptors can be tested by measuring the amount of cAMP accumulated in heart and lung tissues or in CHO-K1 cells (Minneman *et al.*, 1979; Sato *et al.*, 1996; Joseph *et al.*, 2003).

The importance of the adrenergic receptors in normal metabolic functioning of the cell has been proved by generating various knockout mice. Studies have shown that α_{1A}-adrenoceptor knockout mice develop hypotension (Rokosh and Simpson, 2002). Moreover, overexpression of this receptor resulted in increased cardiac contraction (Lin *et al.*, 2001). α_{1B}-adrenoceptor knockout mice become hyperinsulinemic and have high glycogen stores. These mice are also susceptible to obesity (Cotecchia *et al.*, 2002). α_{1C}-adrenoceptor knockout mice developed hypotension but exhibited a resistance to salt-induced hypertension (Tanoue *et al.*, 2002; Chalothorn *et al.*, 2003). However, α_{2C}-adrenoceptor knockout mice have disrupted the presynaptic inhibition of norepinephrine release (Hein *et al.*, 1999). A Gly389Arg (G389R) mutation in the cytoplasmic C-terminus of β-receptors has been related to enhanced G_s protein activation by the receptor, thus resulting in increased adenylyl cyclase activity (Mason *et al.*, 1999). Another Ser49Gly (549G) mutation in the same receptor has been shown to be associated with decreased heart rates, with Gly/Gly homozygotes having the least heart rate when compared to Ser/Gly heterozygotes. Ser/Ser homozygotes have the highest heart rate (Maqbool *et al.*, 1999; Ranade *et al.*, 2002).

Asthma is a chronic respiratory disorder where airways get lined with mucus and get inflamed (Lilly, 2005). It is a clinical syndrome characterized by recurrent airway obstruction, airway hyperresponsiveness and inflammation of the airways. Many genetic and environmental factors, including mutations in the β_2-adrenergic receptor, are believed to be involved in causing asthma. The 'adrenergic theory of asthma' (put forward by Andor Szentivanyi in 1968) proposes that asthma is primarily caused due to blockage of the β_2-adrenergic receptor in the pulmonary smooth muscle cells (Lockey, 2006). The β_2-adrenergic receptor, expressed in airways of smooth muscle cells, epithelial cells, cholinergic nerve cells and blood vessels, upon agonist binding, interacts with the G_s protein. This interaction stimulates downstream signaling, leading to activation of adenylyl cyclase and subsequent cAMP production. This second messenger, in turn, activates many cytosolic kinases, which induce relaxation of airway smooth muscles by promoting bronchodilation (Lohse, 1993).

Asthma is extremely common, affecting 4–7% of the people worldwide. It affects more men than women. Prevalence is higher in people less than 18 years of age. It commonly occurs in males before puberty and in females after puberty. Based on severity of the disease, asthma is classified as mild intermittent, mild persistent, moderate persistent and severe persistent. However, sometimes it is mistaken for chronic obstructive pulmonary disease (COPD). Both multi-genetic and environmental factors play a major role in the predisposition of this disease. Linkage analysis studies have shown the role of two genes, ADAM33 on chromosome 20 and PhF11 on chromosome 11, which stimulate smooth muscles of the airway and fibroblast proliferation and regulate cytokine production, in asthma. Other susceptible genes include those for T-helper 2 cells (T_{H2}) and their cytokines (IL-4, -5 and -9). Acetylcholine, histamines, kinins, neuropeptides, leukotrienes, lipoxins, nitric oxide and platelet-activating factor act as mediators of acute asthmatic response. Of these, acetylcholine acts by stimulating the M_3 muscarinic receptors, causing constriction of airway smooth muscles.

Specific arginine-to-glycine (R16G), glutamine-to-glutamate (Q27E) and threonine-to-isoleucine (T164I) mutations of the β_2-adrenergic receptor lead to varied polymorphisms that affect downstream signaling by the receptor (Liggett, 1997). While R16G mutation leads to a receptor that is rapidly downregulated upon agonist binding, the Q27E mutation makes the receptor resistant to agonist-mediated downregulation. T164I produces a receptor that has altered coupling efficiency to adenylyl cyclase (Liggett, 1997). The T-helper 2 cells, eosinophils, mast cells and other CD_4^+ subtypes and neutrophils form an extensive imflammatory infiltrate in the airway smooth muscles, leading to hypertrophy of the smooth muscles. This results in increased reactivity to allergens, infections, irritants, parasympathetic stimulation and other bronchoconstrictive triggers, also causing release of pro-inflammatory neuropeptides such as substance P, neurokinin A and calcitonin-gene related peptide. Diagnosis is by laboratory-based tests like pulmonary function findings, blood gas analysis, radiographic findings, sputum and electrocardiographic findings. Till date there is no preventive measure for asthma. Treatment for this disease is aimed at resolving airway obstruction and inflammation. Current treatment methods for asthma include avoiding triggers such as pollen, pets, aspirin, and so on. Medical treatment includes usage of short-acting β-receptor agonists such as salmeterol, formoterol, and so on, or prescribing bronchodilators such as a high dosage of glucocorticoids along with long-acting β-receptor agonists like salbutamol, levalbuterol, and so on.

Lutenizing Hormone-Chorionic Gonadotropin Receptors and Familial Male-Limited Precocious Puberty

The lutenizing hormone-chorionic gonadotropin (LH-CG) receptor, also known as lutenizing hormone (LH) receptor or lutropin receptor, is involved in normal and abnormal reproductive hormone functioning. In the ovary, this receptor is necessary for follicular maturation and ovulation, while in testis it is necessary for testosterone production and regulation of spermatogenesis. Many loss-of-function mutations of this receptor lead to infertility in females and pseudohermaphroditism in males.

The lutropin receptor is a member of the rhodopsin superfamily and is found in membranes of testis, ovary and uterus. The gene for this receptor has been mapped to 2p21 (Minegishi *et al*., 1990). It codes for a 674-amino-acid-long protein with a molecular weight of 85–95 kDa, based on the extent of glycosylation (Ascoli *et al*., 2002). Like other glycoprotein hormone receptors, lutropin receptor also has a huge, heavily glycosylated extracellular N-terminal region that is responsible for hormone binding specificity and affinity. This N-terminus also has leucine-rich repeats, about 25 residues long (Moyle *et al*., 1995; Couture *et al*., 1996). These repeats form a horseshoe with β-strands, forming a cleft for binding the hormone. This receptor binds to LH with pIC_{50} of 9.9–10.9 and to chorionic gonadotropin (CG) with pK_d 9.9–11.8 (Jia *et al*., 1991; Müller *et al*., 2003).

The lutropin receptor binds the hormone at its extracellular N-terminal region and also probably its extracellular loops. This binding leads to a conformational change in the receptor by facilitating rearrangement of its TM domains, allowing the cytoplasmic loops and the C-terminus to couple with the cognate G protein and hence transduce signals intracellularly (Hoflack *et al*., 1993; Jiang *et al*., 1995; Moyle *et al*., 1995). Activation of lutropin receptor by the LH and CG leads to coupling of the receptor with G_s protein. This leads to activation of adenylyl cyclase, thus leading to accumulation of cAMP. Transduction of downstream signaling involves the activation of many steroidogenic enzymes via the protein kinase A pathway (Gilchrist *et al*., 1996). The lutropin receptor can also stimulate production of inositol triphosphates by activating phospholipase C and coupling to G_i or G_o proteins (Kühn and Gudermann, 1999).

Many mutations have been reported in these receptors that alter its function. So far only two nonsense mutations have been reported in this receptor, Cys545Stop (C545stop) and Arg554Stop (R554stop). These receptors failed to couple to their cognate G proteins. Two other mutations, Ala593Pro (A593P) and Ser616Tyr (S166Y), have detrimental effects on lutropin receptor function. Ser^{616}, in TM7, lies in the same region as other residues important for normal functioning of the receptor. Substitution mutation of this residue leads to a disruption of the TM domains, thus altering proper folding, expression and trafficking of the receptor.

Male-limited precocious puberty is also known as familial sexual precocity or gonadotropin-independent testotoxicosis. It refers to the appearance of early puberty, as early as 4 years of age in males (Shenker *et al.*, 1993). There is accelerated maturity in patients due to early development of secondary sexual characters (Schöneberg *et al.*, 2004). Under normal conditions, gonadotropin-releasing hormone from the hypothalamus acts on pituitary gland and, hence, stimulates secretion of the gonadotropins LH and FSH. LH then signals the Leydig cells in testes of males to stimulate androgen production, which is responsible for the development of secondary sexual characters. LH binds to the LH-CG receptor present on Leydig cells, thus activating it. The activated receptor binds to G_s protein and hence induces testosterone biosynthesis by further downstream signaling (Brunner and Otten, 1999; Root, 2000).

Many heterozygous mutations in the LH-CG receptor are the cause of familial male precocious puberty. These activating mutations of the receptor lead to amino acid substitutions, mainly in TM5, TM6 and intracellular loop 3 of LH-CG receptor. The most important and widely studied is the aspartate-to-glycine (D578G) mutation in this receptor (Kremer *et al.*, 1995; Shenker *et al.*, 1993). Replacing this Asp with residues having longer or shorter side chains leads to a constitutively active receptor, implying that Asp has side chains of the correct length required for hydrogen bonding with the hormone. These mutations bring about a conformational change in the receptor, leading to its constitutive activation, i.e., the mutated receptor mimics the activated receptor, binds to G_s and induces downstream signaling, leading to production of testosterone (Babovic-Vuksanovic, 1994). However, there can be other diseased conditions also which can lead to male precocious puberty by inducing excessive testosterone production. Leydig cell adenomas are caused due to certain somatic gain-of-function mutations in the LH-CG receptor. These cells are hormone-producing testicular tumors (Liu *et al.*, 1999; Richter-Unruh *et al.*, 2002). Similarly, human CG-secreting germ cell tumors also cause male precocious puberty. This has been attributed to the fact that the β-subunit of human CG shares extensive structural homology with LH. The excess CG binds to the LH-CG receptor, thus stimulating production of testosterone (Englund *et al.*, 1991). Treatment of this disease is by administering steroidogenesis inhibitors such as ketoconazole or competitive inhibitors of androgen receptor function such as spironolactone (Holland *et al.*, 1985; Laue *et al.*, 1989).

Arginine Vasopressin Receptors, Nephrogenic Diabetes Insipidus and Hyponatremia

Vasopressin receptors are also known as arginine vasopressin receptors (AVPRs). These receptors bind the antidiuretic hormone (ADH) vasopressin as their ligand and are responsible for the regulation of osmolality and body fluid volume. These receptors have been implicated in diseases like nephrogenic diabetes insipidus (NDI) and hyponatremia, which are related to kidney functioning and collecting water via the renal ducts. There are three subtypes of vasopressin receptors in humans: AVP_{1A}, AVP_{1B} and AVP_2 receptors (Birnbaumer, 2000). Characteristic features of these three receptor subtypes have been tabulated (Table 7.11). Like other members of this family, the vasopressin receptors are also stabilized by disulfide bonding and palmitoylation of cysteines in the second and third extracellular loops and two conserved cysteines in the C-terminus, respectively (Ovchinnikov *et al.*, 1988; O'Dowd *et al.*, 1989). Also, glycosylation of V_{1A} and V_2 receptors has been shown to play a major role in proper folding and trafficking of the receptor (Pávó and Fahrenholz 1990; Thibonnier *et al.* 1993). However, there are other reports that conflict with the role of these posttranslational modifications in the life cycle of the receptor (Sadeghi *et al.*, 1995, 1997; Innamorati *et al.*, 1996).

Table 7.11 *Vasopressin Receptor Subtypes, Ligand Binding Affinities and Diseases Implicated*

Subtype	*Expression*	*Chromosomal Location*	*Length*	*Ligand Binding Affinity*	*Disease Implicated*	*References*
AVP_{1A}	Liver, smooth muscles of blood vessels and most of the peripheral tissues	12q14–q14	418	4.2–5.6	Hypertension Hyponatremia Congestive heart failure Hyperplasia	Thibonnier *et al.*, 1994 Thibonnier *et al.*, 2000 Mouillac *et al.*, 1995
AVP_{1B}	Adenohypo-physeal region	1q32	424	–	–	Sugimoto *et al.*, 1994
AVP_2	Kidney	Xq28	371	–	Nephrogenic diabetes insipidus	Jard, 1988 Birnbaumer *et al.*, 1992 Seibold *et al.*, 1992 van den Ouweland *et al.*, 1992

Though crystal structure of the vasopressin receptors is not yet available, molecular modeling studies have shown that the ligand, vasopressin, binds in a cleft formed by the TMs (TM2–TM7), about 15° below the extracellular surface (Mouillac *et al.*, 1995). Mutagenesis studies have further shown that conserved Gln residues in TM2, TM3, TM4 and TM6 and a conserved Lys in TM3 are involved in interaction with the ligand (Mouillac *et al.*, 1995; Hausmann *et al.*, 1996). Photoaffinity labeling studies have shown the importance of certain residues present in the extracellular loops in binding the ligand. A specific Tyr^{115} in the extracellular loop 1, when mutated, drastically increases the affinity of the receptor for its ligand (Chini *et al.*, 1995).

Once the V_2 receptor binds vasopressin, it gets activated and in turn activates G_s protein toward its intracellular domain. The activated G protein stimulates adenylyl cyclase to generate intracellular cAMP and hence mediate the actions of the ADH (Orloff and Handler, 1967). In contrast to this receptor, the V_1 receptor follows a different mechanism to transduce its signal intracellularly. Upon activation by the ligand, the V_1 receptor activates the G_q/G_{11} family of proteins, which in turn regulate thc activity of phospholipase C (Michell *et al.*, 1979). Moreover, other studies show that the V_1 receptor might also act by stimulating phospholipases A_2 and D leading to an increase in intracellular Ca^{2+} levels and acidification of the cell by activating Na^{+2}/H^+ exchange channels (Briley *et al.*, 1994).

Nephrogenic diabetes insipidus (NDI) is a condition where large volumes of urine are passed due to inability of the renal tubules to collect water in response to the ADH arginine vasopressin (Chapple *et al.*, 2001). It is the inability to concentrate urine due to impaired renal tubule response to the ADH vasopressin, accompanied by polyuria and polydypsia. Thus, the kidney produces large volumes of hypotonic urine due to loss of its concentrating ability. This leads to dehydration and electrolyte imbalance. NDI can be inherited or can be secondary to renal disorders. It is characterized by polyuria, dehydration and hypernatremia. It can be diagnosed by measuring changes in osmolarity of urine after water deprivation and/or administering vasopressin exogenously. It is inherited as an X-linked trait, but is rarely recessive. While homozygotes are completely unresponsive to the ADH, heterozygotes exhibit reduced or impaired response to the ADH. Acquired NDI results when medulla and distal nephrons are damaged, making the kidneys insensitive to ADH and impairing its urine-concentrating ability.

This disease is caused due to >190 *loss-of-function* mutations in the V_2 arginine vasopressin receptor. Males are much more affected than females, as it is an X-linked disorder (Chapple *et al.*, 2001). Binding of arginine vasopressin to the V_2 receptor leads to increased permeability of the renal cells. However, some forms of NDI are also caused due to defective mutations in the aquaporin 2 water channel (Robben *et al.*, 2006). Due to inactivation mutations, the AVPR2 does not respond to the ADH arginine vasopressin (Schöneberg *et al.*, 2004). Most of the mutations in this receptor lead to intracellular retention of the receptor or defective production due to defective biosynthesis (Chapple *et al.*, 2001). Some of the mutations lead to the accelerated degradation of the receptor. For example, a single insertion of a glycine (G^{804}) leads to a frameshift at codon 245 producing a receptor truncated at intracellular loop 3. An Arg113Trp mutation leads to reduced cell surface expression of the V_2 receptor, affecting its ligand binding ability and G protein coupling (Bichet *et al.*, 1993; Birnbaumer *et al.*, 1994).

Excessive reabsorption of water leads to decreased plasma sodium levels. This condition is called *hyponatremia*. While there may be multiple reasons for hyponatremia, such as low blood volume, hypothyroidism and adrenal insufficiency, the most common cause of hyponatremia is increased levels of the ADH vasopressin. Vasopressin causes water retention, and low blood volume stimulates vasopressin release (Rosenthal *et al.*, 2007). Treatment for hyponatremia includes restriction of water intake, administering intravenous saline or drugs such as the *vaptans* (Decaux *et al.*, 2008). Vaptans are a new class of drugs known as 'antidiuretic hormone receptor antagonists', which act by blocking the V_2 vasopressin receptor. Commonly used vaptans include conivaptan, tolvaptan, relcovaptan, mozavaptan, satavaptan and lixivaptan (Ghali *et al.*, 2005). While conivaptans act on V_{1a} and V_2 receptors, other vaptans act mainly on V_2 receptors. Most of the vaptans are also being studied as a potential cure for heart diseases.

Angiotensin Receptors and Diabetic Nephropathy

Angiotensin is a multifunctional peptide hormone that binds to angiotensin receptors to mediate its action on target cells such as vascular tissue, heart, kidney and brain. Hence, overactivity of these receptors has been implicated in diseases such as congestive heart failure, coronary ischemia and renal insufficiency (Dzau, 1994; Marshall *et al.*, 2006). The gene mapped to 3q21-q25 codes for the 359-amino-acid-long AT_1 receptor in humans (Bergsma *et al.*, 1992; Curnow *et al.*, 1992; Davies *et al.*, 1994), while the 363-amino-acid-long AT_2 receptor has been mapped to Xq22-q23 (Koike *et al.*, 1994; Tissir *et al.*, 1995). These receptors belong to the rhodopsin superfamily of GPCRs and form an important part of the renin–angiotensin system. The two distinct types of angiotensin receptors, namely AT_1 and AT_2, are classified based on their pharmacological properties, ligand binding affinities and transduction mechanisms (de Gasparo and Bottari *et al.*, 1995; de Gasparo and Husain *et al.*, 1995). More recently the AT_3 and AT_4 subtypes have also been discovered, but they are still very poorly understood. Almost all of the functions of angiotensin, such as vasoconstriction, release of aldosterone, activation of sympathetic transmission and cell growth, are via the AT_1 receptor while the AT_2 receptor is involved in antiproliferation, apoptosis, differentiation and vasodilation (Timmermans *et al.*, 1992, 1993; Horiuchi, 1996; Csikos *et al.*, 1998).

Recently, Duvernay *et al.* (2004) have shown that the C-terminus of AT_1 receptors carries a signal for export of the receptor from ER and proper trafficking to the cell surface. Mutants lacking the C-terminal region completely were trapped in the ER and did not traffic to the cell surface. Alanine-scanning mutagenesis studies have revealed the important role played by Phe^{309} and Leu^{316}-Leu^{317} in the $F(X)_6LL$ motif in cell surface expression of the functional receptor. Like other GPCRs, even AT receptors have conserved cysteines in their extracellular domains, which are necessary for stabilizing the tertiary structure. In addition, TM regions and also the extracellular loops are important for ligand binding (Hunyady *et al.*, 1996). Angiotensin II binds both AT receptors with equal affinity of pIC_{50} 9.6–10.0 (de Gasparo and Whitebread, 1994).

The AT_1 and AT_2 receptors are the best studied and are activated by angiotensin II. The activated receptor couples to G_q/G_{11} or G_i/G_o proteins to stimulate phospholipase C, resulting in increase of intracellular Ca^{2+} levels. This in turn activates downstream effectors like protein kinases. Upon stimulation of G_i/G_o by the receptor, adenylyl cyclase is inhibited, but other effector molecules like tyrosine kinase are activated (Catt *et al.*, 1993; de Gasparo and Bottari, 1995; Griendling *et al.*, 1997). They use two intracellular second messengers like inositol triphosphate and diacylglycerol (Capponi, 1996; Griendling *et al.*, 1996). Functionality of AT_1 receptor is checked by measuring the amount of aldosterone released upon induction of the receptor by angiotensin II in bovine adrenal glomerulosa cells (Criscione *et al.*, 1993). The assay method developed for AT_2 receptors employs rat kidney and heart where the amount of nitric oxide and cGMP produced are measured as a result of activation of this receptor (Siragy and Carey, 1996, 1997; Gohlke *et al.*, 1998). Another crude assay for the AT_2 receptor measures the amount of radio-labeled thymidine incorporated and subsequent apoptosis in rats upon activation of this receptor (Dudley and Summerfelt, 1993; Yamada *et al.*, 1996; Horiuchi *et al.*, 1997).

Renal or *diabetic nephropathy* is a condition where chronic diabetes causes renal angiopathy. It is also known as *Kimmelstiel–Wilson syndrome* and *intercapillary glomerulonephritis*. It has been proved earlier that hypertension, renal diseases and angiotensin receptors are correlated (Adler *et al.*, 2000). The metabolic sequelae of hypoglycemia are a major cause of diabetic nephropathy. However, apart from angiotensin receptor, other genetic, hemodynamic and metabolic factors are also involved in causing this disease. It is a polygenic disease and mutations in the gene coding for angiotensin-converting enzyme (ACE) have been extensively related to it. Genetic defects in lipid metabolism, such as polymorphisms in apolipoprotein E (ApoE), have also been implicated in this disease. Genes related to transforming growth factor and matrix metalloproteinase 9 have also been related to this disease.

Studies have shown that administering ACE inhibitors or AT_1 receptor blockers that interfere with the angiotensin–renin system has some beneficial effects as they act by lowering the systemic blood pressure. Hence, new antihypertensive and renal therapies focus on blocking these receptors. AT_1 receptor blockers or angiotensin II receptor antagonists are much more popular than ACE inhibitors since these antagonists act by completely blocking production of angiotensin II from angiotensin I by both ACE-dependent and ACE-independent pathways, for example, the renin–angiotensin pathway. These AT_1 receptor antagonists form a new class of drugs, called *sartans*. Saralasin was the first AT_1 receptor antagonist developed in 1971 but was not very popular since oral administration of this drug was not possible and it lacked receptor subtype specificity in its mode of action. Sartans are more preferred since they have very few adverse side effects.

DRUGS ACTING ON GPCRs

It was in the early twentieth century when Paul Ehrlich proposed that drugs act via specific 'chemoreceptors' to exert their pharmacological effect that led to the discovery, identification and functional characterization of GPCRs. Today this largest family of cell surface receptors is a major target for drugs, almost 50% of the drugs being prescribed target GPCRs. Also, drugs targeting GPCRs are some of the most popular drugs (even compared to non-GPCR targeting drugs). This huge attention and success of GPCR-targetting drugs is mainly due to the fact that GPCRs form one of the most important classes of proteins in the body that are ubiquitous in nature, occurrence and function. Cloning of human GPCR genes has added up to this vast drug-based therapy, increasing the scope of effective drug discovery. A key factor in developing drugs that target GPCRs is the ability to design small molecules that have very high degree of potency and selectivity. The highly specific selectivity of receptors is due to their extensive diversity in terms of binding sites across families and isoforms, tissue-specific expression and localization and, finally, physiological function of the receptor. This selectivity forms the basis for high potency of the drugs for these receptors. The current market trend shows that a vast number of these drugs are specifically targeted toward the rhodopsin family of GPCRs such as the adrenergic, serotonergic, dopaminergic, histaminergic and muscarinic receptors, probably due to the ubiquitous nature and huge effect that these receptors have in proper metabolic functioning of the human body.

Ubiquitous distribution of these receptors makes the drug discovery process of GPCRs all the more difficult and time consuming. The first step of drug discovery process requires prioritization, selection and compound library screening of GPCR targets. Bioinformatics approaches, receptor localization, druggability and target validation lead to effective prioritization of the drug target. Once done, the next step involves rational drug design for lead optimization (Kenakin, 2003). This involves extensive *in vitro* and *in vivo* target-based drug screening for desired pharmacological action with minimal side effects. GPCR target discovery and validation is the basic step that involves identification and characterization of the receptor including cloning, expression and high-throughput screening of the target, which form the basis for compound optimization. However, this process of target identification and validation should be considered with great caution and detail since there tend to appear many false negatives that may mislead the entire process. With the decoding of the human genome, many GPCR sequences are now available even as filtering valid GPCR sequences is a task. This is where bioinformatics approaches come into play. Hidden Markov models and other such computational methods that provide a statistical representation of the genomic sequences make this step much easier (Karchin *et al*., 2002; Menzaghi *et al*., 2002).

GPCR localization along with its tissue-level expression in case of healthy and diseased states is another important factor to be considered while designing the drug. An ideal GPCR for such pharmacological action would be one that has high-level expression in one tissue and comparatively very low-level expression in other tissues, since targeting a ubiquitously expressed receptor is definitely prone to many adverse side effects. '*In situ* hybridization' and reverse transcription-polymerase chain reaction (RT-PCR) are two successful techniques that have shed light on localization and expression patterns of many GPCRs (Schena *et al.*, 1995). Once the target receptor has been tracked down, druggability of the receptor and target validation become important steps. Target validation can be done by using various animal models to study the receptor–drug interaction and also to check any side effects produced thereof. Sequence-specific antisense oligonucleotides that target the mRNA of the target GPCR also help in the process of target validation (Van Oekelen *et al.*, 2003). However, the sequence-independent effect and restricted internalization of the oligonucleotides, makes the use of *si*RNA for target validation a better choice (Dorsett and Tuschl, 2004; Jain, 2004; Sioud, 2004).

Target discovery, localization and validation lead to the druggability of the receptor. This involves consideration of various factors such as the receptor selectivity, distribution, structure, endogenous ligands, metabolic properties and the pharmacological effects the drug will have on the receptor. Virtual screening methods allow selection of drugs from a huge database of compounds, by modeling the receptor–drug interaction *in silico* (Palczewski *et al.*, 2000; Bissantz *et al.*, 2003; Bleicher *et al.*, 2004). Lead optimization then makes it possible to screen the compounds selected, based on the above factors, for *in vitro* interaction and effect studies with the target GPCR. This involves rational drug design and synthesis of those chemical compounds for screening. Binding assays that tell us about the potency of the drug on the receptor and also the nature of binding (competitive, non-competitive and uncompetitive) and the number of binding sites recognized by the drug on the receptor play a major role in lead optimization. *In vitro* functional assays that measure the activity of native receptors followed by *in vivo* animal studies to assess the efficacy and potency of the drug in diseased conditions involve the next step (Sioud, 2007). Once all the above steps have been completed successfully, it is now time to synthesize the chemical compound, keeping in mind certain 'favorable' specific chemical groups and structures with respect to the receptor. Some of these involve benzodiazepines, biphenyls, indoles, piperidines and xanthines. Moreover, the 'Rule of Five' should also be kept in mind while synthesizing the compound. This rule states that for a drug to be effective on a GPCR, it must possess at least two of the following properties: a molecular weight of less than 500 kDa, fewer than five hydrogen bond donors, fewer than 10 hydrogen bond acceptors and a log P below 5. This rule has chemical optimization of many lead compounds (Hardy and Peet, 2004).

Apart from the well-known and well-studied GPCRs, orphan GPCRs are also gaining widespread importance in the field of drug discovery. About 160 orphan GPCRs spread across three GPCR families are currently being studied as targets for drugs. A reverse pharmacological approach is used to screen a library of probable ligands for the orphan receptor. H_3 histamine and LTB_4 leukotriene receptors have been identified by this method (Kamohara *et al.*, 2000; Lovenberg *et al.*, 2000). Another approach is called the orphan receptor strategy. This involves exposure of the recombinantly expressed orphan receptor to a variety of tissue extracts and the signaling responses are measured (Civelli *et al.*, 2006). Once a positive response is elicited the extract is fractionated and characterized for the perfect ligand. This approach has helped deorphan the OLR1 receptor whose ligand was found to be norciceptin or orphanin FQ (Meunier *et al.*, 1995). The following section discusses some of the major classes of GPCR-targeted drugs that have crossed all the above criteria and were introduced into the market successfully as therapeutics for many major human diseases and disorders.

Neuroleptics

Conventional antipsychotics used for treatment typically act by blocking the dopamine D_2 receptor. The potency of these drugs can be classified between high, intermediate or low. High-potency antipsychotics have high affinity for dopamine D_2 receptor but low affinity for α-adrenergic and muscarinic receptors. Low-potency antipsychotics, on the other hand, have low affinity for D_2 receptor and relatively high affinity for α-adrenergic and muscarinic receptors. Some of the conventional antipsychotics include aliphatic phenothiazines (chlorpromazine), piperidines (thioridazine), piperazines (trifluoperazine, fluphenazine, perphenazine), dibenzoxazepines (loxapine), dihydroindolones (molindone), thioxanthenes (thiothixene), butyrophenones (halperidol) and diphenylbutylpiperidines (pimozide). However, these conventional drugs produce severe side effects such as sedation, cognitive blunting, dystonia and muscle stiffness, tremors, weight gain and elevated prolactin levels.

Phenothiazines were the first antipsychotics to be introduced into the market (Fig. 7.7). Drugs belonging to this class share the same structural feature of phenothiazine ring but differ in chemical groups at the R_1 and R_2 positions, C_2 and C_{10}. Generally, a negatively charged electrophilic group is attached to C_2 to facilitate stronger binding to the dopamine receptor. Based on these substitutions, phenothiazines are classified as aliphatic phenothiazines, piperadines and piperazines. Aliphatic phenylthiazines have a dimethylamide group attached to C_{10} and a chlorine atom attached to C_2. Members of this class include chlorpromazine, promazine, methotrimeprazine and triflupromazine. Piperadine phenothiazines have a piperidine ring attached to their C_{10}. They are more specific in receptor selectivity, especially D_2 dopamine receptor, than aliphatic phenothiazines. Thioridazine and mesoridazine belong to this class of drugs. Piperazine phenothiazines have a piperazine ring attached to C_{10}. They exhibit the strongest and maximum potency against D_2 receptors and very low potency to muscarinic, histaminergic and adrenergic receptor systems. Fluphenazine, perphenazine, thiopropazate, acetophenazine, thioproperazine and trifluperazine belong to this class. Other classes of antipsychotics include thioxanthenes, butyrophenones, dihydroindoles, diphenylbutylpiperadines and dibenzoxapines. Thioxanthenes, like thiothixene, are structurally and pharmacologically similar to piperazine phenothiazines. Butyrophenones have a piperidine ring with a carbonyl-substituted *p*-fluorobenzene ring. Haloperidol, the most widely known antipsychotic drug so far, belongs to this class. This class of drugs is highly specific for dopamine receptors and show very little affinity toward muscarinic, histaminergic and adrenergic receptors. Dibenzoxapines have a seven-member central ring with a piperazine side chain and chlorine atom at R_2. It exhibits significant antagonism for dopaminergic and serotonergic receptors. Loxapine and its metabolite amoxapine belong to this class of drugs. Dihydroindoles have a structure similar to indoleamines like serotonin. Molindone is the only dihydroindole that is not associated with weight gain and seizures. Diphenylbutylpiperadines, like pimozide, are known to possess the highest potency for dopamine D_2 receptors among all known conventional antipsychotics. These conventional antipsychotics are administered either orally or intramuscularly (Sadock and Sadock, 2000). Peak plasma levels are achieved within 1–4 h of administration in case of oral administration and slightly faster (30–60 min) in case of intramuscular administration (Maxmen and Ward, 1995). The high lipophilic nature of these antipsychotics leads to their excessive distribution in the brain rather than plasma. These drugs are metabolized in the liver with the help of different enzymes and undergo transformations such as glucuronidation, oxidation, reduction and methylation. They are readily metabolized by hydroxylation and demethylation to more soluble forms that pass through the kidney easily. The half-life of these drugs varies from 18 to 40 h; the excretion occurs through urine and feces, and sometimes also via sweat, tears and saliva (Arana and Rosenbaum, 2000).

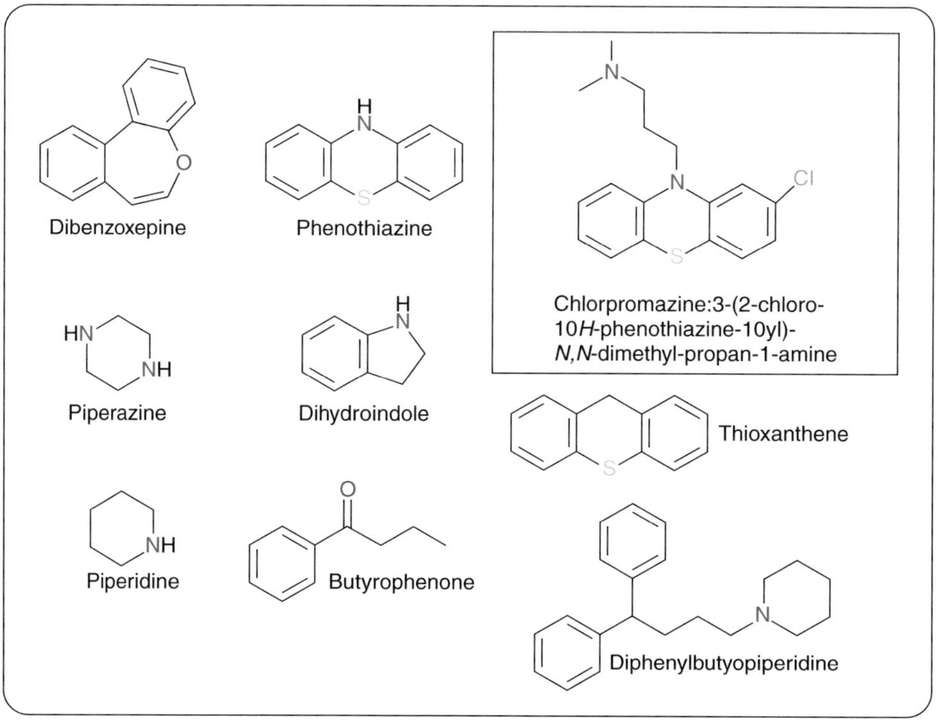

Fig. 7.7 *Conventional Antipsychotics*

(Phenothiazines (e.g., chlorpromazine) belong to the thiazine class of heterocyclic compounds and are one of the first neuroleptics to be introduced in the market. Other chemical structures that have given birth to many conventional antipsychotics are also illustrated.)

Chlorpromazine was the first antipsychotic drug developed; it was synthesized by Paul Charpentier in 1950. It was approved by FDA in 1954 to treat psychiatric disorders. However, it is not approved for use in adults with dementia. It acts as an antagonist for many postsynaptic receptors such as dopamine, serotonin, histamine, adrenergic and muscarinic acetylcholine receptors (Yamada *et al.*, 1995; Kusumi *et al.*, 2000). Hence, it is used to treat schizophrenia and control mental illnesses and depression (Oades *et al.*, 2000; Wu *et al.*, 2005). It is also used as a part of tetanus treatment and to control nausea and vomiting. Chemically, it is a dimethylamine derivative of phenothiazine with an aliphatic side chain and is designated as 2-chloro-10-[3-(dimethylamino)propyl]-phenothiazine.

It also exerts sedative and antiemetic activities. Its sedative property is attributed to the chlorine atom attached to C_2 and its high anticholinergic, anti-adrenergic and antihistaminic activities. Chlorpromazine (structural formula $C_{17}H_{19}ClN_2S$; molecular weight 319 g mol^{-1}) is administered as an injection (Baxter Healthcare Corporation) intravenously or as a tablet orally (Sandoz Inc. and Upsher-Smith Laboratories Inc.). Like other phenothiazines, chlorpromazine is a lipophilic molecule that binds to membrane lipids and proteins. About 90–95% of this drug is found in the plasma, with about 85% of it being bound to the plasma protein, albumin (Arana and Rosenbaum, 2000; Rukhadze *et al.*, 2001; Silva *et al.*, 2004). Moreover, chlorpromazine is also known to cross the blood–brain barrier and accumulate more in the brain than in plasma. Chlorpromazine also crosses the placenta and is excreted in milk; hence, administration of this drug to pregnant women is avoided (Guze and Baxter, 1985). Only about 30–35% of this drug is available for systemic circulation with peak concentrations achieved between 1 and 4 h of administration. Due to its high lipophilicity and high membrane-binding capacity, it has a huge half-life of 16–30 h and can also be detected in urine for several months after discontinuation of the drug (Baldessarini, 2001).

Chlorpromazine is highly effective against dopamine D_2 receptors and up to an extent against D_3 and D_5 receptors. Blocking of the receptor activity by chlorpromazine leads to reduced neurotransmitter effect. However, since dopamine cannot bind to its receptor, there occurs an initial increase in dopamine production resulting in increased dopaminergic neural activity. Slowly the levels of dopamine drop and dopamine is removed from the neural cleft causing significant decrease in neural activity and continued blocking of the dopamine receptors. Chlorpromazine is also a presynaptic inhibitor of dopamine reuptake and hence a potent antidepressant and antiparkinsonian drug (Lacoursiere and Spohn, 1989; Reynolds, 1989; Baldessarini, 2001). Cytochrome P450 family of enzymes, especially CYP2D6 and CYP1A2, aldehyde oxidase and cholinesterase are necessary for metabolism of chlorpromazine. Upto 1% of the unchanged drug is excreted in the urine. However, its metabolism in the liver generates up to 168 different metabolites. Though most of these metabolites do not have any potent activity, some molecules such as 7-hydroxychlorpromazine, mesoridazine, 9-hydroxyrisperidone and a few other N-demethylated metabolites are metabolically active (Williams and Parke, 1964).

Chlorpromazine has been shown to promote or reduce the activity of many other drugs. It increases the activity of antidepressants that act on the central nervous system, such as barbiturates, tranquilizers, narcotics and antihistamines. It also intensifies the action of antihypertensives and anticholinergics. Hence, a dose reduction of either chlorpromazine or the other drug is suggested in such cases. SSRIs and certain barbiturates inhibit cytochrome P450 enzymes that are essential for metabolism of chlorpromazine and hence should not be administered with this drug. Due to its activity on so many receptor systems, chlorpromazine is generally referred to as a 'dirty drug'. Most of its side effects are due to its anticholinergic activities and include sedation, slurred speech, dry mouth, urine retention, constipation, seizures, weight gain, impaired glucose tolerance and, at times, even photosensitivity. Other severe side effects include leukopenia (reduction in number of white blood cells), agranulocytosis, color blindness, partial to complete blindness and pigmentation of the cornea. In some cases, it leads to reduced blood pressure, cardiac arrests and, ultimately, death.

Second-generation antipsychotics are the newer long-acting atypical antipsychotic drugs such as olanzapine, risperidone, quetiapine, ziprasidone and clozapine (Fig. 7.8). They act by blocking both dopamine and serotonin receptor systems and hence are also called *dopamine–serotonin antagonists*.

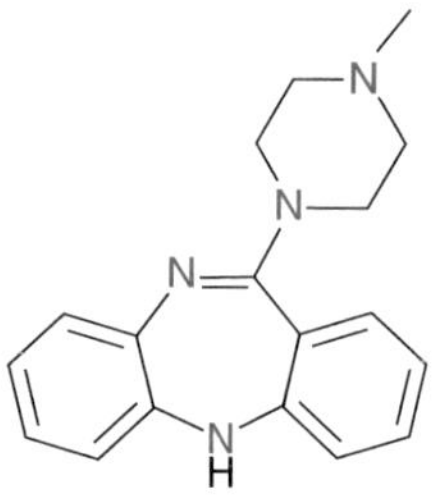

Clozapine: 8-chloro-11-(4-methyl-1-piperazinyl)-5*H*-dibenzo(b,e)(1,4)diazepine

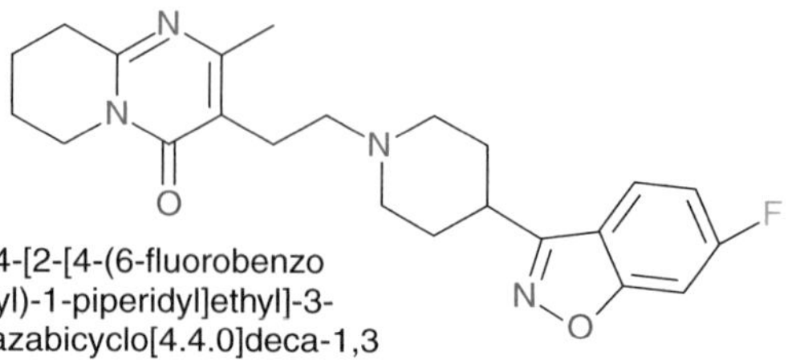

Risperidone: 4-[2-[4-(6-fluorobenzo [d]isoxazol-3-yl)-1-piperidyl]ethyl]-3-methyl-2,6-diazabicyclo[4.4.0]deca-1,3 -dien-5-one

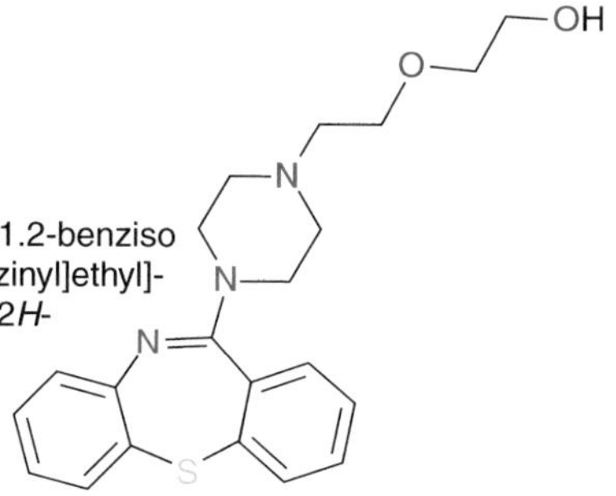

Ziprasidone: 5-[2-[4-(1.2-benziso thiazol-3-yl)-1-piperazinyl]ethyl]-6-chloro-1,3-dihydro-2*H*-indol-2-one

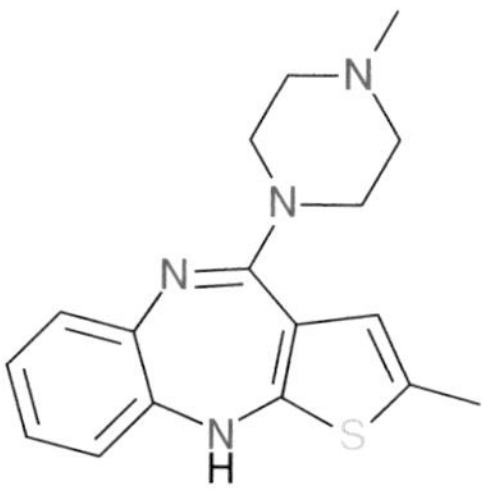

Olanzapine: 2-methyl-4-(4-methyl-1-piperazinyl)-10*H*-thienol[2,3-b][1,5] benzodiazaepine

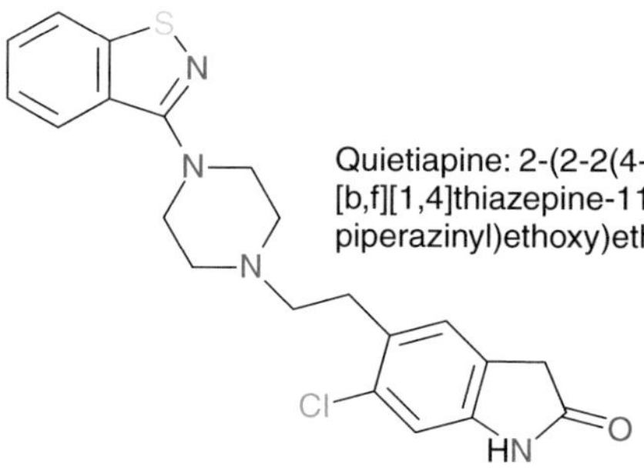

Quietiapine: 2-(2-2(4-dibenzo [b,f][1,4]thiazepine-11-yl-1-piperazinyl)ethoxy)ethanol

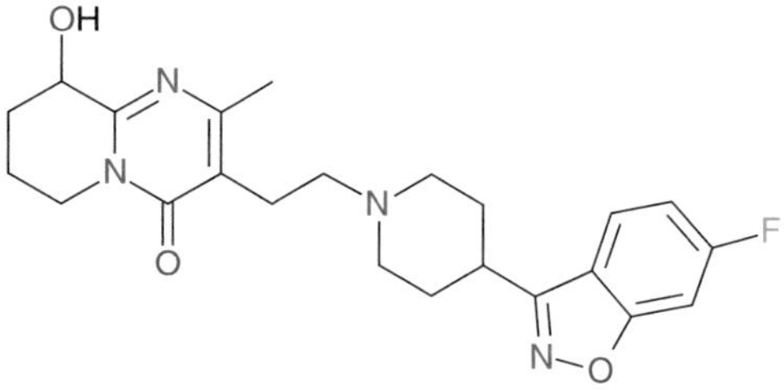

Paliperidone: 3-[2-[4-(6-fluorobenzo [d]isozazol-3-yl)-1piperidyl)ethyl]-7-hydroxy-4-methyl-1,5-diazabicyclo[4.4.0] deca-3,5-dien-2-one

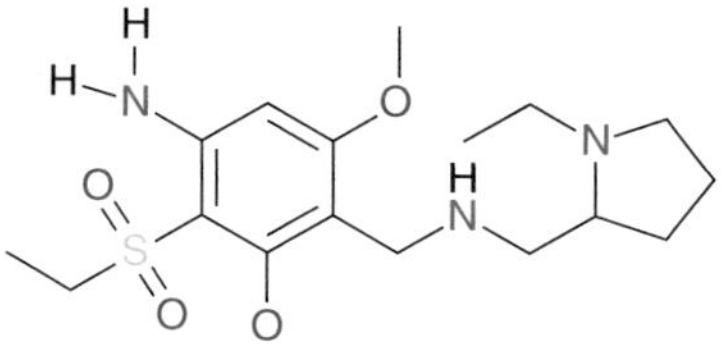

Amisulpride: 4-amino-*N*-[(1-ethyl pyrrolidin-2-yl)methyl]-5-ethylsulfon -2-methoxy-benzamide

Fig. 7.8 ***Second-Generation Antipsychotics are 'Atypical' Antipsychotics Mainly Implicated in the Treatment of Many Psychiatric Disorders***

(They mainly act as serotonin receptors agonists and have very little affinity for dopamine receptors, which attributes to their very few adverse side effects compared to conventional antipsychotics.)

They alleviate positive symptoms and lessen negative symptoms. These drugs are called atypical due to their reduced side-effect spectrum, which differs from that of the traditional antipsychotics used. These newer drugs have less motor system side effects but have long-term, though lower, risks of dyskinesias. Moreover, unlike the conventional antipsychotics that have broad-spectrum dopamine receptor-blocking properties, these newer class of antipsychotics have variable effects on dopamine receptor and neurochemical systems, like serotonin. Risperidone has been shown, *in vitro*, to be possessing 20 times higher affinity for 5-HT_{2A} receptors than for D_2 receptors. Clozapine was developed in the 1960s and was believed to act as an antidepressant due to its tricyclic structure, but it proved to be a potent antipsychotic. It is the only drug known to be effective in about 50% of the patients resistant to conventional antipsychotics. Clozapine is a dibenzodiazepine with strong anticholinergic properties in addition to serotonin-blocking properties. It blocks D_2 and D_1 receptors with equal efficiency. Though this drug does not exhibit any extrapyramidal side effects, it can cause fatal agranulocytosis. Olanzapine blocks 5-HT_2 receptors along with dopamine D_1, D_2 and D_4 receptors. It also exhibits anticholinergic and α_1-blocking properties. Quetiapine has actions similar to clozapine but has reduced agranulocytosis. Prolonged use of this drug has also been implicated in cataracts. Ziprasidone is the newest antipsychotic drug that affects both positive and negative symptoms of schizophrenia. However, though it has very low rates of extrapyramidal effects, it can cause akathisia.

Clozapine was first synthesized in 1958 but it was in 1960 that its use as an antipsychotic came to light. However, initial studies showed the development of agranulocytosis in patients being treated with this drug, which led to a delay in its approval by the FDA (1990) (Griffith and Saamerli, 1975). Clozapine is now used as a potent antipsychotic to treat patients who are resistant to treatment with conventional antipsychotic (Kane *et al.*, 1988). Unlike these conventional drugs, clozapine has very little extrapyramidal side effects. Chemically, clozapine is designated as 3-chloro-6-(4-methylpiperazin-1-yl)-5*H*-benzo[*c*][1,5]benzodiazepine and has the structural formula $C_{18}H_{19}ClN_4$ (molecular weight 326.8 g/mol). Clozapine has a seven-membered cyclic ring and belongs to a group of tricyclic antipsychotic drugs called *dibenzapines*. These antipsychotic dibenzapines have loxapine-like groups called dibenzoxazapines and clozapine-like groups called dibenzodiazapines. Clozapine peaks plasma levels within an hour of oral administration and reaches a steady state within a week of administration. It has an elimination half-life of about 12 h. About 27–47% of unchanged clozapine is available for systemic circulation.

Like conventional antipsychotics, clozapine also undergoes first-pass metabolism in the liver. In addition to cytochrome P450 1A2 and 2D6 enzymes, P450 3A3 is also involved in metabolizing clozapine in the liver (Buur-Rasmussen and Brosen, 1999). Hence, agents such as fluvoxamine, theophylline and ciprofloxacin inhibit the activity of cytochrome P450 class of enzymes and thus such patients will need much lesser amounts of clozapine for effective treatment, whereas smokers, in whom cytochrome P450 enzymes are hyperactive, will require a much higher dose of clozapine for the same efficiency of drug action (Heeringa *et al.*, 1999; Rostami-Hodjegan *et al.*, 2004). About 80% of the administered clozapine appears in urine and feces as transformed metabolites, while only about 5% of unchanged clozapine appears in the urine. The two main metabolites of clozapine are a result of demethylation and oxidation of the terminal nitrogen in the piperazine side chain of clozapine and are excreted much more rapidly from the body than clozapine.

The unique ability of clozapine to act as an antipsychotic without any extrapyramidal side effects can be attributed to its low occupancy of the D_2 receptor and also its higher affinity for receptors other than the D_2 receptors. Studies with positron emission tomography (PET) have shown that while conventional antipsychotics are active when about 80% of the D_2 receptors are occupied by this drug, just about 20–45% of clozapine-bound D_2 receptors are sufficient to mediate the drug action (Farde *et al.*, 1992; Miller, 1996). Unlike conventional antipsychotics, clozapine has very little affinity for D_2 receptors when compared to its affinity for serotonin 5-HT_{1C} and 5-HT_{2A} receptors. Moreover, clozapine and other second-generation antipsychotics bind to the D_2 receptors with lesser affinity and dissociate from the receptor very easily in presence of dopamine, thus allowing normal dopaminergic neuronal transmission (Kapur and Seeman, 2001; Seeman, 2002). Owing to all these reasons, clozapine is preferred over conventional antipsychotics. Also, clozapine, administered in cases of acute schizophrenia, has been found to also decrease the aggressive behavior in such individuals. Clozapine can be assayed for, in the plasma, by combining high-performance liquid chromatography with ultraviolet (UV) detection (Edno *et al.*, 1997). Another assay method makes use of radio-labeled receptors to detect this drug in the plasma (Odou *et al.*, 1996). Apart from the beneficial medicinal uses of clozapine, there also occur serious side effects when administered in higher doses. Clozapine causes constipation, muscle stiffness, drooling, tremors, hyperglycemia and weight gain (Wirshing *et al.*, 1999). Seizures have been observed in 5–10% of patients treated with clozapine (Welch *et al.*, 1994). Sedation is another most serious side effect of clozapine (Angermeyer *et al.*, 2001). Agranulocytosis has been reported in about 1% of patients who take clozapine for the first time. It is also responsible for hypotension and adverse cardiovascular and respiratory effects.

Olanzapine was first used as an antipsychotic in 1995 (Baldwin and Montgomery, 1995) and was approved by the FDA in 1997 (manufactured and marketed by Eli Lilly and Co.). Olanzapine is a thienobenzodiazepine derivative and is structurally similar to clozapine. It is chemically represented as 2-methyl-4-(4-methylpiperazin-1-yl)-5*H*-thieno[3,2-*c*][1,5]benzodiazepine ($C_{17}H_{20}N_4S$; m.w. 312.4 g/mol). It is has affinity for dopamine D_2, D_3, D_4 and D_5, serotonin 5-HT_{2A}, muscarinic, histamine H_1 and α_1-adrenergic receptors. Unlike conventional antipsychotics and like clozapine, olanzapine also has decreased extrapyramidal side effects, which is attributed to its nonspecific dopamine receptor selectivity. Moreover, it also acts a 5-HT_{2A} receptor antagonist. Since serotonergic systems are dependent on dopaminergic systems, this further adds up to its reduced extrapyramidal side effects (Bymaster *et al.*, 1996). Olanzapine is well absorbed and well metabolized in the body. It attains peak plasma levels within 4–6 h of oral administration (Kassahun *et al.*, 1997). About 40% of it undergoes first-pass metabolism immediately and is not available for systemic circulation. Moreover, the bioavailability of olanzapine in the body is not affected by food (Kassahun *et al.*, 1997; Callaghan *et al.*, 1999; Zyprexa, 2004). *In vitro* studies have shown that about 93% of olanzapine is protein bound, mostly to albumin or α_1-acid glycoprotein (Kassahun *et al.*, 1997).

Olanzapine is extensively metabolized in the liver to 10 different metabolites, but mostly to 10-*N*-glucuronide and 4′-*N*-desmethylolanzapine (Macias *et al.*, 1998). Cytochrome P450 1A2 enzyme is primarily responsible for metabolism of olanzapine in the liver (Ring *et al.*, 1996). Mean half-life of olanzapine is about 36 h. However, there occurs about 25–30% decreased clearance rate in women and elderly when compared to men (Patel *et al.*, 1995, 1996; Callaghan *et al.*, 1999). Like all other second-generation drugs, olanzapine is also an atypical drug with minimal side effects, especially extrapyramidal effects. This is implied from the ratio of the drug affinity for serotonin receptors and that for dopamine receptors. The higher is this ratio, due to increased affinity of the drug for serotonin receptors compared to dopamine D_2 receptor, the drug seems to have minimal extrapyramidal side effects, while lower the ratio, due to increased affinity of the drug for D_2 receptors, there seems to be an increase in extrapyramidal effects (Meltzer *et al.*, 1989; Kapur *et al.*, 1998).

Quetiapine was developed in 1984 and is pharmacologically similar to, but is much safer than, clozapine and olanzapine. It was approved by the USFDA in 1997 for treatment of schizophrenia and more recently for the treatment of bipolar disorder. It is currently being marketed by AstraZeneca and Orion Pharma. Like olanzapine, quetiapine has higher and stronger affinity for serotonin 5-HT_{2A} receptor than the dopamine D_2 receptor, which is considered to be the most important factor for its safer use compared to clozapine (Richelson and Souder, 2000). It also acts as an antagonist for adrenergic and histamine receptors. Chemically, it is called 2-[2-(4-benzo[*b*][1,5]benzothiazepin-6-ylpiperazin-1-yl)ethoxy]ethanol with the structural formula $C_{21}H_{25}N_3O_2S$ (m.w. 383 g/mol). Quetiapine is also rapidly absorbed within 1–2 h when administered orally (Goldstein, 1999). The average half-life of this drug is 6 h, but it binds to 5-HT_{2A} and D_2 receptors for much longer (Gefvert *et al.*, 1998; Goldstein, 1999; Seroquel, 2001). About 83% of this drug is protein bound and only about 6% of the orally administered dose is available for systemic absorption. Quetiapine is metabolized by the cytochrome P450 3A4 enzyme in the liver by sulfoxidation and oxidation (Goldstein, 1999). Almost all of the metabolites of this drug are inactive. However, metabolism of this drug is 40% slower in the case of elderly, implying the need for a lesser dose in these patients (Goldstein, 1999).

Quetiapine has very high affinity for 5-HT_{2C} receptors and moderate affinity for 5-HT_{1A} receptors, but very low affinity for D_2 receptors. This low D_2 receptor antagonism is believed to play a positive role in the mode of action of quetiapine, without any side effects (Goldstein, 1996; Kinon and Lieberman, 1996; Seeman and Tallerico, 1998; Richelson and Souder, 2000; Goldstein, 2002). PET and single-photon emission computed tomography studies have shown that clinical effects are observed when just 30–40% of D_2 receptors are occupied by this drug (Kapur, Zipursky, Jones, Shammi *et al.*, 2000). Conventional drugs, on the other hand, occupy about 70% of these D_2 receptors and hence are believed to produce extrapyramidal side effects (Kapur, Zipursky, Jones, Remington *et al.*, 2000). This low occupancy of D_2 receptors with quetiapine is one of the main reasons for almost no extrapyramidal side effects. Moreover, quetiapine binds to about 75% of 5-HT_{2A} receptors. Just like clozapine, olanzapine and quetiapine also have similar interactive effects with other drugs. Moreover, like other neuroleptics, olanzapine and quetiapine have their own share of side effects like aggressiveness, sedation, dryness, insomnia, urinary retention, orthostatic hypotension, low blood pressure and weight gain.

Dopamine agonists are drugs that directly activate the dopamine receptors in the basal ganglia. They are administered orally and usually used as monotherapy, though rarely sufficient as such for a few years. Though they can be used at all stages of the disease, they are particularly useful during later stages of the disease when the effect of levodopa decreases and symptoms start to resurface on and off more frequently. However, using these drugs with small amounts of levodopa effectively delays emergence of dyskinesias and reduces frequency of symptoms showing up on and off, probably because dopamine agonists are able to stimulate dopamine receptors much longer than levodopa alone does. This type of stimulation is physiologic and preserves the receptor better. Recent research supports the fact that dopamine agonists have a neuroprotective effect since dopamine agonists decrease dopamine turnover and reduce oxidative stress when they stimulate dopamine receptors.

These drugs also scavenge hydroxyl, superoxide and nitric oxide radicals by inducing upregulation of the free radical–scavenging enzyme, superoxide dismutase. Certain dopamine agonists also enhance the growth and survival of dopaminergic neurons, *in vitro*. Moreover, they also relax smooth muscles, unlike levodopa. However, negative side effects such as sedation, nausea, orthostatic hypotension, confusion, delirium and psychosis are observed with the usage of dopamine agonists. Lowering concentrations of levodopa that is administered with these drugs may, to a certain extent, minimize the adverse effects of these drugs. Three new dopamine agonists, cabergoline, pramipexole and ropinirole, were added to bromocriptine and pergolide in 1997 (Fig. 7.9). Though cabergoline is a potent D_2 receptor agonist, it has not been approved yet by the FDA for treating Parkinson's in the United States. Pramipexole and ropinirole differ from the two conventional dopamine agonists, bromocriptine and pergolide, in that they are purely D_3 and D_2 receptor agonists, respectively. The non-ergoline structure of these two drugs reduces their side-effect profile by lowering risk for complications such as peptic ulcers, vasoconstriction and pulmonary disorders.

Bromocriptine and *pergolide* are semisynthetic ergoline alkaloids that are potent D_2 receptor agonists used to treat pituitary tumors and Parkinson's disease. Both these drugs are rapidly absorbed

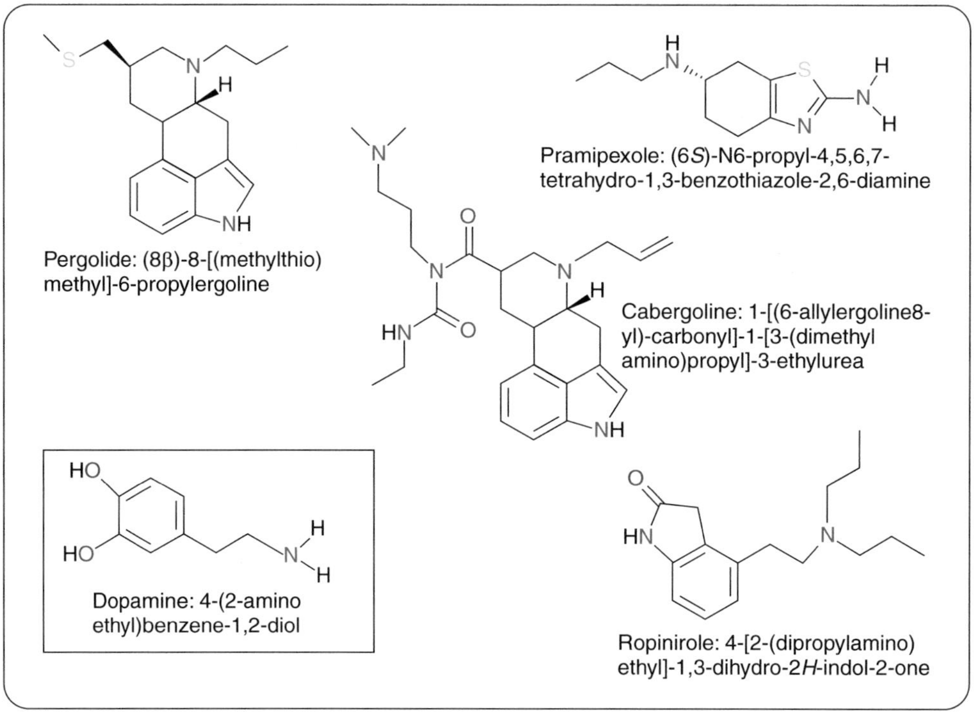

Fig. 7.9 ***Dopamine Agonists Mimic Effects of the Neurotransmitter, Dopamine, to Activate the Dopamine Receptors***

(These drugs are used to treat diseases like Parkinson's and certain pituitary tumors. While pergolide is currently not available in market, pramipexole, ropinirole and cabergoline are newer dopamine agonists.)

by the body and undergo first-pass metabolism in liver (Boyd, 1995; Schade *et al.*, 2007). Hence, only about 30–50% of the administered drug is available for biological action. Peak concentrations are achieved within 2–3 h of oral administration. Pergolide has a half-life of about 27 h. While bromocriptine has an affinity ratio of 2:1 for D_3 versus D_2 receptors, pergolide has a 5:1 affinity for the same receptors. Moreover, these two drugs are also used in conjunction with antidepressants since they enhance the activity of these drugs.

Cabergoline is also an ergot derivative with the chemical name 1-[(6-allylergolin-8β-yl)-carbonyl]-1-[3-(dimethylamino)propyl]-3-ethylurea and the structural formula $C_{26}H_{37}N_5O_2$ (m.w. 451 g/mol). It is used as a second-line agent to treat Parkinson's when bromocriptine is ineffective. About 40–45% of the drug is bound to plasma proteins in the blood and about 30–60% of it is available for systemic absorption. It is unique in having the longest elimination half-life of about 65–110 h. Cabergoline has high affinity for D_2 receptors but also exhibits very low affinity for D_1, adrenergic and serotonin receptors. Cabergoline is extensively metabolized in the liver by the cytochrome P450 class of enzymes and is excreted via urine.

Pramipexole is a non-ergoline benzothiazole-derived dopamine agonist. Chemically, it is called (6*R*)-*N*′-propyl-4,5,6,7-tetrahydro-1,3-benzothiazole-2,6-diamine and has the structural formula $C_{10}H_{17}N_3S$ (m.w. 211 g/mol). It is rapidly absorbed by the body and reaches peak plasma concentrations within 2 h of oral administration. It has a half-life of about 8 h. About 90% of the drug is metabolized and excreted in the urine. While this drug has 20 times more affinity for D_3 than D_2 receptors, unlike ergoline-derived drugs, it does not have any affinity for non-dopamine receptors such as the adrenergic and serotonin receptors. Since only about 15% of this drug is protein bound, more than 90% of it is available for biological action. Pramipexole acts by stimulating dopamine receptors in the striatum, thus restoring dopamine signaling in the synapses. However, certain depressant effects of this drug are due to its binding to the dopamine D_2 receptor (Mierau *et al.*, 1995).

Ropinirole is similar to pramipexole and is a non-ergoline derivative with maximum affinity for D_3 receptors and no affinity for D_1 receptors. It is chemically represented as 4-[2-(dipropylamino) ethyl]-1,3-dihydroindol-2-one and has the structural formula $C_{16}H_{24}N_2O$ (m.w. 260 g/mol). It is rapidly absorbed by the body and reaches peak plasma concentrations within 2 h of oral administration. About 40% of the drug is bound to plasma proteins, and, hence, just about 50% of it is available biologically for systemic absorption. It has a mean half-life of about 6 h. Its mode of action is similar to that of pramipexole and acts by stimulating D_3 receptors in the striatum. It is extensively metabolized by the cytochrome P450 1A2 enzyme in the liver by despropylation and hydroxylation. Most of its metabolites are inactive (Eden *et al.*, 1991; Tompson and Vearer, 2007). In addition to dopamine agonists, anticholinergic drugs such as benzotropine and trihexyphenidyl can also be used during early stages of the disease. Antihistamines like diphenhydramine and orphenadrine, which also have anticholinergic properties, are effective in treating tremors. Anticholinergic tricyclic antidepressants such as amitryptyline may be used along with levodopa for additive effects.

Sartans

Sartans are a class of drugs that modulate the renin–angiotensin system to treat hypertension and diabetic nephropathy. Some of them have also been implicated in congestive heart failure. Valsartan, candesartan, telmisartan, losartan, irbesartan and olmesartan are some of the important members of this drug family, of which only valsartan and candesartan are approved by the FDA for treatment of heart failure (Fig. 7.10). Losartan is the first Angiotensin II receptor blocker (ARB) to be introduced in the market. It is marketed by Merck & Co. under the trade name Cozaar. It is a competitive, selective AT_1 receptor antagonist and is mainly used to treat hypertension. Valsartan is another important ARB that has been implicated in the treatment of hypertension, congestive heart failure and myocardial infarction (Julius *et al.*, 2004; Verma and Strauss, 2004). It is marketed by Novartis under the trade name Diovan in the United States and by Cipla as Valtan and by Torrent Pharmaceuticals as Valzaar in India. Telmisartan is marketed under different trade names such as Pritor or Kinzal (Bayer Schering Pharma), Micardis (Boehringer Ingelheim), Telma (Glenmark Pharma), Telday (Torrent Pharmaceuticals) and Teleact D by (Ranbaxy). It has been approved by the FDA only for the treatment of hypertension. This drug is known for its longest half-life among all available ARBs. In addition to regulating the renin–angiotensin system, it also modulates peroxisome proliferator-activated receptor-γ (PPAR-γ), which is a key regulator of insulin and glucose metabolism (Benson *et al.*, 2004). Irbesartan is another AT_1 receptor antagonist, marketed as Aprovel, Karvea and Avapro by Sanofi-Aventis and Bristol-Meyers jointly. It is commonly used to treat hypertension but probably is also involved in delaying diabetic nephropathy (Lewis *et al.*, 2001). Olmesartan, marketed as Benicar and Olmetec by Daichii Sankyo and Forest Laboratories, regulates high blood pressure by blocking angiotensin II from binding to the AT_1 receptor. It lowers blood pressure by vasodilation. Moreover, due to its affinity for vitamin D receptor, olmesartan is also known to have immunomodulatory properties (Liu *et al.*, 2006; Marshall *et al.*, 2006). Candesartan is marketed by AstraZeneca and Takeda Pharmaceuticals as Blopress, Atacand, Ratacand and Amias. It is mainly used for the treatment of heart failure (Pfeffer *et al.*, 2003). It is also being studied for the treatment of Alzheimer's and dementia. It reduces inflammation by suppressing oxidative stress and preserving brain antioxidant capacity (Ozacmak *et al.*, 2007). Table 7.12 summarizes the important properties of sartans.

Biochemically, there are three functional groups that are necessary for the functional activity of angiotensin receptor blockers: imidazole ring binds to amino acids in helices III (Ser^{109}) and VII (Asn^{295}) of the AT_1 receptor; biphenyl-methyl group binds to residues in helices III (Val^{108}), VI (Trp^{253} and His^{256}) and VII (Arg^{281}, Phe^{300} and Phe^{301}); and tetrazole group interacts with residues in helices IV (Arg^{167}) and V (Lys^{199}) (de Gasparo *et al.*, 2000; Clément *et al.*, 2005). Since most of these angiotensin receptor antagonists have the same pharmacophore, their difference in pharmacological activity is due to different substituents in the basic structure. A lipophilic substituent like a linear alkyl group at position 2 on the imidazole ring, along with a biphenyl-methyl group, helps in interacting with hydrophobic pockets on the receptor. Similarly, an acidic group like tetrazole at position 1 on biphenyl-methyl moiety will help in binding to a basic residue in the receptor, thus making the drug a potent antagonist (Yanagiasawa *et al.*, 1996). Based on these principles, the various sartans have been designed and developed. The imidazole ring of losartan has been replaced with an acylated amino acid, valine, to produce valsartan (Burnier and Brunner, 2000). The hydroxymethyl group of losartan has been replaced with a carbonyl group leading to a new drug, irbesartan, that has much longer receptor binding properties when compared to losartan (Yanagiasawa *et al.*, 1996; Brunier and Brunner, 2000; Aulakh *et al.*, 2007). In case of telmisartan, the tetrazole group has been replaced by

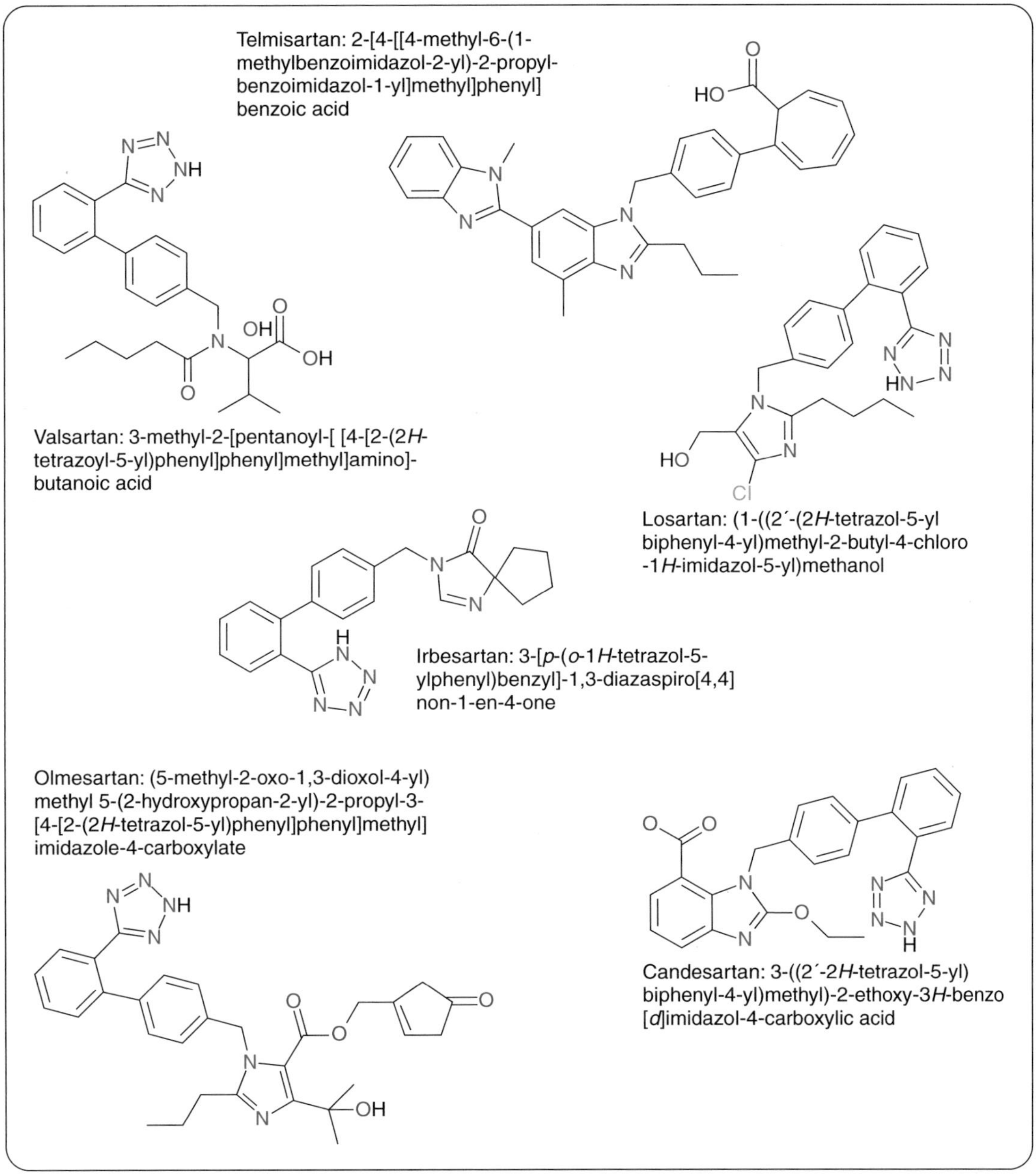

Fig. 7.10 ***Sartans are Angiotensin II Receptor Antagonists Mainly Used for the Treatment of Hypertension, Diabetic Nephropathy and Congestive Heart Failure***

(Sartans act by directly binding to the AT receptors, thus inhibiting their activation.)

Table 7.12 *Specific Class of AT1 Receptor Antagonists Called Sartans and Their Characteristic Features*

Drug	*AT_1R Binding Affinity*	*Half-life (hours)*	*Protein Binding (%)*	*Bioavailability (%)*	*Metabolism*
Candesartan	9.5–9.7	9	>99	15	Hepatic: CYP2C9; CYP11B9
Losartan	8.4–8.8	2	98.7	33	Hepatic: CYP2C9; CYP3A4
Valsartan	8.8–9.0	6	95	25	Hepatic: CYP2C9
Telmisartan	8.4	11–15	90–95	70	–
Irbesartan	8.7–8.8	24	>99	42–58	Hepatic: CYP2C9
Olmesartan	8.1	14–16	>99	29	–
Eprosartan	8.4–8.8	2	98	13	–

carboxylic acid, and this renders the drug more potent than its tetrazole-containing analogues (Aulakh *et al.*, 2007). Eprosartan is a unique ARB since the biphenyl-methyl group has been replaced with carboxy benzyl group, making it to bind the receptor with much more affinity and avidity. However, the physiological and biochemical implications of this drug are yet to be defined.

Losartan was the first AT_1 receptor antagonist developed based on imidazole structure and also the first sartan to be introduced into the market. It is currently marketed by Merck and Co. under the tradename Cozaar. [2-butyl-4-chloro-1-({4-[2-(2*H*-1,2,3,4-tetrazol-5-yl)phenyl]phenyl}methyl)-1*H*-imidazol-5-yl]methanol or losartan has the structural formula $C_{22}H_{23}ClN_6O$ (m.w. 422.9 g/mol). Chemically, losartan is imidazole derivative with a diphenyl tetrazol side chain that is considered important for binding the AT_1 receptors efficiently. The binding affinity (IC_{50}) of this drug for the AT_1 receptor is about 8.7–7.4 (Timmermans *et al.*, 1993; de Gasparo and Whitebread, 1994).

Losartan is actively metabolized in the liver by the cytochrome P450 class of enzymes, CYP450 3A4 and CYP450 2C9. The 5-hydroxymethyl group on imidazole ring is oxidized by these enzymes to produce the most active metabolite of losartan, E-3174. Almost about 14% of the administered dose of losartan is converted to E-3174 in the liver. About 33% of the drug is available for systemic absorption. While losartan achieves its peak plasma concentrations within 1 h of oral administration, E-3174 achieves the same in 3–4 h of oral administration. While the average half-life of losartan is 2 h, that of its metabolite E-3174 is 6–9 h. Losartan cannot be estimated in the blood plasma after 10 h of administration while E-3174 persists in the plasma for up to 24 h after administration of the drug. This implies that the long-term effects of losartan might be mediated by its stronger metabolite, E-3174. Losartan and E-3174 are extremely protein bound, especially albumin in the blood plasma, about 98.7% and 99.8%, respectively. While losartan and E-3174 have high affinities for AT_1 receptor than AT_2 receptor, E-3174 is 10–40-fold more potent than losartan. Moreover, losartan is a reversible competitive inhibitor of AT_1 receptor while E-3174 is a reversible noncompetitive inhibitor of the same receptor. Moreover, food intake slows the absorption of losartan while absorption of its metabolite E-3174 remains unaffected in such conditions. Losartan has a 10-fold lesser affinity for AT_1 receptor when compared to the natural agonist, angiotensin II. However, this drug has 3000-fold higher affinity for AT_1 receptor than AT_2 receptor but E-3174 has 30,000-fold higher affinity for AT_1 receptor than AT_2 receptor. Hence, E-3174 is much more strong, potent and stable than losartan and is probably the agent through which losartan mediates its effects. Losartan is, thus, a unique drug that inhibits the receptor in a competitive and noncompetitive manner simultaneously.

Only 4% of the orally administered dose of losartan is excreted unchanged in the urine, while 6% of its active metabolite is found in urine. While 60% of the orally administered losartan is excreted in feces and the 35% in urine, about 50% of intravenously administered losartan is excreted in feces and about 40% in urine. Losartan is believed to delay the progression of diabetic nephropathy in hypertensive patients and of renal diseases in diabetic patients. Randomized, placebo-controlled, multicenter clinical trials were conducted on about 1513 patients diagnosed with diabetic nephropathy worldwide. Patients were administered 50–100 mg of losartan daily for an average of 3.4 years. About 16% reduction in risks developed due to progressing of the disease was observed. Moreover, losartan also reduced proteinuria by an average of 30% within the first three months of start of the therapy. There was also a significant decrease in the decline of glomerular filtration rate, about 13%. Hence, losartan is indicated for the treatment of diabetic nephropathy in patients with type 2 diabetes and hypertension (Dahlöf *et al.*, 2002). Losartan is also found to downregulate the expression of tumor growth factor-β (TGF-β) receptors in diabetic rats and has been correlated to its nephro-protective activity (Habashi *et al.*, 2006).

Valsartan is a non-peptide, orally active highly specific noncompetitive antagonist of AT_1 receptor. It was mainly used for the treatment of hypertension, congestive heart failure and myocardial infarction. It is chemically described as (2*S*)-3-methyl-2-[pentanoyl-[[4-[2-(2H-tetrazol-5-yl)phenyl] phenyl]methyl]amino]butanoic acid and has the empirical formula $C_{24}H_{29}N_5O_3$ (m.w. 435.5 g/mol). It is currently being marketed in the United States by Novartis under the brand name Diovan and in India by Cipla as Valtan and by Torrent Pharmaceuticals as Valtan. Valsartan is a tetrazol-biphenyl-valine derivative. This drug binds to the AT_1 receptor with an affinity (IC_{50}) of 9.0–8.8 (Verheijen *et al.*, 2000). Valsartan has 30,000-fold higher affinity for AT_1 receptor than for AT_2 receptor.

Orally administered valsartan is absorbed rapidly by the body and reaches a peak plasma concentration within 2 h of administration. This drug has an average half-life of about 6 h. About 25% of the drug is available for biological activity. However, intake of food reduces the absorption rate of the drug by almost 45%. About 95% of the drug binds to plasma protein albumin. Valsartan is actively metabolized by the cytochrome P450 2C9 enzyme in the liver. Unlike losartan, valsartan does not have any active metabolites. Most of the orally administered valsartan, up to 85%, is excreted by feces and very little in urine. Only about 20% of the administered dose is recovered as metabolites, the major one being valeryl 4-hydroxy valsartan. Hence, most of the excreted drug is the parent compound. The hypertensive effects of valsartan were first studied in a group of seven placebo-controlled patients for 4–12 weeks. The administered dose of valsartan was 10–320 mg/day. It took about 4 weeks for effective traetment by valsartan, but long-term follow-up studies showed that this treatment was effective for upto 2 years (Julius *et al.*, 2004). A recent study by Qu *et al.* (2008) has shown that valsartan improved cardiac function in rabbits with heart failure, probably by inducing expression of the enzymes protein kinase A, protein phosphatase 1-α and myocardial sarcoplasmic reticulum calcium adenodine triphosphatase.

Candesartan is marketed as a prodrug candesartan cilexetil by AstraZeneca and Takeda Pharmaceuticals. This prodrug, cyclohexyl 1-hydroxyethyl carbonate ester, is converted to the active drug during absorption from the gastrointestinal tract by ester hydrolysis. Of all the current angiotensin receptor antagonists available in the market, candesartan has the highest affinity for the AT_1 receptors, IC_{50} being 9.7–9.5 (Vanderheyden *et al.*, 1999). It exhibits about 80-fold higher and 10-fold higher affinity for AT_1 receptor compared to losartan and its active metabolite, E-3174, respectively. Chemically, candesartan is 2-ethoxy-3-[[4-[2-(2*H*-tetrazol-5-yl)phenyl]phenyl]methyl] benzimidazole-4-carboxylic acid represented as $C_{24}H_{20}N_6O_3$ (m.w. 440.4 g/mol). Candesartan is administered as a prodrug to increase its bioavailability and rate of absorption. In spite of this it has a poor absorption rate of 15–40% only. It reaches its peak plasma concentration within 3–5 h of oral administration. Unlike losartan and valsartan, food intake does not affect the absorption of candesartan. More than 99% of the drug is bound to serum proteins and does not penetrate red blood cells. Candesartan is actively metabolized in the liver by the cytochrome P450 11B2 and 2C9 enzymes. Candesartan is O-de-ethylated to form an inactive metabolite. However, the prodrug is metabolized in the intestinal walls. The drug has a mean half-life of 10 h. Most of the unchanged drug is excreted via the biliary route (~70%).

Eprosartan was the first non-biphenyl tetrazole to be synthesized. It is a potent AT_1 receptor antagonist and is tolerated better in elderly than conventional ACE inhibitors (Ruilope *et al.*, 2001). It was mainly used for treatment of high blood pressure and hypertension. Eprosartan is chemically designated as 4-[[2-butyl-5-[(*E*)-3-hydroxy-3-oxo-2-(thiophen-2-ylmethyl)prop-1-enyl]imidazol-1-yl]methyl]benzoic acid ($C_{23}H_{24}N_2O_4S$; m.w. 424.5 g/mol). It has an affinity of pIC_{50} 8.8–8.4 for the AT_1 receptors. Eprosartan acts by blocking binding of angiotensin II to the AT_1 receptor in vascular smooth muscle causing vascular dilation. Moreover, it also acts by inhibiting norepinephrine production, thus reducing the blood pressure. About 15% of the orally administered eprosartan is available for biological activity. It has a mean half-life of 5–7 h. More than 98% of the drug is plasma protein bound. The enzymes involved in metabolism of this drug are not known yet. While most of the drug is eliminated unchanged, biliary elimination is maximum.

Telmisartan is a potent non-biphenyl tetrazole ARB. Chemically, it is represented as 4′-[(1,4′-dimethyl-2′-propyl[2,6′-bi-1*H*-benzimidazol]-1′-yl)methyl]-[1,1′-biphenyl]-2-carboxylic acid with the empirical formula $C_{33}H_{30}N_4O_2$ (m.w. 514.6 g/mol). Like other sartans, telmisartan is also highly specific for AT_1 receptors and has about 3000-fold higher affinity for this receptor than the AT_2 receptor. Telmisartan has an affinity (IC_{50}) of 8.4 for the AT_1 receptor (McClellan and Markham, 1998). Upon oral administration, telmisartan reaches peak plasma concentrations within 1 h. It is the ARB with the longest half-life of 24 h, and hence administration of a small dose once a day is sufficient for its efficient activity. About 40% of the orally administered dose is available for systemic absorption. However, bioavailability of this drug is dose dependent as is evident from the studies. Administration of 40 mg/day leaves 48% of the drug for biological activity, while the administration of 160 mg/day leaves about 62% of the drug for systemic absorption. Intake of food reduces the rate of absorption by 6%. More than 99.5% of this drug is bound to serum albumin and α1-acid glycoprotein. Telmisartan is active as such and is metabolized to its inactive acyl glucuronide. However, the enzymes involved in metabolizing this drug are not known yet. Telmisartan and its metabolites are completely eliminated by the biliary system (feces) (McClellan and Markham, 1998). Clinical trial studies with telmisartan were demonstrated in six placebo-controlled subjects. The patients were administered 20–160 mg of this drug per day. The antihypertensive activity of this drug was observed within 3 h of administration. However, in some cases, it took about 4 weeks to be effective. Moreover, the effect of telmisartan was persistent for about a year (McGill and Reilly, 2001).

Olmesartan, just like candesartan, is marketed as a prodrug, olmesartan medoxomil, by Daiichi Sankyo Ltd. The prodrug is ester-hydrolyzed to the active olmesartan during absorption in the gastrointestinal tract (Warner and Jarvis, 2002). Olmesartan, unlike losartan, does not have any active metabolite. Olmesartan medoxomil is described chemically as 2,3-dihydroxy-2-butenyl 4-(1-hydroxy-1-methylethyl)-2-propyl-1-[*p*-(*o*-1*H*-tetrazol-5-ylphenyl)benzyl]imidazole-5-carboxylate, cyclic 2,3-carbonate with the empirical formula $C_{29}H_{30}N_6O_6$ (m.w. 558.5 g/mol). This drug also has a higher affinity for AT_1 receptor and binds to this receptor with an affinity of pIC_{50} 8.1 (Koike *et al.*, 2001). However, it has 12,500-fold higher affinity for AT_1 receptor than AT_2 receptor. Olmesartan reaches peak plasma concentration within 1–2 h of oral administration and is not affected by food. About 26% of this drug is available for systemic absorption and has a mean half-life of about 13 h. More than 99% of the drug is bound to plasma proteins and does not enter the red blood cells. The key enzymes involved in the metabolism of this drug are not known and no metabolites of this drug have been observed so far. More than 50% of the drug is eliminated in feces and the rest in urine.

Vaptans

Vaptans are popularly known as vasopressin receptor antagonists. Vasopressin receptors are responsible for vasoconstriction and free water absorption. Hence, they are implicated in myocardial infarction, nephrogenic diabetes insipidus and hyponatremia. Antagonism of V_1 and V_2 receptors leads to vasodilation and aquaresis, respectively. Vaptans, also known as 'antidiuretic hormone receptor antagonists', act by blocking the vasopressin receptors. Commonly used vaptans include conivaptan, tolvaptan, relcovaptan, mozavaptan, satavaptan and lixivaptan (Fig. 7.11) (Ghali *et al.*, 2005). While conivaptans act on V_{1a} and V_2 receptors, other vaptans act mainly on V_2 receptors. Most of the vaptans are also being studied as a potential cure for heart diseases. Conivaptan was approved by the FDA in 2004 to treat hyponatremia. Conivaptan is a non-peptide dual arginine vasopressin receptor antagonist (Zoler, 2005). This drug acts by exerting antagonistic activity at vasopressin receptors, which leads to the inhibition of excessive vasopressin secretion. This increases water secretion, which leads to fluid loss and decrease in urinary osmolality (Fernandez-Varo *et al.*, 2003). A study involving 74 patients who were administered with 40–80 mg/day of conivaptan to treat hyponatremia concluded that this drug caused an increase in aquaretic effect (secretion of fluids while retaining electrolytes), thus leading to an increase in serum sodium levels and plasma osmolality. There was also a decrease in urine osmolality and urinary sodium (Ghali *et al.*, 2005). Mozavaptan (trade name Physuline) is another vasopressin receptor antagonist that is being marketed by Otsuka Pharmaceutical Co. Ltd., Japan and was approved by FDA in 2006 to treat hyponatremia. Satavaptan (developed by Sanofi-Aventis as V_2 vasopressin receptor antagonist under the trade name Aquilda), tolvaptan and relcovaptan are still awaiting FDA approval.

Conivaptan is a non-peptide V_1/V_2 dual antagonist and was approved by FDA in 2004 to treat hyponatremia (Zoler, 2005). It is marketed by Astellas Pharma US, Inc. under the brand name Vaprisol. It is represented chemically as *N*-[4-(2-methyl-4,5-dihydro-3*H*-imidazo[5,4-*d*][1]benzazepine-6-carbonyl)phenyl]-2-phenylbenzamide and has the structural formula $C_{32}H_{26}N_4O_2$ (m.w. ~ 498g/mol). It is rapidly absorbed by the body and reaches peak plasma concentrations within 2–3 h of oral administration. However, administration by the intramuscular injection is comparatively slow and

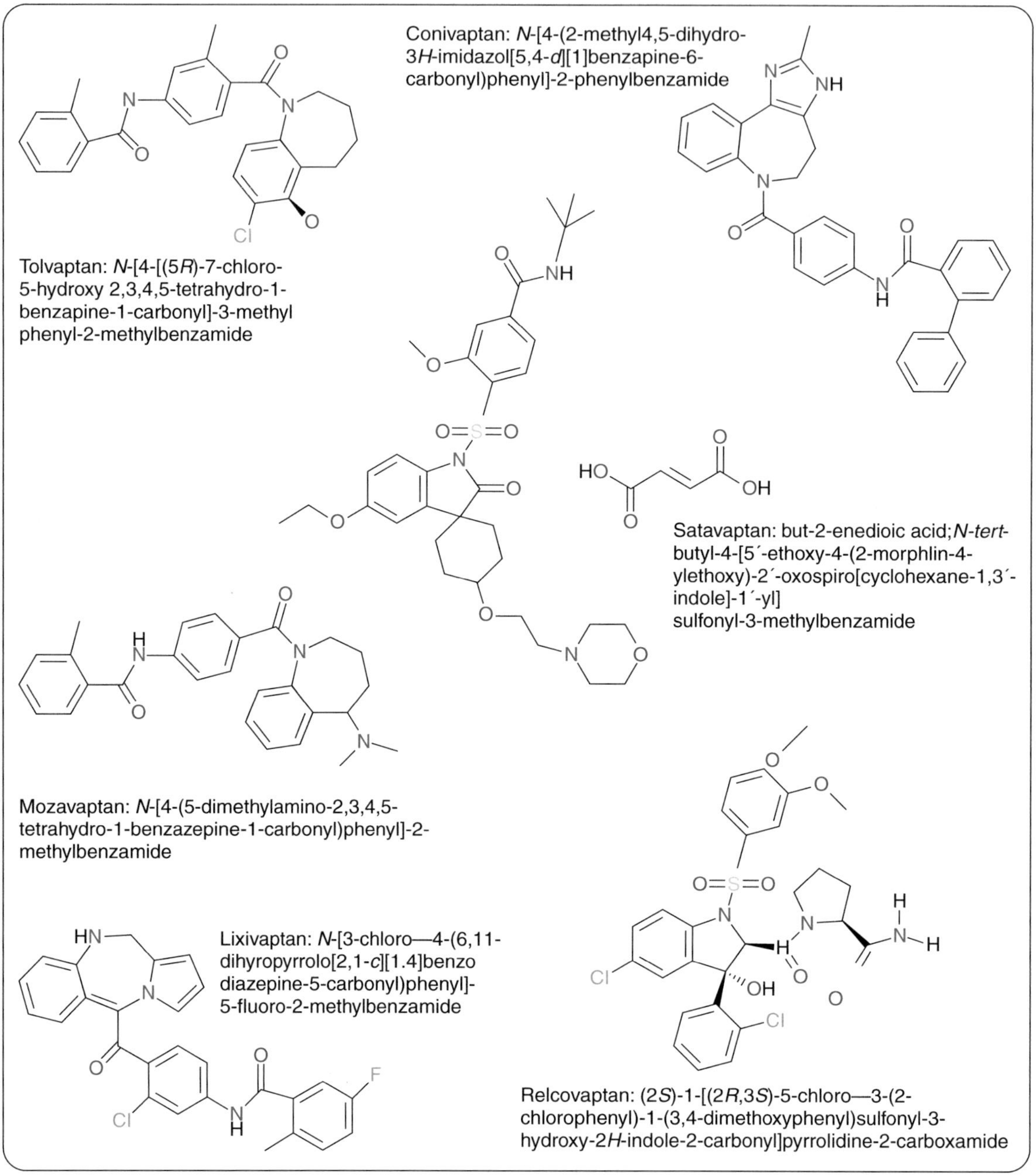

Fig. 7.11 ***Vaptans are Vasopressin Receptor Antagonists that are Implicated in the Treatment of Hyponatremia or Low Sodium Levels and Vasoconstriction***

(Vaptans are also used in the treatment of myocardial infarctions and nephrogenic diabetes insipidus. They are still under consideration for their use in congestive heart failures.)

reaches peak plasma concentrations only in 1–2 days. About 99% of the drug binds to plasma proteins and has a mean half-life of 5 h. This drug is actively metabolized in the liver by the cytochrome P450 3A4 enzymes. The metabolites of this drug, however, show 50–100% affinity for V_2 receptors and less than 50% affinity for V_{1a} receptors.

Conivaptan has nanomolar affinity for the V_{1a} and V_2 receptors *in vitro*. This interaction between conivaptan and the vasopressin receptors *in vivo* in the renal collecting ducts results in aquaresis or excretion of free water. This drug acts by exerting antagonistic activity at vasopressin receptors, which leads to the inhibition of excessive vasopressin secretion and, hence, reduced interaction between the receptor and vasopressin (Udelson *et al.*, 2001). This increases water secretion, which leads to fluid loss and decrease in urinary osmolality, thereby correcting sodium and water imbalance (Fernandez-Varo *et al.*, 2003). A study involving 74 patients who were administered with 40–80 mg/day of conivaptan to treat hyponatremia concluded that this drug caused an increase in aquaretic effect (secretion of fluids while retaining electrolytes), thus leading to an increase in serum sodium levels and plasma osmolality. There was also a decrease in urine osmolality and urinary sodium (Ghali *et al.*, 2005). Overdosage of conivaptan is related to headaches, confusion, insomnia, hypertension, orthostatic hypotension, dehydration, constipation, diarrhea and vomiting. Drugs, such as ketoconazole, clarithromycin, ritonavir and indinavir, that inhibit CYP450 3A4 enzyme activity result in increased conivaptan levels in the blood (Tahara *et al.*, 2005).

Tolvaptan is a competitive V_2 receptor antagonist awaiting FDA approval. It is mainly used for the treatment of hyponatremia. Moreover, this drug does not have any adverse side effects such as hypotension and hypokalemia and no adverse effects on the kidney (Shoaf *et al.*, 2005). Chemically, tolvaptan is represented as *N*-[4-[(5*R*)-7-chloro-5-hydroxy-2,3,4,5-tetrahydro-1-benzazepine-1-carbonyl]-3-methylphenyl]-2-methylbenzamide having the structural formula $C_{26}H_{25}ClN_2O_3$ (m.w. ~ 448 g/mol).

Mozavaptan (trade name Physuline) is another vasopressin receptor antagonist, which is marketed by Otsuka Pharmaceutical Co. Ltd., Japan and was approved by FDA in 2006 to treat hyponatremia. *Satavaptan* (developed by Sanofi-Aventis as V_2 vasopressin receptor antagonist under the trade name Aquilda), tolvaptan and relcovaptan are still awaiting FDA approval.

α- and β-Agonists and Antagonists

α-Agonists are sympathomimetic agents that have effects similar to adrenaline and noradrenaline. They are subdivided into α_1-agonists and α_2-agonists. While α_1-agonists activate phospholipase C leading to an increase in intracellular inositol triphosphate, α_2-agonists, on the other hand, inhibit adenylyl cyclase, leading to a decrease in intracellular calcium. α_1-agonists act as potent vasoconstrictors, vasopressors and nasal decongestants. Methoxamine, methylnorepinephrine, oxymetazoline and phenylephrine are potent α_1-agonists while clonidine, guanfacine, guanabenz and guanoxabenz are potent α_2-agonists (Figures 7.12 and 7.13).

Methoxamine is a non-catecholamine α_1-adrenoceptor agonist used to induce vasoconstriction of skin and blood vessels. It is chemically designated as 2-amino-1-(2,5-dimethoxyphenyl)propan-1-ol and has the structural formula $C_{11}H_{17}NO_3$ (m.w. 211.2 g/mol). It binds to α_{1A}-adrenoceptor with the highest affinity of pK_i 5.0–5.2 (Shibata *et al.*, 1995; Taniguchi *et al.*, 1999). It has moderate affinity for α_{1D}-adrenoceptor and least for α_{1B}-adrenoceptor as pK_i 4.9 and pK_i 4.0, respectively (Shibata *et*

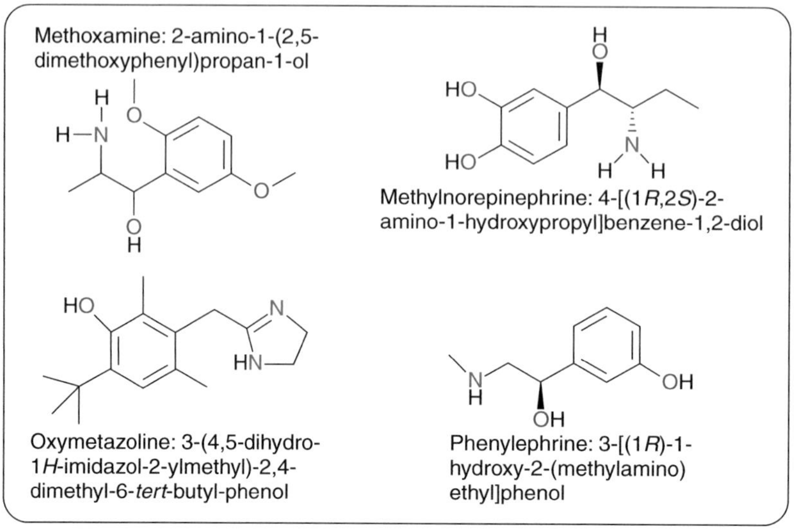

Fig. 7.12 ***α_1-Agonists are Sympathomimetic Agents that Act by Mimicking the Effects of Adrenaline and Noradrenaline on α_1-Adrenergic Receptors***

(They are potent vasoconstrictors and nasal decongestants. They activate the receptors, which in turn activate phospholipase C leading to release of inositol triphosphates.)

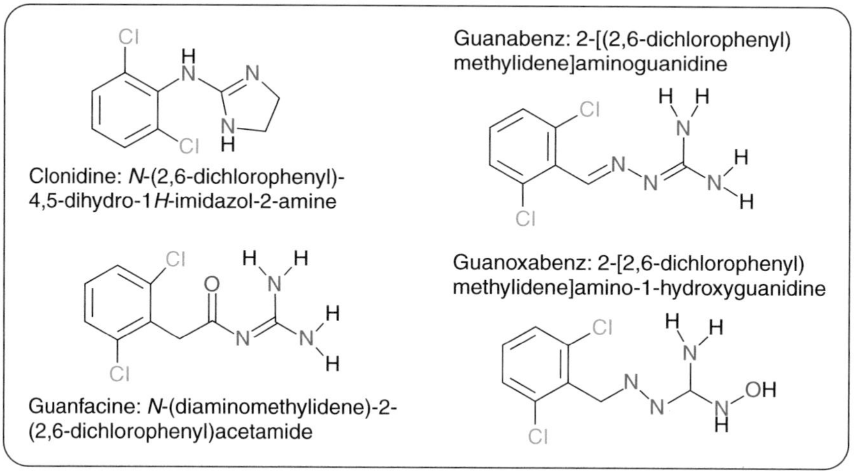

Fig. 7.13 ***α_2-Agonists Act on α_2-Adrenergic Receptors to Activate them***

(They act by inhibiting the activity of adenylyl cyclase leading to a decrease in intracellular calcium.)

al., 1995). Although methoxamine is known to undergo hepatic metabolism, the enzymes involved and the active metabolites of the drug produced as a result of metabolism are not known. Upon oral administration, methoxamine starts acting within 15–20 min while its action is evident in 2 min upon administration intravenously.

Oxymetazoline is a selective complete α_1-agonist and a partial α_2-agonist. It is normally used locally in the eye or the nose as a vasoconstrictor. Chemically, it is represented as 6-*tert*-butyl-3-(4,5-dihydro-1*H*-imidazol-2-ylmethyl)-2,4-dimethylphenol ($C_{16}H_{24}N_2O$; molecular weight 260.3 g/mol). This drug has equal affinity for α_{1A}- and α_{2A}-receptors, pK_i 8.0–8.2 (Obika *et al.*, 1995; Shibata *et al.*, 1995; Taniguchi *et al.*, 1999). However, it acts as a partial agonist and has an affinity of pK_i 6.3–6.8 for the α_{1B}-, α_{1D}-, α_{2C}- and α_{2D}-receptors (Obika *et al.*, 1995; Shibata *et al.*, 1995). It is a sympathomimetic drug that downregulates the receptors. Oxymetazoline acts by inducing vasoconstriction that leads to decrease in conjuctival congestion in the eyes. It also produces congestion in nasal blood vessels resulting in decreased blood flow and nasal congestion. Irrespective of the route of administration, oxymetazoline is absorbed well by the systemic circulation.

Phenylephrine is a prototypical α_1-agonist indicated in treatment of congestions and low blood pressure. It is also used to dilate pupils. It is chemically designated as 3-[(1*R*)-1-hydroxy-2-methylaminoethyl]phenol and has the structural formula $C_9H_{13}NO_2$ (molecular weight 167.2 g/mol). It acts as a full agonist for α_{1B}- and α_{1D}-receptors and has a pIC_{50} of 6.3–7.5 but has a much lower affinity for the α_{1A}-receptor (Minneman *et al.*, 1994; Ford *et al.*, 1997). This drug brings about a contraction of pupillary dilatory muscle and smooth muscles in the arterioles of conjuctiva and peripheral vasoconstriction. It decreases nasal congestion by acting on α_1-receptors in the arterioles of nasal mucosa, thus resulting in nasal constriction. About 95% of the drug is bound to plasma proteins and has a half-life of 2–3 h. Bioavailability of the drug is very low due to first-pass metabolism in the liver. This drug is metabolized by monoamine oxidases in the gut and liver. The drug is eliminated mainly via urine.

Clonidine was first developed in 1970s and is a strong α_2-receptor agonist. It is used in treatment of certain types of neuropathic pain, opioid detoxification, sleep hyperhidrosis, anesthesia and hypertension. Its IUPAC nomenclature is *N*-(2,6-dichlorophenyl)-4,5-dihydro-1*H*-imidazol-2-amine ($C_9H_9Cl_2N_3$; molecular weight 230 g/mol). Clonidine acts by stimulating adrenergic receptors in the brain, resulting in reduced sympathetic outflow and thus leading to reduced blood pressure and heart rate. It has a high affinity for α_{2A}- and α_{2B}-receptors (pK_i 6.7–9.2) but a low affinity for α_2-receptor (pK_i 6.0–7.8) (Jasper *et al.*, 1998; Peltonen *et al.*, 1998; Pihlavisto *et al.*, 1998). Clonidine is well absorbed by the body and has a mean half-life of 15 h. Only 30% of the drug is bound to serum plasma proteins and hence it has a high bioavailability of 65% for systemic circulation. Though the enzymes involved in its metabolism are not known yet, it is known that this drug is metabolized mainly in the liver and *p*-hydroxyclonidine is its major inactive metabolite. Almost 50% of the unchanged drug is eliminated in urine within 24 h of administration (Hossmann *et al.*, 1980).

Guanfacine is a phenylacetyl-derived, centrally acting α_2-receptor agonist mainly used as an antihypertensive agent. Chemically, guanfacine is designated as *N*-(diaminomethylidene)-2-(2,6-dichlorophenyl)acetamide and has the empirical formula $C_9H_9Cl_2N_3O$ (m.w. 246 g/mol). It has the highest affinity for α_{2A}-receptor (pK_i 7.2) and moderate affinity for the other two subtypes of α_2-receptors (pK_i 5.8–6.5) (Jasper *et al.*, 1998). It acts by stimulating the α_2-adrenoceptors, resulting in a decrease in sympathetic nerve impulses from the vasomotors to heart and blood vessels. Upon oral administration, guanfacine reaches peak plasma concentrations within 4 h. It is absorbed very rapidly and completely in the body and almost 80% of the drug is available for systemic circulation. About 70% of the drug is bound to plasma proteins and has a long half-life of 17 h. This drug is actively metabolized by the liver cytochrome P450 enzymes, CYP2C9 and CYP2C19. It is hydroxylated to its inactive metabolite, 3-hydroxyguanfacine, which is primarily eliminated in urine. About 30% of the drug is eliminated unchanged in urine.

Guanabenz is an orally active, central α-agonist of the α_2-type receptor and mainly indicated in the treatment of hypertension. It is structurally similar to clonidine and acts by relaxing the blood vessels. It combines the aminoguanidine side chain of guanethidine with the substituted benzene ring of clonidine. This drug is chemically represented as 2-[(2,6-dichlorophenyl)methylideneamino] guanidine ($C_8H_8Cl_2N_4$; m.w. 231 g/mol). This drug has almost 1300-fold higher affinity for the α_2-receptors than the α_1-receptors. Guanabenz is rapidly absorbed by the body and almost 75% of the drug is available for systemic absorption. More than 90% of the drug is bound to plasma proteins and has a mean half-life of 7–14 h. The drug attains its peak plasma concentration within 2–3 h of oral administration. It is actively metabolized in the liver and undergoes hydroxylation, followed by glucuronidation. Only about 2% of the unchanged drug is recovered in urine.

Drugs that block the activity of α-receptors are indicated in the treatment of high blood pressure. These drugs, called α-antagonists, have limited clinical significance. Phenoxybenzamine, phentolamine and prazosin are the representative members of this class of drugs (Fig. 7.14). *Phenoxybenzamine* is a nonselective α-antagonist that links the presynaptic α_2-receptors to the postsynaptic α_1-receptors. It binds covalently to the receptors and blockade is irreversible and noncompetitive. The blocked receptors have to be recycled and new receptors replaced. It induces hypotension by decreasing peripheral resistance but might also increase heart rate due to blockade of the presynaptic receptors. In contrast to phenoxybenzamine, phentolamine is a competitive blocker of the α_1- and α_2-receptors. It is similar to phenoxybenzamine in its mode of action. It relaxes the vascular smooth muscles, thus reducing blood pressure. Prazosin is a competitive selective α_1-antagonist that acts by relaxing arterial smooth muscles resulting in lowering of blood pressure. Unlike phenoxybenzamine and phentolamine, prazosin has much fewer side effects and hence is preferred over the other two drugs.

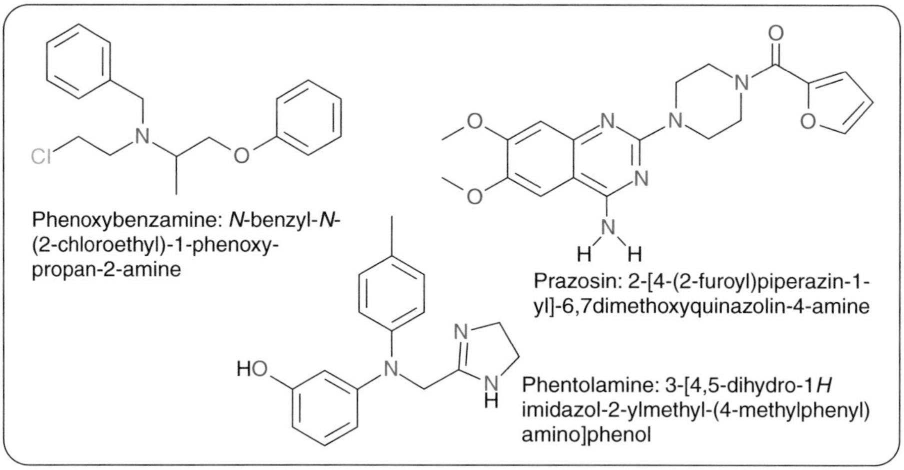

Fig. 7.14 ***α-Antagonists Block the Activity of α-Adrenergic Receptors and are Implicated in Conditions of High Blood Pressure***

(These drugs are not very popular since they have very limited clinical significance.)

β-Agonists or β-adrenergics act by relaxing the bronchial smooth muscles, decrease mast cell degranulation and histamine release, increase mucociliary clearance and inhibit microvascular leakage into the air passage. By far, they are the best drugs available for relieving sudden asthmatic attacks. These bronchodilators stimulate β-adrenergic receptors to widen airway passages. β-Agonists can be short or long acting. While short-acting β_2-agonists such as albuterol start acting immediately and are effective for 6–8 h, long-acting drugs, on the other hand, are active for about 12 h and used in cases of moderate to severe asthma. Moreover, long-acting β-agonists also modulate the effect of corticosteroids, thus decreasing their effective dosage. However, tachycardia and tremor are the most common adverse effects associated with β-agonists.

β-Agonists are drugs that act as agonists for β-adrenergic receptors and hence are used in treatment of cardiac diseases, asthma and COPD (Fig. 7.15). Dobutamine is a β_1-adrenoceptor agonist developed by Eli Lilly and Co. to treat cardiac shock and cardiac failure. It is a sympathomimetic drug that acts by stimulating the β_1-adrenoceptor in the sympathetic nervous system. It stimulates the receptor, thus helping in increased contractability of the heart and cardiac output. Isoprenaline or isoproterenol is another sympathomimetic drug that acts on both β_1- and β_2-adrenoceptors. It is being used to treat cardic failures and asthma. Salbutamol or albuterol is a short-acting β-agonist used as a bronchodilator in case of asthma. It is marketed by GlaxoSmithKline as Ventolin or Ventorlin, as Asthalin by Cipla, as Proventil by Schering-Plough and as ProAir by Teva. It was approved by the FDA in 1980 for treating acute asthma. Fenoterol was developed by Boehringer-Ingelheim and is marketed as Berotec. Its acts on β-adrenoceptors and opens up airway passages in asthmatic patients. Formoterol or eformoterol is a long-acting β-agonist used in the treatment of asthma and COPD. It is marketed as Foradil/Foradile by Novartis, Oxis by AstraZeneca, Atock by Astellas and Perforomist by Dey. It was approved by the FDA in 2005 to treat asthma. It relaxes smooth muscles of the airway passage in lungs. Once diffused into the plasma membrane, it is released back so that it can interact with β-adrenoceptors, and hence is long acting, up to 12 h. Orciprenaline or metaproterenol is a selective β_2-adrenergic receptor agonist that stimulates receptors of the smooth muscles in lungs and uterus. It is marketed as Alotec, Alupent, Metaprel and Novasmasol. Salmeterol is a long-acting β_2-agonist that is used to treat asthma and COPD. It is sold as Advair and Seretide. It was developed by GlaxoSmithKline and approved by the FDA in 2005. It acts like other β-agonists by relaxing smooth muscles in the airway passages. Terbutaline, marketed as Brethine, Bricanyl or Brethaire, is a selective β_2-agonist that is used to treat asthma. It is a fast-acting bronchodilator. It also being examined for its potential use as a drug to prevent contractions during pregnancy. Clenbuterol is also a β_2-agonist that is used as a decongestant and bronchodilator. It stimulates the central nervous system and hence increases the blood pressure, oxygen transport and rates at which fat and protein are utilized in the body. It was approved by the FDA in 2006 for treatment of asthma. It is also being studied as a potential weight reduction pill.

Formoterol is another long-acting β_2-agonist used to treat asthma and COPD. Its IUPAC nomenclature is *N*-[2-hydroxy-5-[1-hydroxy-2-[1-(4-methoxyphenyl)propan-2-ylamino]ethyl]phenyl] formamide represented as $C_{19}H_{24}N_2O_4$ (m.w. 344.4 g/mol). It has 200-fold higher affinity for β_2-receptors when compared to that for the β_1-receptors. Formoterol reaches maximum plasma concentration within 5–10 min of inhalation. Sixty to sixty-five percent of the drug is bound to human serum plasma proteins, of which about 30–40% of it is bound to the serum albumin. It has a mean half-life of 12–13 h. Formoterol is majorly metabolized by four cytochrome P450 enzymes—CYP2D6,

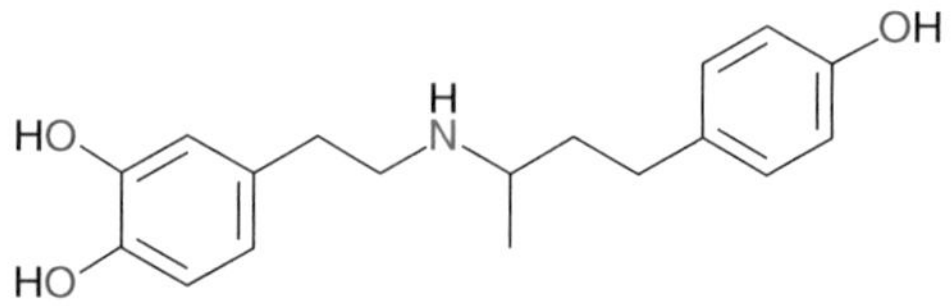

Dobutamine: 4-[2-[4-(4-hydroxyphenyl) butan-2-ylamino]ethyl]benzene-1,2-diol

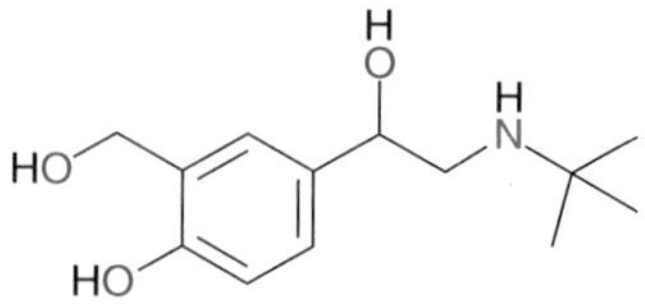

Salbutamol: 4-[2(*tert*-butylamino)-1-hydroxyethyl]-2-(hydroxymethyl)phenol

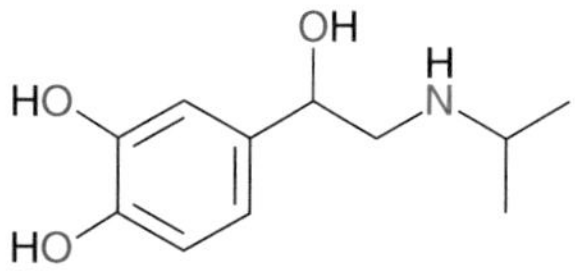

Isoprenaline: 4-[1-hydroxy-2-(1-methyl ethylamino)ethyl] benzene-1,2-diol

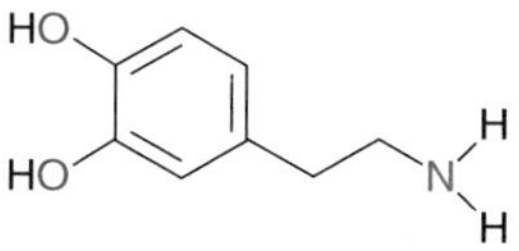

Dopamine: 4-(2-aminoethyl) benzene-1,2-diol

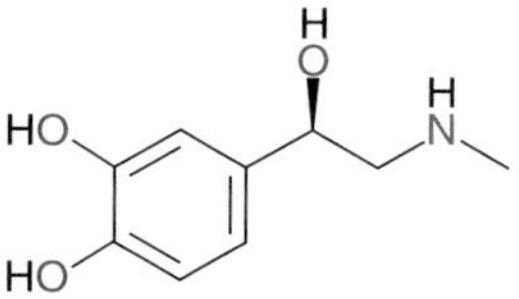

Epinephrine: (*R*)-4-(1-hydroxy -2-(methylamino)ethyl) benzene-1,2-diol

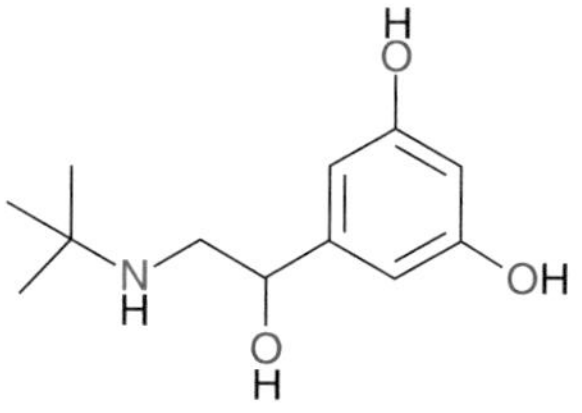

Terbutalines: 5-(1-hydroxy-2-*tert*-butylamino-ethyl) benzene-1,3-diol

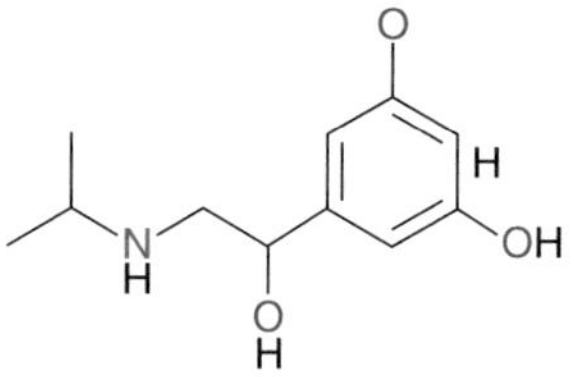

Orciprenaline: 5-[1-hydroxy-2-(1-methyl ethylamine)ethyl]benzene-1,3-diol

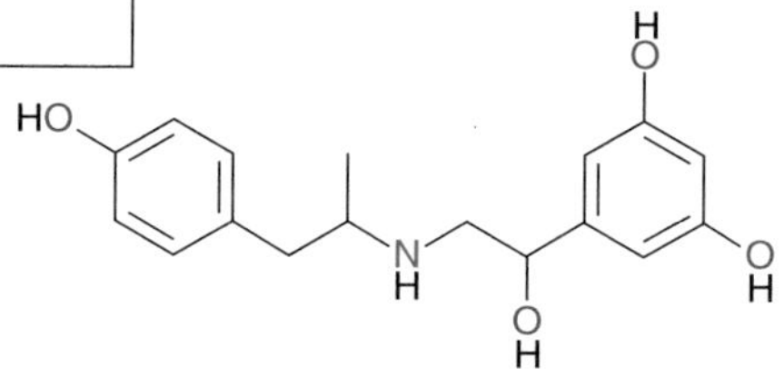

Fenoterol: (*RS*)-1-(3,5-dihydroxyphenyl) -2-(*RS*)-2-(4-hydroxyphenyl)-1-methyl ethylamino]ethanol

Clenbuterol: 1-(4-amino-3,5-dichloro-phenyl)-2-(*tert*-butylamino)ethanol

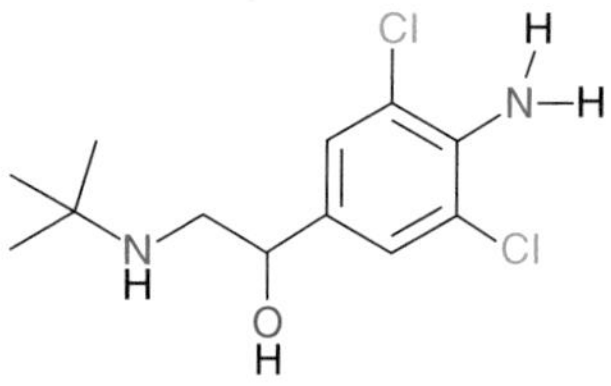

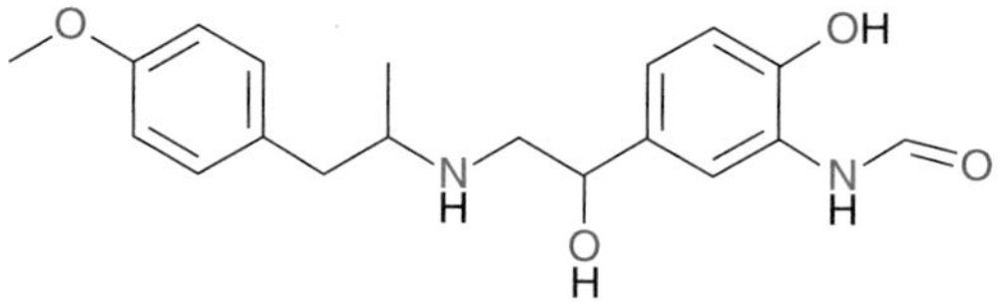

Formoterol: *N*-[2-hydroxy-5-[1-hydroxy-2-[1-(4-methoxyphenyl)propan-2-ylamino]ehtyl] phenyl]formamide

Fig. 7.15 ***β-Agonists, also known as β-Adrenergics, Act by Activating the β-Adrenoceptors and are Potent Bronchodilators***

(They relax bronchial smooth muscles, decrease histamine release and increase mucociliary clearance, thus widening air passages. Till date, they are the best available drugs for treating sudden asthmatic attacks. They may be long-acting or short-acting drugs.)

CYP2C19, CYP2C9 and CYP2A6—which are majorly responsible for O-demethylation of the drug. However, the major metabolic pathway of formeterol is glucuronidation of the phenolic or aliphatic hydroxyl group and O-demethylation followed by glucuronide conjugation of these hydroxyl groups. Minor secondary metabolic pathways include sulfate conjugation and deformylation. Most of the drug and its metabolites are eliminated in urine.

Salbutamol or albuterol is a short-acting β_2-agonist used to treat bronchospasms in case of asthma and COPD. It is a non-catecholamine drug available only as an inhaler. Inhaled albuterol has much fewer side effects than if administered. Chemically, albuterol is represented as 4-[2-(*tert*-butylamino)-1-hydroxyethyl]-2-(hydroxymethyl)phenol having the empirical formula $C_{13}H_{21}NO_3$ (m.w. 239.3 g/mol). This drug acts as a partial agonist of the β_2-receptor with an affinity of pK_i 5.8–6.1 (Isogaya *et al.*, 1999; Baker, 2005). Salbutamol is longer acting than isoprenaline or dobutamine, since it is not prone to rapid enzymatic degradation. Due to inhalation, the systemic absorption of salbutamol is very low. It reaches its peak plasma concentrations within 2–4 h of administration. It has a half-life of about 1.6 h. This drug is hydrolyzed by esterases in cardiac tissue to its active metabolite colterol. The drug is also conjugatively metabolized to salbutamol 4′-*O*-sulfate. Almost 75% of the drug is eliminated within 24 h of inhalation. About 30% of the drug is eliminated unchanged while 45% of it is eliminated as metabolites.

Isoprenaline (also known as isoproterenol) is a catecholamine-based synthetic derivative of noradrenaline. It is a sympathomimetic β-agonist acting on β_1- and β_2-receptors equally. It is chemically designated as 3,4-dihydroxy-α-[(isopropylamino)methyl] benzyl alcohol with the structural formula $C_{11}H_{17}NO_3$ (m.w. 247.7 g/mol). Isoprenaline binds to β_1-receptor with an affinity of pK_i 6.6–7.0 while it binds to β_2-receptor with a comparatively low affinity of pK_i 6.4. It has much lower affinity for the α-adrenergic receptors and almost no affinity for β_3-receptor (Frielle *et al.*, 1987; Sato *et al.*, 1996). This drug acts by stimulating adenyl cyclase thus increasing cAMP levels intracellularly. This, in turn, leads to the relaxation of bronchial smooth muscles and inhibits the release of mediators of hypersensitivity from cells, especially the mast cells. Isoprenaline is rapidly absorbed and metabolized by the body. It is metabolized primarily in the liver by the catechol-*O*-methyltransferase enzymes. The major metabolite after intravenous administration is 3-*O*-methylisoprenaline that exhibits very weak affinity for the β-adrenoceptors. Isoprenaline has a half-life of few minutes when administered parenterally, but a few hours when administered intravenously. Moreover, it is not as readily taken up by the sympathetic neurons as adrenaline or noradrenaline and, hence, has a longer duration of action. But since it is a catecholamine and catecholamines are readily degraded in the human body, especially by enzymes in the gut wall, the activity of isoprenaline is brief and short-lived.

Dobutamine is also a synthetic catecholamine that exhibits higher affinities for the β-adrenoceptors, but also very little affinity for the α_1-adrenergic receptors. It is a sympathomimetic drug used for the treatment of heart failure and cardiogenic shock. Chemically, dobutamine is designated as 4-[2-[4-(4-hydroxyphenyl)butan-2-ylamino]ethyl]benzene-1,2-diol with the empirical formula $C_{18}H_{23}NO_3$ (m.w. 301.3 g/mol). It is better classified as an ionodilator since it exhibits both vasodilator and positive ionotropic properties. This drug acts as a partial agonist for the β-adrenoceptors with an affinity of pK 5.5 for β_1- and β_3-adrenoceptors and an affinity of pK_i 6.4 for β_2-adrenoceptors (Isogaya *et al.*, 1999; Liapakis *et al.*, 2004). This drug acts directly on the β-adrenoceptors of the heart, thus increasing the myocardial contractility and stroke volume leading to enhanced cardiac output. Dobutamine is a very fast-acting drug and attains peak plasma concentrations within 2 min of administration. Hence, the biological effect of dobutamine can be witnessed within 1–2 min of administration. The mean half-life of dobutamine is also very less, 2 min. The metabolism of dobutamine is similar to that of isoprenaline, by catechol-*O*-methyltransferases, to the inactive major metabolite 3-*O*-methyldobutamine. Elimination of dobutamine is by the biliary system.

Xamoterol is a partial β_1-agonist that acts as a cardiac stimulant. It has been shown to improve the diastolic and systolic left ventricular pressure in patients with mild to moderate heart failure. Xamoterol, *N*-[2-[[2-hydroxy-3-(4-hydroxyphenoxy)propyl]amino]ethyl]morpholine-4-carboxamide, has the structural formula $C_{16}H_{25}N_3O_5$ (m.w. 339.3 g/mol). It is a partial agonist of the β_1-adrenoceptor with an affinity of pK_i 7.0 (Isogaya *et al.*, 1999). Due to its extensive hydrophilic nature, the rate of drug absorption from the gastrointestinal tract is very slow. Only about 9% of the drug is available for systemic absorption and biological activity. Upon oral administration, it is rapidly metabolized by sulfate conjugation of the 4-hydro group in the gut wall, while upon intravenous administration it is metabolized by the liver. About 56% of the inactive conjugate in case of oral administration is eliminated in urine (Rang *et al.*, 2003).

Orciprenaline is an orcinol isomer of adrenaline, in which two hydroxyl groups have been moved to adjacent positions on the benzene ring. Orciprenaline or metaproterenol is chemically designated as 5-[1-hydroxy-2-(propan-2-ylamino)ethyl]benzene-1,3-diol and has the empirical formula $C_{11}H_{17}NO_3$ (m.w. 211.2 g/mol). It is a partially selective β_2-agonist and acts by stimulating the β-adrenoceptors to activate adenyl cyclase, thus increasing intracellular cAMP concentrations. Since it is not a catecholamine, it is not subject to rapid degradation by sulfokinase in gut wall and catechol *O*-methyltransferases elsewhere, and, hence, it is much more stable than isoprenaline-like drugs. Moreover, since the hydroxyl groups are still present, the drug is still polar enough to enter the brain and, hence, does not cause insomnia like other drugs such as ephedrine. About 3% of the drug is absorbed as is by the lungs, while oral administration makes nearly 40% of the drug available for systemic absorption. The drug has a half-life of about 6 h and is majorly metabolized by enzymes in the gastrointestinal tract and hepatic system. However, the exact enzymes involved are not yet clear.

Salmeterol is a long-acting β_2-agonist prescribed for the treatment of asthma and COPD. It is chemically represented as 2-(hydroxymethyl)-4-[1-hydroxy-2-[6-(4-phenylbutoxy)hexylamino] ethyl]phenol and has the structural formula $C_{25}H_{37}NO_4$ (m.w. 415.5 g/mol). It is a complete agonist of the β_2-adrenoceptor and binds to the receptor with an affinity of pK_i 8.8 (Baker, 2005). It acts for about 12 h when compared to the 4 h activity of salbutamol and also has 50-fold higher affinity for the receptor compared to salbutamol. The long lipophilic side chains of salmeterol bind to the receptor, thus activating it constantly, in the lungs and bronchiolar smooth muscles. This causes relaxation of the smooth muscles in bronchi, vasodilation and, hence, increased airflow into the lungs (Salpeter *et al.*, 2006). While small therapeutic doses of salmeterol are undetected in the plasma, higher concentrations of the inhaled drug appear within 5–45 min of inhalation, with mean peak concentration achieved within 20 min of inhalation. More than 96% of the drug is bound to serum proteins and has a mean half-life of 5.5 h. Aliphatic oxidation of the drug by cytochrome P450 3A4 to α-hydroxysalmeterol occurs in human liver microsomes. The drug is extensively metabolized by hydroxylation since no unchanged drug is detected in urine or feces.

β-Antagonists, also called as β-blockers or symptolytic agents, act by binding reversibly or irreversibly to the β-adrenoceptors, thus preventing receptor-mediated intracellular effects. These drugs have been variously indicated in management and treatment of cardiac arrythmias, arterial hypertension, coronary heart disease (including secondary protection after myocardial infarction), congestive heart failure, hyperthyroidism, migraine and even glaucoma. β-Blockers block the activity of endogenous catecholamines such as adrenaline and noradrenaline on the adrenergic receptors. They reduce the effects of excitement and physical exertion on heart by blocking the normal epinephrine-mediated sympathetic actions, but only in excited cardiac cells. They do not act on resting cells. Propanolol was the first clinically useful β-blocker to be recognized. Other members of this family include acebutolol, bisoprolol, atenolol, esmolol, labetalol, carvedilol and metoprolol (Fig. 7.16).

Proponalol: [2-hydroxy-3-(naphthalen-1-yloxy)propyl](propan-2-yl)amine

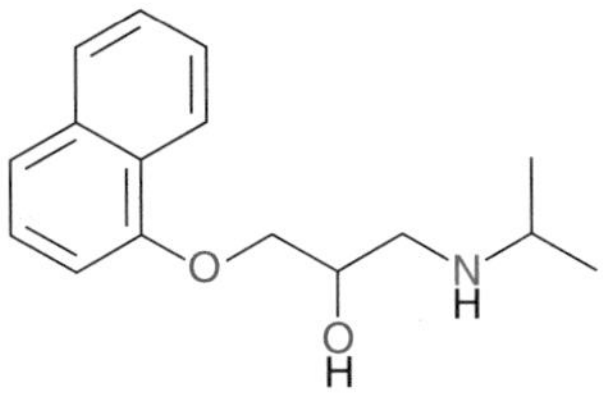

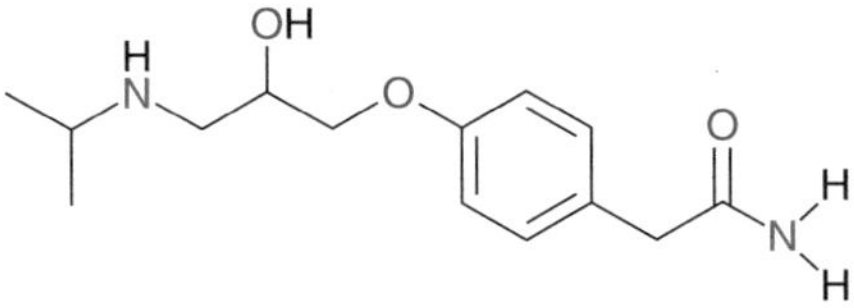

Atenolol: 2-4-[2-hydroxy-3-(propan-2-ylamino)propoxy]phenylacetamide

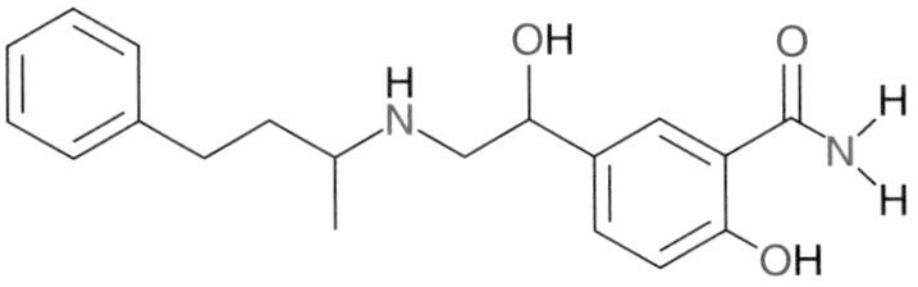

Labetalol: 2-hydroxy-5-1-hydroxy-2-[(4-phenylbutan-2-yl)amino]ethylbenzamide

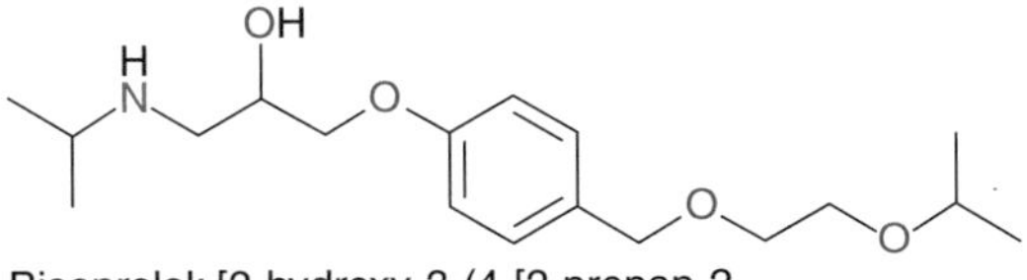

Bisoprolol: [2-hydroxy-3-(4-[2-propan-2-yloxyl)ethoxy]methylphenoxy)propyl](propan-2-yl)amine

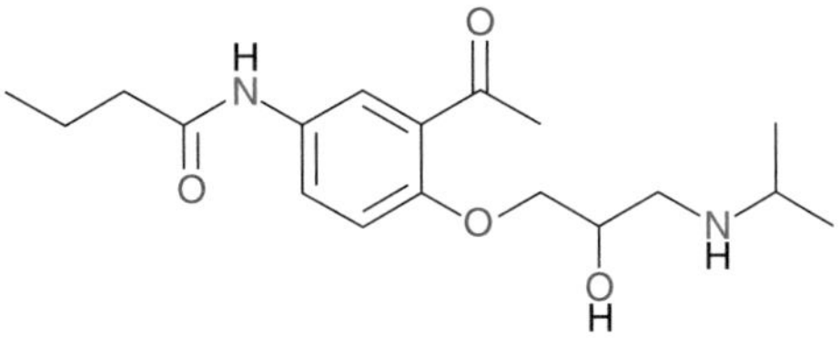

Acebutolol: *N*-3-acetyl-4-[2-hydroxy-3-(propan-2-ylamino)propoxy]phenylbutanamide

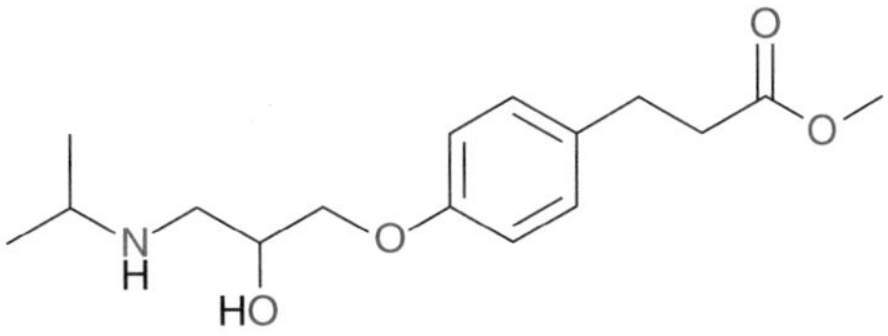

Esmolol: methyl 3-4-[2-hydroxy-3-(propan-2-ylamino)propoxyl]phenylpropanoate

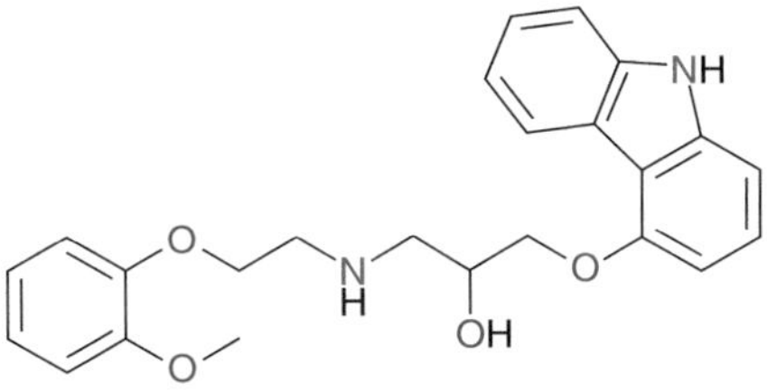

Carvedilol: [3-(9*H*-carbazol-4-yloxy)-2-hydroxypropyl][2-(2-methoxyphenoxy)ethyl]amine

Fig. 7.16 ***β-Antagonists, Popularly Known as β-Blockers, are Symptolytic Agents that Bind to β-Adrenoceptors to Inhibit their Activity***

(They are variously implicated in treatment of arterial hypertension, migraine, glaucoma and congestive heart failures.)

Propanolol is a non-selective β-blocker and the only drug approved for treating migraine in children. It is a highly lipophilic molecule implicated in treatment of hypertension, glaucoma, myocardial infarction, hyperthyroidism and angina pectoris. It is chemically designated as 1-naphthalen-1-yloxy-3-(propan-2-ylamino)propan-2-ol and has the structural formula $C_{16}H_{21}NO_2$ (m.w. 259.3 g/mol). Propanolol is a racemic mixture of the *R*(+)- and the *S*(–)-enantiomers. The *S*(–)-enantiomer is 100 times more potent than the *R*(+)-enantiomer in blocking the adrenoceptors. Also, clearance of the *S*(–)-enantiomer is much slower than the *R*(+)-enantiomer. It has a strong affinity for β_1-receptor and binds with an affinity of pK_i 8.2–8.9 (Louis *et al.*, 1999; Joseph *et al.*, 2004; Baker, 2005). However, this drug has the highest affinity (pK_i 9.1–9.5) for β_2-receptors (Isogaya *et al.*, 1999; Louis *et al.*, 1999; Baker, 2005). It has the least affinity of pK_i 6.3–7.2 for β_3-receptors (Louis *et al.*, 1999; Popp *et al.*, 2004). Propanolol exerts its antihypertensive activities by decreasing cardiac output, inhibiting renin release from the kidneys and decreasing sympathetic nerve conduction from vasomotors to brain cells. Due to its anesthetic property, it has a membrane-stabilizing ability, which has been implicated in treatment of cardiac arrythmias. However, the exact mechanism of this action is not clear yet.

Propanolol is almost completely absorbed after oral administration, but due to first-pass metabolism in the liver, only 25% of the drug administered is available for systemic circulation. This drug has a half-life of 4 h. About 90% of the drug is bound to the plasma proteins albumin and α1-acid glycoprotein and the binding is enantiomer specific. While the *S*(–)-enantiomer is bound to α1-acid glycoprotein, the *R*(+)-enantiomer is majorly bound to serum albumin. Propanolol is rapidly metabolized by aromatic hydroxylation, N-dealkylation and direct glucuronidation. The major metabolites include propranolol glucuronide, naphthyloxylactic acid and glucuronic acid and sulfate conjugates of 4-hydroxy propranolol. Metabolism is majorly mediated by cytochrome P450 CYP2D6, CYP2C19 and CYP1A2 enzymes in the liver.

Acebutolol is a hydrophilic cardioprotective β-blocker with very mild intrinsic sympathomimetic activity. It is chemically designated as *N*-[3-acetyl-4-[2-hydroxy-3-(propan-2-ylamino)propoxy] phenyl]butanamide and has the structural formula $C_{18}H_{28}N_2O_4$ (m.w. 336.4 g/mol). It is a more potent antagonist of the β_1-receptor than of the β_2-receptor. It blocks β_1-receptor at a dose 50–100-fold lesser than that required by β_2-blockers to block the corresponding receptor. This drug reduces the resting heart rate and cardiac output during rest and after exercise. It also reduces systolic and diastolic blood pressures while resting and also post-exercise. Acebutolol is rapidly absorbed by the gastrointestinal tract and undergoes first-pass metabolism. Bioavailability of the drug for systemic absorption is 40%. The major metabolite is an *N*-acetyl derivative called diacetolol, and is pharmacologically active and equipotent as acebutolol. The time taken by acebutolol to reach peak plasma concentrations is 2.5 h while that of diacetolol is 3.5 h. The half-life of acebutolol is 3–4 h while that of diacetolol is 8–13 h. Since acebutolol and diacetolol are hydrophilic molecules, only minimal quantities are detected in the cerebrospinal fluid. Also, only about 26% of the drug is bound to serum plasma proteins. About 60% of the drug is eliminated via the biliary pathway while the rest is eliminated through urine.

Antidepressants

SSRIs inhibit reuptake of serotonin or 5-HT and include citalopram, escitalopram, fluoxetine, fluvoxamine, paroxetine and sertraline (Fig. 7.17). These drugs induce synthesis of more 5-HT to stimulate the postsynaptic 5-HT receptors, by preventing the reuptake of presynaptic 5-HT. SSRIs are not subtype specific and hence not only stimulate 5-HT_1 receptors with antidepressant and anti-anxiolytic effects but also stimulate 5-HT_2 and 5-HT_3 receptors, causing anxiety, insomnia, sexual dysfunction, nausea and headache. Another disadvantage of using SSRIs is that there occurs an initial increase in severity of the symptoms, even leading to life-threatening suicidal tendencies. Fluoxetine and fluvoxamine have also been shown to inhibit certain cytochrome P450 enzymes, leading to fatal drug interactions.

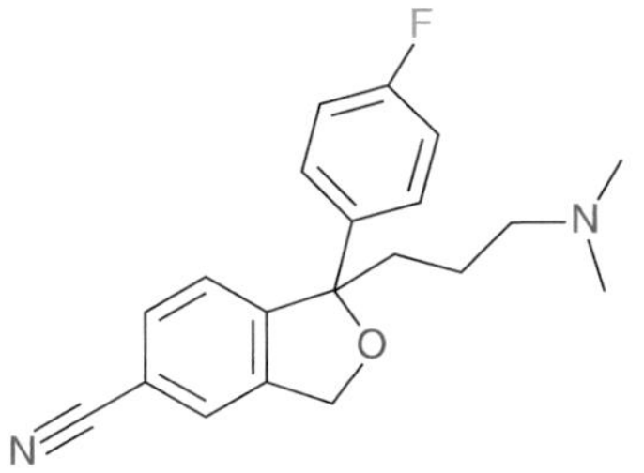

Citalopram: 1-[3-(dimethylamino)propyl-1-(4-fluorophenyl)-1,3-dihydroisobenzofuran-5-carbonitrile

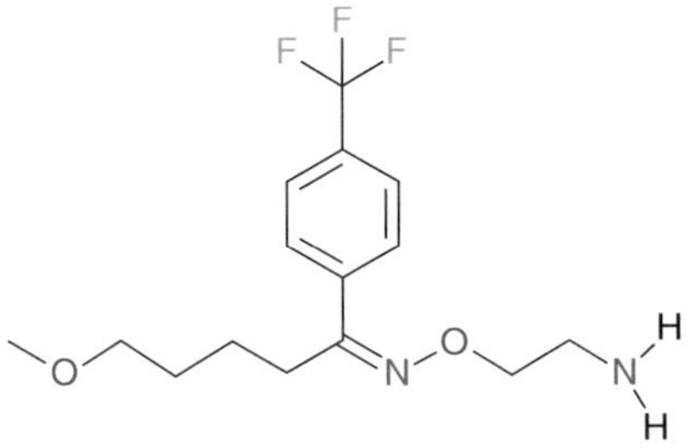

Fluvoxamine: (*Z*)-5-methoxy-1-[4-(trifluoromethyl)phenyl]pentan-1-one *O*-2-aminoethyl oxime

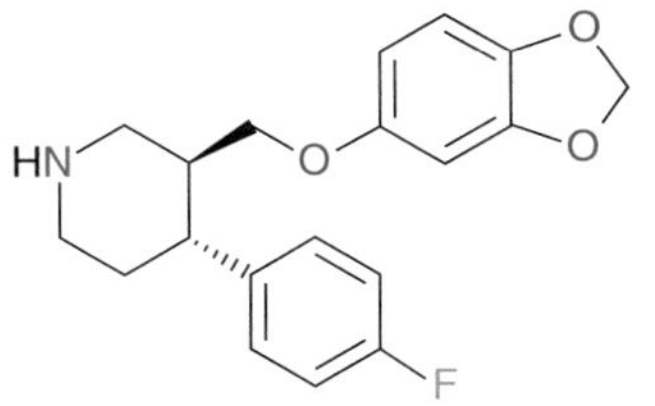

Paroxetine: (3*S*, 4*R*)-3-([benzo[*d*][1,3]dioxol-5-yloxyl]methyl)-4-(4-fluorophenyl)piperidine

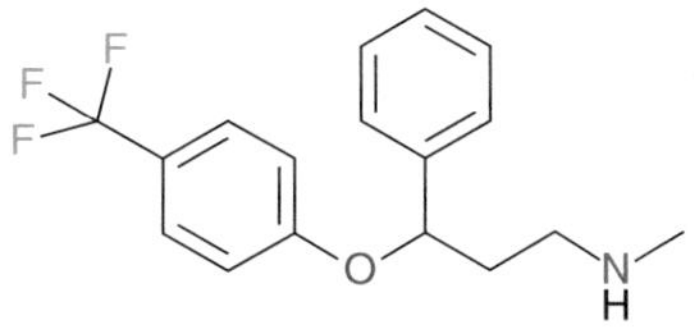

Fluoxetine: *N*-methyl-3-phenyl-3-[4-(trifluoromethyl)phenoxy]propan-1-amine

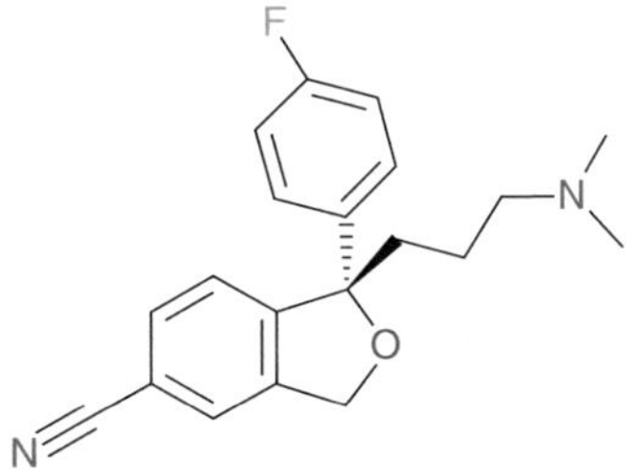

Escitalopram: (*S*)-1-[3-(dimethylamino) propyl]-1-(4-fluorophenyl)-1,3-dihydroiso benzofuran-5-carbonitrile

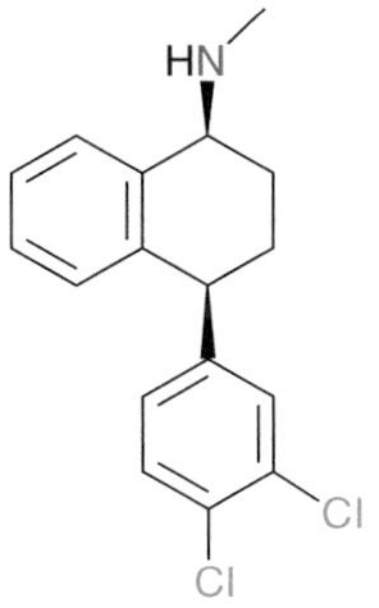

Sertraline: (1*S*,4*S*)-4-(3,4-dichlorophenyl)-*N*-methyl-1,2,3,4-tetrahydronaphthalen-1-amine

Fig. 7.17 ***SSRIs, Selective Serotonin Reuptake Inhibitors, are AntiDepressants Used for Treatment of Depression, Anxiety and Other Personality Disorders***

(They inhibit the reuptake of serotonin or 5-hydroxytryptamine from the synapses, thus inducing the synthesis of more serotonin.)

Citalopram, a racemic bicyclic phthalene derivative, is an antidepressant that acts on serotonin receptors. It was first described in 1977 when it was found to be a potent inhibitor of serotonin reuptake (Hyttel, 1977, 1978). However, it was later discovered that much of the activity of citalopram is due to its *S*(–)-enantiomer, *S*-citalopram. Citalopram has a stereocenter to which a flurophenyl group and an *N,N*-dimethyl-3-aminopropyl group are bound. Due to this chirality the molecule exists in two enantiomeric forms, *S*(–)-citalopram and *R*(+)-citalopram. *S*-Citalopram has been found to be 167 times more potent than *R*-citalopram at inhibiting serotonin reuptake in rat brain (Hyttel *et al.*, 1992). Citalopram was intially sold as an enantiomeric mixture containing equal concentrations of both the enantiomers. However, after it was discovered that most of the effects of this drug are mainly due to its *S*-enantiomer, it is now sold in its pure *S*-enantiomeric form as *escitalopram*. This drug, being highly lipophilic, is sold as a salt of oxalate that makes it easily absorbable by the body. Chemically, citalopram is designated as 1-(3-dimethylaminopropyl)-1-(4-fluorophenyl)-3*H*-2-benzofuran-5-carbonitrile and has the structural formula $C_{20}H_{21}FN_2O$ (m.w. 324.3 g/mol). Citalopram is used to treat the symptoms of major depression, social anxiety disorder and panic disorder. Citalopram is also known to inhibit reuptake of monoamine and inhibits reuptake of dopamine at very high concentrations (Hyttel, 1977; Owens *et al.*, 2001). It acts by blocking reuptake of serotonin by the 5-HT_{1A} receptors at the neuronal membrane. Like other SSRIs, this drug also has very low affinity for histamine, acetylcholine and norepinephrine receptors.

Citalopram is generally well absorbed and has a bioavailability of almost 80% (Baumann and Larsen, 1995). About 50% of the drug is bound to serum plasma proteins. It undergoes very little first-pass metabolism and has a very long half-life of almost 35 h (Joffe *et al.*, 1998). The drug achieves its peak plasma concentrations within 2–4 h of oral administration (Kragh-Sorensen *et al.*, 1981). Citalopram undergoes active metabolism by the hepatic cytochrome P450 class of enzymes—2C19, 3A4 and 2D6. These enzymes demethylate citalopram to its major metabolite, mono-desmethylcitalopram (Kobayashi *et al.*, 1997; Rochat *et al.*, 1997; von Moltke *et al.*, 1999). Mono-desmethylcitalopram is further demethylated by CYP2D6 enzyme to di-desmethylcitalopram (Sindrup *et al.*, 1993; von Moltke *et al.*, 1999). Compared to citalopram, mono-desmethylcitalopram is 4 times less potent as an SSRI but 11 times more potent as serotonin reuptake inhibitor (Hyttel, 1982). The major and minor metabolites of citalopram have half-lives of 50 and 100 h, respectively (Kragh-Sorensen *et al.*, 1981; Overø, 1982).

Fluoxetine is a serotonin reuptake inhibitor used as an antidepressant and in treatment of bulimia nervosa and obsessive compulsive disorder. Chemically it is represented as *N*-methyl-3-phenyl-3-[4-(trifluoromethyl)phenoxy]propan-1-amine ($C_{17}H_{18}F_3NO$; m.w. 309.3 g/mol). The antidepressant, anti-obsessive-compulsive and anti-bulimic properties are due to its direct effect on CNS to inhibit uptake of serotonin. Fluoxetine has a bioavailability index of 72% and reaches its peak plasma concentrations within 6–8 h of oral administration. Almost 95% of the drug is bound to serum plasma proteins, especially albumin and α1-glycoprotein. It has a mean half-life of 1–3 days. It is well metabolized by the liver cytochrome P450 CYP2D6 enzyme to its active metabolite norfluoxetine by demethylation (Wong *et al.*, 1974). The active metabolite of fluoxetine also has potency similar to fluoxetine. Fluoxetine is a racemic mixture of *S*-fluoxetine and *R*-fluoxetine. Both enantiomers are equally potent (Wong *et al.*, 1995).

Fluvoxamine is another member of this class that is mainly used to treat obsessive compulsive disorder. It is one of the first SSRIs to be introduced in the market. Chemically, it is designated as 5-methoxy-4′-(trifluoromethyl)valerophenone-(*E*)-*O*-(2-aminoethyl)oxime and has the empirical formula $C_{15}H_{21}F_3N_2O_2$ (m.w. 434.4 g/mol). It acts by inhibiting serotonin uptake in brain neurons. It has no significant affinity for histaminergic, α- or β-adrenergic, muscarinic or dopaminergic receptors. About 50% of the drug is available for systemic absorption. More than 75% of the drug is bound to albumin and has an half-life of 15 h. It is actively metabolized in the liver by many cytochrome P450 class of enzymes. These enzymes include 2C19, 1A2, 2C9, 2D6 and 1A1. Apart from these enzymes, monoamine oxidase is also involved in its metabolism. Of the nine metabolites identified, the most active one is fluvoxamine acid. Other major metabolites include an N-acetylated analog and fluvoxethanol. All of the metabolites along with the parent drug are eliminated mainly in the urine (Hyttel, 1993).

Serotonin modulators or 5-HT blockers selectively block 5-HT$_2$ receptors and inhibit reuptake of 5-HT and norepinephrine. This class of drugs, also known as serotonin receptor antogonists, includes nefazodone, trazodone and mirtazapine (Fig. 7.18). Unlike SSRIs, serotonin modulators exhibit only antidepressant and anti-anxiolytic effects and do not cause sexual dysfunction. However, nefazodone has been shown to be interfering with drug-metabolizing liver enzymes and causes liver failure. Trazodone, though related to nefazodone, does not inhibit presynaptic reuptake of serotonin and has been shown to cause postural hypotension as an α-adrenergic blocker. Moreover, it is very sedating, thus limiting its dosage as an antidepressant. Mirtazapine, a tetracyclic piperazinoazepin, on the other hand, inhibits serotonin reuptake presynaptically and also blocks α_2-adrenergic receptors, 5-HT$_2$ and 5-HT$_3$ receptors and increases release of norepinephrine and serotonin. It has the most efficient serotonergic function without any sexual dysfunction, nausea or adverse cardiac effects. Moreover,

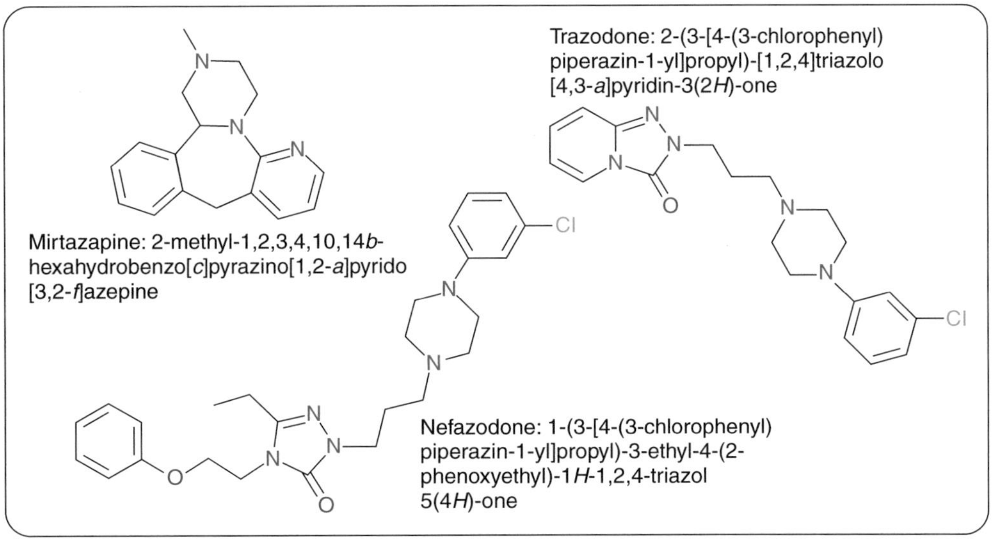

Fig. 7.18 ***Serotonin Receptor Antagonists or 5-HT Blockers Inhibit Reuptake of Serotonin and Norepinephrine from the Synapses by Binding to and Blocking the Serotonin Receptors***

(They are preferred over SSRIs since they exhibit only antidepressant and anti-anxiolytic effects and do not have any of the adverse side effects observed with SSRIs.)

it also has minimal interaction with drug-metabolizing enzymes in the liver. It is generally well tolerated, except for sedation and slight weight gain.

Trazodone is a second-generation antidepressant that acts by blocking reuptake of serotonin by the synapses. It has a very high bioavailability and a mean half-life of 3–6 h. It is quickly absorbed by the body and reaches its peak plasma concentration within 1 h of oral administration. Ninety to ninety-five percent of the drug is bound to plasma proteins. It is actively metabolized by cytochrome CYP450 3A4 and 2D6 enzymes (Jauch *et al.*, 1976).

Nefazodone is closely related to trazodone and acts by blocking postsynaptic 5-HT_{2A} receptors and presynaptic serotonin reuptake. Chemically it is represented as 2-[3-[4-(3-chlorophenyl)-1-piperazinyl]propyl]-5-ethyl-2,4-dihydro-4-(2-phenoxyethyl)-3*H*-1,2,4-triazol-3-one ($C_{25}H_{32}ClN_5O_2$; m.w. 470 g/mol). Nefazodone is rapidly and completely absorbed but also extensively metabolized in the body. Twenty percent of the drug is bioavailable for systemic circulation and reaches peak plasma concentrations within 2 h of oral administration. It has a half-life of 2–4 h. Nefazodone is N-dealkylated and aliphatic- and aromatic-hydroxylated by enzymes in the liver to its metabolites hydroxynefazodone, *meta*-chlorophenylpiperazine and a triazole-dione metabolite. Of these three metabolites, only hydroxynefazodone has pharmacological activity similar to that of nefazodone. While nefazodone also antagonizes α_1-adrenergic receptors, producing sedation, muscle relaxation and many cardiovascular effects, its affinity for benzodiazepine and cholinergic, dopaminergic, histaminic and β- or α_2-adrenergic receptors is not significant (Sánchez and Hyttel, 1999).

Serotonin-norpepinephrine reuptake inhibitors include venlafaxine (a phenyethylamine) and duloxetine (Fig. 7.19). These drugs have dual 5-HT and norepinephrine modes of action and do not

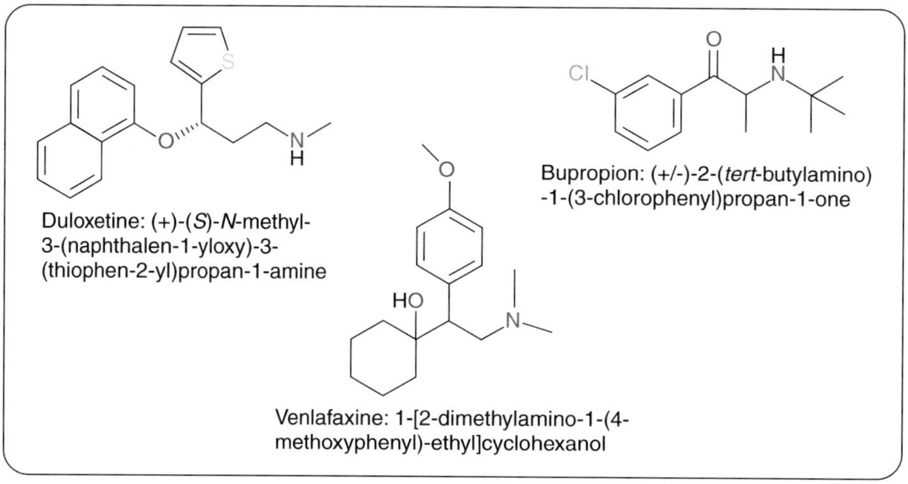

Fig. 7.19 ***Serotonin-Norepinephrine Reuptake Inhibitors and Dopamine-Norepinephrine Reuptake Inhibitors Act by Preventing Reuptake of Serotonin and Dopamine, Respectively, in Addition to Norepinephrine. Hence, they are Dual-Acting Drugs and Act Similar to Serotonin Receptor Antagonists.***

(While venlafaxine and duloxetine belong to the former class, buproprion is the only member of the latter class.)

have the side effects of SSRIs. Patients with severe depression somehow seem to respond better to venlafaxine. Moreover, this drug does not interact with any of the drug-metabolizing enzymes from the liver. However, nausea and certain withdrawal symptoms such as irritability and anxiety are common. Duloxetine is similar to venlafaxine in mode of action and severity of side effects. Dopamine-norepinephrine reuptake inhibitors somehow favor catecholaminergic, dopaminergic and noradrenergic systems, but not the serotonergic system. Bupropion is the only drug in this class so far, and has been shown to help treat patients with attention-deficit hyperactivity disorder and cocaine dependence (Fig. 7.19). Though it does not cause sexual dysfunction and has no adverse cardiac effects, it does exhibit severe side effects such as hypertension, seizures and interaction with certain hepatic enzymes. It may also result in dose-dependent reversible memory loss.

Heterocyclic antidepressants include tricyclic (tertiary amines such as amitriptyline and imipramine and their secondary metabolites nortriptyline and desipramine), modified tricyclic and tetracyclic antidepressants. These drugs act by increasing the availability of norepinephrine by blocking 5-HT reuptake in the presynaptic cleft. Desipramine and nortriptyline have greater effects on norepinephrine reuptake systems while amitriptyline has a greater effect on serotonergic systems. However, their long-term use downregulates $\alpha 1$-adrenergic receptors in the postsynaptic membrane. These drugs are now rarely used since their overdose causes toxicity and severe side effects resulting due to blocking of muscarinic, histaminic and $\alpha 1$-adrenolytic actions. They also have strong anticholinergic properties. Drugs such as maprolitine and clomipramine lower the threshold for seizures. Other heterocyclics include doxepin, protriptyline and trimipramine (Fig. 7.20).

FUTURE PERSPECTIVES

Cell surface receptors and their corresponding signal transduction mechanisms were never in such spotlight as they are today. GPCR-mediated signaling pathways have been implicated in an alarmingly huge number of diseases. These diseases are a result of the numerous mutations occurring in GPCRs that cause abnormal folding of the protein and its subsequent retention in the ER. Moreover, GPCR mutations that lead to normal protein synthesis and folding might cause loss of function by impairing receptor activation upon agonist binding or G protein coupling. On the other hand, gain-of-function mutations cause constitutive activation of the receptor, leading to constant downstream signaling. There exist enough data today to establish a correlation between polymorphisms of GPCRs, their abnormal signal transduction pathways and particular phenotypic expression. All these data including molecular bases of diseases involving GPCRs provide an insight and open up a whole new world of clinical and pharmaceutical science of GPCR-based drug discovery.

Advances in molecular genetics, sequencing, analysis of polymorphisms in DNA sequences and other new approaches for rapid identification and functional characterization of receptors lead to the establishment of molecular targets for highly specific drug action. GPCR-based drug discovery holds great promise since drugs with therapeutic activities that have been screened and validated taking into account the numerous receptor subtypes also into consideration will exhibit very high molecular specificity. This great enhancement in specificity of the drug for its target will result in very little or almost no adverse side effects. Also, decoding the biochemistry involved in receptor subtype–ligand interaction will aid in discovering drugs that can target specific conformations of the receptors.

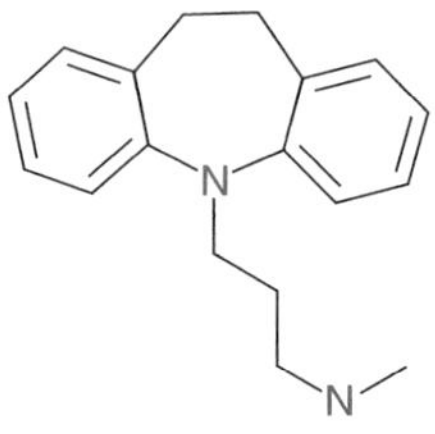

Imapramine: 3-(10,11-dihydro-5*H*-dibenzo[*b,f*]azepine-5-yl)-*N,N*-dimethyl propan-1-amine

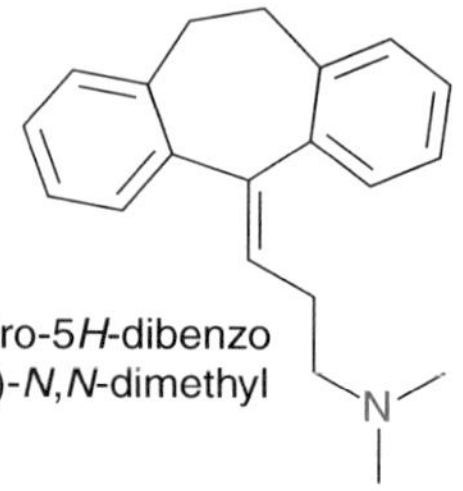

Amitriptyline: 3-(10,11-dihydro-5*H*-dibenzo [*a,d*]cycloheptane-5-ylidene)-*N,N*-dimethyl -1-propanamine

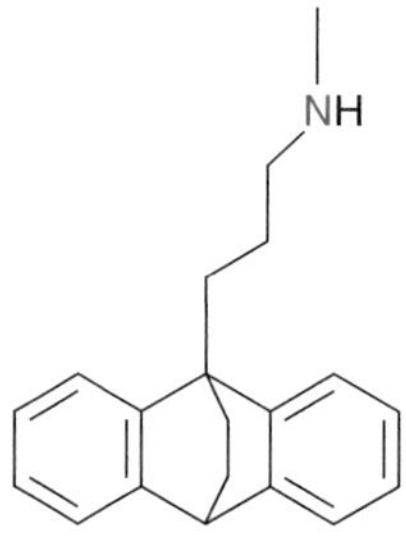

Maprolitine: *N*-methyl-9,10-ethano anthracene-9(10*H*)-propanamine

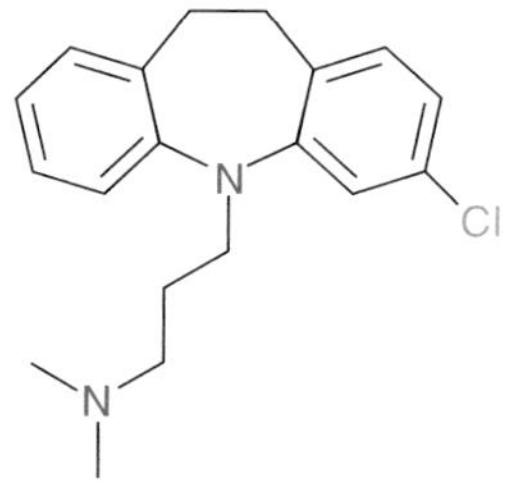

Clomipramine: 3-(3-chloro-10,11-dihydro-5*H*-dibenzo-[*b,f*]azepin-5-yl)-*N,N*-dimethylpropan-1-amine

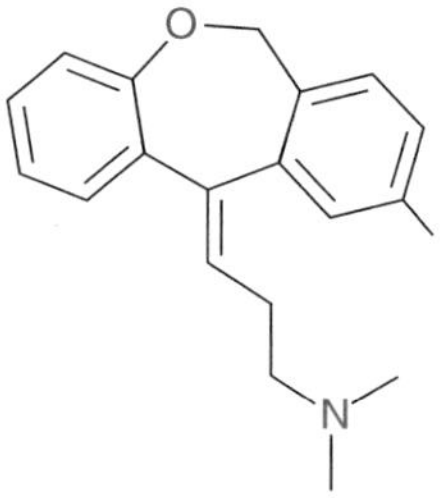

Doxepine: 3-(dibenzo[*b,e*]oxepin-11(6*H*)-ylidene-*N,N*-dimethylpropan -1-amine

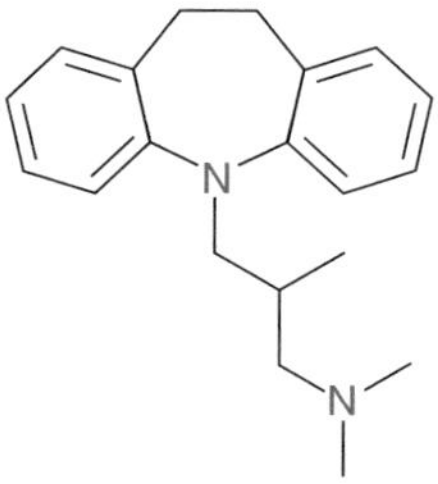

Trimipramine: 3-(10,11-dihydro-5*H*-dibenzo[*b,f*]azepin-5-yl)-*N,N*,2-trimethyl propan-1-amine

Fig. 7.20 ***Heterocyclic Antidepressants include Tricyclic, Modified Tricyclic and Tetracyclic Antidepressants***

(They increase the availability of norepinephrine by preventing its' reuptake in presynaptic receptors. However, they are not very popular due to the adverse side effects attached to their administration.)

However, this field of GPCR-targeted drug discovery has crossed all initial barriers and reached a stage where its major current challenge would be to identify agonists and antagonists for the orphan GPCRs, if and when implicated in diseased conditions (e. g., constitutively activated receptors).

The application of a combination of conventional and advanced modern molecular techniques will accelerate the process of deorphaning GPCRs, their sequencing, analyzing polymorphisms in genes coding for these receptors, constructing their biochemical pathways based on proteins and other effector molecules that interact with the receptors and finally their implication in specific diseased conditions. All this will proportionately speed up the process of drug target discovery, validation and lead optimization, thus contributing to the expanding clinical, medical and pharmaceutical therapy-based science.

REFERENCES

AbdAlla, S., Zaki, E., Lother, H., Quitterer, U. (1999). Involvement of the amino terminus of B_2 receptor in an agonist-induced receptor dimerization. *Journal of Biological Chemistry* **274**:26079–26084.

Abdulaev, N.G. (2003). Building a stage for interhelical play in rhodopsin. *Trends in Biochemical Sciences* **28**:399–402.

Adan, R.A., Szklarczyk, A.W., Oosterom, J., Brakkee, J.H., Nijenhuis, W.A., Schaaper, W.M., Meloen, R.H., Gispen, W.H. (1999). Characterization of melanocortin receptor ligands on cloned brain melanocortin receptors and on grooming behavior in the rat. *European Journal of Pharmacology* **378(3)**:249–258.

Adham, N., Kao, H.T., Schecter, L.E., Bard, J., Olsen, M., Urquhart, D., Durkin, M., Hartig, P.R., Weinshank, R.L., Branchek, T.A. (1993). Cloning of another human serotonin receptor (5-HT1F): a fifth 5-HT1 receptor subtype coupled to the inhibition of adenylate cyclase. *Proceedings at the National Academy of Sciences U.S.A.* **90(2)**:408–412.

Adham, N., Bard, J.A., Zgombick, J.M., Durkin, M.M., Kucharewicz, S., Weinshank, R.L., Branchek, T.A. (1997). Cloning and characterization of the guinea pig 5-HT1F receptor subtype: a comparison of the pharmacological profile to the human species homolog. *Neuropharmacology* **36(4–5)**:569–576.

Adler, A.I., Stratton, I.M., Neil, H.A.W., Yudkin, J.S., Matthews, D.R., Cull, C.A., Wright, A.D., Turner, R.C., Holman, R.R. (2000). Association of systolic blood pressure with macrovascular and microvascular complications of type 2 diabetes (UKPDS 36): Prospective observational study. *British Medical Journal* **321(7258)**:412–419.

Ahlquist, R.P. (1948). A study of adrenotropic receptors. *American Journal of Physiology* **153(3)**:586–600.

Ahuja, S.K., Murphy, P.M. (1996). The CXC chemokines growth-regulated oncogene (GRO) α, GROβ, GROγ, neutrophil-activating peptide-2, and epithelial cell-derived neutrophil-activating peptide-78 are potent agonists for the type B, but not the type A, human interleukin-8 receptor. *Journal of Biological Chemistry* **271(34)**:20545–20550.

Ai, L-S., Liao, F. (2002). Mutating the four extracellular cysteines in the chemokine receptor CCR6 reveals their differing roles in receptor trafficking, ligand binding, and signaling. *Biochemistry* **41(26)**:8332–8341.

Akamizu, T., Ikuyama, S., Saji, M., Kosugi, S., Kozak, C., McBride, O.W., Kohn, L.D. (1990). Cloning, chromosomal assignment, and regulation of the rat thyrotropin receptor: expression of the gene is regulated by thyrotropin, agents that increase cAMP levels, and thyroid autoantibodies. *Proceedings of the National Academy of Sciences USA* **87(15)**:5677–5681.

Akamizu, T., Inoue, D., Kosugi, S., Kohn, L.D., Mori, T. (1994). Further studies of amino acids (268–304) in thyrotropin (TSH)-lutropin/chorionic gonadotropin (LH/CG) receptor chimeras: Cysteine-301 is important in TSH binding and receptor tertiary structure. *Thyroid* **4(1)**:43–48.

Albert, P.R., Sajedi, N., Lemonde, S., Ghahremani, M.H. (1999). Constitutive G(i2)-dependent activation of adenylyl cyclase type II by the 5-HT1A receptor. Inhibition by anxiolytic partial agonists. *Journal of Biological Chemistry* **274(50)**:35469–35474.

Allegeier, A., Offermanns, S., Van Sande, J., Spicher, K., Schultz, G., Dumont, J. (1994). The human thyrotropin receptor activates G-proteins Gs and Gq/11. *Journal of Biological Chemistry* **269(19)**:13733–13735.

Amat, M., Benjamin, C.F., Williams, L.M., Prats, N., Terricabras, E., Beleta, J., Kunkel, S.L., Godessart, N. (2006). Pharmacological blockade of CCR1 ameliorates murine arthritis and alters cytokine networks in vivo. *British Journal of Pharmacology* **149(6)**:666–675.

Angermeyer, M.C., Löffler, W., Müller, P., Schulze, B., Priebe, S. (2001). 'Patients and relatives' assessment of clozapine treatment. *Psychological Medicine* **31(3)**:509–517.

Aramori, I., Ferguson, S.S., Bieniasz, P.D., Zhang, J., Cullen, B., Cullen, M.G. (1997). Molecular mechanism of desensitization of the chemokine receptor CCR-5: Receptor signaling and internalization are dissociable from its role as an HIV-1 co-receptor. *EMBO Journal* **16(15)**:4606–4616.

Arana, G.W., Rosenbaum, J.F. (2000). *Handbook of Psychiatric Drug Therapy*. Philadelphia, PA: Lippincott Williams and Wilkins.

Arias, D.A., Navenot, J-M., Zhang, W-b., Broach, J., Peiper, S.C. (2003). Constitutive activation of CCR5 and CCR2 induced by conformational changes in the conserved TXP motif in transmembrane helix 2. *Journal of Biological Chemistry* **278(38)**:36513–36521.

Aronica, E., Dickson, D.W., Kress, Y., Morrison, J.H., Zukin, R.S. (1998). Non-plaque dystrophic dendrites in Alzheimer hippocampus: A new pathological structure revealed by glutamate receptor immunocytochemistry. *Neuroscience* **82(4)**:979–991.

Arora, K.K., Sakai, A., Catt, K.J. (1995). Effects of second intracellular loop mutations on signal transduction and internalization of the gonadotropin-releasing hormone receptor. *Journal of Biological Chemistry* **270(39)**:22820–22826.

Ascoli, M., Fanelli, F., Segaloff, D.L. (2002). The lutropin/choriogonadotropin receptor, a 2002 perspective. *Endocrine Reviews* **23(2)**:141–174.

Aulakh, G.K., Sodhi, R.K., Singh, M. (2007). An update on non-peptide angiotensin reeptor antagonists and related RAAS modulators. *Life Sciences* **81(8)**:615–639.

Baba, M., Imai, T., Nishimura, M., Kakizaki, M., Takagi, S., Hieshima, K., Nomiyama, H., Yoshie, O. (1997). Identification of CCR6, the specific receptor for a novel lymphocyte-directed CC chemokine LARC. *Journal of Biological Chemistry* **272(23)**:14893–14898.

Baba, M., Nishimura, O., Kanzaki, N., Okamoto, M., Sawada, H., Iizawa, Y., Shiraishi, M., Aramaki, Y., Okonogi, K., Ogawa, Y., Meguro, K., Fujino, M. (1999). A small-molecule, nonpeptide CCR5 antagonist with highly potent and selective anti-HIV-1 activity. *Proceedings of the National Academy of Sciences USA* **96(10)**:5698–5703.

Babovic-Vuksanovic, D., Donaldson, M.D., Gibson, N.A., Wallace, A.M. (1994). Hazards of ketoconazole therapy in testotoxicosis. *Acta Paediatrica* **83(9)**:994–997.

Baker, J.G. (2005). The selectivity of beta-adrenoceptor antagonists at the human beta1, beta2 and beta3 adrenoceptors. *British Journal of Pharmacology* **144(3)**:317–322.

Baldessarini, R.J. (2001). Drugs and the treatment of psychiatric disorders: Depression and anxiety disorders. *In* Goodman and Gilman's The Pharmacological Basis of Therapeutics, Hardman, J.G., limbird, L.E, Gilman, A.G. (Eds.) 10th Edition, pp. 447–499. United States of America, The McGraw Hill Companies.

Baldwin, D.S., Montgomery, S.A. (1995). First clinical experience with olanzapine (LY 170053): Results of an open-label safety and dose-ranging studies in patients with schizophrenia. *International Clinical Psychopharmacology* **10(4)**:239–244.

Ballesteros, J.A., Shi, L., Javitch, J.A. (2001). Structural mimicry in G-protein coupled receptors: Implications of the high-resolution structure of rhodopsin for structure–function analysis of rhodopsin-like receptors. *Molecular Pharmacology* **60(1)**:1–19.

Ban, T., Kosugi, S., Kohn, L.D. (1992). Specific antibody to the thyrotropin receptor identifies multiple receptor forms in membranes of cells transfected with wild-type receptor complementary deoxyribonucleic acid: Characterization of their relevance to receptor synthesis, processing, structure, and function. *Endocrinology* **131(2)**:815–829.

Barak, L.S., Oakley, R.H., Laporte, S.A., Caron, M.G. (2001). Constitutive arrestin-mediated desensitization of a human vasopressin receptor mutant associated with nephrogenic diabetes insipidus. *Proceedings of the National Academy of Sciences* U.S.A. **98(1)**:93–98.

Barak, L.S., Wilbanks, A.M., Caron, M.G. (2003). Constitutive desensitization: A new paradigm for G protein-coupled receptor regulation. *Assay and Drug Development Technologies* **1(2)**:339–346.

Barlic, J., Andrews, J.D., Kelvin, A.A., Bosinger, S.E., DeVries, M.E., Xu, L., Dobransky, T., Feldman, R.D., Ferguson, S.S.G., Kelvin, D.J. (2000). Regulation of tyrosine kinase activation and granule release through β-arrestin by CXCR1. *Nature Immunology* **1(3)**:227–233.

Barlic, J., Khandaker, M.S., Mahon, E., Andrews, J., DeVries, M.E., Mitchell, G.B., Rahimpour, R., Tan, C.M., Ferguson, S.S.G., Kelvin, D.J. (1999). β-Arrestins regulate interleukin-8-induced CXCR1 internalization. *Journal of Biological Chemistry* **274(23)**:16287–16294.

Barnett-Norris, J., Lynch, D., Reggio, P.H. (2005). Lipids, lipid rafts and caveolae: Their importance for GPCR signaling and their centrality to the endocannabinoid system. *Life Sciences* **77(14)**:1625–1639.

Basmaciogullari, S., Pacheco, B., Bour, S., Sodroski, J. (2006). Specific interaction of CXCR4 with CD4 and CD8α: Functional analysis of the CD4/CXCR4 interaction in the context of HIV-1 envelope glycoprotein-mediated membrane fusion. *Virology* **353(1)**:52–67.

Baumann, P., Larsen, F. (1995). The pharmacokinetics of citalopram. *Reviews in Contemporary Pharmacotherapy* **6**:287–295.

Beeley, N.R.A., Sage, C. (2003). GPCRs: An update on structural approaches to drug discovery. *Targets* **2(1)**:19–25.

Befort, K., Tabbara, L., Kling, D., Maigret, B., Keiffer, B.L. (1996). Role of aromatic transmembrane residues of the delta opioid receptor in ligand recognition. *Journal of Biological Chemistry* **271(17)**:10161–10168.

Benson, S.C., Pershadsingh, H.A, Ho, C.I., Chittiboyina, A., Desai, P., Pravenec, M., Qi, N., Wang, J., Avery, M.A., Kurtz, T.W. (2004). Identification of telmisartan as a unique angiotensin II receptor antagonist with selective PPARgamma-modulating activity. *Hypertension* **43(5)**:993–1002.

Berendsen, H.H. (1995). Interactions between 5-hydroxytryptamine receptor subtypes: Is a disturbed receptor balance contributing to the symptomatology of depression in humans? *Pharmacology and Therapeutics* **66(1)**:17–37.

Bergen, A.W., van den Bree, M.B., Yeager, M., Welch, R., Ganjei, J.K., Haque, K., Bacanu, S., Berrettini, W.H., Grice, D.E., Goldman, D., Bulik, C.M., Klump, K., Fichter, M., Halmi, K., Kaplan, A., Strober, M., Treasure, J., Woodside, B., Kaye, W.H. (2003). Candidate genes for anorexia nervosa in the 1p33-36 linkage region: Serotonin 1D and delta opioid receptor loci exhibit significant association to anorexia nervosa. *Molecular Psychiatry* **8(4)**:397–406.

Berger, E.A., Murphy, P.M., Farber, J.M. (1999). Chemokine receptors as HIV-1 coreceptors: Roles in viral entry, tropism and disease. *Annual Review of Immunology* **17**:657–700.

Bergsma, D.J., Ellis, C., Kumar, C., Nuthulaganti, P., Kersten, H., Elshourbagy, N., Griffin, E., Stadel, J.M., Aiyar, N. (1992). Cloning and characterization of a human angiotensin II type 1 receptor. *Biochemical and Biophysical Research Communications* **183(3)**:989–995.

Bermack, J.C., Li, M., Bullock, C., Zhou, Q.Y. (2001). Regulation of transport of the dopamine D1 receptor by a new membrane-associated ER protein. *Nature Cell Biology* **3(5)**:492–498.

Berson, E.L., Rosner, B., Sandberg, M.A., Dryja, T.P. (1991). Ocular findings in patients with autosomal dominant retinitis pigmentosa and a rhodopsin gene defect (Pro-23-His). *Archives of Ophthalmology* **109(1)**:92–101.

Berson, E.L., Rosner, B., Sandberg, M.A., Hayes, K.C., Nicholson, B.W., Weigel-DiFranco, C., Willett, W., Felix, J.S., Laties, A.M. (1993). A randomized trial of vitamin A and vitamin E supplementation for retinitis pigmentosa. *Archives of Ophthalmology* **111(6)**:761–772.

Bhatnagar, A., Williams, D.L., Gray, J.A., Woods, J., Benovic, J.L., Roth, B.L. (2001). The dynamin-dependent, arrestin-independent internalization of 5-hydroxytryptamine 2A (5-HT_{2A}) serotonin receptors reveals differential sorting of arrestins and 5-HT_{2A} receptors during endocytosis. *Journal of Biological Chemistry* **276(11)**:8269–8277.

Bhatnagar, A., Sheffler, D.J., Kroeze, W.K., Compton-Toth, B., Roth, B.L. (2004). Caveolin-1 interacts with 5-HT_{2A} serotonin receptors and profoundly modulates the signaling of selected $G\alpha_q$-coupled protein receptors. *Journal of Biological Chemistry* **279(33)**:34614–34623.

Bhowmick, N., Huang, J., Puett, D., Isaacs, N.W., Lapthorn, A.J. (1996). Determination of residues important in hormone binding to the extracellular domain of the luteinizing hormone/chorionic gonadotropin receptor by site-directed mutagenesis and modeling. *Molecular Endocrinology* **10(9)**:1147–1159.

Bichet, D.G., Arthus, M.F., Lonergan, M., Hendy, G.N., Paradis, A.J., Fujiwara, T.M., Morgan, K., Gregory, M.C., Rosenthal, W., Didwania, A., Antaramian, A., Birnbaumer, M. (1993). X-linked nephrogenic diabetes insipidus mutations in North America and the Hopewell hypothesis. *Journal of Clinical Investigation* **92(3)**:1262–1268.

Bickford, L.C., Mossessova, E., Goldberg, J. (2004). A structural view of the COPII vesicle coat. *Current Opinion in Structural Biology* **14(2)**:147–153.

Biebermann, H., Krude, H., Elsner, A., Chubanov, V., Gudermann, T., Grüters, A. (2003). Autosomal-dominant mode of inheritance of a melanocortin-4 receptor mutation in a patient with severe early-onset obesity is due to a dominant-negative effect caused by receptor dimerization. *Diabetes* **52(12)**:2984–2988.

Birkett, J.T., Arranz, M.J., Munro, J., Osbourn, S., Kerwin, R.W., Coliier, D.A. (2000). Association analysis of the 5-HT5A gene in depression, psychosis and antipsychotic response. *Neuroreport* **11(9)**:2017–2020.

Birnbaumer, M., Seibold, A., Gilbert, S., Ishido, M., Barberis, C., Antaramian, A., Brabet, P., Rosenthal, W. (1992). Molecular cloning of the receptor for human antidiuretic hormone. *Nature* **357(6376)**:333–335.

Birnbaumer, M., Gilbert, S. Rosenthal, W. (1994). An extracellular congenital nephrogenic diabetes insipidus mutation of the vasopressin receptor reduces cell surface expression, affinity for ligand and coupling to the Gs/adenylyl cyclase system. *Molecular Endocrinology* **8(7)**:886–894.

Birnbaumer, M. (2000). Vasopressin receptors. *Trends in Endocrinology and Metabolism* **11(10)**:406–410.

Bissantz, C., Bernard, P., Hibert, M., Rognan, D. (2003). Protein-based virtual screening of chemical databases: II. Are homology models of G-protein coupled receptors suiTable targets? *Proteins* **50(1)**:5–25.

Blanpain, C., Migeotte, I., Lee, B., Vakili, J., Doranz, B.J., Govaerts, C., Vassart, G., Doms, R.W., Parmentier, M. (1999). CCR5 binds multiple CC-chemokines: MCP-3 acts as a natural antagonist. *Blood* **94(6)**:1899–1905.

Bleicher, K.H., Green, L.G., Martin, R.E., Rogers-Evans, M. (2004). Ligand identification for G-protein-coupled receptors: a lead generation perspective. *Current Opinion in Chemical Biology* **8(3)**:287–296.

Blondel, O., Gastineau, M., Dahmoune, Y., Langlois, M., Fischmeister, R. (1998). Cloning, expression and pharmacology of four human 5-hydroxytryptamine 4 receptor isoforms produced by alternative splicing in the carboxyl terminus. *Journal of Neurochemistry* **70(6)**:2252–2261.

Boess, F.G., Monsma, F.J.Jr., Meyer, V., Zwingelstein, C., Sleight, A.J. (1997). Interaction of tryptamine and ergoline compounds with threonine 196 in the ligand binding site of the 5-hydroxytryptamine6 receptor. *Molecular Pharmacology* **52(3)**:515–523.

Bonomi, M., Busnelli, M., Persani, L., Vassart, G., Costagliola, S. (2006). Structural differences in the hinge region of the glycoprotein hormone receptors: Evidence from the sulfated tyrosine residues. *Molecular Endocrinology* **20(12)**:3351–3363.

Bouvier, M., Loisel, T.P., Hebert, T. (1995). Dynamic regulation of G-protein coupled receptor palmitoylation: Potential role in receptor function. *Biochemical Society Transactions* **23(3)**:577–581.

Boyd, A. (1995). Bromocriptine and psychosis: A literature review. *Psychiatric Quarterly* **66(1)**:87–95.

Brady, J.D., Rich, T.C., Le, X., Stafford, K., Fowler, C.J., Lynch, L., Karpen, J.W., Brown, R.L., Martens, J.R. (2004). Functional role of lipid raft microdomains in cyclic nucleotide-gated channel activation. *Molecular Pharmacology* **65(3)**:503–511.

Brelot, A., Heveker, N., Pleskoff, O., Sol, N., Alizon, M. (1997). Role of the first and third extracellular domains of CXCR-4 in human immunodeficiency virus coreceptor activity. *Journal of Virology* **71(6)**:4744–4751.

Briley, E., Lolait, S., Axelrod, J., Felder, C. (1994) The cloned vasopressin V1a receptor stimulated phospholipase A2, phospholipase C and phospholipase D through activation of receptor-operated calcium channels. *Neuropeptides* **27(1)**:63–74.

Brookmeyer, R., Gray, S., Kawas, C. (1998). Projections of Alzheimer's disease in the United States and the public health impact of delaying disease onset. *American Journal of Public Health* **88(9)**:1337–1342.

Brown, D.A., London, E. (1998). Functions of lipid rafts in biological membranes. *Annual Review of Cell and Developmental Biology* **14**:111–136.

Brown, J.H., Makman, M.H. (1973). Stimulation by dopamine of adenylate cyclase in retinal homogenates and of adenosine-3′:5′-cyclic monophosphate formation in intact retina. *Proceedings of the National Academy of Sciences USA* **69(3)**:539–543.

Brown, P. (1994). Understanding the inner voices. *New Scientist* **143**:26–31.

Brunner, H.G., Otten, B.J. (1999). Precocious puberty in boys. *New England Journal of Medicine* **341(23)**:1763–1765.

Bruno, J.F., Whittaker, J., Song, J.F., Berelowitz, M. (1991). Molecular cloning and sequencing of a cDNA encoding a human alpha 1A adrenergic receptor. *Biochemical Biophysical Research Communications* **179(3)**:1485–1490.

Bunge, S., Wedemann, H., David, D., Terwilliger, D.J., Van Den Born, L.I., Aulehla-Scholz, C., Samanns, C., Horn, M., Ott, J., Schwinger, E., Schinzel, A., Denton, M.J., Gal, A. (1993). Molecular analysis and genetic mapping of the rhodopsin gene in families with autosomal dominant retinitis pigmentosa. *Genomics* **17(1)**:230–233.

Burford, N.T., Wang, D., Sadee, W. (2000). G-protein coupling of mu-opioid receptors (OP3): elevated basal signaling activity. *Biochemistry Journal* **348(Pt 3)**:531–537.

Burger, M., Burger, J.A., Hoch, R.C., Oades, Z., Takamori, H., Schraufstatter, I.U. (1999). Point mutation causing constitutive signaling of CXCR2 leads to transforming activity similar to Kaposi's sarcoma Herpesvirus-G protein-coupled receptor. *Journal of Immunology* **163(4)**:2017–2022.

Burnier, M., and Brunner, H.R. (2000). Angiotensin II receptor antagonists. *Lancet* **355(9204)**:637–645.

Burns, C.M., Chu, H., Rueter, S.M., Hutchinson, L.K., Canton, H., Sanders-Bush, E., Emeson, R.B. (1997). Regulation of serotonin-2C receptor G-protein coupling by RNA editing. *Nature* **387(6630)**:303–308.

Buur-Rasmussen, B., Brosen, K. (1999). Cytochrome P450 and therapeutic drug monitoring with respect to clozapine. *European Neuropsychopharmacology* **9(6)**:453–459.

Bylund, D.B., Eikenberg, D.C., Hieble, J.P., Langer, S.Z., Lefkowitz, R.J., Minneman, K.P., Molinoff, P.B., Ruffolo, R.R. Jr., Trendelenburg, A.U. (1994). International Union of Pharmacology nomenclature of adrenoceptors. *Pharmacological Reviews* **46(2)**:121–136.

Bylund, D.B., Ray-Prenger, C. (1989). Alpha-2A and alpha-2B adrenergic receptor subtypes: Attenuation of cyclic AMP production in cell lines containing only one receptor subtype. *Journal of Pharmacology and Experimental Therapeutics* **251(2)**:640–644.

Bymaster, F., Calligaro, D.O., Falcone, J.F., Marsh, R.D., Moore, N.A., Tye, N.C., Seeman, P., Wong, D.T. (1996). Radioreceptor binding profile of the atypical antipsychotic olanzapine. *Neuropsychopharmacology* **14(2)**:87–96.

Callaghan, J.T., Bergstrom, R.F., Ptak, L.R., Beasley, C.M. (1999). Olanzapine: Pharmacokinetic and pharmacodynamic profile. *Clinical Pharmacokinetics* **37(3)**:177–193.

Capponi, A.M. (1996). Distribution and signal transduction of angiotensin II AT1 and AT2 receptors. *Blood Pressure. Supplement* **2**:41–46.

Carlsson, A., Lindqvist, M., Magnusson, T. (1957). 3,4-Dihydroxyphenylalanine and 5-hydroxytryptophan as reserpine antagonists. *Nature* **180(4596)**:1200.

Carlsson, A., Lindqvist, M., Magnusson, T., Walbeck, B. (1958). On the presence of 3-hydroxytyramine in brain. *Science* **127(3296)**:471.

Cartier, L., Dubois-Dauphin, M., Hartley, O., Irminger-Finger, I., Krause, K.H. (2003). Chemokine-induced cell death in CCR5-expressing neuroblastoma cells. *Journal of Neuroimmunology* **145(1–2)**:27–39.

Castensson, A., Emilsson, L., Sunderberg, R., Jazin, E. (2003). Decrease of serotonin receptor 2C in schizophrenia brains identified by high-resolution mRNA expression analysis. *Biological Psychiatry* **54(11)**:1212–1221.

Catt, K.J., Sandberg, K., Balla, T. (1993). Angiotensin II receptor and signal transduction mechanisms. In: Raizada, M.K., Phillips, M.I., Sumners, C. (eds), *Cellular and molecular biology of the renin–angiotensin system*, pp. 307–356. Boca Raton, FL: CRC Press.

Cetani, F., Tonacchera, M., Vassart, G. (1996). Differential effects of NaCl concentration on the constitutive activity of the thyrotropin and the luteinizing hormone/chorionic gonadotropin receptors. *FEBS Letters* **378(1)**:27–31.

Chhajlani, V., Wikberg, J.E.S. (1992). Molecular cloning and expression of the human melanocyte stimulating hormone receptor cDNA. *FEBS Letters* **309(3)**:417–420.

Chhajlani, V., Muceniece, R., Wikberg, J.E.S. (1993). Molecular cloning of a novel human melanocortin receptor. *Biochemical and Biophysical Research Communications* **195(2)**:866–873.

Chalmers, D.T., Lopez, J.F., Akil, H., Watson, S.J. (1993). Molecular aspects of the stress axis and serotonergic function in depression. *Clinical Neuroscience* **1**:122–128.

Chalothorn, D., McCune, D.F., Edelmann, S.E., Tobita, K., Keller, B.B., Lasley, R.D., Perez, D.M., Tanoue, A., Tsujimoto, G., Post, G.R., Piascik, M.T. (2003). Differential cardiovascular regulatory activities of the alpha 1B- and alpha 1D-adrenoceptor subtypes. *Journal of Pharmacology and Experimental Therapeutics* **305(3)**:1045–1053.

Chan, D., Kim, P. (1998). HIV entry and its inhibition. *Cell* **93(5)**:681–684.

Chapple, J.P., Grayson, C., Hardcastle, A.J., Saliba, R.S., Spuy, J., Cheetham, M.E. (2001). Unfolding retinal dystrophies: A role for molecular chaperones? *Trends in Molecular Medicine* **7(9)**:414–421.

Charo, I.F., Myers, S.J., Herman, A., Franci, C., Connolly, A.J., Coughlin, S.R. (1994). Molecular cloning and functional expression of two monocyte chemoattractant protein 1 receptors reveal alternative splicing of the carboxyl terminal tails. *Proceedings of the National Academy of Sciences U.S.A.* **91**:2752–2756.

Chatterton, J.E., Awobuluyi, M., Premkumar, L.S., Takahashi, H.,Talantova, M., Shin, Y., Cui, J., Tu, S., Sevarino, K.A., Nakanishi, N., Tong, G., Lipton, S.A., Zhang, D.. (2002). Excitatory glycine receptors containing the NR3 family of NMDA receptor subunits. *Nature* **415**:793–798.

Chelikani, P., Hornak, V., Eilers, M., Reeves, P.J., Smith, S.O., RajBhandary, U.L., Khorana, H.G. (2007). Role of group-conserved residues in the helical core of beta2-adrenergic receptor. *Proceedings of the National Academy of Sciences USA* **104(17)**:7027–7032.

Chen, C.-R., Tanaka, K., Chazenbalk, G.D., McLachlan, S.M., Rapoport, B. (2001). A full biological response to autoantibodies in Graves' disease requires a disulfide-bonded loop in the thyrotropin receptor N-terminus homologous to a laminin EGF-like domain. *Journal of Biological Chemistry* **276(18)**:14767–14772.

Chen, G., Jayawickreme, C., Way, J., Armour, S., Queen, K., Watson, C., Ignar, D., Chen, W., Kenakin, T.P. (1999) Constitutive receptor systems for drug discovery. *Journal of Pharmacological and Toxicological Methods* **42(4)**:199–206.

Chini, B., Mouillac, B., Ala, Y., Balestre, M.N., Trumpp-Kallmeyer, S., Hoflack, J., Elands, J., Hibert, M., Manning, M., Jard, S., Barberis, C. (1995). Tyr 115 is the key residue for determining agonist selectivity in the V1a vasopressin receptor. *EMBO Journal* **14(10)**:2176–2182.

Chini, B., Parenti, M. (2004). G-protein coupled receptors in lipid rafts and caveolae: How, when and why they go there? *Journal of Molecular Endocrinology* **32(2)**:325–338.

Choe, H., Farzan, M., Sun, Y., Sullivan, N., Rollins, B., Ponath, P.D., Wu, L., Mackay, C.R., LaRosa, G., Newman, W., Gerard, N., Gerard, C., Sodroski, J. (1996). The beta-chemokine receptors CCR3 and CCR5 facilitate infection by primary HIV-1 isolates. *Cell* **85(7)**:1135–1148.

Chou, C.C., Fine, J.S., Pugliese-Sivo, C., Gonsiorek, W., Davies, L., Deno, G., Petro, M., Schwarz, M., Zavodny, P.J., Hipkin, R.W. (2002). Pharmacologicla characterization of the chemokine receptor, hCCR1 in a sTable transfectant and differentiated HL-60 cells: antagonism of hCCR1 activation by MIP-1β. *British Journal of Pharmacology* **137(5)**:663–665.

Chun, M., Liyanage, U.K., Lisanti, M.P., Lodish, H.F. (1994). Signal transduction of a G protein-coupled receptor in caveolae: Colocalization of endothelin and its receptor with caveolin. *Proceedings of the National Academy of Sciences U.S.A.* **91(24)**:11728–11732.

Civelli, O., Saito, Y., Wang, Z., Nothacker, H., Reinscheid, R.K. (2006). Orphan GPCRs and their ligands. *Pharmacology and Therapeutics* **110**:525–532.

Clément, M., Martin, S.S., Beaulieu, M., Chamberland, C., Lavigne, P., Leduc, R. (2005). Determining the environment of the ligand binding pocket of the angiotensin II hAT1 receptor using methionine proximity assay. *Journal of Biological Chemistry* **280(29)**:27121–27129.

Cocchi, F., DeVico, A.L., Garzino-Demo, Arya, S.K., Gallo, R.C., Lusso, P. (1995). Identification of RANTES, MIP-1α, and MIP-1β as the major HIV-suppressive factors produced by CD8+ T cells. *Science* **270(5243)**:1811–1815.

Cody, J.D., Reveles, X.T., Hale, D.E., Lehman, D., Coon, H., Leach, R. (1999). Haplosufficiency of the melanocortin-4 receptor gene in individuals with deletions of 18q. *Human Genetics* **105(5)**:424–427.

Coleman, R.A., Smith, W.L., Narumiya, S. (1994). International Union of Pharmacology classification of prostanoid receptors: Properties, distribution and structure of the receptors and their subtypes. *Pharmacological Reviews* **46(2)**:205–229.

Combadiere, C., Ahuja, S.K., Van Damme, J., Tiffany, H.L., Gao, J-L., Murphy, P.M. (1995). Monocyte chemoattarctant protein-3 is a functional ligand at CC chemokine receptors 1 and 2b. *Journal of Biological Chemistry* **270(50)**:29671–29675.

Combadiere, C., Ahuja, S.K., Tiffany, H.L., Murphy, P.M. (1996). Cloning and functional expression of CC CKR5, a human monocyte CC chemokine receptor selective for MIP-1(alpha), MIP-1(beta), and RANTES. *Journal of Leukocyte Biology* **60(1)**:147–152.

Combadiere, C., Gao, J., Tiffany, H.L., Murphy, P.M. (1998). Gene cloning, RNA distribution and functional expression of mCX3CR1, a mouse chemotactic receptor for the CX3C fractalkine. *Biochemical and Biophysical Research Communications* **253(3)**:728–732.

Compan, V., Zhou, M., Grailhe, R., Gazzara, R.A., Martin, R., Gingrich, J.,Dumuis, ABrunner, D., Bockaert, J., Hen, R. (2004). Attenuated response to stress and novelty and hypersensitivity to seizures in 5-HT_4 receptor knock-out mice. *Journal of Neuroscience* **24(2)**:412–419.

Concepcion, F., Mendez, A., Chen, J. (2002). The carboxyl-terminal domain is essential for rhodopsin transport in rod photoreceptors. *Vision Research* **42**:417–426.

Conner, A.C., Simms, J., Hay, D.L., Mahmoud, K., Howitt, S.G., Wheatley, M., Poyner, D.R. (2004). Heterodimers and family-B GPCRs: RAMPs, CGRP and adrenomedullin. *Biochemical Society Transactions* **32(Pt 5)**:843–846.

Cormier, E.G., Persuh, M., Thompson, D.A.D., Lin, S.W., Sakmar, T.P., Olson, W.C., Dragic, T. (2000). Specific interaction of CCR5 amino-terminal domain peptides containing sulfotyrosines with HIV-1 envelope glycoprotein gp120. *Proceedings of the National Academy of Sciences USA* **97(11)**:5762–5767.

Costagliola, S., Panneels, V., Bonomi, M., Koch, J., Many, M.C., Smits, G., Vassart, G. (2002). Tyrosine sulfation is required for agonist recognition by glycoprotein hormone receptors. *EMBO Journal* **21(4)**:504–513.

Costagliola, S., Vassart, G. (2000). Monoclonal antibodies against human TSHR with strong TBII and TBAB activities recognize a linear epitope modified by a posttranslational modification (Abstract). In: *Proceedings of the 12th International Thyroid Congress Kyoto Japan*, p. O–597, Japan Endocrine Society.

Cotecchia, S., Björklöf, K., Rossier, O., Stanasila, L., Greasley, P., Fanelli, F. (2002). The alpha1b-adrenergic receptor subtype: Molecular properties and physiological implications. *Journal of Receptor and Signal Transduction Research* **22(1–4)**:1–16.

Couet, J., Li, S., Okamoto, T., Ikezu, T., Lisanti, M.P. (1997). Identification of peptide and protein ligands for the caveolin-scaffolding domain. Implications for the interaction of caveolin with caveolae-associated proteins. *Journal of Biological Chemistry* **272(10)**:6525–6533.

Coughlin, S.R. (1994). Expanding horizons of receptors coupled to G-proteins: Diversity and disease. *Current Opinion in Cell Biology* **6(2)**:191–197.

Couture, L., Naharisoa, H., Grebert, D., Remy, J-J., Pajot-Augy, E., Bozon, V., Haertle, T., Salesse, R. (1996). Peptide and immunochemical mapping of the ectodomain of the porcine LH receptor. *Journal of Molecular Endocrinology* **16(1)**:15–25.

Coyle, J.T., Tsai, G. and Goff, D. (2003). Converging evidence of NMDA receptor hypofunction in the pathophysiology of schizophrenia. *Annals of the New York Academy of Sciences* **1003**:318–27.

Creese, I., Burt, D.R., Snyder, S.H. (1976). Dopamine receptor binding predicts clinical and pharmacological potencies of antischizophrenic drugs. *Science* **192(4238)**:481–483.

Crisanti, P., Omri, B., Hughes, E.J., Meduri, G., Hery, C., Clauser, E., Jacquemin, C., Saunier, B. (2001). The expression of thyrotropin receptor in the brain. *Endocrinology* **142(2)**:812–822.

Criscione, L., de Gasparo, M., Bühlmayer, P., Whitebread, S., Ramjoué, H.P.R., Wood, J. (1993). Pharmacological profile of valsartan: A potent, orally active, nonpeptide antagonist of the angiotensin-II AT1-receptor subtype. *British Journal of Pharmacology* **110(2)**:761–771.

Csikós, T., Chung, O., Unger, T. (1998). Receptors and their classification: Focus on angiotensin II and the AT2 receptor. *Journal of Human Hypertension* **12(5)**:311–318.

Cull-Candy, S., Brickley, S., Farrant, M. (2001). NMDA receptor subunits: Diversity, development and disease. *Current Opinion in Neurobiology* **11(3)**:327–335.

Curnow, K.M., Pascoe, L., White, P. (1992). Genetic analysis of the human type-1 angiotensin II receptor. *Molecular Endocrinology* **6(7)**:1113–1118.

D'Aniello, A., Lee, J.M., Petrucelli, L., Di Fiore, M.M. (1998). Regional decreases of free D-aspartate levels in Alzheimer's disease. *Neuroscience Letters* **250(2)**:131–134.

Dahlöf, B., Devereux, R.B., Kjeldsen, S.E., Julius, S., Beevers, G., de Faire, U., Fyhrquist, F., Ibsen, H., Kristiansson, K., Lederballe-Pedersen, O., Lindholm, L.H., Nieminen, M.S., Omvik, P., Oparil, S., Wedel, H. (2002). Cardiovascular morbidity and mortality in the losartan intervention for endpoint reduction in hypertension study (LIFE): A randomised trial against atenolol. *Lancet* **359(9311)**:995–1003.

Dairaghi, D.J., Fan, R.A., McMaster, B.E., Hanley, M.R., Schall, T.J. (1999). HHV8-encoded vMIP-1selectively engages chemokine receptor CCR8. Agonist and antagonist profiles of viral chemokines. *Journal of Biological Chemistry* **274(31)**:21569–21574.

Dal Toso, R., Somme, B., Ewert, M., Herb, A., Prichett, D.B., Bach, A., Shivers, B.D., Seeburg, P.H. (1989). The dopamine D2 receptor: Two molecular forms generated by alternative splicing. *EMBO Journal* **8(13)**:4025–4034.

Damaj, B.B., McColl, S.R., Neote, K., Songqing, N., Ogborn, K.T., Hébert, C.A., Naccache, P.H. (1996). Identification of G-protein binding sites of the human interleukin-8 receptors by functional mapping of the intracellular loops. *FASEB Journal* **10(12)**:1426–1434.

Damian, M., Martin, A., Mesnier, D., Pin, J., Banères, J. (2006). Asymmetric conformational changes in a GPCR dimer controlled by G-proteins. *EMBO Journal* **25(24)**:5693–5702.

Daugherty, B.L., Siciliano, S.J., DeMartino, J.A., Malkowitz, L., Sirotina, A., Springer, M.S. (1996). Cloning, expression and characterization of the human eosinophil eotaxin receptor. *Journal of Experimental Medicine* **183(5)**:2349–2354.

Davies, E., Bonnardeaux, A., Lathrop, G.M., Corvol, P., Clauser, E., Soubrier, F. (1994). Angiotensin II (type-1) receptor locus: CA repeat polymorphism and genetic mapping. *Human Molecular Genetics* **3(5)**:838.

de Gasparo, M., Bottari, M., Levens, N.R. (1995). Characteristics of angiotensin II receptors and their role in cell and organ physiology. In: Laragh, J.H., Brenner, B.M. (eds), *Hypertension: Pathophysiology, Diagnosis, and Management, Vol. 1*, pp. 1695–1720. New York: Raven Press.

de Gasparo, M., Catt, K.J., Inagami, T., Wright, J.W., Unger, T. (2000). International Union of Pharmacology: XXIII. The angiotensin II receptors. *Pharmacological Reviews* **52(3)**:415–472.

de Gasparo, M., Husain, A., Alexander, W., Catt, K.J., Chiu, A.T., Drew, M., Goodfriend, T., Harding, J.W., Inagami, T., Timmermans, P.B. (1995). Proposed update of angiotensin receptor nomenclature. *Hypertension* **25(5)**:924–927.

de Gasparo, M., Whitebread, S. (1994). Heterogeneity of angiotensin receptor subtypes. In: Timmermanns, P.B.M.W.M., Wexler, R.R. (eds), *Medicinal chemistry of the renin–angiotensin system*, pp. 269–294. Amsterdam: Elsevier.

De Kloet, E.R., Rosenfel, P., Van Eekelen, J.A.M., Sutanto, W., Levine, S., (eds) (1988) Stress, glucocorticoids and development. In: *Progress in Brain Research*, pp. 101–120. Amsterdam: Elsevier.

De Kloet, E.R., Vreugdenhil, E., Oitzl, M.S., Joëls, M. (1998). Brain corticosteroid receptor balance in health and disease. *Endocrine Reviews* **19(3)**:269–301.

Decaux, G., Soupart, A., Vassart, G. (2008). Non-peptide arginine vasopressin antagonists: The vaptans. *Lancet* **371(9624)**:1624–1632.

Delgado, M.B., Clark-Lewis, I., Loetscher, P., Langen, H., Thelen, M., Baggiolini, M., Wolf, M. (2001). Rapid inactivation of stromal cell-derived factor-1 by cathepsin G associated with lymphocytes. *European Journal of Immunology* **31(3)**:699–707.

Desai, M.A., Burnett, J.P., Mayne, N.G., Schoepp, D.D. (1995). Cloning and expression of human metabotropic glutamate receptor 1 alpha: enhanced coupling on co-transfection with a glutamate transporter. *Molecular Pharmacology* **48(4)**:648–657.

Del Tredici, A.L., Schiffer, H.H., Burstein, E.S., Lameh, J., Mohell, N., Hacksell, U., Brann, M.R., Weiner, D.M. (2004). Pharmacology of polymorphic variants of the human 5-HT1A receptor. *Biochemical Pharmacology* **67(3)**:479–490.

Dionne, I.J., Garant, M.J., Nolan, A.A., Pollin, T.I., Lewis, D.G., Shuldiner, A.R., Poehlman, E.T. (2002). Association between obesity and a polymorphism in the beta(1)-adrenoceptor gene (Gly389Arg ADRB1) in Caucasian women. *International Journal of Obesity and Related Metabolic Disorders* **26(5)**:633–639.

Dinulescu, D.M., Cone, R.D. (2000). Agouti and agouti-related protein: Analogies and contrasts. *Journal of Biological Chemistry* **275(10)**:6695–6698.

Dobner, T., Wolf, I., Emrich, T., Lipp, M. (1992). Differentiation-specific expression of a novel G protein-coupled receptor from Burkitt's lymphoma. *European Journal of Immunology* **22(11)**:2795–2799.

Dong, C., Filipeanu, C.M., Duvernay, M.T., Wu, G. (2007). Regulation of G protein-coupled receptor export trafficking. *Biochimica et Biophysica Acta* **1768(4)**:853–870.

Dong, C., Zhou, F., Fugetta, E.K., Filipeanu, C.M., Wu, G. (2008). Endoplasmic reticulum export of adrenergic and angiotensin II receptors is differentially regulated by Sar1 GTPase. *Cell Signaling* **20(6)**:1035–1043.

Doranz, B.J., Grovit-Ferbas, K., Sharron, M.P., Mao, S.H., Goetz, M.B., Daar, E.S., Doms, R.W., O'Brien, W.A. (1997). A small-molecule inhibitor directed against the chemokine receptor CXCR4 prevents its use as an HIV-1 coreceptor. *Journal of Experimental Medicine* **186(8)**:1395–1400.

Dorsett, Y., Tuschl, T. (2004). siRNAs: Applications in functional genomics and potential as therapeutics. *Nature Reviews Drug Discovery* **3(4)**:318–329.

Doss, R.C., Perkins, J.P., Harden, T.K. (1981). Recovery of beta-adrenergic receptors following long-term exposure of astrocytoma cells to catecholamine. *Journal of Biological Chemistry* **256(23)**:12281–12286.

D'Souza-Li, L., Canaff, L., Janicic, N., Cole, D.E., Hendy, G.N. (2001). An acceptor splice site mutation in the calcium-sensing receptor (CASR) gene in familial hypocalciuric hypercalcemia and neonatal severe hyperparathyroidism. *Human Mutation* **18(5)**:411–421.

Dudley, D.T., Summerfelt, R.M. (1993). Regulated expression of angiotensin II (AT2) binding sites in R3T3 cells. *Regulatory Peptides* **44(2)**:199–206.

Dunah, A.W., Sirianni, A.C., Fienberg, A.A., Bastia, E., Schwarzschild, M.A., Standaert, D.G. (2004). Dopamine D1-dependant trafficking of striatal *N*-methyl-D-aspartate glutamate receptors requires Fyn protein tyrosine kinase but not DARPP-32. *Molecular Pharmacology* **65(1)**:121–129.

Dupré, D.J., Baragli, A., Rebois, R.V., Ethier, N., Hébert, T.E. (2007). Signalling complexes associated with adenylyl cyclase II are assembled during their biosynthesis. *Cellular Signaling* **19(3)**:481–489.

Dupré, D.J., Robitaille, M., Ethier, N., Villeneuve, L.R., Mamarbachi, A.M., Hébert, T.E. (2006). Seven transmembrane receptor core signaling complexes are assembled prior to plasma membrane trafficking. *Journal of Biological Chemistry* **281(45)**:34561–34573.

Duprez, L., Parma, J., Costagliola, S., Hermans, J., Van Sande, J., Dumont, J.E., Vassart, G. (1997). Constitutive activation of the TSH receptor by spontaneous mutations affecting the N-terminal extracellular domain. *FEBS Letters* **409(3)**:469–474.

Duvernay, M.T., Filipeanu, C.M., Wu, G. (2005). The regulatory mechanisms of export trafficking of G protein-coupled receptors. *Cellular Signaling* **17(12)**:1457–1465.

Duvernay, M.T., Zhou, F., Wu, G. (2004). A conserved motif for the transport of G protein-coupled receptors from the endoplasmic reticulum to the cell surface. *Journal of Biological Chemistry* **279(29)**:30741–30750.

Dzau, V.J. (1994). Cell biology and genetics of angiotensin in cardiovascular disease. *Journal of Hypertension, Supplement* **12(4)**:S3-10.

Eason, M.G., Kurose, H., Holt, B.D., Raymond, J.R., Liggett, S.B. (1992). Simultaneous coupling of alpha 2-adrenergic receptors to two G-proteins with opposing effects. Subtype-selective coupling of alpha 2C10, alpha 2C4, and alpha 2C2 adrenergic receptors to Gi and Gs. *Journal of Biological Chemistry* **267(22)**:15795–15801.

Eden, R.J., Costall, B., Domeney, A.M., Gerrard, P.A., Harvey, C.A., Kelly, M.E., Naylor, R.J., Owen, D.A., Wright, A. (1991). Preclinical pharmacology of ropinirole (SK&F 101468-A): A novel dopamine D2 agonist. *Pharmacology Biochemistry and Behavior* **38(1)**:147–154.

Edno, L., Combourieu, I., Cazenave, M., Tignol, J. (1997). Assay for quantitation of clozapine and its metabolite *N*-desmethylclozapine in human plasma by high performance liquid chromatography with ultraviolet detection. *Journal of Pharmaceutical and Biomedical Analysis* **16(2)**:311–318.

Eilers, M., Patel, A.B., Liu, W., Smith, S.O. (2002). Comparison of helix interactions in membrane and soluble α-bundle proteins. *Biophysical Journal* **82(5)**:2720–2736.

Emile, L., Mercken, L., Apiou, F., Pradier, L., Bock, M.D., Menager, J., Clot, J., Doble, A., Blanchard, J.C. (1996). Molecular cloning, functional expression, pharmacological characterization and chromosomal localization of the human metabotropic glutamate receptor type 3. *Neuropharmacology* **35**:523–530.

Emorine, L.J., Marullo, S., Briend-Sutren, M.M., Patey, G., Tate, K., Delavier-Kutchko, C., Strosberg, A.D. (1989). Molecular characterization of the human beta 3-adrenergic receptor. *Science* **245(4922)**:1118–1121.

Englund, A.T., Geffner, M.E., Nagel, R.A., Lippe, B.M., Braunstein, G.D. (1991). Pediatric germ cell and human chorionic gonadotropin-producing tumors. Clinical and laboratory features. *American Journal of Diseases of Children* **145(11)**:1294–1297.

Ernst, O.P., Meyer, C.K., Marin, E.P., Henklein, P., Fu, W.Y., Sakmar, T.P., Hofmann, K.P. (2000). Mutation of the fourth cytoplasmic loop of rhodopsin affects binding of transducin and peptides derived from the carboxyl-terminal sequences of transducin alpha and gamma subunits. *Journal of Biological Chemistry* **275(3)**:1937–1943.

Faraone, S., Khan, S. (2006). Candidate gene studies of attention-deficit/hyperactivity disorder. *Journal of Clinical Psychiatry* **67(Suppl 8)**:13–20.

Farde, L., Nordström, A.L., Wiesel, F.A., Pauli, S., Hallidan, C., Sedvall, G. (1992). Positron emission tomographic analysis of central D1 and D2 receptor occupancy in patients treated with classical neuroleptics and clozapine. Relation to extrapyramidal side effects. *Archives of General Psychiatry* **49(7)**:538–544.

Fargin, A., Raymond, J.R., Regan, J.W., Cotecchia, S., Lefkowitz, R.J., Caron, M.G. (1989). Effector coupling mechanisms of the cloned 5-HT1A receptor. *Journal of Biological Chemistry* **264(25)**:14848–14852.

Farooqi, I.S., Keogh, J.M., Yeo, G.S., Lank, E.J., Cheetham, T., O'Rahilly, S. (2003). Clinical spectrum of obesity and mutations in the melanocortin 4 receptor gene. *New England Journal of Medicine* **348(12)**:1085–1095.

Farzan, M., Mirzabekov, T., Kolchinsky, P., Wyatt, R., Cayabyab, M., Gerard, N.P., Gerard, C., Sodroski, J., Choe, H. (1999). Tyrosine sulfation of the amino terminus of CCR5 facilitates HIV-1 entry. *Cell* **96(5)**:667–676.

Feng, Y., Broder, C.C., Kennedy, P.E., Berger, E.A. (1996). HIV-1 entry cofactor: Functional cDNA cloning of a seven-transmembrane, G protein-coupled receptor. *Science* **272(5263)**:872–877.

Ferguson, S.S.G. (2001). Evolving concepts in G-protein coupled receptor endocytosis: The role of receptor desensitization and signaling. *Pharmacological Reviews* **53(1)**:1–24.

Ferguson, S.S.G., Downey, W.E., III, Colaprietro, A.M., Koch, W.J., Caron, M.G. (1996) Role of β-arrestin in mediating agonist-promoted G-protein coupled receptor internalization. *Science* **271(5247)**:363–366.

Fernández-Varo, G., Ros, J., Cejudo-Martin, P., Cano C., Arroyo, V., Riviera, F., Rodes, J., Jimenez, W. (2003). Effect of the V_{1a}/V_2-AVP receptor antagonist, conivaptan, on renal water metabolism and systemic hemodynamics in rats with cirrhosis and ascites. *Journal of Hepatology* **38(6)**:755–761.

Ferrari-Toninelli, G., Bonini, S.A., Cenini, G., Maccarinelli, G., Grilli, M., Uberti, D., Memo, M. (2008). Dopamine receptor agonists for protection and repair in Parkinson's disease. *Cuurent Topics in Medicinal Chemistry* **8(12)**:1089–1099.

Fieger, C.B., Huang, M., Brocklyn, J.R.V., Goetzl, E.J. (2005). Type 1 sphingosine 1-phosphate G protein-coupled receptor signaling of lymphocyte functions requires sulfation of its extracellular amino-terminal tyrosines. *FASEB Journal* **19(13)**:1926–1928.

Fiorica-Howells, E., Hen, R., Gingrich, J., Li, Z., Gershon, M.D. (2002). 5-HT(2A) receptors: location and functional analysis in intestines of wild-type and 5-HT(2A) knockout mice. *American Journal of Physiology and Gastrointestinal Liver Physiology* **282(5)**:G877–893.

Fishburn, C., Bellili, D., David, C., Carmon, S., Fuchs, S. (1993). A novel short isoform of the D3 dopamine receptor generated by alternative splicing in the third cytoplasmic loop. *Journal of Biological Chemistry* **268(8)**:5872–5878.

Fitzgerald, L.W., Iyer, G., Conklin, D.S., Krause, C.M., Marshall, A., Patterson, J.P., Tran, D.P., Jonak, G.J., Hartig, P.R. (1999). Messenger RNA editing of the human serotonin 5-HT2C receptor. *Neuropsychopharmacology* **21(2 Suppl.)**:82S–90S.

Flomen, R., Knight, J., Sham, P., Kerwin, R., Makoff, A. (2004). Evidence that RNA editing modulates splice site selection in the 5-HT2C receptor gene. *Nucleic Acids Research* **32(7)**:2113–2122.

Flor, P.J., Lindauer, K., Püttner, I., Rüegg, D., Lukic, S., Knöpfel, T., Kuhn, R. (1995). Molecular cloning, functional expression and pharmacological characterization of the human metabotropic glutamate receptor type 2. *European Journal of Neuroscience* **7(4)**:622–629

Fong, T.M., Mao, C., MacNeil, T., Kalyani, R., Smith, T., Weinberg, D., Tota, M.R., Van der Ploeg, L.H. (1997). ART (protein product of agouti-related transcript) as an antagonist of MC-3 and MC-4 receptors. *Biochemical and Biophysical Research Communications* **237(3)**:629–631.

Forray, C., Bard, J.A., Wetzel, J.M., Chiu, G., Shapiro, E., Tang, R., Lepor, H., Hartig, P.R., Weinshank, R.L., Branchek, T.A., *et al.* (1994). The alpha 1-adrenergic receptor that mediates smooth muscle contraction in human prostate has the pharmacological properties of the cloned human alpha 1c subtype. *Molecular Pharmacology* **45(4)**:703–708.

Ford, A.P.D.W., Daniels, D.V., Chang, D.J., Gever, J.R., Jasper, J.R., Lesnick, J.D., Clarke, D.E. (1997). Pharmacological pleiotropism of the human recombinant alpha1A-adrenoceptor: implications for alpha1-adrenoceptor classification. *British Journal of Pharmacology* **121(6)**:1127–1135.

Fredricksson, R., Lagerström, M.C., Schiöth, H.B. (2005). Expansion of the superfamily of GPCRs in chordates. *Annals of the New York Academy of Sciences* **1040**:89–94.

Fredricksson, R., Lagerström, M. C., Lundin, L., Schiöth, H. B. (2003). The G-protein-coupled receptors in the human genome form five main families: Phylogenetic analysis, paralogon groups and fingerprints. *Molecular Pharmacology* **63(6)**:1256–1272.

Fremont, V., Zhang, M., Weintraub, B.D., Szkudlinski, M.W. (2001). Novel insights into the molecular mechanism of glycoprotein hormone receptor activation (Abstract). *FASEB Journal* **15**:A175.

Frielle, T., Collins, S., Daniel, K.W., Caron, M.G., Lefkowitz, R.J., Kobilka, B.K. (1987). Cloning of the cDNA for the human beta 1-adrenergic receptor. *Proceedings of the National Academy of Sciences USA* **84(22)**:7920–7924.

Futter, C.E., Pearse, A., Hewlett, L.J., Hopkins, C.R. (1996). Multivesicular endosomes containing internalized EGF–EGF receptor complexes mature and then fuse directly with lysosomes. *Journal of Cell Biology* **132(6)**:1011–1023.

Fuxe, K., Manger, P., Genedani, S., Agnati, L. (2006). The nigrostriatal DA pathway and Parkinson's disease. *Journal of Neural Transmission Supplement* **70**:71–83.

Gage, R.M., Kim, K.A., Cao, T.T., von Zastrow, M. (2001). A transplantable sorting signal that is sufficient to mediate rapid recycling of G protein-coupled receptors. *Journal of Biological Chemistry* **276(48)**:44712–44720.

Galliera, E., Jala, V.R., Trent, J.O., Bonecchi, R., Signorelli, P., Lefkowitz, R.J., Mantovani, A., Locati, M., Haribabu, B. (2004). β-Arrestin-dependent constitutive internalization of the human chemokine decoy receptor D6. *Journal of Biological Chemistry* **279(24)**:25590–25597.

Gallo, R.C., Lusso, P. (1997). Chemokines and HIV-infection. *Current Opinion in Infectious Diseases* **10**:12–17.

Gantz, I., Gantz, I., Miwa, H., Konda, Y., Shimoto, Y., Tashiro, T., Watson, S.J., DelValle, J., Yamada, T. (1993a). Molecular cloning, expression, and gene localization of a fourth melanocortin receptor. *Journal of Biological Chemistry* **268(20)**:15174–15179.

Gantz, I., Konda, Y., Tashiro, T., Shimoto, Y., Miwa, H., Munzert, G., Watson, S.J., DelValle, J., Yamada, T. (1993b). Molecular cloning of a novel melanocortin receptor. *Journal of Biological Chemistry* **268(11)**:8246–8250.

Garin, A., Tarantino, N., Faure, S., Daoudi, M., Lécureuil, C., Bourdais, A., Debré, P., Deterre, P., Combadiere, C. (2003). Two novel fully functional isoforms of CX3CR1 are potent HIV coreceptors. *Journal of Immunology* **171(10)**:5305–5312.

Geddes, J.W., Chang-Chui, H., Cooper, S.M., Lott, I.T., Cotman, C.W. (1986). Density and distribution of NMDA receptors in the human hippocampus in Alzheimer's disease. *Brain Research* **399(1)**:156–161.

Gefvert, O., Bergström, M., Långström, B., Lundberg, T., Lindström, L., Yates, R. (1998). Time-course of central nervous dopamine D2 and 5-HT2 receptor blockade and plasma drug concentrations after discontinuation of quetiapine (seroquel) in patients with schizophrenia. *Psychopharmacology (Berlin)* **135(2)**:119–126.

Geijtenbeek, T.B.H., van Vliet, S.J., van Duijnhoven, G.C.F., Figdor, C.G., van Kooyk, Y. (2001). DC-SIGN, a dentritic cell-specific HIV-1 receptor present in placenta that infects T-cells in trans—A review. *Placenta* **22(Suppl. A)**:S19–23.

George, S.R., O'Dowd, B.F., Lee, S.P. (2002). G-protein coupled receptor oligomerization and its potential for drug discovery. *Nature Reviews Drug Discovery* **1(10)**:808–820.

Gether, U. (2000). Uncovering molecular mechanisms involved in activation of G-protein coupled receptors. *Endocrine Reviews* **21(1)**:90–113.

Gether, U., Kobilka, B.K. (1998). G protein-coupled receptors: II. Mechanism of agonist activation. *Journal of Biological Chemistry* **273(29)**:17979–17982.

Gether, U., Lin, S., Ghanouni, P., Ballesteros, J.A., Weinstein, H., Kobilka, B.K. (1997). Agonists induce conformational changes in transmembrane domains III and VI of the β_2 adrenoceptor. *EMBO Journal* **16(22)**:6737–6747.

Ghali, J.K., Koren, M.J., Taylor, J.R., Brooks-Asplund, E., Fan, K., Long, W.A., Smithe, N. (2005). Efficacy and safety of oral conivaptan: A V_{1A}/V_2 vasopressin receptor antagonist, assessed in a randomized, placebo-controlled trial in patients with euvolemic or hypervolemic hyponatremia. *Journal of Clinical Endocrinology and Metabolism* **91(6)**:2145–2152.

Ghanouni, P., Steenhuis, J.J., Farrens, D.L., Kobilka, B.K. (2001). Agonist-induced conformational changes in the G-protein-coupling domain of the β_2 adrenergic receptor. *Proceedings of the National Academy of Sciences USA* **98(11)**:5997–6002.

Gilchrist, R.L., Ryu, K.S., Ji, I., Ji, T.H. (1996). The luteinizing hormone/chorionic gonadotropin receptor has distinct transmembrane conductors for cAMP and inositol phosphate signals. *Journal of Biological Chemistry* **271(32)**:19283–19287.

Giros, B., Sokoloff, P., Martres, M-P., Riou, J-F., Emorine, L.J., Schwartz, J.C. (1989). Alternative splicing directs the expression of two D2 dopamine receptor isoforms. *Nature* **342(6252)**:923–926.

Gohlke, P., Pees, C., Unger, T. (1998). Angiotensin AT2 receptor stimulation increases aortic cyclic GMP in SHRSP by a kinin-dependent mechanism. *Hypertension* **31(1 Pt 2)**:349–355.

Goldstein, J. (1996). Pre-clinical profile of seroquel (quetiapine): An atypical anti-psychotic with clozapine-like pharmacology, In: Holliday, S.G., Ancill, R.J., MacEwan, G.W. (eds), *Schizophrenia: Breaking down the Barriers*, pp. 177–208. London: Wiley.

Goldstein, J. (1999). Quetiapine fumarate (seroquel): A new atypical anti-psychotic. *Drugs of Today (Barcelona)* **35**:193–210.

Goldstein, J.M. (2002). Mechanism of action of quetiapine, a modulator of dopamine at the D2 receptor. Nov2–7, In: *Presentation at the Society for Neuroscience*, Orlando, FL.

Gosling, J., Monteclaro, F.S., Atchison, R.E., Arai, H., Tsou, C-L., Goldsmith, M.A., Charo, I.F. (1997). Molecular uncoupling of C–C chemokine receptor 5-induced chemotaxis and signal transduction from HIV-1 coreceptor activity. In: *Proceedings of the National Academy of Sciences USA* **94(10)**:5061–5066.

Gouldson, P.R., Snell, C.R., Bywater, R.P., Higgs, C., Reynolds, C.A. (1998). Domain swapping in G-protein coupled receptor dimers. *Protein Engineering* **11(12)**:1181–1193.

Govaerts, C., Blanpain, C., Deupi, X., Ballet, S., Ballesteros, J.A., Wodak, S.J., Vassart, G., Pardo, L., Parmentier, M. (2001). The T*X*P motif in the second transmembrane helix of CCR5. A structural determinant of chemokine-induced activation. *Journal of Biological Chemistry* **276(16)**:13217–13225.

Grailhe, R., Grabtree, G.W., Hen, R. (2001). Human 5-HT(5A) receptors: the 5-HT(5A) receptor is functional but the 5-HT(5B) receptor was lost during mammalian evolution. *European Journal of Pharmacology* **418(3)**:157–167.

Graves, P.N., Davies, T.F. (2000). New insights into the thyroid-stimulating hormone receptor. The major antigen of Graves' disease. *Endocrinology and Metabolism Clinics of North America* **29(2)**:267–286.

Graves, R.J. (1835/1940). New observed affection of the thyroid gland in females. (Clinical lectures.) *London Medical and Surgical Journal (Renshaw)* **7**:516–517. Reprinted in *Medical Classics* **5**:33–36.

Gray, J.A., Bhatnagar, A., Gurevich, V.V., Roth, B.L. (2003). The interaction of a constitutively active arrestin with the arrestin-insensitive 5-HT(2A) receptor induces agonist-independent internalization. *Molecular Pharmacology* **63(5)**:961–972.

Green, S.A., Turki, J., Innis, M., Liggett, S.B. (1994). Amino-terminal polymorphisms of the human β_2-adrenergic receptor impart distinct agonist-promoted regulatory properties. *Biochemistry* **33(47)**:9414–9419.

Greenamyer, J.T., Penney, J.B., D'Amato, C.J., Young, A.B. (1987). Dementia of the Alzheimer's type: Changes in hippocampal l-[^{3}H]glutamate binding. *Journal of Neurochemistry* **48(2)**:543–551.

Greenamyer, J.T., Penney, J.B., Young, A.B., D'Amato, C.J., Hicks, S.P., Shoulson, I. (1985). Alterations in l-glutamate binding in Alzheimer's and Huntington's diseases. *Science* **227(4693)**:1496–1499.

Griendling, K.K., Lassègue, B., Alexander, R.W. (1996). Angiotensin receptors and their therapeutic implications. *Annual Reviews in Pharmacology and Toxicology* **36**:281–306.

Griendling, K.K., Ushiofukai, M., Lassègue, B., Alexander, R.W. (1997). Angiotensin II signaling in vascular smooth muscle—new concepts. *Hypertension* **29(1 Pt 2)**:366–373.

Griffith, R.W., Saamerli, K. (1975). Clozapine and agranulocytosis. *Lancet* **2(7936)**:657.

Grossmann, M., Szkudlinski, M.W., Wong, R., Dias, J.A., Ji, T.H., Weintraub, B.D. (1997). Substitution of the seat-belt region of the thyrotropin (TSH)-subunit with the corresponding regions of choriogonadotropin or follitropin confers luteotropic, but not follitropic activity to chimeric TSH. *Journal of Biological Chemistry* **272(24)**:15532–15540.

Gu, D., Ge, D., Snieder, H., He, J., Chen, S., Huang, J., Li, B., Chen, R., Qiang, B. (2006). Association of [alpha]1A adrenergic receptor gene variants on chromosome 8p21 with human stage 2 hypertension. *Journal of Hypertension* **24(6)**:1057–1064.

Gurevich, V.V., Gurevich, E.V. (2006). The structural basis of arrestin-mediated regulation of G-protein coupled receptors. *Pharmacology and Therapeutics* **110(3)**:465–502.

Gürkan, C., Stagg, S.M., Lapointe, P., Balch, W.E. (2006). The COPII cage: Unifying principles of vesicle coat assembly. *Nature Reviews Molecular Cellular Biology* **7(10)**:727–738.

Guzé, B.H., Baxter, L.R., Jr. (1985). Current concepts: Neuroleptic malignant syndrome. *New England Journal of Medicine* **313(3)**:163–166.

Habashi, J.P., Judge, D.P., Holm, T.M., Cohn, R.D., Loeys, B.L., Cooper, T.K., Myers, L., Klein, E.C., Liu, G., Calvi, C., Podowski, M., Neptune, E.R., Halushka, M.K., Bedja, D., Gabrielson, K., Rifkin, D.B., Carta, L., Ramirez, F., Huso, D.L., Dietz, H.C. (2006). Losartan, an AT1 antagonist, prevents aortic aneurysm in a mouse model of Marfan syndrome, and preserves muscle tissue architecture in DMD mouse models. *Science* **312(5770)**:117–121.

Hager, J., Hansen, L., Vaisse, C., Vionnet, N., Philippi, A., Poller, W., Velho, G., Carcassi, C., Contu, L., Julier, C., Cambien, F., Passa, P., Lathrop, M., Carcassi, C., Kindsvogel, W., Demenais, F., Nishimura, E., Froguel, P. (1995). A missense mutation in the glucagon receptor gene is associated with non-insulin-dependant diabetes mellitus. *Nature Genetics* **9(3)**:299–304.

Hague, C., Chen, Z., Uberti, M., Minneman, K.P. (2003). Alpha1-adrenergic receptor subtypes: Non-identical triplets with different dancing partners. *Life Science* **74(4)**:411–418.

Hamblin, M.W. and Metcalf, M.A. (1991). Primary structure and functional characterization of a human 5-HT$_1$D-type serotonin receptor. *Molecular Pharmacology* **40(2)**:143–148.

Hamel, E., Fan, E., Linville, D., Ting, V., Villemure, J.G., Chia, L.S. (1993). Expression of mRNA for the serotonin 5-hydroxytryptamine1D beta receptor subtype in human and bovine cerebral arteries. *Molecular Pharmacology* **44(2)**:242–246.

Hammond, C., Helenius, A. (1995). Quality control in the secretory pathway. *Current Opinion in Cell Biology* **7(4)**:523–529.

Han, M., Smith, S.O., Sakmar, T.P. (1998). Constitutive activation of opsin by mutation of methionine 257 on transmembrane helix 6. *Biochemistry* **37(22)**:8253–8261.

Hanyaloglu, A.C., Vrecl, M., Kroeger, K.M., Miles, L.E., Qian, H., Thomas, W.G., Eidne, K.A. (2001). Casein kinase II sites in the intracellular C-terminal domain of the thyrotropin-releasing hormone receptor and chimeric gonadotropin-releasing hormone receptors contribute to β-arrestin-dependent internalization. *Journal of Biological Chemistry* **276(21)**:18066–18074.

Hardy, L.W., Peet, N.P. (2004). The multiple orthogonal tools approach to define molecular causation in the validation of druggable targets. *Drug Discovery Today* **9(3)**:117–126.

Hargrave, P.A., Hamm, H.E., Hofmann, K.P. (1993). Interaction of rhodopsin with G-protein, transducin. *Bioessays* **15(1)**:43–50.

Hasegawa, Y., Higuchi, S., Matsushita, S., Miyaoka, H. (2002). Association of a polymorphism of the serotonin 1B receptor gene and alcohol dependence with inactive aldehyde dehydrogenase-2. *Journal of Neural Transmission* **109(4)**:513–521.

Hashimoto, T., Inazawa, J., Okamoto, N., Tagawa, Y., Bessho, Y., Honda Y., Nakanishi, S. (1997). The whole nucleotide sequence and chromosomal localization of the gene for human metabotropic glutamate receptor subtype 6. *European Journal of Neuroscience* **9(6)**:1226–1235.

Hashimoto, M., Rockenstein, E., Crews, L., Masliah, E. (2003). Role of protein aggregation in mitochondrial dysfunction and neurodegeneration in Alzheimer's and Parkinson's diseases. *Neuromolecular Medicine* **4(1–2)**:21–36.

Haugen, B.R., Pacini, F., Reiners, C., Schlumberger, M., Ladenson, P.W., Sherman, S.I., Cooper, D.S., Graham, K.E., Braverman, L.E., Skarulis, M.C., Davies, T.F., DeGroot, L.J., Mazzaferri, E.L., Daniels, G.H., Ross, D.S., Luster, M., Samuels, M.H., Becker, D.V., Maxon, H.R., Cavalieri, R.R., Spencer, C.A., McEllin, K., Weintraub, B.D., Ridgway, E.C. (1999). A comparison of recombinant human thyrotropin and thyroid hormone withdrawal for the detection of thyroid remnant or cancer. *Journal of Clinical Endocrinology and Metabolism* **84(11)**:3877–3885.

Hausmann, H., Richters, A., Kreienkamp, H., Meyerhof, W., Mattei, H., Lederis, K., Zwiers, H., Richter, D. (1996). Mutational analysis and molecular modeling of the nonapeptide hormone binding domains of the [Arg8] vasotocin receptor. *Proceedings of the National Academy of Sciences USA* **93(14)**:6907–6912.

Hawi, Z., Dring, M., Kirley, A., Foley, D., Kent, L., Craddock, N., Asherson, P., Curran, S., Gould, A., Richards, S., Lawson, D., Pay, H., Turic, D., Langley, K., Owen, M., O'Donovan, M., Thapar, A., Fitzgerald, M., Gill, M. (2002). Serotonergic system and attention deficit hyperactivity disorder (ADHD): A potential susceptibility locus at the 5-HT(1B) receptor gene in 273 nuclear families from a multi-centre sample. *Molecular Psychiatry* **7(7)**:718–725.

Hawkins, L.M., Prybylowski, K., Chang, K., Moussan, C., Stephenson, F.A., Wenthold, R.J. (2004). Export from the endoplasmic reticulum of assembled *N*-methyl-d-aspartic acid receptors is controlled by a motif in the C terminus of the NR2 subunit. *Journal of Biological Chemistry* **279(28)**:28903–28910.

Hebert, T.E., Moffet, S., Morello, J.P., Loisel, T.P., Bichet, D.G., Barrett, C., Bouvier, M. (1996). A peptide derived from β_2-adrenergic receptor transmembrane domains inhibits both receptor dimerization and activation. *Journal of Biological Chemistry* **271**:16384–16392.

Heeringa, M., Beurskens, R., Schouten, W., Verduijn, M.M. (1999). Elevated plasma levels of clozapine after concomitant use of fluvoxamine. *Pharmacy World and Science* **21(5)**:243–244.

Hein, L., Altman, J.D., Kobilka, B.K. (1999). Two functionally distinct 2-adrenergic receptors regulate sympathetic neurotransmission. *Nature* **402**:181–118.

Heise, C.E., Pahuja, A., Hudson, S.C., Mistry, M.S., Putnam, A.L., Gross, M.M., Gootlieb, P.A., Wade, W.S., Kiankarimi, M., Schwarz, D., Crowe, P., Zlotnik, A., Alleva, D.G. (2005). Pharmaclogical characterization of CXC chemokine receptor 3 ligands and a small molecule antagonist. *Journal of Pharmacology and Experimental Therapeutics* **313(3)**:1263–1271.

Hernández, F., Avila, J. (2007). Tauopathies. *Cell and Molecular Life Sciences* **64(17)**:2219–2233.

Hernanz-Falcón, P., Rodríguez-Frade, J.M., Serrano, A., Juan, D., del Sol, A., Soriano, S.F., Roncal, F., Gómez, L., Valencia, A., Martínez, A.C., Mellado, M. (2004). Identification of amino acid residues crucial for chemokine receptor dimerization. *Nature Immunology* **5(2)**:216–223.

Herrmann, S-M., Nicaud, V., Tiret, L., Evans, A., Kee, F., Ruidavets, J-B., Arveiler, D., Luc, G., Morrison, C., Hoehe, M.R., Paul, M., Cambien, F. (2002). Polymorphisms of the [beta]2-adrenoceptor (ADRB2) gene and essential hypertension: the ECTIM and PEGASe studies. *Journal of Hypertension* **20(2)**:229–235.

Hessel, E., Müller, P., Herrmann, A., Hofmann, K.P. (2001). Light-induced reorganization of phospholipids in rod disc membranes. *Journal of Biological Chemistry* **276(4)**:2538–2543.

Hesselgesser, J., Ng, H.P., Liang, M., Zheng, W., May, K., Bauman, J.G., Monahan, S., Islam, I., Wei, G.P., Ghannam, A., Taub, D.D., Rosser, M., Snider, R.M., Morrissey, M.M., Perez, H.D., Horuk, R. (1998). Identification and characterization of small molecule functional antagonists of the CCR1 chemokine receptor. *Journal of Biology Chemistry* **273(25)**:15687–15692.

Hieble, J.P., Ruffolo, R.R., Jr. (1996). Subclassification and nomenclature of alpha-1 and alpha-2 adrenoceptors. *Progress in Drug Research* **47**:81–130.

Hilairet, S., Foord, S.M., Marshall, F.H., Bouvier, M. (2001). Protein–protein interaction and not glycosylation determines the binding selectivity of heterodimers between the calcitonin receptor-like receptor and the receptor activity-modifying proteins. *Journal of Biological Chemistry* **276(31)**:29575–29581.

Hinney, A., Hohmann, S., Geller, F., Vogel, C., Hess, C., Wermter, A.K., Brokamp, B., Goldschmidt, H., Siegfried, W., Remschmidt, H., Schäfer, H., Gudermann, T., Hebebrand, J. (2003). Melanocortin-4 receptor gene: Case-control study and transmission disequilibrium test confirm that functionally relevant mutations are compatible with a major gene effect for extreme obesity. *Journal of Clinical Endocrinology and Metabolism* **88(9)**:4258–4267.

Hlavackova, V., Goudet, C., Kniazeff, J., Zikova, A., Maurel, D., Vol, C., Trojanova, J., Prézeau, L., Pin, J., Blahos, J. (2005). Evidence for a single heptahelical domain being turned on upon activation of a dimeric GPCR. *EMBO Journal* **24(3)**:499–509.

Ho, G., MacKenzie, R.G. (1999). Functional characterization of mutations in melanocortin-4 receptor associated with human obesity. *Journal of Biological Chemistry* **274(50)**:35816–35822.

Hoermann, R., Schumm-Draeger, P.M., Mann, K. (1992). Antagonists of the human TSH receptor: *In vitro* and *in vivo* studies of their functional and immunological effects. *Experimental and Clinical Endocrinology* **100(1–2)**:36–40.

Hoflack, J., Hibert, M.F., Trumpp-Kallmeyer, S., Bidart, J-M. (1993). Three-dimensional models of gonado-thyrotropin hormone receptor transmembrane domain. *Drug Design Discovery* **10(2)**:157–171.

Holland, F.J., Fishman, L., Bailey, J.D., Fazekas, A.T. (1985). Ketoconazole in the management of precocious puberty not responsive to LHRH-analogue therapy. *New England Journal of Medicine* **312(16)**:1023–1028.

Holmes, W.E., Lee, J., Kuang, W.J., Rice, G.C., Wood, W.I. (1991). Structure and functional expression of a human interleukin-8 receptor. *Science* **253(5025)**:1278–1280.

Homey, B., Wang, W., Soto, H., Buchanan, M.E., Wiesenborn, A., Catron, D., Muller, A., McClanahan, T. K., Dieu-Nosjean, M. C., Orozco, R., Ruzicka, T., Lehmann, P., Oldham, E., Zlotnik, A. (2000). Cutting edge: The orphan chemokine receptor G protein-coupled receptor-2 (GPR-2, CCR10) binds the skin-associated chemokine CCL27 (CTACK/ALP/ILC). *Journal of Immunology* **164(7)**:3465–3470.

Horiuchi, M. (1996). Functional aspects of angiotensin type 2 receptor. *Advances in Experimental Medicine and Biology* **396**:217–224.

Horiuchi, M., Hayashida, W., Kambe, T., Yamada, T., Dzau, V.J. (1997). Angiotensin type 2-receptor dephosphorylates Bcl2 by activating mitogen-activated protein kinase phosphatase-1 and induces apoptosis. *Journal of Biological Chemistry* **272**:19022–19026.

Hossmann, V., Maling, T.J., Hamilton, C.A., Reid, J.L., Dollery, C.T. (1980). Sedative and cardiovascular effects of clonidine and nitrazepam. *Clinical Pharmacology and Therapeutics* **28(2)**:167–176.

Hu, C.W., Hoffman, B.B. (1993). Cycloheximide induces the alpha 1B adrenergic receptor gene by activation of transcription in DDT1 MF-2 smooth muscle cells. *Molecular Pharmacology* **44(6)**:1105–1112.

Huang, X-E., Hamajima, N., Saito, T., Matsuo, K., Mizutani, M., Iwata, H., Iwase, T., Miura, S., Mizuno, T., Tokudome, S., Tajima, K. (2001). Possible association of β2- and β3-adrenergic receptor gene polymorphisms with susceptibility to breast cancer. *Breast Cancer Research* **3(4)**:264–269.

Huang, Y.Y., Oquendo, M.A., Friedman, J.M., Greenhill, L.L., Brodsky, B., Malone, K.M., Khait, V., Mann, J.J. (2003). Substance abuse disorder and major depression are associated with the human 5-HT1B receptor gene (HTR1B) G861C polymorphism. *Neuropsychopharmacology* **28(1)**:163–169.

Huggins, D.J., Grant, G.H. (2005). The function of the amino terminal domain in NMDA receptor modulation. *Journal of Molecular Graphics and Modeling* **23(4)**:381–388.

Hummel, M., Unterwald, E. (2002). D1 dopamine receptor: A putative neurochemical and behavioral link to cocaine action. *Journal of Cell Physiology* **191(1)**:17–27.

Hunyady, L., Balla, T., Catt, K.J. (1996). The ligand binding site of the angiotensin AT1 receptor. *Trends in Pharmacological Sciences* **17(4)**:135–140.

Huszar, D., Lynch, C.A., Fairchild-Huntress, V., Dunmore, J.H., Fang, Q., Berkemeier, L.R., Gu, W., Kesterson, R.A., Boston, B.A., Cone, R.D., Smith, F.J., Campfield, L.A., Burn, P., Lee, F. (1997). Targeted disruption of the melanocortin-4 receptor results in obesity in mice. *Cell* **88(1)**:131–141.

Hyttel, J. (1977). Neurochemical characterization of a new potent and selective serotonin uptake inhibitor: Lu10-171. *Psychopharmacology (Berlin)* **51(3)**:225–233.

Hyttel, J. (1978). Effect of a specific 5-HT uptake inhibitor, citalopram (Lu 10-171), 3*H*-5-HT uptake in rat brain synaptosomes *in vitro*. *Psychopharmacology (Berlin)* **60(1)**:13–18.

Hyttel, J. (1982). Citalopram- Pharmacological profile of specific serotonin uptake inhibitor with anti-depressant activity. *Progress in Neuro-psychopharmacology and Biological Psychiatry* **6(3)**:277–295.

Hyttel, J., Bøgesø, K.P., Perregaard, J., Sánchez, C. (1992). The pharmacological effect of citalopram residues in the (S)-(+)-enantiomer. *Journal of Neural Transmission—General Section* **88(2)**:157–160.

Hyttel, J. (1993). Comparative pharmacology of selective serotonin re-uptake inhibitors (SSRIs). *Nordic Journal of Psychiatry* **47(s30)**:5–12.

Ikonomovic, M.D., Katsuyoshi, M., Peter, D., Ronald, H., Roxanne, S., David, A. (1997). The loss of GluR2(3) immunoreactivity precedes neurofibrillary tangle formation in the entorhinal cortex and hippocampus of Alzheimer brains. *Journal of Neuropathology and Experimental Neurology* **56**:1018–1027.

Imai, T., Chantry, D., Raport, C.J., Wood, C.L., Nishimura, M., Godiska, R., Yoshie, O., Gray, P.W. (1998). Macrophage-derived chemokine is functional ligand for the CC chemokine receptor 4. *Journal of Biological Chemistry* **273(3)**:1764–1768.

Inamura, F., Arimoto, I., Fujiyoshi, Y., Doi, T. (2000). W276 mutation in the endothelin receptor subtype B impairs G_q coupling but not G_i or G_o couling. *Biochemistry* **39(4)**:686–692.

Innamorati, G., Sadeghi, H., Birnbaumer, M.A. (1996) Fully active nonglycosylated V2 vasopressin receptor. *Molecular Pharmacology* **50(3)**:467–473.

Isele, J., Sakmar, T.P., Siebert, F. (2000). Rhodopsin activation affects the environment of specific neighboring phospholipids: An FTIR study. *Biophysical Journal* **79(6)**:3063–3071.

Isogaya, M., Sugimoto, Y., Tanimura, R., Tanaka, R., Kikkawa, H., Nagao, T., Kurose, H. (1999). Binding pockets of the beta(1)- and beta(2)-adrenergic receptors for subtype-selective agonists. *Molecular Pharmacology* **56(5)**:875–885.

Jankovic, J. (2008). Parkinson's disease: Clinical features and diagnosis. *Journal of Neurology, Neurosurgery and Psychiatry* **79(4)**:368–376.

Jansen, K.L., Faull, R.L., Dragunow, M., Synek, B.L. (1990). Alzheimer's disease: Changes in hippocampal *N*-methyl-d-aspartate, quisqualate, neurotensin, adenosine, benzodiazepine, serotonin and opioid receptors—An autoradiographic study. *Neuroscience* **39(3)**:613–627.

January, B., Seibold, A., Whaley, B., Hipkin, R.W., Lin, D., Schonbrunn, A., Barber, R., Clark, R.B. (1997). β_2-adrenergic receptor desensitization, internalization, and phosphorylation in response to full and partial agonists. *Journal of Biological Chemistry* **272(38)**:23871–23879.

Jard, S. (1988). Mechanisms of action of vasopressin and vasopressin antagonists. *Kidney International Supplement* **34**:S38–42.

Jasper, J.R., Lesnick, J.D., Chang, L.K., Yamanishi, S.S., Chang, T.K., Hsu, S.A.O., Daunt, D.A., Bonhaus, D.W., Eglen, R.M. (1998). Ligand efficacy and potency at recombinant alpha 2 adrenergic receptors—Agonist-mediated [^{35}S]GTPgammaS binding. *Biochemical Pharmacology* **55(7)**:1035–1043.

Jauch, R., Kopitar, Z., Prox, A., Zimmer, A. (1976). Pharmacokinetics and metabolism of trazodone in man (in German). *Arzneimittelforschung* **26**(11):2084–2089.

Jain, K.K. (2004). RNAi and siRNA in target validation. *Drug Discovery Today* **9(7)**:307–309.

Jia, X.C., Oikawa, M., Bo, M., Tanaka, T., Ny, T., Boime, I., Hsueh, A.J. (1991). Expression of human luteinizing hormone (LH) receptor: Interaction with LH and chorionic gonadotropin from human but not equine, rat, and ovine species. *Molecular Endocrinology* **5**:759–768.

Jiang, X., Dreano, M., Buckler, D.R., Cheng, S., Ythier, A., Wu, H., Hendrickson, W.A, Tayar, N.E. (1995). Structural predictions for the ligand-binding region of glycoprotein hormone receptors and the nature of hormone–receptor interactions. *Structure* **3(12)**:1341–1353.

Joffe, P., Larsen, F.S., Pederson, V., Ring-Larsen, H., Aaes-Jørgensen T., Sidhu, J. (1998). Single-dose pharmacokinetics of citalopram in patients with moderate renal insufficiency or hepatic cirrhosis compared with healthy subjects. *European Journal of Clinical Pharmacology* **54(3)**:237–242.

Johnson, B.G., Wright, R.A., Arnold, M.B., Wheeler, W.J., Ornstein, P.L., Schoepp, D.D. (1999). [^{3}H]-LY341495 as a novel antagonist radioligand for group II metabotropic glutamate (mGlu) receptors: characterization of binding to membranes of mGlu receptor subtype expressing cells. *Neuropharmacology* **38(10)**:1519–1529.

Jones, K.A., Borowsky, B., Tamm, J.A., Craig, D.A., Durkin, M.M., Dai, M., Yao, W., Johnson, M., Gunwaldsen, C., Huang, L., Tang, C., Shen, Q., Salon, J.A., Morse, K., Laz, T., Smith, K.E., Nagarathnam, D., Noble, S.A., Branchek, T.A., Gerald, C. (1998). GABA(B) receptors function as a heteromeric assembly of the subunits GABA(B)R1 and GABA(B)R2. *Nature* **396(6712)**:674–679.

Joseph, S.S., Lynham, J.A., Colledge, W.H., Kaumann, A.J. (2004). Binding of (–)-[3*H*]-CGP12177 at two sites in recombinant human beta 1-adrenoceptors and interaction with beta-blockers. *Naunyn Schmiedeberg's Archives in Pharmacology* **369(5)**:525–532.

Joseph, S.S., Lynham, J.A., Molenaar, P., Grace, A. A., Colledge, W. H., Kaumann, A.J. (2003). Intrinsic sympathomimetic activit of (–)-pindolol mediated through a (–)-propranolol-resistant site of the beta 1-adrenoceptor in human atrium and recombinant receptors. *Naunyn Schmiedeberg's Archives in Pharmacology* **368(6)**:496–503.

Julius, S., Kjeldsen, S.E., Weber, M., Brunner, H.R., Ekman, S., Hansson, L., Hua, T., Laragh, J., McInnes, G.T., Mitchell, L., Plat, F., Schork, A., Smith, B., Zanchetti, A. (2004). Outcomes in hypertensive patients at high cardiovascular risk treated with regimens based on valsartan or amlodipine: The VALUE randomised trial. *Lancet* **363(9423)**:2022–2031.

Kajava, A.V., Vassart, G., Wodak, S.J. (1995). Modeling of the three-dimensional structure of proteins with the typical leucine-rich repeats. *Structure* **3(9)**:867–877.

Kamitani, S. and Sakata, T. (2001). Glycosylation of human CRLR and Asn123 is required for ligand binding and signaling. *Biochimica Biophysica Acta—Molecular and Cell Research* **1539(1–2)**:131–139.

Kamohara, M., Takasaki, J., Matsumoto, M., Saito, T., Ohishi, T., Ishii, H., Furuichi, K. (2000). Molecular cloning and characterization of another leukotriene B4 receptor. *Journal of Biological Chemistry* **275(35)**:27000–27004.

Kane, J., Honigfeld, G., Singer, J., Meltzer, H. (1988). Clozapine for the treatment-resistant schizophrenic: A double-blind comparison with chlorpromazine. *Archives of General Psychiatry* **45(9)**:789–796.

Kapas, S., Cammas, F.M., Hinson, J.P., Clark, A.J. (1996). Agonist and receptor binding properties of adrenocorticotropin peptides using the cloned mouse adrenocorticotropin receptor expressed in a stably transfected HeLa cell line. *Endocrinology* **137(8)**:3291–3294.

Kapur, S., Seeman, P. (2001). Does fast dissociation from the dopmaine D2 receptor explain the action of atypical antipsychotics?: A new hypothesis. *American Journal of Psychiatry* **158(3)**:360–369.

Kapur, S., Zipursky, R., Jones, C., Shammi, C.S., Remington, G., Seeman, P. (2000). A positron emission tomography study of quetiapine in schizophrenia: A preliminary finding of an antipsychotic effect with only transiently high dopamine D2 receptor occupancy. *Archives of General Psychiatry* **57(6)**:553–559.

Kapur, S., Zipursky, R., Jones, C., Remington, G., Houle, S. (2000). Relationship between dopamine D2 occupancy, clinical response, and side-effects: A double blind PET study of first episode schizophrenia. *American Journal of Psychiatry* **157(4)**:514–520.

Kapur, S., Zipursky, R.B., Remington, G., Jones, C., DaSilva, J., Wilson, A.A., Houle, S. (1998). 5-HT2 and D2 receptor occupancy of olanzapine in schizophrenia: A PET investigation. *American Journal of Psychiatry* **155(7)**:921–928.

Karchin, R., Karplus, K., Haussler, D. (2002). Classifying G-protein coupled receptors with support vector machines. *Bioinformatics* **18(1)**:147–159.

Kassahun, K., Mattiuz, E., Nyhart, E., Jr., Obermeyer, B., Gillespie, T., Murphy, A., Goodwin, R.M., Tupper, D., Callaghan, J.T., Lemberger, L. (1997). Disposition and biotransformation of the antipsychotic agent olanzapine in humans. *Drug Metabolism and Disposition* **25(1)**:81–93.

Katzin, W.E., Fishleder, A.J., Tubbs, R.R. (1989). Investigation of the clonality of lymphocytes in Hashimoto's thyroiditis using immunoglobulin and T-cell receptor gene probe. *Clinical Immunology and Immunopathology* **51(2)**:264–274.

Kaumann, A.J. and Levy, F.O. (2006). 5-hydroxytryptamine receptors in the human cardiovascular system. *Pharmacology and Therapeutics* **111(3)**:674–706.

Kaupmann, K., Malitschek, B., Schuler, V., Heid, J., Froestl, W., Beck, P., Mosbacher, J., Bischoff, S., Kilik, A., Shigemoto, R., Karschin, A., Bettler, B. (1998). $GABA_{(B)}$-receptor subtypes assemble into functional heteromeric complexes. *Nature* **396(6712)**:683–687.

Kawate, N., Menon, K.M. (1994). Palmitoylation of luteinizing hormone/human choriogonadotropin receptors in transfected cells. Abolition of palmitoylation by mutation of Cys-621 and Cys-622 residues in the cytoplasmic tail increases ligand-induced internalization of the receptor. *Journal of Biological Chemistry* **269(48)**:30651–30658.

Kebabian, J.W., Petzold, G.L., Greengard, P. (1972). Dopamine-sensitive adenylate cyclase in caudate nucleus of rat brain, and its similarity to the 'dopamine receptor'. *Proceedings of the National Academy of Sciences USA* **69(8)**:2145–2149.

Keen, T.J., Inglehearn, C.F., Leslfit, D.H., Bashir, R., Jay, M., Bird, A.C., Jay, B., Battacharya, S.S. (1991). Autosomal dominant retinitis pigmentosa: Four new mutations in rhodopsin, one of them in the retinal attachment site. *Genomics* **11(1)**:199–205.

Kenakin, T.P. (2003). The secret lives of GPCRs. *Drug Discovery Today* **8(15)**:674.

Kidd, A., Okita, N., Row, V.V., Volpé, R. (1980). Immunologic aspects of Graves' and Hashimoto's diseases. *Metabolism* **29(1)**:80–99.

Kiefer, L.L., Veal, J.M., Mountjoy, K.G., Wilkison, W.O. (1998). Melanocortin receptor binding determinants in the agouti protein. *Biochemistry* **37(4)**:991–997.

Kienast, T., Heinz, A. (2006). Dopamine and the diseased brain. *CNS and Neurological Disorders and Drug Targets* **5(1)**:109–131.

Kifor, O., Kifor, I., Moore, F.D., Jr., Butters, R.R., Jr., Brown, E.M. (2003). m-Calpain colocalizes with the calcium-sensing receptor (CaR) in caveolae in parathyroid cells and participates in degradation of the CaR. *Journal of Biological Chemistry* **278(33)**:31167–31176.

Kinon, B.J., Lieberman, J.A. (1996). Mechanisms of action of atypical anti-psychotic drugs: A critical analysis. *Psychopharmacology (Berlin)* **124(1–2)**:2–34.

Knight, A.R., Misra, A., Quirk, K., Benwell, K., Revell, D., Kennett, G., Bickerdike, M. (2004). Pharmacological characterization of the agonist radioligand binding site of $5\text{-}HT_{2A}$, $5\text{-}HT_{2B}$, and $5\text{-}HT_{2C}$ receptors. *Nauyn-Schmiedeberg's Archives of Pharmacology* **370(2)**:114–123.

Kobayashi, K., Chiba, K., Yagi, T., Shimada, N., Taniguchi, T., Horie, T., Tani, M., Yamamoto, T., Ishizaki, T., Kuroiwa, Y. (1997). Identification of cytochrome P450 isoforms involved in citalopram N-demethylation by human liver microsomes. *Journal of Pharmacology and Experimental Therapeutics* **280(2)**:927–933.

Kobilka, B.K., Matsui, H., Kobilka, T.S., Ynag-Feng, T.L., Francke, U., Caron, M.G., Lefkowitz, R.J., Regan, J.W. (1987). Cloning, sequencing, and expression of the gene coding for the human platelet alpha 2-adrenergic receptor. *Science* **238(4827)**:650–656.

Kohen, R., Metcalf, M.A., Khan, N., Druck, T., Huebner, K., Lachowicz, J.E., Meltzer, H.Y., Sibley, D.R., Roth, B.L., Hamblin, M.W. (1996). Cloning, characterization, and chromosomal localization of a human 5-HT6 serotonin receptor. *Journal of Neurochemistry* **66(1)**:47–56.

Kohler, B., Biebermann, H., Krohn, H.P., Dralle, D., Finke, R., gruters, A. (1996). A novel germline mutation in the TSH receptor gene causing nonautoimmune congenital hyperthyroidism. *International Congress of Endocrinology*, San Francsico, 1996 Abstract 1:P-946.

Kohn, L.D., Saji, M., Akamizu, T., Ikuyama, S., Isozaki, O., Kohn, A.D., Santisteban, P., Chan, J.Y., Bellur, S., Rotella, C.M. (1989). Receptors of the thyroid: The thyrotropin receptor is only the first violinist of a symphony orchestra. *Advances in Experimental Medicine and Biology* **261**:151–209.

Kohn, L.D., Shimura, H., Shimura, Y., Hidaka, A., Giuliani, C., Napolitano, G., Ohmori, M., Laglia, G., Saji. M. (1995). The thyrotropin receptor. *Vitamins and Hormones* **50**:287–384.

Koike, G., Horiuchi, M., Yamada, T., Szpirer, C., Jacob, H.J., Dzau, V.J. (1994). Human type 2 angiotensin II receptor gene cloned, mapped to the X chromosome, and its mRNA is expressed in the human lung. *Biochemical and Biophysical Research Communications* **203(3)**:1842–1850.

Koike, H., Sada, T., Mizuno, M. (2001). *In vitro* and *in vivo* pharmacology of olmesartan medoxomil, an angiotensin II type AT1 receptor antagonist. *Journal of Hypertension* **19(1)**:S3–14.

Konradi, C., Heckers, S. (2003). Molecular aspects of glutamate dysregulation: Implications for schizophrenia and its treatment. *Pharmacology and Therapeutics* **97**:153–179.

Kosugi, S., Akamizu, T., Takai, O., Prabhakar, B.S., Kohn, L.D. (1991). The extracellular domain of the TSH receptor has an immunogenic epitope reactive with Graves' IgG but unrelated to receptor function as well as determinants having different roles for high affinity TSH binding and the activity of thyroid-stimulating autoantibodies. *Thyroid* **1(4)**:321–330.

Kosugi, S., Ban, T., Akamizu, T., Valente, W., Kohn, L.D. (1993). Use of thyrotropin receptor (TSHR) mutants to detect stimulating TSHR antibodies in hypothyroid patients with idiopathic myxedema, who have blocking TSHR antibodies. *Journal of Clinical Endocrinology and Metabolism* **77(1)**:19–24.

Kosugi, S., Sugawa, H., Mori T. (1996). TSH receptor and LH receptor. *Endocrine Journal* **43**:595–604.

Kragh–Sørensen, P., Overø, K.F., Peterson, O.L., Jensen, K., Parnas, W. (1981). The kinetics of citalopram: Single and multiple dose studies in man. *Acta Pharmacologica et Toxicologica (Copenhagen)* **48(1)**:53–60.

Kremer, H., Kraaij, R., Toledo, S.P.A., Post, M., Fridman, J.B., Hayashida, C.Y., van Reen, M., Milgrom, E., Ropers, H.-H., Mariman, E., Themmen, A.P.N., Brunner, H.G. (1995). Male psuedohermaphroditism due to a homozygous missense mutation of the lutenising hormone receptor gene. *Nature Genetics* **9(2)**:160–164.

Kristiansen, K. (2004). Molecular mechanisms of ligand binding, signaling and regulation within the superfamily of G-protein-coupled receptors: molecular modeling and mutagenesis approaches to receptor structure function. *Pharmacology and Therapeutics* **103(1)**:21–80.

Krobert, K.A., Bach,. T., Syversveen, T., Kvingdegal, A.M., Levy, F.O. (2001). The cloned human 5-HT7 receptor splice variants: a comparative characterization of their pharmacology, function and distribution. *Naunyn Schmiedeberg's Archives of Pharmacology* **363(6)**:620–632.

Kroeze, W.K., Kristiansen, K., Roth, B.L. (2002). Molecular biology of serotonin receptors—Structure and function at the molecular level. *Current Topics in Medicinal Chemistry* **2(6)**:507–528.

Kühn, B., and Gudermann, T. (1999). The luteinizing hormone receptor activates phospholipase C via preferential coupling to Gi2. *Biochemistry* **38**:12490–12498.

Kurland, L., Melhus, H., Karlsson, J., Kahan, T., Malmqvist, K., Ohman, P., Nyström, F., Högg, A., Lind, L. (2002). Polymorphisms in the angiotensinogen and angiotensin II type 1 receptor gene are related to change in left ventricular mass during antihypertensive treatment: results from the Swedish Irbesartan left ventricular hypertrophy investigation versus Atenolol (SILVHIA) trial. *Journal of Hypertension* **20(4)**:657–663.

Kursar, J.D., Nelson, D.L., Wainscott, D.B., Baez, M. (1994). Molecular cloning, functional expression, and mRNA tissue distribution of the human 5-hydroxytryptamine2B receptor. *Molecular Pharmacology* **46(2)**:227–234.

Kusumi, I., Takahashi, Y., Suzuki, K., Kameda, K., Koyama, T. (2000). Differential effects of subchronic treatments with atypical antipsychotic drugs on dopamine D2 and serotonin 5-HT2A receptors in the rat brain. *Journal of Neural Transmission* **107(3)**:295–302.

Kuwasako, K., Shimekake, Y., Masuda, M., Nakahara, K., Yoshida, T., Kitaura, M., Kitamura, K., Eto, T., Sakata, T. (2000). Visualization of the calcitonin receptor-like receptor and its receptor activity-modifying proteins during internalization and recycling. *Journal of Biological Chemistry* **275(38)**:29602–29609.

Lacoursiere, R.B., Spohn, H.E. (1989). Chorpromazine In: Reynolds, J. (ed.), *Martindale: The Extra Pharmacopoeia*, 29th ed., pp. 722–725. London: The Pharmaceutical Press.

Lagane, B., Ballet, S., Planchenault, T., Balabanian, K., Le Poul, E., Blanpain, C., Percherancier, Y., Staropoli, I., Vassart, G., Oppermann, M., Parmentier, M., Bachelerie, F. (2005). Mutation of the DRY motif reveals different structural requirements for the CC chemokine receptor 5-mediated signaling and receptor endocytosis. *Molecular Pharmacology* **67(6)**:1966–1976.

Lahti, A.C., Weiler, M.A., Tamara, M.B.A., Parwani, A., Tamminga, C.A. (2001). Effects of ketamine in normal and schizophrenic volunteers. *Neuropsychopharmacology* **25(4)**:455–467.

Lam, S., Shen, Y., Nguyen, T., Messier, T.L., Brann, M., Comings, D., George, S.R.. O'Dowd, B.F. (1996). A serotonin receptor gene (5HT1A) variant found in a Tourette's syndrome patient. *Biochemical and Biophysical Research Communications* **219(3)**:853–858.

Lanctot, P.M., Leclerc, P.C., Clément, M., Auger-Messier, M., Escher, E., Leduc, R., Guillemette, G. (2005). Importance of N-glycosylation positioning for cell-surface expression, targeting, affinity and quality control of the human AT_1 receptor. *Biochemical Journal* **390 (Pt 1)**:367–376.

Laue, L., Kenigsberg, D., Pescovitz, O.H., Hench, K.D., Barnes, K.M., Loriaux, D.L., Cutler, G.B. (1989). Treatment of familial male precocious puberty with spironolactone and testolactone. *New England Journal of Medicine* **320(8)**:496–502.

Laugwitz, K., Allegeier, A., Offermanns, S., Spicher, K., Sande, J.V., Dumont, J.E., Schultz, G. (1996). The human thyrotropin receptor: A heptahelical receptor capable of stimulating members of all four G protein families. *Proceedings of the National Academy of Sciences USA* **93(1)**:116–120.

Launay, J.M., Birraux, G., Bondoux, D., Callebert, J., Choi, D.S., Loric, S., Maroteaux, L. (1996). Ras involvement in signal transduction by the serotonin 5-HT2B receptor. *Journal of Biological Chemistry* **271(6)**:3141–3147.

Laurie, D.J., Schoeffter, P., Wiederhold, K.H., Sommer, B. (1997). Cloning, distribution and functional expression of the human mGlu6 metabotropic glutamate receptor. *Neuropharmacology* **36(2)**:145–152

Lee, B., Horuk, R., Rice, G.C., Bennett, G.L., Camerato, T., Wood, W.I. (1992). Characterization of two high affinity human interleukin-8 receptors. *Journal of Biological Chemistry* **267**:16283–16287.

Lee, B., Doranz, B.J., Rana, S., Yi, Y., Mellado, M., Frade, J.M., Martinez, A.C., O'Brien, S.J., Dean, M., Collman, R.G., Doms, R.W. (1998). Influence of the CCR2-V64I polymorphism on human immunodeficiency virus type 1 coreceptor activity and on chemokine receptor function of CCR2b, CCR3, CCR5, and CXCR4. *Journal of Virology* **72(9)**:7450–7458.

Leech, C.J., Faber, J.E. (1996). Different alpha-adrenoceptor subtypes mediate constriction of arterioles and venules. *American Journal of Physiology* **270(2 Pt 2)**:H710–722.

Legler, D.F., Loetscher, M., Roos, R.S., Clark-Lewis, I., Baggiolini, M., Moser, B. (1998). B cell-attracting chemokine 1, a human CXC chemokine expressed in lymphoid tissues, selectively attracts B lymphocytes via BLR1/CXCR5. *Journal of Experimental Medicine* **187(4)**:655–660.

Lelias, J.M., Kaghad, M., Rodriguez, M., Chalon, P., Bonnin, J., Dupre, I., Delpech, B., Bensaid, M., LeFur, G., Ferrara, P., Caput, D. (1993). Molecular cloning of a human β3-adrenergic receptor cDNA. *FEBS Lett.* **324(2)**:127–130.

Leuthäuser, K., Gujer, R., Aldecoa, A., McKinney, R.A., Muff, R., Fischer, J.A., Born, W. (2000). Receptor-activity-modifying protein 1 forms heterodimers with two G-protein-coupled receptors to define ligand recognition. *Biochemical Journal* **351 (Pt 2)**:347–351.

Levy, F.O., Holtgreve-Grez, H., Taskén, K., Solberg, R., Ried, T., Gudermann, T. (1994). Assignment of the gene encoding the 5-HT_{1E} serotonin receptor (S31) (Locus HTR1E) to human chromosome 6q14-q15. *Genomics* **22(3)**:637–640.

Lewis, E.J., Hunsicker, L.G., Clarke, W.R., Berl, T., Pohl, M.A., Lewis, J.B., Ritz, E., Atkins, R.C., Rohde, R., Raz, I. (2001). Renoprotective effect of the angiotensin-receptor antagonist irbesartan in patients with nephropathy due to type 2 diabetes. *New England Journal of Medicine* **345(12)**:851–860.

Leysen, J.E., Gommeren, W., Heylen, L., Luyten, W.H., Van de Weyer, I., Vanhoenacker, P., Haegeman, G., Schotte, A., van Gompel, P., Wouters, R., Lesage, A.S. (1996). Alniditan, a new 5-hydroxytryptamine1D agonist and migraine-abortive agent: ligand-binding properties of human 5-hydroxytryptamine1D alpha, human 5-hydroxytryptamine1D beta, and calf 5-hydroxytryptamine1D receptors investigated with [3H]5-hydroxytryptamine and [3H]alniditan. *Molecular Pharmacology* **50(6)**:1567–1580.

Li, J., and Lee, A.S. (2006). Stress induction of GRP78/BiP and its role in cancer. *Current Molecular Medicine* **6(1)**:45–54.

Li, J-L., Canham, R.M., Vongpatanasin, W., Leonard, D., Auchus, R.J., Victor, R.G. (2006). Do allelic variants in α2A and α2C adrenergic receptors predispose to hypertension in blacks? *Hypertension* **47(6)**:1140–1146.

Li, T., Franson, W.K., Gordan, J.W., Berson, E.L., Dryja, T.P. (1995). Constitutive activation of phototransduction by K296E opsin is not a cause of photoreceptor degeneration. *Proceedings of the National Academy of Sciences USA* **92(8)**:3551–3555.

Liao, F., Rabin, R.L., Smith, C.S., Sharma, G., Nutman, T.B., Farber, J.M. (1999). CC-Chemokine receptor 6 is expressed on diverse memory subsets of T cells and determines responsiveness to macrophage inflammatory protein 3α. *Journal of Immunology* **162**:186–194.

Liao, F., Alderson, R., Su, J., Ullrich, S.J., Kreider, B.L., Farber, J.M. (1997). STRL22 is a receptor for the CC chemokine MIP-3α. *Biochemical Biophysical Research Communications* **236(1)**:212–217.

Liapakis, G., Chan, W.C., Papadokostaki, M., Javitch, J.A. (2004). Synergistic contributions of the functional groups of epinephrine to its affnity and efficacy at the beta(2)-adrenergic receptor. *Molecular Pharmacology* **65**:1181–1190.

Liggett, S.B. (1997). Polymorphisms of the β_2-adrenergic receptor and asthma. *American Journal of Respiratory and Critical Care Medicine* 156:S156–162.

Lilly, C.M. (2005). Diversity of asthma: Evolving concepts of pathophysiology and lessons from genetics. *Journal of Allergy and Clinical Immunology* **115**:S526–531.

Limbird, L.E., De Meyts, P., Lefkowitz, R.J. (1975). β-adrenergic receptors: Evidence for negative co-operativity. *Biochemical and Biophysical Research Communications* **64**:1160–1168.

Lin, F., Owens, W.A., Chen, S., Stevens, M.E., Kesteven, S., Arthur, J.F., Woodcock, E.A., Feneley, M.P., Graham, R.M. (2001). Targeted alpha (1A) overexpression induces enhanced cardiac contractility but not hypertrophy. *Circulatory Research* **89**:343–350.

Lin, S.L., Setya, S., Johnson-Farley, N.N., Cowen, D.S. (2002). Differential coupling of 5-HT(1) receptors to G proteins of the G(i) family. *British Journal of Pharmacology* **136**:1072–1078.

Lipton, S.A. (2006). Paradigm shift in neuroprotection by NMDA receptor blockade: memantine and beyond. *Nature Reviews Drug Discovery* **5**:160–170.

Lisman, J.E., Coyle, J.T., Green, R.W., Javitt, D.C., Benes, F.M., Heckers, S., Grace, A.A. (2008). Circuit-based framework for understanding neurotransmitter and risk gene interactions in schizophrenia. *Trends in Neuroscience* **31**:234–242.

Liu, G., Duranteau, L., Carel, J.C., Monroe, J., Doyle, D.A., Shenker, A. (1999). Leydig-cell tumors caused by an activating mutation of the gene encoding the luteinizing hormone receptor. *New England Journal of Medicine* **341**:1731–1736.

Liu, P.T., Stenger, S., Li, H., Wenzel, L., Tan, B.H., Krutzik, S.R., Ochoa, M.T., Schauber, J., Wu, K., Meinken, C., Kamen, D.L., Wagner, M., Bals, R., Steinmeyer, A., Zugel, U., Gallo, R.L., Eisenberg, D., Hweison, M., Hollis, B.W., Adams, J.S., Bloom, B.R., Modlin, R.L. (2006). Toll-like receptor triggering of a vitamin D-mediated human antimicrobial response. *Science* **311**:1770–1773.

Liu, Q., Schonbrunn, A. (2001). Agonist-induced phosphorylation of somatostatin receptor subtype 1(Sst1): Relationship to desensitization and internalization. *Journal of Biological Chemistry* **276**:3709–3717.

Liu, R., Paxton, W.A., Choe, S., Ceradini, D., Martin, S.R., Horuk, R., MacDonald, M.E., Stuhlmann, H., Koup, R.A., Landau, N.R. (1996). Homozygous defect in HIV-1 coreceptor accounts for resistance of some multiply-exposed individuals to HIV-1 infection. *Cell* **86**:367–377

Liu, Y., Zhang, J. (2000). Recent developments in NMDA receptors. *Chinese Medical Journal* **113(10)**:948–956.

Lockey, R. (2006). Andor Szentivanyi, MD, May 4, 1925–October 22, 2005. *Journal of Allergy and Clinical Immunology* **117**:32–33.

Loetscher, M., Geiser, T., O'Reilly, T., Zwahlen, R., Baggiolini, M., Moser, B. (1994). Cloning of a human seven-transmembrane domain receptor, LESTR, that is highly expressed in leukocytes. *Journal of Biological Chemistry* **269(1)**:232–237.

Loetscher, M., Amara, A., Oberlin, E., Brass, N., Legler, D.F., Loetscher, P., D'Apuzzo, M., Meese, E., Rousset, D., Virelizier, J-L., Baggiolini, M., Arenzana-Seisdedos, F., Moser, B. (1997). TYMSTR, a putative chemokine receptor selectively expressed in activated T cells, exhibits HIV-1 coreceptor function. *Current Biology* **7(9)**:652–660.

Loetscher, M., Loetscher, P., Brass, N., Meese, E., Moser, B. (1998a). Lymphocyte-specific chemokine receptor CXCR3: regulation, chemokine binding and gene localization. *Eur. J. Immunol.* **28(11)**:3696–3705.

Loetscher, P., Gong, J.H., Dewald, B., Baggiolini, M., Clark-Lewis, I. (1998b). N-terminal peptides of stromal cell-derived factor-1 with CXCchemokine receptor 4 agonist and antagonist activities. *Journal of Biological Chemistry* **273(35)**:22279–22283.

Lohse, M.J. (1993). Molecular mechanisms of membrane receptor desensitization. *Biochimica et Biophysica Acta* **1179(2)**:171–188.

Lohse, M.J., Andexinger, S., Pitcher, J., Trukawinski, S., Codina, J., Faure, J.P., Caron, M.G., Lefkowitz, R.J. (1992). Receptor-specific desensitization with purified proteins. Kinase dependance and receptor specificity of β-arrestin and arrestin in the β_2-adrenergic receptor and rhodopsin systems. *Journal of Biological Chemistry* **267**:8558–8564.

López, J.F., Chalmers, D., Little, K.Y., Watson, S.J. (1998). Regulation of $5HT_{1a}$ receptor, glucocorticoid and mineralocorticoid receptor in rat and human hippocampus: Implications for the neurobiology of depression. *Biological Psychiatry* **43(8)**:547–573.

Loric, S., Maroteaux, L., Kellermann, O., Launay, J.M. (1995). Functional serotonin-2B receptors are expressed by a teratocarcinoma-derived cell line during serotoninergic differentiation. *Molecular Pharmacology* **47(3)**:458–466.

Louis, S.N., Nero, T.L., Iakovidis, D., Jackman, G.P., Louis, W.J. (1999). LK 204-545, a highly selective beta1-adrenoceptor antagonist at human beta-adrenoceptors. *European Journal of Pharmacology* **367(2–3)**:431–435.

Lovenberg, T.W., Pyati, J., Chang, H., Wilson, S.J., Erlander, M.G. (2000). Cloning of rat histamine H_3 receptor reveals distinct species pharmacological profiles. *Journal of Pharmacology and Experimental Therapeutics* **293(3)**:771–778.

Lubrano-Berthelier, C., Durand, E., Dubern, B., Shapiro, A., Dazin, P., Weill, J., Ferron, C., Froguel, P., Vaisse, C. (2003). Intracellular retention is a common characteristic of childhood obesity-associated MC4R mutations. *Human Molecular Genetics* **12(2)**:145–153.

Lusso, P. (2006). HIV and the chemokine system: 10 years later. *EMBO Journal* **25(3)**:447–456.

Lüttichau, H.R., Clark-Lewis, I., Jensen, P.Ø., Moser, C., Gerstoft, J., Schwartz, T.W. (2003). A highly selective CCR2 chemokine agonist encoded by human herpesvirus 6. *Journal of Biological Chemistry* **278(13)**:10928–10933.

Ma, Q., Jones, D., Borghesani, P.R., Segal, R.A., Nagasawa, T., Kishimoto, T., Bronson, R.T., Springer, T.A. (1998). Impaired B-lymphopoiesis, myelopoiesis, and derailed cerebellar neuron migration in CXCR4- and SDF-1-deficient mice. *Proceedings of the National Academy of Sciences USA* **95(16)**:9448–9453.

Macias, W.L., Bergstrom, R.F., Cerimele, B.J., Kassahun, K., Tatum, D.E., Callaghan, J.T. (1998). Lack of effect of olanzapine on the pharmacokinetics of a single aminophylline dose in healthy men. *Pharmacotherapy* **18(6)**:1237–1248.

MacNeil, D.J., Howard, A.D., Guan, X., Fong, T.M., Nargund, R.P., Bednarek, M.A., Goulet, M.T., Weinberg, D.H., Strack, A.M., Marsh, D.J., Chen, H.Y., Shen, C.P., Chen, A.S., Rosenblum, C.I., MacNeil, T., Tota,

M., MacIntyre, E.D., Van der Ploeg, L.H. (2002). The role of melanocortins in body weight regulation: Opportunities for the treatment of obesity. *European Journal of Pharmacology* **440(2–3)**:141–157.

Maggio, R., Barbier, P., Colelli, A., Salvadori, F., Demontis, G., Corsini, G.U. (1999). G protein-linked receptors: Pharmacological evidence for the formation of heterodimers. *Journal of Pharmacology and Experimental Therapeutics* **291(1)**:251–257.

Maggio, R., Vogel, Z., Wess, J. (1993). Coexpression studies with mutant muscarinic/adrenergic receptors provide evidence for intermolecular 'cross-talk' between G-protein-linked receptors. *Proceedings of the National Academy of Sciences USA* **90(7)**:3103–3107.

Makoff, A., Pilling, C., Hrrington, K., Emson, P. (1996). Human metabotropic glutamate receptor type 7: molecular cloning and mRNA distribution in CNS. *Brain Research: Molecular Brain Research* **40(1)**:165–170.

Maqbool, A., Hall, A.S., Ball, S.G., Balmforth, A.J. (1999). Common polymorphisms of beta1-adrenoceptor: Identification and rapid screening assay. *Lancet* **353(9156)**:897.

Marchese, A., Docherty, J.M., Nguyen, T., Heiber, M., Cheng, R., Heng, H.H.Q., Tsui, L-C., Shi, X., George, S.R., O'Dowd, B.F. (1994). Cloning of human genes encoding novel G protein-coupled receptors. *Genomics* **23(3)**:609–618.

Marchese, A., Benovic, J.L. (2001). Agonist-promoted ubiquitination of the G protein-coupled receptor CXCR4 mediates lysosomal sorting. *Journal of Biological Chemistry* **276(49)**:45509–45512.

Marchese, A., Raiborg, C., Santini, F., Keen, J.H., Stenmark, H., Benovic, J.L. (2003).The E3 ubiquitin ligase AIP4 mediates ubiquitination and sorting of the G protein-coupled receptor CXCR4. *Developmental Cell* **5(5)**:709–722.

Marin, E.P., Krishna, A.G., Sakmar, T.P. (2001). Rapid activation of transducin by mutations distant from the nucleotide-binding site. Evidence for a mechanistic model of receptor-catalyzed nucleotide exchange by G proteins. *Journal of Biological Chemistry* **276(29)**:27400–27405.

Marin, E.P., Krishna, A.G., Zvyaga, T.A., Isele, J., Siebert, F., Sakmar, T.P. (2000). The amino terminus of the fourth cytoplasmic loop of rhodopsin modulates rhodopsin–transducin interaction. *Journal of Biological Chemistry* **275(3)**:1930–1936.

Marshall, T.G., Lee, R.E., Marshall, F.E. (2006). Common angiotensin receptor blockers may directly modulate the immune system via VDR, PPAR and CCR2b. *Theoretical Biology and Medical Modelling* **10**:1–33.

Mason, D.A., Moore, J.D., Green, S.A., Liggett, S.B. (1999). A gain-of-function polymorphism in a G-protein coupling domain of the human beta1-adrenergic receptor.*Journal of Biological Chemistry* **274(18)**:12670–12674.

Martí, S.B., Cichon, S., Propping, P., Nöthen, M. (2002). Human metabotropic glutamate receptor 2 gene (GRM2): chromosomal sublocalization (3p21.1–p21.2) and genomic organization. *American Journal of Medical Genetics* **114(1)**:12–14.

Maxmen, J., Ward, N. (1995). *Psychotropic Drugs Fast Facts*, 2nd ed. New York: WW Norton.

McAllister, G., Charlesworth, A., Snodin, C., Beer, M.S., Noble, A.J., Middlemiss, D.N., Iversen, L.L., Whiting, P. (1992). Molecular cloning of a serotonin receptor from human brain (5HT1E): a fifth 5HT1-like subtype. *Proceedings of the National Academy of Sciences U.S.A.* **89(12)**:5517–5521.

McCarthy, S., Mottagui-Tabar, S., Mizuno, Y., Sennblad, B., Hoffstedt, J., Arner, P., Wahlestedt, C., Andersson, B. (2005). Complex, *HTR2C* linkage disequilibrium and promoter associations with body mass index and serum leptin. *Human Genetics* **117(6)**:545–557.

McClellan, K.J., Markham, A. (1998). Telmisartan. *Drugs* **56**:1039–1044.

McDowell, J.H., Kuehn, H. (1977). Light-induced phosphorylation of rhodopsin in cattle photoreceptor membranes: Substrate activation and inactivation. *Biochemistry* **16(18)**:4054–4060.

McGill, J.B., Reilly, P.A. (2001). Telmisartan plus hydrochlorothiazide vs telmisartan or hydrochlorothiazide monotherapy in patients with mild to moderate hypertension: A multi-center randomized, double-blind, placebo-controlled, parallel group trial. *Clinical Therapy* **23**:833–850.

Meltzer, H.Y., Matsubara, S., Lee, J.C. (1989). Classification of typical and atypical antipsychotics on the basis of dopamine D-1, D-2 and serotonin2 pK_i values. *Journal of Pharmacology and Experimental Therapeutics* **251(1)**:238–246.

Mendes, H.F., van der Spuy, J., Chapple, J.P., Cheetham, M.E. (2005). Mechanisms of cell death in rhodopsin retinitis pigmentosa: Implications for therapy. *Trends in Molecular Medicine* **11(4)**:177–185.

Mengistu, M., Lukes, Y.G., Nagy, E.V., Burch, H.B., Carr, F.E., Lahiri, S., Burman, K.D. (1994). TSH receptor gene expression in retroocular fibroblasts. *Journal of Endocrinological Investigations* **17(6)**:437–441.

Menon, S.T., Han, M., Sakmar, T.P. (2001). Rhodopsin: Structural basis of molecular physiology. *Physiological Reviews* **81(4)**:1659–1688.

Menzaghi, F.D.P., Behan, D.P., Chalmers, D.T. (2002). Constitutively activated G-protein coupled receptors: A novel approach to CNS drug discovery. *Current Drug Targets—CNS and Neurological Disorders* **1(1)**:105–121.

Meunier, J.C., Mollereau, C., Toll, L., Suaudeau, C., Moisand, C., Alvinerie, P., Butour, J.L., Guillemot, J.C., Ferrara, P., Monsarrat, B., Mazargull, H., Vassart, G., Parmentler, M., Costentin, J. (1995). Isolation and structure of the endogenous agonist of opioid receptor-like ORL1 receptor. *Nature* **377(6549)**:532–535.

Mialet, J., Dahmoune, Y., Lezoualc'h, F., Berque-Bestel, I., Eftekhari, P., Hoebeke, J., Sicsic, S., Langlois, M., Fischmeister, R. (2000). Exploration of the ligand binding site of the human 5-HT4 receptor by site-directed mutagenesis and molecular modeling. *British Journal of Pharmacology* **130(3)**:527–538.

Michell, R.H., Kirk, C.J., Billah, M.M. (1979). Hormonal stimulation of phosphatidylinositol breakdown with particular reference to the hepatic effects of vasopressin. *Biochemical Society Transactions* **7(5)**:861–865.

Michelotti, G.A., Price, D.T., Schwinn, D.A. (2000). Alpha-1 adrenergic receptor regulation: Basic science and clinical implications. *Pharmacology and Therapeutics* **88(3)**:281–309.

Mierau, J., Schneider, F., Ensinger, H., Chio, C., Lajiness, M., Huff, R. (1995). Pramipexole binding and activation of cloned and expressed dopamine D2, D3 and D4 receptors. *European Journal of Pharmacology* **290(1)**:29–36.

Mihara, K., Kondo, T., Suzuki, A., Yasui-Furukori, N., Ono, S., Sano, A., Koshiro, K., Otani, K., Kaneko, S. (2003). Relationship between functional dopamine D2 and D3 receptors gene polymorphisms and neuroleptic malignant syndrome. *American Journal of Medical Genetics B: Neuropsychiatry and Genetics* **117(1)**:57–60.

Miller, D.D. (1996). The clinical use of clozapine plasma concentrations in the management of treatment-refractory schizophrenia. *Annals of Clinical Psychiatry* **8(2)**:99–109.

Milligan, G., Lopez-Giminez, J., Wilson, S., Carillo, J.J. (2004). Selectivity in oligomerization of G-protein coupled receptors. *Seminars in Cell and Developmental Biology* **15(3)**:263–268.

Minakami, R., Katsuki, F., Sugiyama, H. (1993). A variant of metabotropic glutamate receptor subtype 5: an evolutionally conserved insertion with no termination codon. *Biochemical Biophysical Research Communications* **194(2)**:622–627.

Minakami, R., Katsuki, F., Yamamoto, T., Nakamura, K., Sugiyama, H. (1994). Molecular cloning and functional expression of two isoforms of human metabotropic glutamate receptor subtype 5. *Biochemical Biophysical Research Communications* **199(3)**:1136–1143.

Minegishi, T., Nakamura, K., Takakura, Y., Miyamoto, K., Hasegawa, Y., Ibuki, Y., Igarashi, M., Minegish, T. [corrected to Minegishi, T.]. (1990). Cloning and sequencing of human LH/hCG receptor cDNA. *Biochemical and Biophysical Research Communications* **172(3)**:1049–1054.

Minneman, K.P., Hegstrand, L.R., Molinoff, P.B. (1979). The pharmacological specificity of beta-1 and beta-2 adrenergic receptors in rat heart and lung *in vitro*. *Molecular Pharmacology* **16(1)**:21–33.

Minneman, K.P., Theroux, T.L., Hollinger, S., Han, C., Esbenshade, T.A. (1994). Selectivity of agonists for cloned ±1-adrenergic receptor subtypes. *Molecular Pharmacology* **46(5)**:929–936.

Mirzadegan, T., Diehl, F., Ebi, B., Bhakta, S., Polsky, I., McCarley, D., Mulkins, M., Weatherhead, G.S., Lapierre, J-M., Dankwardt, J., Morgans, D., Jr., Wilhelm, R., Jarnagin, K. (2000). Identification of the binding site for a novel class of CCR2b chemokine receptor antagonists: Binding to a common chemokine receptor motif within the helical bundle. *Journal of Biological Chemistry* **275(33)**:25562–25571.

Mitchell, D.C., Niu, S.L., Litman, B.J. (2003). Enhancement of G protein-coupled signaling by DHA phospholipids. *Lipids* **38(4)**:437–443.

Mochizuki, D., Yuyama, Y., Tsujita, R., Komaki, H., Sagai, H. (1992). Cloning and expression of the human 5-HT1B-type receptor gene. *Biochemical Biophysical Research Communications* **185(2)**:517–523.

Moench, S.J., Moreland, J., Stewart, D.H., Dewey, T.G. (1994). Fluorescence labeling of the palmitoylation sites of rhodopsin. *Biochemistry* **33(19)**:5791–5796.

Monsma, F.J., McVittie, L D., Gerfen, C R., Mahan, L C., Sibley, D.R. (1989). Multiple D2 dopamine receptors produced by alternative RNA splicing. *Nature* **342(6252)**:926–929.

Moore, S., Jaeschke, H., Kleinau, G., Neumann, S., Costanzi, S., Jiang, J., Childress, J., Raaka, B.M., Colson, A., Paschke, R., Krause, G., Thomas, C.J., Gershengorn, M.C.(2006). Evaluation of small molecule modulators of the luteinizing hormone/choriogonadotropin and thyroid stimulating hormone receptors: Structure activity relationships and selective binding patterns. *Journal of Medicinal Chemistry* **49(13)**:3888–3896.

Morello, J.P., Bichet, D.G. (2001). Nephrogenic diabetes insipidus. *Annual Reviews of Physiology* **63**:607–630.

Morello, J.P., Salahpour, A., Petaja-Repo, U.E., Laperriere, A., Lonergan, M., Arthus, M., Nabi, I.R., Bichet, D.G., Bouvier, M. (2001). Association of calnexin with wild type and mutant AVPR2 that cause nephrogenic diabetes insipidus. *Biochemistry* **40(23)**:6766–6775.

Moro, O., Lameh, J., Sadee, W. (1993). Serine- and threonine-rich domain regulates internalization of muscarinic cholinergic receptors. *Journal of Biological Chemistry* **268(10)**:6862–6865.

Morris, A.J., Malbon, C.G. (1999). Physiological regulation of G-protein linked signaling. *Physiological Reviews* **79(4)**:1373–1430.

Mouillac, B., Chini, B., Balestre, M.N., Elands, J., Trumpp-Kallmeyer, S., Hoflack, J., Hibert, M., Jard, S., Barberis, C. (1995). The binding site of neuropeptide vasopressin V1a receptor. Evidence for a major localization within transmembrane regions. *Journal of Biological Chemistry* **270(43)**:25771–25777.

Mountjoy, K.G., Kong, P.L., Taylor, J.A., Willard, D.H., Wilkison, W.O. (2001). Melanocortin receptor-mediated mobilization of intracellular free calcium in HEK293 cells. *Physiological Genomics* **5(1)**:11–19.

Mountjoy, K.G., Mortrud, M.T., Low, M.J., Simerly, R.B., Cone, R.D. (1994). Localization of the melanocortin-4 receptor (MC4-R) in neuroendocrine and autonomic control circuits in the brain. *Molecular Endocrinology* **8(10)**:1298–1308.

Mountjoy, K.G., Robbins, L.S., Mortrud, M.T., Cone, R.D. (1992). The cloning of a family of genes that encode the melanocortin receptors. *Science* **257(5074)**:1248–1251.

Moyle, W.R., Campbell, R.K., Rao, S.N.V., Ayad, N.G., Bernard, M.P., Han, Y., Wang, Y. (1995). Model of human chorionic gonadotropin and lutropin receptor interaction that explains signal transduction of the glycoprotein hormones. *Journal of Biological Chemistry* **270(34)**:20020–20031.

Muciaccia, B., Padula, F., Vicini, E., Gandini, L., Lenzi, A., Stefanini, M. (2005). Beta-chemokine receptors 5 and 3 are expressed on the head region of human spermatozoon. *FASEB Journal* **19(14)**:2048–2050.

Müller, T., Gromoll, J., Simoni, M. (2003). Absence of exon 10 of the human luteinizing hormone (LH) receptor impairs LH, but not human chorionic gonadotropin action. *Journal of Clinical Endocrinology and Metabolism* **88(5)**:2242–2249.

Murdoch, C. and Finn, A. (2000). Chemokine receptors and their role in inflammation and infectious diseases. *Blood* **95(10)**:3032–3043.

Murphy, P.M., Tiffany, H.L. (1991). Cloning of complementary DNA encoding a functional human interleukin-8 receptor. *Science* **253(5025)**:1280–1283.

Murphy, B.E.P., Dhar, V., Ghadirian, A.M., Chouinard, G., Keller, R. (1991). Response to steroid suppression in major depression resistant to antidepressant therapy. *Journal of Clinical Psychopharmacology* **11(2)**:121–126.

Mutel, V., Ellis, G.J., Adam, G., Chaboz, S., Nilly, A., Messer, J., Bleuel, Z., Metzler, V., Malherbe, P., Schlaeger, E.J., Roughley, B.S., Faull, R.L., Richards, J.G. (2000). Characterization of [(3)H]quisqualate binding to recombinant rat metabotropic glutamate 1a and 5a receptors and to rat and human brain sections. *Journal of Neurochemistry* **75(6)**:2590–2601.

Nagasawa, T., Hirota, S., Tachibana, K., Takakura, N., Nishikawa, S., Kitamura, Y., Yoshida, N., Kikutani, H., Kishimoto, T. (1996). Defects of B-cell lymphopoiesis and bone-marrow myelopoiesis in mice lacking the CXC chemokine PBSF/SDF-1. *Nature* **382(6592)**:635–638.

Nakanishi, S. (1992). Molecular diversity of glutamate receptors and implications for brain function. *Science* **258(5082)**:597–603.

Nakhai, B., Nielsen, D.A., Linnoila, M., Goldman, D.B. (1995). Two naturally occurring amino acid substitutions in the human 5-HT1A receptor: Glycine 22 to serine 22 and isoleucine 28 to valine 28. *Biochemical and Biophysical Research Communications* **210(2)**:530–536.

Namkung, Y., Sibley, D.R. (2004). Protein kinase C mediates phosphorylation, desensitization and trafficking of the D_2 dopamine receptor. *Journal of Biological Chemistry* **279(47)**:49533–49541.

Napier, C., Sale, H., Mosley, M., Rickett, G., Dorr, P., Mansfield, R., Holbrook, M. (2005). Molecular cloning and radioligand binding characterization of the chemokine receptor CCR5 from rhesus macaque and human. *Biochemical Pharmacology* **71(1–2)**:163–172.

Nardese, V., Longhi, R., Polo, S., Sironi, F., Arcelloni, C., Paroni, R., DeSantis, C., Sarmientos, P., Rizzi, M., Bolognesi, M., Pavone, V., Lusso, P. (2001). Structural determinants of CCR5 recognition and HIV-1 blockade in RANTES. *Nature Structural Biology* **8(7)**:611–615.

Nebel, I.T., Trultsch, B., Paschke, R. (1999). TSH receptor mutation database. *Journal of Clinical Endocrinology and Metabolism* **84(6)**:2263.

Nebigil, C.G., Choi, D.S., Dierich, A., Hickel, P., Le Meur, M., Messaddeq, N., Launay, J. M., Maroteaux, L. (2000). Serotonin 2B receptor is required for heart development. *Proceedings of the National Academy of Sciences USA* **97(17)**:9508–9513.

Nebigil, C.G., Hickel, P., Messaddeq, N., Vonesch, J.L., Douchet, M.P., Monassier, L., György, K., Matz, R., Andriantsitohaina, R., Manivet, P., Launay, J.M., Maroteaux, L. (2001). Ablation of serotonin 5-HT(2B) receptors in mice leads to abnormal cardiac structure and function. *Circulation* **103(24)**:2973–2979.

Nebigil, C.G., Jaffré, F., Messaddeq, N., Hickel, P., Monassier, L., Launay, J.M., Maroteaux, L. (2003). Overexpression of the serotonin 5-HT2B receptor in heart leads to abnormal mitochondrial function and cardiac hypertrophy. *Circulation* **107(25)**:3223–3229.

Neumann, S., Kleinau, G., Costanzi, S., Moore, S., Jiang, J., Raaka, B.M., Thomas, C.J., Krause, G., Gershengorn, M.C. (2008). A low-molecular-weight antagonist for the human thyrotropin receptor with therapeutic potential for hyperthyroidism. *Endocrinology* **149(12)**:5945–5950.

Newmann-Tancredi, A., Wootton, R., Strange, P.G. (1992). High-level sTable expression of recombinant 5-HT_{1A} 5-hydroxytryptamine receptors in Chinese Hamster Ovary cells. *Biochemical Journal* **285(Pt 3)**:933–938.

Newmann-Tancredi, A., Chaput, C., Gavaudan, S., Verrièle, L., Millan, M. (1998). Agonist and antagonist actions of (–) pindolol at recombinant human serotonin 1A (5-HT_{1A}) receptors. *Neuropsychopharmacology* **18(5)**:395–398.

Ng, G.Y.K., O' Dowd, B.F., Lee, S.P., Chung, H.T., Brann, M.R., Seeman, P., George, S.R. (1996). Dopamine D2 receptor dimers and receptor-blocking peptides. *Biochemical and Biophysical Research Communications* **227(1)**:200–204.

Nibbs, R., Graham, G., Rot, A. (2003). Chemokines on the move: Control by the chemokine 'interceptors' Duffy blood group antigen and D6. *Seminars in Immunology* **15(5)**:287–294.

Nichols, D.E., Nichols, C.D. (2008). Serotonin receptors. *Chemical Reviews* **108(5)**:1614–1641.

Nijenhuis, W.A., Garner, K.M., van Rozen, R.J., Adan, R.A. (2003). Poor cell surface expression of human melanocortin-4 receptor mutations associated with obesity. *Journal of Biological Chemistry* **278(25)**:22939–22945.

Nikbin, N., Edwards, C., Reynolds, C.A. (2003). G-protein coupled receptor dimerization. *Iranian Journal of Pharmacology and Therapeutics* **2**:1–11.

Niswender, C.M., Copeland, S.C., Herrick-Davis, K., Emeson, R.B., Sanders-Bush, E. (1999). RNA editing of the human serotonin 5-hydroxytryptamine 2C receptor silences constitutive activity. *Journal of Biological Chemistry* **274(14)**:9472–9478.

Niu, S.L., Mitchell, D.C., Lim, S.Y., Wen, Z.M., Kim, H.Y., Salem Jr. N., Litman, B.J. (2004). Reduced G protein-coupled signaling efficiency in retinal rod outer segments in response to *n*-3 fatty acid deficiency, *Journal of Biological Chemistry* **279(30)**:31098–31104.

Noda, H., Miyaji, Y., Nakanishi, A., Konishi, F., Miki, Y. (2007). Frequent reduced expression of alpha-1B-adrenergic receptor caused by aberrant promoter methylation in gastric cancers. *British Journal of Cancer* **96(2)**:383–390.

Oades, R.D., Rao, M.L., Bender, S., Sartory, G., Muller, B.W. (2000). Neuropsychological and conditioned blocking performance in patients with schizophrenia: Assessment of the contribution of neuroleptic dose, serum levels and dopamine D2-receptor occupancy. *Behavioral Pharmacology* **11(3–4)**:317–330.

Oakley, R.H., Laporte, S.A., Holt, J.A., Barak, L.S., Caron, M.G. (1999). Association of beta-arrestin with G-protein coupled receptors during clathrin-mediated endocytosis dictates the profile of receptor resensitization. *Journal of Biological Chemistry* **274(45)**:32248–32257.

Obika, K., Shibata, K., Horie, K., Foglar, R., Kimura, K., Tsujimoto, G. (1995). NS-49, a novel alpha-1a adrenoceptor selective agonist characterization using recombinant human alpha-1 adrenoceptors. *Europen Journal of Pharmacology* **291(3)**:327–334.

Oda, Y., Sanders, J., Evans, M., Kiddie, A., Munkley, A., James, C., Richards, T., Wills, J., Furmaniak, J., Smith, B.R. (2000). Epitope analysis of the human thyrotropin (TSH) receptor using monoclonal antibodies. *Thyroid* **10(12)**:1051–1059.

Odou, P., Frimat, B., Fontaine, B., Luyckx, M., Brunet, C., Robert, H., Dine, T., Gressier, B., Cazin, M., Cazin, J.C. (1996). Determination of clozapine in serum by radioreceptor assay versus high-performance liquid chromatography: Possible detection of hydroxy-metabolites. *Journal of Clinical Pharmacy and Therapy* **21(5)**:337–342.

O'Dowd, B., Hnatowich, M., Caron, M., Lefkowitz, R., Bouvier, M. (1989). Palmitoylation of the human α_2-adrenergic receptor. Mutation of Cys341 in the carboxyl tail leads to an uncoupled nonpalmitoylated form of the receptor. *Journal of Biological Chemistry* **264(13)**:7564–7569.

Oh, S.B., Endoh, T., Simen, A.A., Ren, D., Miller, R.J. (2002). Regulation of calcium currents by chemokines and their receptors. *Journal of Neuroimmunology* **123(1–2)**:66–75.

Ohmura, T., Oshita, M., Kigoshii, S., Muramatsu, I. (1992). Identification of alpha-1-adrenoceptor subtypes in the rat vas deferens: Binding and functional studies. *British Journal of Pharmacology* **107(3)**:697–704.

Ohnishi, S., Takano, K. (2004). Amyloid fibrils from the viewpoint of protein folding. *Cell and Molecular Life Sciences* **61(5)**:511–524.

Okada, T., Palczewski, K. (2001). Crystal structure of rhodopsin: Implications for vision and beyond. *Current Opinion in Structural Biology* **11(4)**:420–426.

Okazaki, R., Chikatsu, N., Nakatsu, M., Takeuchi, Y., Ajima, M., Miki, J., Fujita, T., Arai, M., Totsuka, Y., Tanaka, K., Fukumoto, S. (1999). A novel activating mutation in calcium-sensing receptor gene associated with a family of autosomal dominant hypocalcemia. *Journal of Clinical Endocrinology and Metabolism* **84(1)**:363–366.

Oksche, A., Rosenthal, W. (1998). The molecular basis of nephrogenic diabetes insipidus. *Journal of Molecular Medicine* **76(5)**:326–337.

Onali, P., Schwartz, J.P. (1983). Inhibition of VIP-sensitive adenylate cyclase by dopamine in rat anterior pituitary. *Advances in Biochemical Psychopharmacology* **36**:199–207.

Oosterom, J., Nijenhius, W.A.J., Schaaper, W.M.M., Slootstra, J., Meleon, R.H., Gispen, W.H.H., Burbach, J.P.H., Adan, R.A.H. (1999). Conformation of the core sequence in melanocortin peptides directs selectivity for the melanocortin MC_3 and MC_4 receptors. *Journal of Biological Chemistry* **274(24)**:16853–168860.

Oppermann, M. (2004). Chemokine receptor CCR5: Insights into structure, function, and regulation. *Cellular Signaling* **16(11)**:1201–1210.

Orloff, J., Handler, J. (1967) The role of adenosine 3′,5′-phosphate in the action of antidiuretic hormone. *American Journal of Medicine* **42(5)**:757–768.

Orsini, M.J., Parent, J-L., Mundell, S.J., Benovic, J.L. (1999). Trafficking of the HIV coreceptor CXCR4. Role of arrestins and identification of residues in the C-terminal tail that mediate receptor internalization. *Journal of Biological Chemistry* **274(43)**:31076–31086.

Ostrom, R.S., Insel, P.A. (2004). The evolving role of lipid rafts and caveolae in G protein-coupled receptor signaling: Implications for molecular pharmacology. *British Journal of Pharmacology* **143(2)**:235–245.

Ovchinnikov, Y.A., Abdulaev, N.G., Bogachuk, A.S. (1988) Two adjacent cysteine residues in the C-terminal cytoplasmic fragment of bovine rhodopsine are palmitoylated. *FEBS Letters* **230(1–2)**:1–5.

Overø, K.F. (1982). Kinetics of citalopram in man: Plasma levels in patients. *Progress in Neuro-psychopharmacology and Biological Psychiatry* **6(3)**:311–318.

Overton, M.K., Blumer, K.J. (2000). G-protein coupled receptors function as oligomers *in vivo*. *Current Biology* **10(6)**:341–344.

Owens, M.J., Knight, D.L., Nemeroff, C.B. (2001). Second generation SSRIs: Human monoamine transporter binding profile of escitalopram and R-fluoxetine. *Biological Psychiatry* **50(5)**:345–350.

Ozacmak, V., Sayan, H., Cetin, A., Akyildiz-Igdem, A. (2007). AT1 receptor blocker candesartan-induced attenuation of brain injury of rats subjected to chronic cerebral hypoperfusion. *Neurochemical Research* **32(8)**:1314–1321.

Palczewski, K., Buczylko, J., Kaplan, M.W., Polans, A.S., Crabb, J.W. (1991). Mechanism of rhodopsin kinase activation. *Journal of Biological Chemistry* **266(20)**:12949–12955.

Palczewski, K., Kumasaka, T., Hori, T., Behnke, C.A., Motoshima, H., Fox, B.A., Le Trong, I., Teller, D.C., Okada, T., Stenkamp, R.E., Yamamoto, M., Miyano, M. (2000). Crystal structure of rhodopsin: A G protein-coupled receptor. *Science* **289(5480)**:739–745.

Paoletti, P., Neyton, J. (2007). NMDA receptor subunits: Function and pharmacology. *Current Opinion in Pharmacology* **7(1)**:39–47.

Parker, E.M., Grisel, D.A., Iben, L.G., Shapiro, R.A. (2006). A single amino acid difference accounts for the pharmacological distinctions between the rat and human 5-hydroxytryptamine$_{1B}$ receptors. *Journal of Neurochemistry* **60(1)**:380–383.

Parma, J., Duprez, L., Van Sande, J., Cochaux, P., Gervy, C., Mockel, J., Dumont, J., Vassart, G. (1993). Somatic mutations in the thyrotropin receptor gene cause hyperfunctioning thyroid adenomas. *Nature* **365(6447)**:649–651.

Paschke, R., Geenen, V. (1995). Messenger RNA expression for a TSH receptor variant in the thymus of a two-year-old child. *Journal of Molecular Medicine* **73(11)**:577–580.

Paschke, R., Van Sande, J., Parma, J., Vassart, G. (1996). The TSH receptor and thyroid diseases. *Clinical Endocrinology and Metabolism* **10(1)**:9–27.

Pastan, I., Roth, J., Macchia, V. (1966). Binding of hormone to tissue: The first step in polypeptide hormone action. *Proceedings of the National Academy of Sciences USA* **56(6)**:1802–1809.

Patel, B.R., Curtz, D.L., Callaghan, J.T., Beasley C.M., Jr., Cerimele, B.J., Bergstrom, R.F. (1996). Effects of smoking and gender on population pharmacokinetics of olanzapine in a Phase III clinical trial (abstract). *Pharmacological Research* **13(suppl. 9)**:S408.

Patel, B.R., Nyhart, E.H., Callaghan, J.T. (1995). Combined population pharmacokintic analysis of olanzapine in healthy volunteers (abstract). *Pharmacological Research* **12**:S360.

Paul, S., Park, H., Filipek, S., Wells, J.W., Palczewski, K. (2004). Oligomerization of G-protein coupled receptors: Past, present and future. *Biochemistry* **43(50)**:15643–15656.

Pávó, I., Fahrenholz, F. (1990). Differential inactivations of vasopressin receptor subtypes in isolated membranes and intact cells by *N*-ethylmaleimide. *FEBS Letters* **272(1–2)**:205–208.

Peltonen, J.M., Pihlavisto, M., Scheinin, M. (1998). Subtype-specific stimulation of [^{35}S]GTPγS binding by recombinant alpha-2 adrenoceptors. *European Journal of Pharmacology* **355(2–3)**:275–279.

Percherancier, Y., Planchenault, T., Valenzuela-Fernandez, A., Virelizier, J-L., Arenzana-Seisdedos, F., Bachelerie, F. (2001). Palmitoylation-dependent control of degradation, life span, and membrane expression of the CCR5 receptor. *Journal of Biological Chemistry* **276(34)**:31936–31944.

Perez, D.M. (2003). The evolutionarily triumphant G-protein coupled receptor. *Molecular Pharmacology* **63(6)**:1202–1205.

Petty, M.A., Elands, J., Johnson, M.P., Linnik, M.D., Hamel, E., Moskowitz, M.A., Lee, W.S., McCarty, D.R., Hibert, M., Baron, B.M. (1997). The selectivity of MDL 74,721 in models of neurogenic versus vascular components of migraine. *European Journal of Pharmacology* **336(2–3)**:127–136.

Pfeffer, M., Swedberg, K., Granger, C., Held, P., McMurray, J., Michelson, E., Olofsson, B., Ostergren, J., Yusuf, S., Pocock, S. (2003). Effects of candesartan on mortality and morbidity in patients with chronic heart failure: The CHARM-Overall programme. *Lancet* **362(9386)**:759–766.

Pierce, K.L., Premont, R.T., Lefkowitz, R.J. (2002). Seven-transmembrane receptors. *Nature Reviews Molecular Cell Biology* **3(9)**:639–650.

Pihlavisto, M., Sjöholm, B., Scheinin, M., Wurster, S. (1998). Modulation of agonist binding to recombinant human alpha-2 adrenoceptors by sodium ions. *Biochimica et Biophysica Acta—Molecular Cell Research* **1448(1)**:135–146.

Pin, J-P., Duvoisin, R. (1995). The metabotropic glutamate receptors: Structure and functions. *Neuropharmacology* **34(1)**:1–26.

Pin, J.P., Kniazeff, J., Liu, J., Binet, V., Goudet, C., Rondard, P., Prézeau, L. (2005). Allosteric functioning of dimeric class C G-protein-coupled receptors. *FEBS Journal* **272(12)**:2947–2955.

Pippig, S., Andexinger, S., Lohse, M.J. (1995). Sequestration and recycling of beta 2-adrenergic receptors permit receptor resensitization. *Molecular Pharmacology* **47(4)**:666–676.

Pitcher, J.A., Payne, E.S., Csortos, C., DePaoli, R.A., Lefkowitz, R.J. (1995). The G-protein coupled receptor phosphatase: A protein phosphatase type 2A with a distinct sub-cellular distribution and substrate specificity. *Proceedings of the National Academy of Sciences USA* **92(18)**:8343–8347.

Pizzolato, G., Chierichetti, F., Rossato, A., Briani, C., Dam, M., Borsato, N., Saitta, B., Zanco, P., Ferlin, G., Battistin, L. (1993). Dopamine receptor SPET imaging in Parkinson's disease: A[^{123}I]-IBZM and [^{99}mTc]-HM-PAO study. *European Neurology* **33**:143–148.

Politowska, E., Kazmierkiewicz, R., Wiegand, V., Fahrenholz, F., Ciarkowski, J. (2001). Molecular modelling study of the role of cholesterol in the stimulation of the oxytocin receptor. *Acta Biochimica Polonica* **48(1)**:83–93.

Popp, B.D., Hutchinson, D.S., Evans, B.A., Summers, R.J. (2004). Stereoselectivity for interactions of agonists and antagonists at mouse, rat and human beta 3-adrenoceptors. *European Journal of Pharmacology* **484(2–3)**:323–331.

Porcellini, A., Ciullo, I., Laviola, L., Amabile, G., Fenzi, G., Avvedimento, V.E. (1994). Novel mutations of thyrotropin receptor gene in thyroid hyperfunctioning adenomas. *Journal of Clinical Endocrinology and Metabolism* **79(2)**:657–661.

Post, R.M. (1992). Transduction of psychosocial stress into the neurobiology of recurrent affective disorder. *American Journal of Psychiatry* **149(8)**:999–1010.

Power, C.A., Church, D.J., Meyer, A., Alouani, S., Proudfoot, A.E.I., Clark-Lewis, I., Sozzani, S., Mantovani, A., Well,s T.N.C. (1997). Cloning and characterization of a specific receptor for the novel CC chemokine MIP-3α from lung dendritic cells. *Journal of Experimental Medicine* **186(6)**:825–835

Pranzatelli, M.R. (1992). Serotonin receptor ontogeny: Effects of agonists in 1-day-old rats. *Pharmacology, Biochemistry and Behavior* **43(4)**:1273–1277.

Prinster, S.C., Holmqvist, T.G., Hall, R.A. (2006). α_{2C}-Adrenergic receptors exhibit enhanced surface expression and signaling upon association with β_2-adrenergic receptors. *Journal of Pharmacology and Experimental Therapeutics* **318(3)**:974–981.

Prossnitz, E.R. (2004). New role for arrestins in post-endocytic trafficking of G-protein coupled receptors. *Life Sciences* **75**:893–899.

Qanbar, R., Bouvier, M. (2003) Role of palmitoylation/depalmitoylation reactions in G-protein coupled receptor function. *Pharmacological Therapy* **97(1)**:1–33.

Qu, F.C., Liu, C.H., Jiang, B. (2008). Effects of valsartan on sarcoplasmic reticulum calcium adenodine triphosphatase, protein kinase A and protein phosphatase 1 alpha in a rabbit model of heart failure. *Zhonghua Xin Xue Guan Bing Za Zhi* **36(9)**:790–793.

Quillent, C., Oberlin, E., Braun, J., Rousset, D., Gonzalez-Canali, G., Metais, P., Montagnier, L., Virelizier, J-L., Arenzana-Seisdedos, F., Beretta, A. (1998). HIV-1-resistance phenotype conferred by combination of two separate inherited mutations of *CCR5* gene. *Lancet* **351(9095)**:14–18.

Quist, J.F., Barr, C.L., Schachar, R., Roberts, W., Malone, M., Tannock, R., Basile, V.S., Beitchman, J., Kennedy, J.L. (2003). The serotonin 5-HT1B receptor gene and attention deficit hyperactivity disorder. *Molecular Psychiatry* **8(1)**:98–102.

Rajeswaran, W.G., Hocart, S.J., Murphy, W.A., Taylor, J.E., Coy, D.H. (2001). Highly potent and subtype selective ligands derived by *N*-methyl scan of a somatostatin antagonist. *Journal of Medicinal Chemistry* **44(8)**:1305–1311.

Ramarao, C.S., Denker, J.M., Perez, D.M., Gaivin, R.J., Riek, P.P., Graham, R.M. (1992). Genomic organization and expression of the human alpha 1B-adrenergic receptor. *Journal of Biological Chemistry* **267(30)**:21936–21945.

Rana, B.K., Shiina, T., Insel, P.A. (2001) Genetic variations and polymorphisms of G- protein coupled receptors: Functional and therapeutic implications. *Annual Review of Pharmacology and Toxicology* **41**:593–624.

Ranade, K., Jorgenson, E., Sheu, W.H., Pei, D., Hsiung, C.A., Chiang, F.T., Chen, Y.D., Pratt, R., Olshen, R.A., Curb, D, Cox, D.R., Botstein, D., Risch, N. (2002). A polymorphism in the beta 1 adrenergic receptor is associated with resting heart rate. *American Journal of Human Genetics* **70(4)**:935–942.

Rang, H.P., Dale, M.M., Ritter, J.M. (2003). Noradrenergic transmission. In: *Pharmacology*, pp. 163. Edinburgh, UK: Churchill Livingstone.

Rapoport, B., Chazenbalk, G.D., Jaume, J.C., McLachlan, S.M. (1998). The thyrotropin (TSH) receptor: Interaction with TSH and autoantibodies. *Endocrine Reviews* **19(6)**:673–716.

Rasmussen, H.B., Timm, S., Wang, A.G., Soeby, K., Lublin, H., Fenger, M., Hemmingsen, R. Werge, T. (2006) Association between the CCR5 32-bp deletion allele and late onset of schizophrenia. *American Journal of Psychiatry* **163(3)**:507–511.

Rasmussen, S.G., Choi, H.J., Rosenbaum, D.M., Kobilka, T.S., Thian, F.S., Edwards, P.C., Burghammer, M., Ratnala, V.R., Sanishvili, R., Fischetti, R.F., Schertler, G.F., Weis, W.I., Kobilka, B.A. (2007). Crystal structure of the human beta 2 adrenergic G-protein-coupled receptor. *Nature* **450(7168)**:383–387.

Rees, S.B., McLachlan, S.M., Furmaniak, J. (1988). Autoantibodies to the thyrotropin receptor. *Endocrine Reviews* **9**:106–121.

Rees, S., den Daas, I., Foord, S., Goodson, S., Bull, D., Kilpatrick, G., Lee, M. (1994). Cloning and characterization of the human 5-HT_{5A} serotonin receptor. *FEBS Letters* **355(3)**:242–246.

Regan, J.W., Kobilka, T.S., Yang-Feng, T.L., Caron, M.G., Lefkowitz, R.J., Kobilka, B.K. (1988). Cloning and expression of a human kidney cDNA for an alpha 2-adrenergic receptor subtype. *Proceedings of the National Academy of Sciences U.S.A.* **85(17)**:6301–6305.

Ren, Q., Kurose, H., Lefkowitz, R.J., Cotecchia, S. (1993). Constitutively active mutants of the alpha 2-adrenergic receptor. *Journal of Biological Chemistry* **268(22)**:16483–16487.

Represa, A,, Tremblay, E., Ben-Ari, Y. (1989). Transient increase of NMDA-binding sites in human hippocampus during development. *Neuroscience Letters* **99(1–2)**:61–66.

Reynolds, J. (ed.) (1989). *Martindale: The Extra Pharmacopoeia*, 29th ed. London: The Pharmaceutical Press.

Rhee, M.H., Nevo, I., Levy, R., Vogel, Z. (2000). Role of the highly conserved Asp-Arg-Tyr motif in signal transduction of the CB_2 cannabinoid receptor. *FEBS Letters* **466(2–3)**:300–304.

Richardson, R.M., Marjoram, R.J., Barak, L.S., Snyderman, R. (2003). Role of the cytoplasmic tails of CXCR1 and CXCR2 in mediating leukocyte migration, activation, and regulation. *Journal of Immunology* **170(6)**:2904–2911.

Richelson, E., Souder, T. (2000). Binding of antipsychotic drugs to human brain receptors focus on newer generation compounds. *Life Sciences* **68(1)**:29–39.

Richter–Unruh, A., Wessels, H.T., Menken, U., Bergmann, M., Schmittmann-Ohters, K., Schaper, J., Tappeser, S., Hauffa, B.P. (2002). Male LH-independent sexual precocity in a 3.5-year-old boy caused by a somatic activating mutation of the LH receptor in a Leydig cell tumor. *Journal of Clinical Endocrinology and Metabolism* **87(3)**:1052–1056.

Ring, B.J., Catlow, J., Lindsay, T.J., Gillespie, T., Roskos, L.K., Cerimele, B.J., Swanson, S.P., Hamman, M.A., Wrighton, S.A. (1996). Identification of the human cytochromes P450 responsible for the *in vitro* formation of the major oxidative metabolites of the antipsychotic agent olanzapine. *Journal of Pharmacology and Experimental Therapeutics* **276(2)**:658–666.

Richelson, E., Souder, T. (2000). Binding of anti-psychotic drugs to human brain receptors focus on newer generation compounds. *Life Sciences* **68(1)**:29–39.

Robben, J.H., Knoers, N.V., Deen, P.M. (2006). Cell biological aspects of the vasopressin type-2 receptor and aquaporin 2 water channel in nephrogenic diabetes insipidus. *American Journal of Physiology—Renal Physiology* **291(2)**:F257–F270.

Robert, J., Clauser, E., Petit, P.X., Ventura, M.A. (2005). A novel C-terminal motif is necessary for the export of the vasopressin V1b/V3 receptor to the plasma membrane. *Journal of Biological Chemistry* **280(3)**:2300–2308.

Robinson, P.R., Buczylko, J., Ohguro, H., Palzewski, K. (1994). Opsins with mutations at the site of chromophore attachment constitutively activate transducin but are not phosphorylated by rhodopsin kinase. *Proceedings of the National Academy of Sciences USA* **91(12)**:5411–5415.

Rochat, B., Amey, M., Gillet, M., Meyer, U.A., Baumann, P. (1997). Identification of three cytochrome P450 isozymes involved in N-demethylation of citalopram enantiomers in human liver microsomes. *Pharmacogenetics* **7(1)**:1–10.

Roitt, I.M., Doniach, D., Campbell, P.N., Hudson, V.R. (1956). Autoantibodies in Hashimoto's disease (lymphadenoid goitre). *Lancet* **2**:820–822.

Rokosh, D.G., Simpson, P.C. (2002). Knockout of the alpha 1 A/C adrenergic receptor subtype: The alpha 1 A/C is expressed in resistance arteries and is required to arterial blood pressure. *Proceedings of the National Academy of Sciences USA* **99(14)**:9474–9479.

Root, A.W. (2000). Precocious puberty. *Pediatrics in Review* **21**:10–19.

Rosenfeld, R.D., Zeni, L., Welcher, A.A., Narhi, L.O., Hale, C., Marasco, J., Delaney, J., Gleason, T., Philo, J.S., Katta, V., Hui, J., Baumgartner, J., Graham, M., Stark, K.L., Karbon, W.(1998). Biochemical, biophysical, and pharmacological characterization of bacterially expressed human agouti-related protein. *Biochemistry* **37(46)**:16041–16052.

Rosenthal, S.M., Gitelman, S.E., Vargas, G.A., Feldman, B.J. (2007). Gain-of-function mutations in the V2 vasopressin receptor. *Hormone Research* **67(Suppl. 1)**:121–125.

Rostami-Hodjegan, A., Amin, A.M., Spencer, E.P., Lennard, M.S., Tucker, G.T., Flanagan, R.J. (2004). Influence of dose, cigarette smoking, age, sex, and metabolic activity on plasma clozapine concentrations: A predictive model and nomograms to aid clozapine dose adjustment and to assess compliance in individual patients. *Journal of Clinical Psychopharmacology* **24(1)**:70–78.

Rousseau-Merck, M.F., Misrahi, M., Loosfelt, H., Atger, M., Milgrom, E., Berger, R. (1990). Assignment of the human thyroid stimulating hormone receptor (TSHR) gene to chromosome 14q31. *Genomics* **8(2)**:233–236.

Ruffing, N., Sullivan, N., Sharmeen, L., Sodroski, J., Wu, L. (1998). CCR5 has an expanded ligand-binding repertoire and is the primary receptor used by MCP-2 on activated T cells. *Cellular Immunology* **189(2)**:160–168.

Ruilope, L., Jäger, B., Prichard, B. (2001). Eprosartan versus enalapril in elderly patients with hypertension: A double-blind, randomized trial. *Blood Pressure* **10(4)**:223–229.

Rukhadze, M.D., Bezarashvili, G.S., Sidamonidze, N.S., Tsagareli, S.K. (2001). Investigation of binding process of chlorpromazine to bovine serum albumin by means of passive and active experiments. *Biomedical Chromatography* **15(6)**:365–373.

Russo, D., Arturi, F., Schlumberger, M., Caillou, B., Monier, R., Filetti, S. (1995). Activating mutations of the TSH receptor in differentiated thyroid carcinomas. *Oncogene* **11(9)**:1907–1911.

Russo, D., Betterle, C., Arturi, F., Chiefari, E., Girelli, M.E., Filetti, S. (2000). A novel mutation in the thyrotropin (TSH) receptor gene causing loss of TSH binding but constitutive receptor activation in a family with resistance to TSH. *Journal of Clinical Endocrinology and Metabolism* **85(11)**:4238–4242.

Russo, D., Chazenbalk, G.D., Nagayama, Y., Wadsworth, H.L., Rapoport, B. (1991). Site-directed mutagenesis of the human thyrotropin receptor: Role of asparagine-linked oligosaccharides in the expression of a functional receptor. *Molecular Endocrinology* **5(1)**:29–33.

Sadee, W., Hoeg, E., Lucas, J., Wang, D. (2001). Genetic variations in human G-protein coupled receptors: Implications for drug therapy. *AAPS PharmSci* **3(3)**:E22.

Sadeghi, H.M., Innamorati, G., Birnbaumer, M. (1995). Functional properties of mutant V2 receptors. In: Saito, T., Kurokawa, K., Yoshida, S. (eds), *Neurohypophysis: Recent Progress of Vasopressin and Oxytocin Research*, pp. 445–451. Amsterdam: Elsevier.

Sadeghi, H.M., Innamorati, G., Dagarag, M., Birnbaumer, M. (1997) Palmitoylation of the V2 vasopressin receptor. *Molecular Pharmacology* **52(1)**:21–29.

Sadock, B.J., Sadock, V. (eds) (2000). *Comprehensive Textbook of Psychopharmacology*. Philadelphia, PA: Lippincott Williams and Wilkins.

Saeki, T., A. Naya. (2003). CCR1 Chemokine receptor antagonist. Current Pharmaceutical Design **9**: 1201–1208.

Salahpour, A., Angers, S., Mercier, J.F., Lagacé, M., Marullo, S., Bouvier, M. (2004). Homodimerization of the β_2-adrenergic receptor as a prerequisite for cell surface targeting. *Journal of Biological Chemistry* **279(32)**:33390–33397.

Salesse, R. (1996). Peptide and immunochemical mapping of the ectodomain of the porcine LH receptor. *Journal of Molecular Endocrinology* **16**:15–25.

Salom, D., Lodowski, D.T., Stenkamp, R.E., Le Trong, I., Golczak, M., Jastrzebska, B., Harris, T., Ballesteros, J.A., Palczewski, K. (2006). Crystal structure of a photoactivated deprotonated intermediate of rhodopsin. *Proceedings of the National Academy of Sciences USA* **103(44)**:16123–16128.

Salpeter, S., Buckley, N., Ormiston, T., Salpeter, E. (2006). Meta-analysis: Effect of long-acting beta-agonists on severe asthma exacerbations and asthma-related deaths. *Annals of Internal Medicine* **144(12)**:904–912.

Samson, M., Labbe, O., Mollereau, C., Vassart, G., Parmentier, M. (1996). Molecular cloning and expression of a new human CC-chemokine receptor gene. *Biochemistry* **35(11)**:3362–3367.

Samson, M., Soularue, P., Vassart, G., Parmentier, M. (1996b). The genes encoding the human CC-chemokine receptorsCC-CKR1 to CC-CKR5 (CMKBR1-CMKBR5) are clustered in the p21.3-p24 region of chromosome 3. *Genomics* **36(3)**:522–526.

Samson, M., Libert, F., Doranz, B.J., Rucker, J., Liesnard, C., Farber, C-M., Saragosti, S., Lapouméroulie, C., Cognaux, J., Forceille, C., Muyldermans, G., Verhofstede, C., Burtonboy, G., Georges, M., Imai, T., Rana, S., Yi, Y., Smyth, R.J., Collman, R.G., Doms, R.W., Vassart, G., Parmentier, M. (1996c). Resistance to HIV-1 infection in Caucasian individuals bearing mutant alleles of the CCR-5 chemokine receptor gene. *Nature* **382(6593)**:722–725.

Sánchez, C., Hyttel, J. (1999). Comparison of the effects of antidepressants and their metabolites on reuptake of biogenic amines and on receptor binding. *Cellular and Molecular Neurobiology* **19(4)**:467–489.

Santini, F., Gaidarov, I., Keen, J.H. (2002). G-protein coupled receptor/arrestin3 modulation of the endocytic machinery. *Journal of Cell Biology* **156(4)**:665–676.

Sato, Y., Kurose, H., Isogaya, M., Nagao, T. (1996). Molecular characterization of pharmacological properties of T-0509 for beta-adrenoceptors. *European Journal of Pharmacology* **315(3)**:363–367.

Savarese, T.M., Wang, C.D., Fraser, C.M. (1992). Site-directed mutagenesis of the rat m1 muscarinic acetylcholine receptor: Role of conserved cysteines in receptor function. *Journal of Biological Chemistry* **267(16)**:11439–11448.

Schade, R., Andersohn, F., Suissa, S., Haverkamp, W., Garbe, E. (2007). Dopamine agonists and the risk of cardiac-valve regurgitation. *New England Journal of Medicine* **356(1)**:29–38.

Schena, M., Shalon, D., Davis, R.W., Brown, P.O. (1995). Quantitative monitoring of gene expression patterns with a complementary DNA microarray. *Science* **270(5235)**:467–470.

Scherer, S.W., Soder, S., Duvoisin, R.M., Huizenga, J.J., Tsui, C.C. (1997). The human metabotropic glutamate receptor 8 (GRM8) gene: a disproportionately large gene located at 7q31.3-q32.1. *Genomics* **44(2)**:232–236.

Schioth, H.B., Muceniece, R., Wikberg, J.E.S., Szardenings, M. (1996). Alternative translation initiation codon for the human melanocortin MC3 receptor does not affect the ligand binding. *European Journal of Pharmacology* **314(3)**:381–384.

Schipani, E., Jensen, G.S., Picus, J., Nissenson, R.A., Gardella, T.A., Juppner, H. (1997). Constitutive activation of the cyclic adenosine 3′,5′-monophosphate signaling pathway by parathyroid hormone (PTH)-related peptide receptors mutated at two loci for Jansen's metaphyseal chondrodysplasia. *Molecular Endocrinology* **11(7)**:851–858.

Schmuck, K., Ullmer, C., Engels, P., Lübbert, H. (1994). Cloning and functional characterization of the human 5-HT_{2B} serotonin receptor. *FEBS Letters* **342(1)**:85–90.

Schneier, F.R., Liebowitz, M.R., Abi-Dargham, A., Zea-Ponce, Y., Lin, S.H., Laruelle, M. (2000). Low dopamine D(2) receptor binding potential in social phobia. *American Journal of Psychiatry* **157(3)**:457–459.

Schoepp, D.D., Conn, P.J. (1993). Metabotropic glutamate receptors in brain function and pathology. *Trends in Pharmacological Sciences* **14(1)**:13–20.

Schoepp, D.D., Jane, D.E., Monn, J.A. (1999). Pharmacological agents acting at subtypes of metabotropic glutamate receptors. *Neuropharmacology* **38(10)**:1431–1476.

Schols, D., Struyf, S., Van Damme, J., Esté, J.A., Henson, G., De Clercq, E. (1997). Inhibition of T-tropic HIV strains by selective antagonization of the chemokine receptor CXCR4. *Journal of Experimental Medicine* **186(8)**:1383–1388.

Schöneberg, T., Schulz, A., Hermsdorf, T., Rőmpler, H., Sangkuhl, K. (2004). Mutant G-protein-coupled receptors as a cause of human diseases. *Pharmacology and Therapeutics* **104(3)**:173–206.

Schorge, S., Colquhoun, D. (2003). Studies of NMDA receptor function and stoichiometry with truncated and tandem subunits. *Journal of Neuroscience* **23(4)**:1151–1158.

Schulz, A., Grosse, R., Schultz, G., Gudermann, T., Schöneberg, T. (2000). Structural implication for receptor oligomerization from functional reconstitution studies of mutant V2 vasopressin receptors. *Journal of Biological Chemistry* **275**:2381–2389.

Schweickart, V.L., Raport, C.J., Godiska, R., Byers, M.G., Eddy, R.L. Jr., Shows, T.B., Gray, P.W. (1994). Cloning of human and mouse EBl1, a lymphoid-specific G-protein-coupled receptor encoded on human chromosome 17q12-q21.2. *Genomics* **23(3)**:643–650.

Schweickart, V.L., Epp, A., Raport, C.J., Gray, P.W. (2000). CCR11 is a functional receptor for the monocyte chemoattractant protein family of chemokines. *Journal of Biological Chemistry* **275(13)**:9550–9556.

Sedvall, G., Farde, L. (1995). Chemical brain anatomy in schizophrenia. *Lancet* **346(8977)**:743–749.

Seeman, P. (2002). Atypical antipsychotics: Mechanism of action. *Canadian Journal of Psychiatry* **47(1)**:27–38.

Seeman, P., Chau–Wong, M., Tedesco, J., Wong, K. (1975). Brain receptors for antipsychotic drugs and dopamine: Direct binding assays. *Proceedings of the National Academy of Sciences USA* **72(11)**:4376–4380.

Seeman, P., Guan, H., Van Tol, H.H. (1993). Dopamine D4 receptors elevated in schizophrenia. *Nature* **365(6445)**:441–445.

Seeman, P., Tallerico, T. (1998). Anti-psychotic drugs which elicit little or no parkinsonism bind more loosely than dopamine to brain D2 receptors, yet occupy high levels of these receptors. *Molecular Psychiatry* **3(2)**:123–134.

Seeman, P., Weinshenker, D., Quirion, R., Srivastava, L.K., Bhardwaj, S.K., Grandy, D.K., Premont, R.T., Sotnikova, T.D., Boksa, P., El-Ghundi, M., O'dowd, B.F., George, S.R., Perreault, M.L., Männistö, P.T., Robinson, S., Palmiter, R.D., Tallerico, T. (2005). Dopamine supersensitivity correlates with D2 high states, implying many paths to psychosis. *Proceedings of the National Academy of Sciences USA* **102(9)**:3513–3518.

Seibert, C., Cadene, M., Sanfiz, A., Chait, B.T., Sakmar, T.P. (2002). Tyrosine sulfation of CCR5 N-terminal peptide by tyrosylprotein sulfotransferases 1 and 2 follows a discrete pattern and temporal sequence. *Proceedings of the National Academy of Sciences USA* **99(17)**:11031–11036.

Seibert, C., Veldkamp, C.T., Peterson, F.C., Chait, B.T., Volkman, B.F., Sakmar, T.P. (2008). Sequential tyrosine sulfation of CXCR4 by tyrosylprotein sulfotransferases. *Biochemistry* **47(43)**:11251–11262.

Seibold, A., Brabet, P., Rosenthal, W., Birnbaumer, M. (1992). Structure and chromosomal localization of the human antidiuretic hormone receptor gene. *American Journal of Human Genetics* **51(5)**:1078–1083.

Seroquel (Quetiapine). (2001). Wilmington DE, AstraZeneca Pharmaceuticals.

Sever, S. (2002). Dynamin function and endocytosis. *Current Opinion in Cell Biology* **14;**463–467.

Shenker, L. Laue, S. Kosugi, J.J. Merendino Jr., Minegishi, T., Cutler, G.B., Jr. (1993). A constitutively activating mutation of the luteinizing hormone receptor in familial male precocious puberty. *Nature* **365(6447)**:652–654.

Shenoy, S.K., Lefkowitz, R.J. (2003). Trafficking patterns of beta-arrestin and G-protein coupled receptors determined by the kinetics of beta-arrestin deubiquitination. *Journal of Biological Chemistry* **278(16)**:14498–14506.

Shibata, K., Foglar, R., Horie, K., Obika, K., Sakamoto, A., Ogawa, S., Tsujimoto, G. (1995). KMD-3213, a novel, potent, alpha 1a-adrenoceptor-selective antagonist: Characterization using recombinant human alpha 1-adrenoceptors and native tissues. *Molecular Pharmacology* **48(2)**:250–258.

Shoaf, S., Elizari, M., Wang, Z., Sekar, K., Grinfeld, G.R., Barbagelata, N.A., Lerman, J., Bramer, S.L., Tronge, J., Orlandi, C. (2005). Tolvaptan administration does not affect steady state amiodarone concentrations in patients with cardiac arrhythmias. *Journal of Cardiovascular Pharmacology and Therapeutics* **10(3)**:165–171.

Sibley, D.R., Strasser, R.H., Caron, M.G., Lefkowitz, R.J. (1985). Homologous desensitization of adenylate cyclase is associated with phosphorylation of the beta-adrenergic receptor. *Journal of Biological Chemistry* **260(7)**:3883–3886.

Silva, D., Cortez, C.M., Louro, S.R. (2004). Quenching of the intrinsic fluorescence of bovine serum albumin by chlorpromazine and hemin. *Brazilian Journal of Medical Biology and Research* **37(7)**:963–968.

Sindrup, S.H., Brosen, K., Hansen, M.G.J, Aaesjorgensen, T., Overø, K.F., Gram, L.F. (1993). Pharmacokinetics of citalopram in relation to the spartein and mephenytoin oxidaton polymorphisms. *Therapeutic Drug Monitoring* **15(1)**:11–17.

Singh, V., and Curtiss, R., III. (1994). Hormonotoxins: The role of positive charge of lysine residue on the immunological, biological and cytotoxic properties of ovine lutropin-S-S-gelonin conjugates. *Molecular and Cellular Biochemistry* **130(1)**:91–101.

Sioud, M. (2004). Therapeutic siRNAs. *Trends in Pharmacological Sciences* **25**:22–28.

Sioud, M. (2007). Main approaches to target discovery and validation. *Methods in Molecular Biology* **360**:1–12.

Siragy, H.M., Carey, R.M. (1996). The subtype-2 (AT2) angiotensin receptor regulates renal cyclic guanosine 3',5'-monophosphate and AT1 receptor-mediated prostaglandin E2 production in conscious rats. *Journal of Clinical Investigation* **97(8)**:1978–1982.

Siragy, H.M., Carey, R.M. (1997). The subtype 2 (AT2) angiotensin receptor mediates renal production of nitric oxide in conscious rats. *Journal of Clinical Investigation* **100(2)**:264–269.

Smith, A.I., Funder, J.W. (1988) Proopiomelanocortin processing in the pituitary, central nervous system, and peripheral tissues. *Endocrine Reviews* **9(1)**:159–179.

Sodhi, M.S., Burnet, P.W.J., Makoff, A.J., Kerwin, R.W., Harrison, P.J. (2001). RNA editing of the 5-HT2C receptor is reduced in schizophrenia. *Molecular Psychiatry* **6(4)**:373–379.

Sokoloff, P., Giros, B., Martres, M.P., Bouthenet, M.L., Schwartz, J.C. (1990). Molecular cloning and characterization of a novel dopamine receptor (D3) as a target for neuroleptics. *Nature* **347(6289)**: 146–151.

Spiro, R.G. (2002). Protein glycosylation: Nature, distribution, enzymatic formation, and disease implications of glycopeptide bonds. *Glycobiology* **12(4)**:43R–56R.

Stam, N.J., Huizen, F.V., Alebeek, C,V., Dijkema, R., Tonnaer, J.A.D.M., Olijve, W. (1992). Genomic organization, coding sequence and functional expression of human 5-HT_2 and 5-HT_{1A} receptor genes. *European Journal of Pharmacology* **227(2)**:153–162.

Stam, N.J., Vanderheyden, P., van Alebeek, C., Klomp, J., de Boer, T., van Delft, A.M., Olijve, W. (1994). Genomic organization and functional expression of the gene encoding the human serotonin 5-HT2c receptor. *European Journal of Pharmacology* **269(3)**:339–348.

Stam, N.J., Roesink, C., Dijcks, F., Garritsen, A., van Herpen, A., Olijve, W. (1997). Human serotonin 5-HT_7 receptor: cloning and pharmacological characterization of two receptor variants. *FEBS Letters* **413(3)**:489–494.

Stam, W.B., Van der Graaf, P.H., Saxena, P.R. (1998). Functional characterisation of the pharmacological profile of the putative alpha1B-adrenoceptor antagonist, (+)-cyclazosin. *European Journal of Pharmacology* **361(1)**:79–83.

Stein, S.A., Oates, E.L., Hall, C.R., Grumbles, R.M., Fernandez, L.M., Taylor, N.A., Puett, D., Jin, S. (1994). Identification of a point mutation in the thyrotropin receptor of the *hyt/hyt* hypothyroid mouse. *Molecular Endocrinology* **8**:129–138.

Stenkamp, R.E., Filipek, S., Driessen, C.A., Teller, D.C., Palczewski, K. (2002). Crystal structure of rhodopsin: a template for cone visual pigments and other G protein-coupled receptors. *Biochimica Biophysica et Acta* **1565(2)**:168–182.

Stephen, D., Bon, C., Holzwarth, J.A., Galvan, M., Pruss, R.M. (1996). Human metabotropic glutamate receptor 1: mRNA distribution, chromosome localization and functional expression of two splice variants. *Neuropharmacology* **35(12)**:1649–1660.

Stephenson, F.A. (2006). Structure and trafficking of NMDA and GABAA receptors. *Biochemical Society Transactions* **34(Pt 5)**:877–881.

Stiles, G.L., Caron, M.G., Lefkowitz, R.J. (1984). Beta-adrenergic receptors: Biochemical mechanisms of physiological regulation. *Physiological Reviews* **64(2)**:661–743.

Stitham, J., Stojanovic, A., Merenick, B. L., O'Hara, K.A., Hwa, J. (2003). The unique ligand-binding pocket for the human prostacyclin receptor: Site-directed mutagenesis and molecular modeling. *Journal of Biological Chemistry* **278(6)**:4250–4257.

Strader, C.D., Sigal, I.S., Dixon, R.A. (1989). Structural basis of beta-adrenergic receptor function. *The FASEB Journal* **3(7)**:1825–1832.

Strizki, J.M., Xu, S., Wagner, N.E., Wojcik, L., Liu, J., Hou, Y., Endres, M., Palani, A., Shapiro, S., Clader, J.W., Greenlee, W.J., Tagat, J.R., McCombie, S., Cox, K., Fawzi, A.B., Chou, C-C., Pugliese-Sivo, C., Davies, L., Moreno, M.E., Ho, D.D., Trkola, A., Stoddart, C.A., Moore, J.P., Reyes, G.R., Baroudy, B.M. (2001). SCH-C (SCH 351125), an orally bioavailable, small molecule antagonist of the chemokine receptor CCR5, is a potent inhibitor of HIV-1 infection *in vitro* and *in vivo*. *Proceedings of the National Academy of Sciences USA* **98(22)**:12718–12723.

Strosberg, A.D. (1997). Structure and function of the β_3-adrenergic receptors. *Annual Reviews in Pharmacology and Toxicology* **37**:421–450.

Su, S.B., Mukaida, N., Wang, J., Nomura, H., Matsushima, K. (1996). Preparation of specific polyclonal antibodies to a C-C chemokine receptor, CCR1, and determination of CCR1 expression on various types of leukocytes. *Journal of Leukocyte Biology* **60(5)**:658–666.

Sugimoto, T., M., Mochizuki, S., Watanabe, Y., Hashimoto, S., Kawashima, H. (1994) Molecuar Cloning and functional expression of a CDNA encoding the human V(1B) Vassopressin receptor. *Journal of Biological Chemistry* **269**:27088–27092.

Sun, Y., Cheng, Z., Ma, L., Pei, G. (2002). β-Arrestin 2 is critically involved in CXCR4-mediated chemotaxis, and this is mediated by its enhancement of p38 MAPK activation. *Journal of Biological Chemistry* **277(51)**:49212–49219.

Sunahara, R.K., Guan, H.C., O'Dowd, B.F., Seeman, P., Laurier, L.., Ng, G., George, S.R., Torchia, J., Van Tol, H.H., Niznik, H.B. (1991). Cloning of the gene for a human dopamine D5 receptor with higher affinity for dopamine than D1. *Nature* **350(6319)**:614–619.

Sundaramurthy, D., Campbell, D.A., Leek, J.P., Markham, A.F., Pieri, L.F. (1998). Assignment of the melanocortin 4 receptor (MC4R) gene to human chromosome band 18q22 by *in situ* hybridisation and radiation hybrid mapping. *Cytogenetics and Cell Genetics* **82(1–2)**:97–98.

Sung, C.H., Davenport, C.M., Hennessey, J.C., Maumenee, I.H., Jacobson, S.G., Heckenlively, J.R., Nowakowski, R., Fishman, G., Gouras, P., Nathans, J. (1991). Rhodopsin mutations in autosomal dominant retinitis pigmentosa. *Proceedings of the National Academy of Sciences USA* **88**:6481–6485.

Szkudlinski, M.W., Fremont, V., Ronin, C., Weintraub, B.D. (2002). Thyroid-stimulating hormone and thyroid-stimulating hormone receptor structure–function relationships. *Physiological Reviews* **82(2)**:473–502.

Szkudlinski, M.W., The, N., Grossmann, M., Tropea, J.E., Weintraub, B.D. (1996). Engineering human glycoprotein hormone superactive analogs. *Nature Biotechnology* **14(10)**:1257–1263.

Tahara, A., Tsukada, J., Tomura, Y., Kusayama, T., Wada, K., Ishii, N., Taniguchi, N., Suzuki, T., Yatsu, T., Uchida, W., Shibasaki, M. (2005). Effects of YM218, a nonpeptide vasopressin V1A receptor-selective antagonist, on human vasopressin and oxytocin receptors. *Pharmacologial Research* **51(3)**:275–281.

Takahashi, K., Tokita, S., Kotani, H. (2003). Generation and characterization of highly constitutive active histamine H3 receptors. *Journal of Pharmacology and Experimental Therapeutics* **307(1)**:213–218.

Takai, D., Yagi, Y., Wakazono, K., Ohishi, N., Morita, Y., Sugimura, T., Ushijima, T. (2001). Silencing of HTR1B and reduced expression of EDN1 in human lung cancers, revealed by methylation-sensitive representational difference analysis. *Oncogene* **20(51)**:7505–7513.

Tang, J., Kaslow, R. A. (2003). The impact of host genetics on HIV infection and disease progression in the era of highly active antiretroviral therapy. *AIDS* **17 (Suppl 4)**:S51–S60.

Taniguchi, T., Inagaki, R., Murata, S., Akiba, I., Muramatsu, I. (1999). Microphysiometric analysis of human alpha 1a-adrenoceptor expressed in Chinese hamster ovary cells. *British Journal of Pharmacology* **127**:962–968.

Tanoue, A., Koba, M., Miyawaki, S., Koshimizu, T.A., Hosoda, C., Oshikawa, S., Tsujimoto, G. (2002). Role of the alpha 1D-adrenergic receptor in the development of salt-induced hypertension. *Hypertension* **40(1)**:101–106.

Tansky, M. F., Pothoulakis, C., Leeman S.E. (2007). Functional consequences of alteration of N-linked glycosylation sites on the neurokinin 1 receptor. *Proceedings of the National Academy of Sciences USA* **104(25)**:10691–10696.

Tao, Y. (2006). Inactivating mutations of G-protein coupled receptors and diseases: Structure–function insights and therapeutic implications. *Pharmacology and Therapeutics* **111(3)**:949–973.

Terillon, S., Bouvier, M. (2004). Roles of G-protein coupled receptor dimerization. From ontogeny to signal regulation. *EMBO Reports* **5**:30–34.

Thibonnier, M., Goraya, T., Berti-Mattera, L. (1993) G protein coupling of human platelet V1 vascular vasopressin receptors. *American Journal of Physiology* **264(5 Pt 1)**:C1336–1344.

Thibonnier, M., Auzan, C., Madhun, Z., Wilkins, P., Berti-Mattera, L., Clauser, E. (1994). Molecular cloning, sequencing and functional expression of a CDNA encoding the human Via vasopressin receptor. *Journal of Biological Chemistry* **269**:3304–3310.

Thibonnier, M., Conarty, D.M., Phesnicher, L. (2000). Mediators of the mitogenic action of human vasopressin receptors. *American Journal of Physiology—Heart and Circulatory Physiology* **279**:H2529–H2539.

Thomas, D.R., Gittins, S.A., Collin, L.L., Middlemiss, D.N., Riley, G., Hagan, J., Gloger, I., Ellis, C.E., Forbes, I.T., Brown, A.M. (1998). Functional characterization of the human cloned 5-HT$_7$ receptor (long form); antagonist profile of SB-258719. *British Journal of Pharmacology* **124(6)**:1300–1306.

Thomsen, C., Pekhletski, R., Haldeman, B., Gilbert, T.A., O'Hara, P., Hampson, D.R. (1997). Cloning and characterization of a metabotropic glutamate receptor, mGluR4b. *Neuropharmacology* **36**:21–30.

Tiberi, M., Jarvie, K.R., Silvia, C., Falardeau, P., Gingrich, J.A., Godinot, N., Bertrand, L., Yang-Feng, T.L., Fremeau, R.T., Jr., Caron, M.G. (1991). Cloning, molecular characterization, and chromosomal assignment of a gene encoding a second D1 dopamine receptor subtype: Differential expression pattern in rat brain compared with the D1A receptor. *Proceedings of the National Academy of Sciences USA* **88(17)**:7491–7495.

Timmermans, P.B., Benfield, P., Chiu, A.T., Herblin, W.F., Wong, P.C., Smith, R.D. (1992). Angiotensin II receptors and functional correlates. *American Journal of Hypertension* **5(12 Pt 2)**:221S–235S.

Timmermans, P.B., Wong, P.C., Chiu, A.T., Herblin, W.F., Benfield, P., Carini, D.J., Lee, R.J., Wexler, R.R., Saye, J.A., Smith, R.D. (1993). Angiotensin II receptors and angiotensin II receptor antagonists. *Pharmacological Reviews* **45**:205–251.

Tissir, F., Rivière, M., Guo, D.F., Tsuzuki, S., Inagami, T., Levan, G., Szpirer, J., Szpirer, C. (1995). Localization of the genes encoding the three rat angiotensin II receptors, Agtr1a, Agtr1b, Agtr2, and the human AGTR2 receptor respectively to rat chromosomes 17q12, 2q24 and Xq34, and the human Xq22. *Cytogenetics and Cell Genetics* **71(1)**:77–80.

Tohgo, A., Pierce, K.L., Choy, E.W., Lefkowitz, R.J., Luttrell, L.M. (2002). β-Arrestin scaffolding of the ERK cascade enhances cytosolic ERK activity but inhibits ERK-mediated transcription following angiotensin $AT1_a$ receptor stimulation. *Journal of Biological Chemistry* **277(11)**:9429–9436.

Toivanen, P., Toivanen, A. (1994). Does *Yersinia* induce autoimmunity? *International Archives of Allergy and Immunology* **104**:107–111.

Tomer, Y., Davies, T. (1993). Infection, thyroid disease, and autoimmunity. *Endocrinology Reviews* **14**:107–120.

Tomlinson, S., Heagerty, A.M., Weetman, A.P., Malik, R.A. (eds) (2008). *Mechanisms of Disease: An Introduction to Clinical Science*, 2nd ed.. Cambridge University Press.

Tompson, D.J., and Vearer, D. (2007). Steady-state pharmacokinetic properties of a 24-hour prolonged-release formulation of ropinirole: Results of two randomized studies in patients with Parkinson's disease. *Clinical Pharmacokinetics* **29(12)**:2654.

Tonacchera, M., Van Sande, J., Cetani, F., Swillens, S., Schvartz, C., Winiszewski, P., Portmann, L., Dumont, J.E., Vassart, G., Parma, J. (1997). Functional characteristics of three new germline mutations of the thyrotropin receptor gene causing autosomal dominant toxic thyroid hyperplasia. *Journal of Clinical Endocrinology and Metabolism* **81(2)**:547–554.

Trejo, J., Coughlin, S.R. (1999). The cytoplasmic tails of protease-activated receptor-1 and substance P receptor specify sorting to lysosomes versus recycling. *Journal of Biological Chemistry* **274(4)**:2216–2224.

Tsai, G. and Coyle, J.T. (2002) Glutametergic mechanisms in schizophrenia. *Annual Reviews in Pharmacology and Toxicology* **42**:165–179.

Tsao, P., Cao, T., von Zastrow, M. (2001). Role of endocytosis in mediating downregulation of G-protein coupled receptors. *Trends in Pharmacological Sciences* **22(2)**:91–96.

Tunaru, S., Lättig, J., Kero, J., Krause, G., Offermanns, S. (2005). Characterization of determinants of ligand binding to the nicotinic acid receptor GPR109A (HM74A/PUMA-G). *Molecular Pharmacology* **68(5)**:1271–1280.

Turner, P.R., O'Connor, K., Tate, W.P., Abraham, W.C. (2003). Roles of amyloid precursor protein and its fragments in regulating neural activity, plasticity and memory. *Progress in Neurobiology* **70(1)**:1–32.

Uberti, M.A., Hague, C., Oller, H., Minneman, K.P., Hall, R.A. (2005). Heterodimerization with β_2-adrenergic receptors promotes surface expression and functional activity of α_{1D}-adrenergic receptors. *Journal of Pharmacology and Experimental Therapeutics* **313(1)**:16–23.

Udelson, J.E., Smith, W.B., Hendrix, G.H., Painchaud, P.A., Ghazzi, M., Thomas, I., Ghali, J.K., Selaru, P., Chanoine, F., Pressler, M.L., Konstam, M.A. (2001). Acute hemodynamic effects of conivaptan, a dual V(1A) and V(2) vasopressin receptor antagonist, in patients with advanced heart failure. *Circulation* **104(20)**:2417–2423.

Uggucioni, M., Mackay, C.R., Ochensberger, B., Loetscher, P., Rhis, S., LaRosa, G.J., Rao, P., Ponath, P.D., Baggiolini, M., Dahinden, C.A. (1997). High expression of the chemokine receptor CCR3 in human blood basophils. Role in activation by eotaxin, MCP-4, and other chemokines. *Journal of Clinical Investigation* **100(5)**:1137–1143.

Uhlenhuth, E. (1927). The anterior lobe of the hypophysis as a control mechanism of the function of the thyroid gland. *British Journal of Experimental Biology* **5**:1–5.

Ulas, J., Cotman, C.W. (1997). Decreased expression of *N*-methyl-d-aspartate receptor 1 messenger RNA in select regions of Alzheimer brain. *Neuroscience* **79(4)**:973–982.

Vaisse, C., Clement, K., Durand, E., Hercberg, S., Guy-Grand, B., Froguel, P. (2000). Melanocortin-4 receptor mutations are a frequent and heterogeneous cause of morbid obesity. *Journal of Clinical Investigation* **106(2)**:253–262.

Valtonen, V.V., Ruutu, P., Varis, K., Ranki, M., Malkamaki, M., Makela, P.H. (1986). Serological evidence for the role of bacterial infections in the pathogenesis of thyroid diseases. *Acta Medica Scandinavica* **219(1)**:105–111.

VanDenBrink, M.A., Vergouwe, M.N., Ophoff, R.A., Naylor, S.L., Dauwerse, H.G., Saxena, P.R., Ferrari, M.D., Frants, P.R. (1998). Chromosomal localization of the 5-HT1F receptor gene: no evidence for involvement in response to sumitriptan in migraine patients. *American Journal of Medical Genetics* **77(5)**:415–420.

Vanderheyden, P.M.L., Fierens, F.L.P., De Backer, J.P., Frayman, N., Vauquelin, G. (1999). Distinction between surmounTable and insurmounTable selective AT1 receptor antagonists by use of CHO-K1 cells expressing human angiotensin II AT1 receptors. *British Journal of Pharmacology* **126(4)**:1057–1065.

Van Oekelen, D., Luyten, W.H., Leysen, J.E. (2003). Ten years of antisense inhibition of brain G-protein-coupled receptor function. *Brain Research Reviews* **42(2)**:123–142.

Van den Ouweland, A.M.W. Dreesen, J.C.F.M., Verdijk, M., Knoers, V.V.A.M., Monnens, L.A.H., Rocchi, M., van Oost, B.A. (1992). Mutations in the vasopressin type 2 receptor gene (AVPR2) associated with nephrogenic dioeletes insipidus. *Nature Genetics* **2**:99–102.

Van Rhee, A.M., Jacobson, K.A. (1996). Molecular architecture of G protein-coupled receptors. *Drug Development and Research* **37**:1–38.

Van Sande, J., Massart, C., Costagliola, S., Allgeier, A., Cetani, F., Vassart, G., Dumont, J.E. (1996). Specific activation of the thyrotropin receptor by trypsin. *Molecular and Cellular Endocrinology* **119(2)**:161–168.

Van Sande, J., Parma, J., Tonacchera, M., Swillens, S., Dumont, J., Vassart, G. (1995). Somatic and germline mutations of the TSH receptor gene in thyroid diseases. *Journal of Clinical Endocrinology and Metabolism* **80**:2577–2585.

Van Tol, H.H.M., Wu, C.M., Guan, H.C., Ohara, K., Bunzow, J.R., Civelli, O., Kennedy, J., Seeman, P., Niznik, H.B., Jovanovic, V. (1992). Multiple dopamine D4 receptor variants in the human population. *Nature* **358(6382)**:149–152.

Vassart, G., Desarnaud, F., Duprez, L., Eggerickx, D., Labbe, O., Libert, F., Mollereau, C., Parma, J., Paschke, R., Tonacchera, M. (1995). The G protein-coupled receptor family and one of its members, the TSH receptor. *Annals of the New York Academy of Sciences* **766**:23–30.

Vassart, G., Dumont, J.E. (1992). The thyrotropin receptor and the regulation of thyrocyte function and growth. *Endocrine Reviews* **13(3)**:596–611.

Vázquez-Prado, J., Casas-González, P., García-Sáinz, J.A. (2003). G protein-coupled receptor cross-talk: Pivotal roles of protein phosphorylation and protein–protein interactions. *Cellular Signaling* **15(6)**:549–557.

Veldkamp, C.T., Seibert, C., Peterson, F.C., De la Cruz, N.B., Haugner 3rd, J.C., Basnet, H., Sakmar, T.P., Volkman, B.F. (2008). Structural basis for CXCR4 sulfotyrosine recognition by the chemokine SDF-1/CXCL-12. *Science Signaling* **1(37)**:ra4.

Verheijen, I., Fierens, F.L., Debacker, J.P., Vauquelin, G., Vanderheyden, P.M. (2000). Interaction between the partially insurmounTable antagonist valsartan and human recombinant angiotensin II type 1 receptors. *Fundamentals of Clinical Pharmacology* **14(6)**:577–585.

Verma, S., Strauss, M. (2004). Angiotensin receptor blockers and myocardial infarction. *British Medical Journal* **329**:1248–1249.

Volpe, R. (1979). Subacute (de Quervain's) thyroiditis. *Clinical Endocrinology and Metabolism* **8**:81–95.

von Basedow, K.A. (1840/1945). Exophthalmus durch Hypertrophie des Zellgewebes in der Augenhöhle. *[Casper's] Wochenschrift für die gesammte Heilkunde*, Berlin, **6**:197–204, 220–228. Partial English translation in: Major, R.H. *Classic Descriptions of Disease*. Springfield, IL: C.C. Thomas.

von Moltke, L.L., Greenblatt, D.J., Grassi, J.M., Granda, B.W., Venkatakrishnan, K., Duan, S.X., Fogelman, S.M., Harmatz, J.S., Shader, R.I. (1999). Citalopram and desmethylcitalopram *in vitro*: Human cytochromes mediating transformation, and cytochrome inhibitory effects. *Biological Psychiatry* **46(6)**:839–849.

von Zastrow, M. (2003). Mechanisms regulating membrane trafficking of G-protein coupled receptors in the endocytic pathway. *Life Sciences* **74(2–3)**:217–224.

Wadsworth, H.L., Chazenbalk, G.D., Nagayama, Y., Russo, D., Rapoport, B. (1990). An insertion in the human thyrotropin receptor critical for high affinity hormone binding. *Science* **249(4975)**:1423–1425.

Waldhoer, M., Fong, J., Jones, R.M., Lunzer, M.M., Sharma, S.K., Kostenis, E., Portoghese, P.S., Whistler, J.L. (2005). A heterodimer-selective agonist shows *in vivo* relevance of G protein-coupled receptor dimers. *Proceedings of the National Academy of Sciences USA* **102(25)**:9050–9055.

Wang, J., Whetsell, M., Klein, J.R. (1997). Local hormone networks and intestinal T cell homeostasis. *Science* **275(5308)**:1937–1939.

Wang, Q., O'Brien, P.J., Chen, C-X., Cho, D-S., C., Murray, J.M., Nishikura, K. (2000). Altered G protein-coupling functions of RNA editing isoform and splicing variant serotonin 2C receptors. *Journal of Neurochemistry* **74**:1290–1300.

Wang, Z., Bilsky, E.J., Porreca, F., Sadee, W. (1994). Constitutive receptor activation as a regulatory mechanism underlying narcotic tolerance and dependance. *Life Science* **54(20)**:PL339–350.

Warner, G.T., Jarvis, B. (2002). Olmesartan medoxomil. *Drugs* **62**:1345–1353.

Weinshank, R.L., Zgombick, J.M., Macchi, M., Adham, N., Lichtblau, H., Branchek, T.A., Hartig, P.R. (1990). Cloning, expression, and pharmacological characterization of a human alpha 2B-adrenergic receptor. *Molecular Pharmacology* **38(5)**:681–688.

Weinshank, R.L., Zgombick, J.M., Macchi, M.J., Branchek, T.A., Hartig, P.R. (1992). Human serotonin 1D receptor is encoded by a subfamily of two distinct genes: 5-HT^{1D} alpha and 5-HT_{1D} beta. *Proceedings of the National Academy of Sciences U.S.A.* **89(8)**:3630–3634.

Welch, J., Manschreck, T., Redmond, D. (1994). Clozapine-induced seizures and EEG changes. *Journal of Neuropsychiatry and Clinical Neuroscience* **6(3)**:250–256.

Weng, Y., Siciliano, S.J., Waldburger, K.E., Sirotina-Meisher, A., Staruch, M.J., Daugherty, B.L., Gould, S.L., Springer, M.S., DeMartino, J.A. (1998). Binding and functional properties of recombinant and exogenous CXCR3chemokine receptors. *Journal of Biological Chemistry* **273**:18288–18291.

Wenzel, B.E., Gutekunst, R., Heesemann, J. (1991). Hashimoto's thyroiditis and enteropathogenic *Yersinia enterocolitica*. In: Scherbaum, W.A., Weinheimer, B., Bogner, U., Bottazzo, G.F. (eds), *Autoimmune Thyroiditis: Approaches towards Its Etiological Differentiation*, pp. 205–210. Berlin: Springer-Verlag.

Wenzel-Seifert, K., Liu, H.Y., Seifert, R. (2002). Similarities and differences in the coupling of human beta 1- and beta 2-adrenoceptors to Gs (alpha) splice variants. *Biochemical Pharmacology* **64**:9–20.

Wess, J. (1998). Molecular basis of receptor/G-protein-coupling selectivity. *Pharmacological Therapy* **80(3)**:231–264.

Wheatley, M., Hawtin, S.R. (1999). Glycosylation of G-protein-coupled receptors for hormones central to normal reproductive functioning: Its occurrence and role. *Human Reproductive Update* **5(4)**:356–364.

White, J.H., Wise, A., Main, M.J., Green, A., Fraser, N.J., Disney, G.H., Barnes, A.A., Emson, P., Foord, S.M., Marshall, F.H. (1998). Heterodimerization is required for the formation of a functional $GABA_{(B)}$ receptor. *Nature* **396(6712)**:679–682.

White, S.H., Ladokhin, A.S., Jayasinghe, S., Hristova, K. (2001). How membranes shape protein structure. *Journal of Biological Chemistry* **276**:32395–32398.

Whitehead, I.P., Zohn, I.E., Der, C.J. (2001). Rho GTPase-dependent transformation by G protein-coupled receptors. *Oncogene* **20(13)**:1547–1555.

Wilbanks, A., Zondlo, S.C., Murphy, K., Mak, S., Soler, D., Langdon, P., Andrew, D.P., Wu, L., Briskin, M. (2001). Expression cloning of the STRL33/BONZO/TYMSTR ligand reveals elements of CC, CXC and CX3C chemokines. *Journal of Immunology* **166(8)**:5145–5154.

Williams, R.T., Parke, D.V. (1964). The metabolic fate of drugs. *Annual Review of Pharmacology* **4**:85–114.

Wirshing, D.A., Wirshing, W.C., Kysar, L., Berisford, M.A. (1999). Novel antipsychotics: Comparison of weight gain liabilities. *Journal of Clinical Psychology* **60(6)**:358–363.

Wong, D.T., Bymaster, F.P., Engleman, E.A. (1995). Prozac (fluoxetine, Lilly 110140), the first selective serotonin uptake inhibitor and an antidepressant drug: Twenty years since its first publication. *Life Sciences* **57(5)**:411–441.

Wong, D.T., Horng, J.S., Bymaster, F.P., Hauser, K.L., Molloy, B.B. (1974). A selective inhibitor of serotonin uptake: Lilly 110140, 3-(*p*-trifluoromethylphenoxy)-*N*-methyl-3-phenylpropylamine. *Life Sciences* **15(3)**:471–479.

Wright, R.A., Arnold, M.B., Wheeler, W.J., Ornstein, P.L., Schoepp, D.D. (2000). Binding of [^{3}H]-(2S,1'*S*,2'*S*)-2-(9—xanthylmethyl)-2-(2'-carboxycycloprrpyl) glycine ([^{3}H]-LY341495) to cell membranes expressing recombinant human group III metabotropic glutamate receptor subtypes. *Nauyn-Schmiedebergs Archives of Pharmacology* **362**:546–554.

Wu, S., Wright, R.A., Rockey, P.K., Burgett, S.G., Arnold, J.S., Rosteck, P.R. Jr., Johnson, B.G., Schoepp, D.D., Belagaje, R.M. (1998). Group III human metabotropic glutamate receptors 4,7 and 8: molecular cloning, functional expression, and comparison of pharmacological properties in RGT cells. *Brain Research: Molecular Brain Research* **53(1–2)**:88–97.

Wu, S., Xing, Q., Gao, R., Li, X., Gu, N., Feng, G., He, L. (2005). Response to chlorpromazine treatment may be associated with polymorphisms of the DRD2 gene in Chinese schizophrenic patients. *Neuroscience Letters* **376(1)**:1–4.

Wuyts, A., Proost, P., Lenaerts, J-P., Ben-Baruch, A., Van Damme, J., Wang, J.M. (1998). Differential usage of the CXC chemokine receptors 1 and 2 by interleukin-8, granulocyte chemotactic protein-2 and epithelial-cell-derived neutrophil attractant-78. *European Journal of Biochemistry* **255(1)**:67–73.

Wyatt, R., Sodroski, J. (1998). The HIV-1 envelope glycoproteins: Fusogens, antigens, and immunogens. *Science* **280(5371)**:1884–1888.

Wyse, B.D., Prior, I.A., Qian, H., Morrow, I.C., Nixon, S., Muncke, C., Kurzchalia, T.V., Thomas, W.G., Parton, R.G., Hancock, J.F. (2003). Caveolin interacts with the angiotensin II type 1 receptor during exocytic transport but not at the plasma membrane. *Journal of Biological Chemistry* **278(26)**:23738–23746.

Yamada, J., Sugimoto, Y., Horisaka, K. (1995). Serotonin2 (5-HT2) receptor agonist 1-(2,5-dimethoxy-4-iodophenyl)-2-aminopropane (DOI) inhibits chlorpromazine- and haloperidol-induced hypothermia in mice. *Biology and Pharmaceutical Bulletin* **18(11)**:1580–1583.

Yamada, T., Horiuchi, M., Dzau, V.J. (1996). Angiotensin II type 2 receptor mediates programmed cell death. *Proceedings of the National Academy of Sciences USA* **93(1)**:156–160.

Yanagiasawa, H., Amemiya, Y., Kanazaki, T., Shimoji, Y., Fujimoto, K., Kitahari, Y. (1996). Nonpeptide angiotensin II receptor antagonists: Synthesis, biological activities, and structure–activity relationships of imidazole-5-carboxylic acids bearing alkyl, alkenyl, and hydroxyalkyl substituents at the 4-position and their related compounds. *Journal of Medicinal Chemistry* **39(1)**:323–338.

Yang-Feng, T.L., Xue, F.Y., Zhong, W.W., Cotecchia, S., Frielle, T., Caron, M.G., Lefkowitz, R.J., Francke, U. (1990). Chromosomal organization of adrenergic receptor genes. *Proceedings of the National Academy of Science U.S.A.* **87(4)**:1516–1520.

Yang-Feng, T.L., Han, H., Lomansey, J.W., Caron, M.G. (1994). Localization of the cDNA for an alpha 1-adrenergic receptor subtype (ADRA1D) to chromosome band 20p13. *Cytogenetics and Cell Genetics* **66(3)**:170–171.

Yang, Y.K., Fong, T.M., Dickinson, C.J., Mao, C., Li, J.Y., Tota, M.R., Mosley, R., Van Der Ploeg, L.H., Gantz, I. (2000). Molecular determinants of ligand binding to the human melanocortin-4 receptor. *Biochemistry* **39(48)**:14900–14911.

Yankner, B.A., Duffy, L.K., Kirschner, D.A. (1990). Neurotrophic and neurotoxic effects of amyloid beta protein: Reversal by tachykinin neuropeptides. *Science* **250(4978)**:279–282.

Yeo, G.S.H., Lank, E.J., Farooqi, I.S., Keogh, J., Challis, B.G., O'Rahilly, S. (2003). Mutations in the human melanocortin-4 receptor gene associated with severe familial obesity disrupts receptor function through multiple molecular mechanisms. *Human Molecular Genetics* **12(5)**:561–574.

Yoshida, T., Imai, T., Heishima, K., Kusuda, J., Baba, M., Kitaura, M., Nishimura, M., Kakizaki, M., Nomiyama, H., Yoshie, O. (1997). Molecular cloning of a novel human CC chemokine EBl1-ligand chemokine that is a specific functional ligand for EBl1, CCR7. *Journal of Biological Chemistry* **272(21)**:13803–13809.

Yoshida, T., Imai, T., Kakizaki, M., Nishimura, M., Takagi, S., Yoshie, O. (1998). Identification of single C motif-1/lymphotactin receptor CXCR1. *Journal of Biological Chemistry* **273**:16551–16554.

Yoshie, O., Zlotnik, A. (2000). Chemokines: A new classification system and their role in immunity. *Immunity* **2**:121–127.

Zaballos, A., Varona, R., Gutiérrez, J., Lind, P., Márquez, G. (1996). Molecular cloning and RNA expression of two new human chemokine-like receptor genes. *Biochemical Biophysical Research Communications* **227(3)**:846–853.

Zaballos, A., Gutierrez, J., Varona, R., Ardavin, C., Marquez, G. (1999). Cutting edge: Identification of the orphan chemokine receptor GPR-9-6 as CCR9, the receptor for the chemokine TECK. *Journal of Immunology* **162**:5671–5675.

Zgombick, J.M., Schechter, L.E., Macchi, M., Hartig, P.R., Branchek, T.A., Weinshank, R.L. (1992). Human gene S31 encodes the pharmacologically defined serotonin 5-hydroxytryptamine1E receptor. *Molecular Pharmacology* **42(2)**:180–185.

Zhang, M., Tong, K.P., Fremont, V., Chen, J., Narayan, P., Puett, D., Weintraub, B.D., Szkudlinski, M.W. (2000). The extracellular domain suppresses constitutive activity of the transmembrane domain of the human TSH receptor: Implications for hormone-receptor interaction and antagonist design. *Endocrinology* **141(9)**:3514–3517.

Zhang, M.L., Sugawa, H., Kosugi, S., Mori, T. (1995). Constitutive activation of the thyrotropin receptor by deletion of a portion of the extracellular domain. *Biochemical and Biophysical Research Communications* **211(1)**:205–210.

Zhang, Z., Austin, S.C., Smyth E.M. (2001). Glycosylation of human prostacyclin receptor: Role in ligand binding and signal transduction. *Molecular Pharmacology* **60(3)**:480–487.

Zhao, J., Ma, L., Wu, Y.L., Wang, P., Hu, W., Pei, G. (1998). Chemokine receptor CCR5 functionally couples to inhibitory G proteins and undergoes desensitization. *Journal of Cellular Biochemistry* **71(1)**:36–45.

Zhou, F., Filipeanu, C.M., Duvernay, M.T., Wu, G. (2006). Cell-surface targeting of α_2-adrenergic receptors-Inhibition by a transport deficient mutant through dimerization. *Cell Signal.* **18(3)**:318–327.

Zoffmann, S., Turcatti, G., Galzi, J., Dahl, M., Chollet, A. (2001). Synthesis and characterization of fluorescent and photoactivaTable MIP-1α ligands and interactions with chemokine receptors CCR1 and CCR5. *Journal of Medicinal Chemistry* **44(2)**:215–222.

Zoler, M.L. (2005). Conivaptan reverses hyponatremia: Based on positive Phase III studies, FDA issued an approvable letter for the sodium-regulating drug (Rx). *Internal Medicine News* **38(4)**:52.

Zyprexa (Olanzapine) Tablets (product information). (2004). Indianapolis, IN, Eli Lilly.

8

Pharmacogenomics of Cardiovascular Drugs

Parshuram J. Sonawane, Bhavani S. Sahu and Nitish R. Mahapatra*

Cardiovascular Genetics Lab, Department of Biotechnology, Indian Institute of Technology Madras, Chennai, India

INTRODUCTION

Pharmacogenomics is a rapidly evolving area aimed at understanding the genetic contribution to interindividual variability in the efficacy and toxicity of drugs. It holds great promise for individualized therapy based on a person's genetic makeup, which will allow selection of medicines that are likely to be the most effective with minimal toxicity. The drug discovery process can also be guided by pharmacogenomics. This chapter reviews the various approaches (candidate gene and genome-wide) and methods (polymorphism discovery techniques) to pharmacogenomics research, with special reference to cardiovascular diseases. The current literature on genetic associations with cardiovascular drug response is discussed. This chapter also describes the ways in which comprehensive genomic data might be utilized for treatment of highly prevalent cardiovascular diseases such as hypertension.

Cardiovascular diseases are the leading causes of mortality affecting ~25–35% people in urban populations worldwide (Gupta *et al.*, 2008; Rosamond *et al.*, 2008). These diseases not only result in an enormous loss of human life, but also lead to a huge health-care cost, tremendous economic and social burden and declining national productivity and quality of life. While the mortality associated with cardiovascular diseases seems to be declining in Western Europe and North America (Muller-Nordhorn *et al.*, 2008; Rosamond *et al.*, 2008), the burden of cardiovascular diseases continues to rise and is expected to be a major cause of death in adults from developing countries (Mathers and

---

*nmahapatra@iitm.ac.in

Loncar, 2006). Notably, South Asians have a greater prevalence of cardiovascular risk factors than the rest of the world (Joshi *et al.*, 2007), and India itself is estimated to have 60% of the world's heart disease patients by 2010 (Xavier *et al.*, 2008).

Numerous studies over the years have established several risk factors for cardiovascular diseases, including hypertension, dyslipidemia and tobacco use. Consequently, antihypertensive (such as angiotensin-converting enzyme [ACE] inhibitors or angiotensin receptor blockers [ARBs] or beta-blockers), cholesterol-lowering (such as 'statins') and other drugs (such as 'thrombolytics') are used for therapeutic interventions. It has been observed that while some individuals may attain the desired therapeutic effects from a particular drug, others may not respond at all and some patients may experience adverse drug reactions (ADRs). Moreover, a dose of a drug may be unsafe in some individuals while it is safe in others. Indeed, in the USA alone, it is estimated that over 2 million people are hospitalized and 100,000 die each year from ADR (Lazarou *et al.*, 1998). Of note, cardiovascular drugs were most often associated with ADR admissions in hospitals for adults and elderly patients in different populations (Passarelli *et al.*, 2005; Kongkaew *et al.*, 2008; Mehta *et al.*, 2008). Thus, there is a significant inter-patient variability in response to the drugs including those used to treat cardiovascular diseases.

Such variability in drug action may be due to various factors that include age, ethnicity, individual genetic makeup and interacting drugs. At present, the clinicians treat their patients with different drugs on a trial-and-error basis to find out the suitable one for a particular patient. Interestingly, recent studies have shown that for a number of drugs, genetic variability plays a very important role for the variable drug response. Therefore, the new area 'pharmacogenomics' is being pursued to have an understanding of the genetic contributions to drug efficacy and toxicity by investigation of the interactions between a putative pharmacological agent and person's genome. The ultimate aim of pharmacogenomics would be to tailor a drug according to a person's genetic makeup. This chapter summarizes the various approaches and methods for research on pharmacogenomics and reviews the current literature on cardiovascular pharmacogenomics.

MECHANISMS OF THE VARIABILITY IN DRUG ACTION: PHARMACOKINETICS AND PHARMACODYMANICS

The variability in drug action may be of two types: *pharmacokinetics* or *pharmacodynamics*. Pharmacokinetic variability refers to variability in delivery of drug to, or removal from, key molecular sites of action that mediate efficacy and/or toxicity. The molecules involved in these processes include both drug-metabolizing enzymes (DMEs; such as members of the cytochrome P450 [CYP] superfamily including CYP2D6 and CYP2C9, *N*-acetyltransferases [NAT2], thiopurine methyltransferase [TPMT] and UDP-glucuronosyltransferases [UDP-GT]) as well as drug transport molecules that mediate drug uptake into, and efflux from, intracellular sites (Roden, 2003; Meyer, 2004). On the other hand, pharmacodynamic variability refers to variable drug effects despite equivalent drug delivery to molecular sites of action that may be caused by variability in the function of the target molecule, at the receptor or post-receptor level (Roden, 2003). It is conceivable that an alteration in the DNA sequence of a gene encoding a DME/drug transporter may change its function and influence the pharmacokinetics of drugs. Similarly, an alteration in the DNA sequence of a gene encoding drug target protein may change its function and influence the pharmacodynamics of drugs. Indeed, a number of studies available in the literature showed that genetic variations (such as single nucleotide polymorphisms [SNPs] or halpotypes) influence the effect of cardiovascular drugs. Highlights of such studies are discussed in the section titled 'Evidences of cardiovascular pharmacogenomics'. The reader may visit the Pharmacogenomics Knowledge Base website (http://www.pharmgkb.org) for additional information.

EVIDENCES OF CARDIOVASCULAR PHARMACOGENOMICS

Several studies have reported the contribution/association of genetic variations on the variable (increased/decreased) response and ADR to cardiovascular drugs. Table 8.1 represents a list of such evidences known thus far. Of note, because there are many genetic association reports in the literature

Table 8.1 *Genes and Genotypes Associated with Response to Cardiovascular Drugs*

Gene(s)	*Genotype(s)*	*Drug Used in Study*	*Variation in Drug Response*
Angiotensin-converting enzyme *(ACE)*	Del/Ins (D/I)	Antiarrhythmic drug (AAD)	D allele is associated with failure to ADD therapy in patients with lone atrial fibrillation
		Hydrochlorothiazide (diuretic)	D allele showed reduced antihypertensive response
		ACE inhibitors	DD genotype associated with decreased proteinurea
Angiotensinogen *(AGT)*	Met235Thr	ACE inhibitor and AT1 receptor antagonist	T allele associated with greater reduction of blood pressure and greater decrease in left ventricular mass with antihypertensive treatment
Angiotensin II receptor type I *(AGTR1)*	A1166 C	Irbesartan (AT1 receptor antagonist)	C allele responded with greater reduction in left ventricular mass
		Losartan (AT1 receptor antagonist)	C allele associated with greater reduction in mean blood pressure
Bradykinin receptor B2 *(BDKRB2)*	C-58T	ACE inhibitors	T allele associated with ACE inhibitor–related cough
β-1 adrenergic receptor *(ADRB1)*	Arg389Gly	Metaprolol (β-blocker)	Arg/Arg homozygote hypertensives displayed greater reduction in blood pressure
β-2 adrenergic receptor *(ADRB2)*	Arg16Gly	Salbutamol, terbutaline (β-agonists)	Systemic infusions of β-agonists resulted in larger vasodilation in subjects homozygous for the Arg16 alleles
Cholesteryl ester transfer protein *(CETP)*	TaqIB polymorphism B1/B2	Pravastatin, atorvastatin (statin)	B1/B1 associated with increased response to pravastatin and atorvastatin

(Contd)

(Table 8.1 Contd)

Gene(s)	*Genotype(s)*	*Drug Used in Study*	*Variation in Drug Response*
Hepatic lipase *(LIPC)*	C-514T	Bezafibrate (lipid-lowering drug)	CC genotype associated with increased lipid-lowering response
Apolipoprotein E *(APOE)*	Epsilon 4	Pravastatin (statin)	Epsilon 4 carriers among myocardial infarction patients associated with a significant benefit in terms of survival
Adducin 1 *(ADD1)*	Gly460Trp	Hydrochlorothiazide (diuretic)	Trp allele associated with increased response to diuretics in hypertensives
Vitamin K epoxide reductase complex 1 *(VKORC1)*	HaplotypeA/ HaplotypeB	Warfarin (anticoagulant)	Haplotype A associated with 2.3-fold less dose requirement
Cytochrome P450 *(CYP2C9, CYP2D6)*	*CYP2C9*2* *CYP2C9*3*	Warfarin (anticoagulant)	Non-wild-type alleles associated with reduced warfarin daily dose requirement.
	*CYP2D6*4*	Metoprolol (β-blocker)	Patients carrying *CYP2D6*4* alleles are at increased risk of bradycardia
		Atorvastatin (statin)	*CYP2D6*4* allele associated with statin-induced muscle events

that either involved very small sample sizes or were not replicated, herein we have included only those pharmacogenomic examples for which there is some evidence of replication. These genetic variations may be classified into two major groups, described in the following subsections.

Drug Target/Pathway Gene Variations

Renin–angiotensin system (RAS) variants. RAS has been well studied for its important role in the pathophysiology of cardiovascular diseases. Angiotensinogen (AGT) is first converted by renin to angiotensin I, which is then converted to angiotensin II by ACE. A majority of the known actions of angiotensin II (AngII), the main effector molecule of RAS pathway, are mediated by AngII type I receptor (AGTR1), including arteriolar vasoconstriction and pressor responses (Baudin, 2005). Because of such profound roles, components of the RAS are important drug targets. Indeed, ACE inhibitors and AGTR1 blockers are used in treatment of several cardiovascular diseases (Schmieder *et al.*, 2007; Siest *et al.*, 2007). ACE inhibitors are the first-line agents in heart failure and are commonly used in hypertension and post-myocardial infarction. However, substantial variability in response to ACE inhibitors among patients has been observed. For example, less than 50% of hypertensive people achieve adequate lowering of blood pressure with ACE inhibitor monotherapy and the success rate is greater in White patients as compared to Black patients (Materson *et al.*, 1995). Such variability in drug response is thought to be contributed by the polymorphisms in the genes encoding the components of RAS. The most well described genetic variations in the RAS are *ACE* I/D (insertion/deletion of a 287-bp DNA segment in intron 16), AGT M235T (substitution of methionine by threonine at 235 codon) and *AGTR1* A1166C (A to C variant at 1166 nucleotide position in 3′-untranslated region [UTR]) polymorphisms (Rigat *et al.*, 1990; Siest *et al.*, 2007). Individuals homozygous for the D allele (DD genotype) have been reported to display almost 2-fold higher serum ACE levels than those homozygous for I allele (II genotype) (Rigat *et al.*, 1990). The D allele (ID and DD genotypes) has been associated with failure to antiarrhythmic drug (ADD) therapy in patients with lone atrial fibrillation—failure of drug response being 5%, 41% and 47% in patients with II, ID and DD genotypes (P <0 .005, II vs. ID/DD), respectively (Darbar *et al.*, 2007). Patients having at least one D allele also showed reduced response to the antihypertensive treatment by the diuretic hydrochlorothiazide that is used as a gold-standard therapy for hypertension (Sciarrone *et al.*, 2003; Jiang *et al.*, 2007). The DD genotype also displayed decreased proteinurea in response to ACE inhibitor treatment for renal disease (Goldstein *et al.*, 2003).

The T allele of AGT M235T polymorphism that displayed higher plasma AGT level (Schunkert *et al.*, 1997) has been associated with enhanced blood pressure reduction as well as greater reduction of left ventricular mass upon treatment with ACE inhibitor and AGTR1 antagonist irbesartan (Hingorani *et al.*, 1995; Kurland *et al.*, 2002). The greater degree of reduction of left ventricular mass by irbesartan was also associated with the C allele of *AGTR1* A1166C polymorphism as compared to the A allele (Kurland *et al.*, 2002). Similarly, carriers of the 1166C allele displayed greater decrease in mean blood pressure when treated with the AGTR1 antagonist losartan (Miller *et al.*, 1999). The RAS genetic polymorphisms may also contribute to ADRs during treatment with ACE inhibitors. For example, about 10% of the patients treated with ACE inhibitors develop dry cough, which is believed to be due to bradykinin accumulation during this therapy (Johnson and Humma, 2002). Of note, a proximal promoter polymorphism (C-58T) has been associated with the ACE inhibitor–related cough (Mukae *et al.*, 2000).

Beta-adrenergic receptor variants. Beta-blockers are frequently used in the treatment of several cardiovascular disease states including hypertension, heart failure and post-myocardial infarction. On the other hand, beta-agonists are used for ionotropic support in critically ill patients and in diagnostic procedures (Johnson and Humma, 2002). The responses to these drugs are mediated by beta-adrenergic receptors 1 and 2 (abbreviated as ADRB1 and ADRB2), which play a pivotal role in regulation of the activity of the sympathetic nervous system. The genetic variants in these receptors that have been consistently associated with drug response are ADRB1 Arg389Gly and ADRB2 Arg16Gly. *In vitro* mutagenesis studies have shown that basal adenylyl cyclase activity is nearly 2-fold higher for the Arg389 than for the Gly389 form and that there are more than 3-fold differences in the maximal beta-agonist stimulated adenylyl cyclase activity between the two variants (Mason *et al.*, 1999). Consistent with these findings, Arg389 homozygote individuals display a higher systolic and diastolic blood pressures as well as higher heart rate (Johnson and Humma, 2002). Thus, the ADRB1 Arg389 variant seemed to be an important determinant of beta-agonist and beta-blocker responses. Indeed, the beta-blocker metoprolol displayed a significantly greater blood pressure reduction in hypertensive patients homozygous for the Arg389 alleles than in patients with the Gly389 alleles (Brodde, 2008a). Similarly, the ADRB2 Arg16 allele has been associated with hypertension in several studies, suggesting functional effects with respect to agonist-mediated actions (Johnson and Humma, 2002). It has also been shown that the Arg16 variant displays greater agonist (viz. salbutamol, terbutaline)- mediated vasodilation than the Gly16 variant (Gratze *et al.*, 1999; Hoit *et al.*, 2000; Brodde, 2008b).

Cholesteryl ester transfer protein, hepatic lipase and apolipoprotein E variants. The relationships between the efficacies of lipid-lowering drugs with polymorphisms in the genes coding for cholesteryl ester transfer protein (CETP), hepatic lipase (LIPC) and apolipoprotein E (APOE) have been well studied in view of the association of polymorphisms in these genes with cardiovascular diseases (Nemeth *et al.*, 1995; Kuivenhoven *et al.*, 1998; Gerdes *et al.*, 2000; Isaacs *et al.*, 2004; Mohrschladt *et al.*, 2005; Chiodini *et al.*, 2007; Kathiresan *et al.*, 2008). Certain polymorphisms in these genes predict the degree of cholesterol lowering as well as the outcomes of lipid-lowering therapy. For example, the *CETP* TaqIB polymorphism (restriction polymorphism TaqIB in intron 1; the presence of the DNA variation was referred to as B1 and its absence as B2) has been shown to be a significant predictor of future cardiovascular events in patients treated with statins (HMG-CoA reductase inhibitors), such that homozygotes for TaqIB1 alleles display a greater response than TaqI B2/B2 carriers (Kuivenhoven *et al.*, 1998; Mohrschladt *et al.*, 2005). A promoter polymorphism (C-514T) in *LIPC* gene was associated with the activity of LIPC and high-density lipoprotein (HDL) levels: the CT and TT genotypes displayed significantly lower LIPC activity and higher HDL levels as compared to the CC genotype (Isaacs *et al.*, 2004). The CC genotype showed a better response to the lipid-lowering drug bezafibrate (an agonist of peroxisome proliferator activator receptor) with a better effect in homozygous CC subjects (Cenarro *et al.*, 2005). The carriers of epsilon4 allele (that contains arginine at 112 and 158 residue positions) of APOE have been associated with a significant beneficial effect in terms of survival from pravastatin treatment in myocardial infarction patients (Chiodini *et al.*, 2007).

Adducin 1 variants. Adducin 1 (ADD1) represents a 'renal hypertensive gene' that modulates the capacity of tubular epithelial cells to transport sodium and hence affects the blood pressure levels (Manunta *et al.*, 1999). Consistently, it has been suggested to play a role in the salt-sensitive form of essential hypertension in view of the significant linkage of the *ADD1* locus with hypertension (Cusi *et al.*, 1997). Indeed, there is a significant association between a Gly460Trp polymorphism in the *ADD1* gene and salt sensitivity in patients with essential hypertension: patients with the Trp460 allele showed greater sensitivity to changes in sodium balance, and heterozygous (Gly/Trp) hypertensive patients displayed a greater fall in mean arterial pressure in response to hydrochlorothiazide treatment, than did wild-type homozygous (Gly/Gly) hypertensive patients (Cusi *et al.*, 1997). Interestingly, patients carrying at least one I allele of *ACE* and one 460Trp allele of ADD1 had the largest mean blood pressure decrease with hydrochlorothiazide treatment. ADD1 Gly460Trp and *ACE* I/D polymorphisms may, therefore, be useful to predict the interindividual degree of response to hydrochlorothiazide (Sciarrone *et al.*, 2003).

VKORC1 (vitamin K epoxide reductase complex, subunit 1) variants. VKORC1, an 18-kDa transmembrane protein of the endoplasmic reticulum, is the target of coumarin anticoagulants. It recycles vitamin K epoxide to the reduced form of vitamin K, an essential cofactor in the formation of several active clotting factors (II, VII, IX and X) through γ-glutamyl carboxylation (Cain *et al.*, 1997). Many studies documented that genetic variants of VKORC1 result in altered sensitivity to the anticoagulant warfarin, requiring lower doses during long-term therapy to avoid adverse effects (Rieder *et al.*, 2005; Li *et al.*, 2006; Takahashi *et al.*, 2006; Scott *et al.*, 2008). For example, in a retrospective study of patients receiving long-term warfarin maintenance therapy, 10 common SNPs were identified in the noncoding regions of the *VKORC1* gene and five major haplotypes were inferred. Among those haplotypes, a low-dose haplotype group A and a high-dose haplotype group B were identified. The mean maintenance dose of warfarin differed significantly among the three haplotype group combinations, at ~2.7 mg/day for A/A, ~4.9 mg/day for A/B and ~6.2 mg/day for B/B genotypes (Rieder *et al.*, 2005). This study also revealed that Asian Americans displayed a higher proportion of group A haplotypes while African Americans a higher proportion of group B haplotypes. It is noteworthy that VKORC1 polymorphisms may, in some cases, contribute to the variation in dose requirement more than variants of the P450 enzyme CYP2C9, which catalyzes the metabolism of warfarin (Schwarz *et al.*, 2008).

Drug-Metabolizing Enzyme Gene Variations

The first phase in the metabolism and elimination of numerous endogenous and exogenous molecules and ingested drugs involves the hepatic cytochrome P450 (CYP) system, wherein the CYP enzymes convert these substances into electrophilic intermediates that are then conjugated by Phase II enzymes (e.g., UDP glucuronosyltransferases, *N*-acetyltransferases) to hydrophilic derivatives and excreted (Nebert, 1997). Genetic variations in these DMEs have long been recognized for their role in drug response variability. Certain polymorphisms may affect drug plasma concentrations and predispose patients to ADR or therapeutic failure despite treatment with usual drug doses (Johnson and Humma, 2002). Indeed, several DME genes have inactivating mutations (leading to absent or nonfunctional protein), which results in the ineffective elimination of the drug causing excessively high (as high as ~10-fold over normal) plasma drug concentrations. In such cases, drugs that have a narrow therapeutic range (a small range in which the drug exerts its efficacy without causing toxicity) can have profound adverse clinical consequences. On the other hand, if the drug has a wide therapeutic range, a marked increase in the plasma drug concentration is well tolerated. Notably, many cardiovascular drugs have wide therapeutic indexes although there are exceptions too (discussed below).

The genetic variations in the CYP family of enzymes have been extensively studied. Notably, the CYP2A6, CYP2C9, CYP2C19 and CYP2D6 enzymes have functional genetic variants with marked differences in allele frequencies among different ethnic populations (Evans and Johnson, 2001). However, the polymorphisms that have consistently associated with cardiovascular drug metabolism are located in the genes coding for the CYP2C9 and CYP2D6 enzymes.

CYP2C9 (cytochrome P450, subfamily 2C, polypeptide 9) variants. Two alleleic variants of *CYP2C9* gene have been identified (in addition to the wild-type *CYP2C9*1* allele): *CYP2C9*2*, where cysteine substitutes for arginine at amino acid position 144, and *CYP2C9*3*, where leucine substitutes for isoleucine at residue 359. Both these allelic variants have impaired hydroxylation of *S*-warfarin (an anticoagulant having ~5-fold greater activity than the *R*-enantiomer) when expressed *in vitro*; the *CYP2C9*3* variant is less than 5% as efficient as the wild-type enzyme, while *CYP2C9*2* shows about 12% of wild-type activity, as a result of the amino acid substitution altering the interaction of the enzyme with cytochrome P450 oxidoreductase (Stubbins *et al.*, 1996; King *et al.*, 2004). Therefore, people carrying *CYP2C9*2* and *CYP2C9*3* alleles are poor metabolizers of *S*-warfarin. Of note, *S*-warfarin has a narrow therapeutic range. Therefore, with a dose of warfarin (which is normal for people carrying wild-type *CYP2C9* alleles), the poor metabolizers will have toxic level of the drug in their plasma. Consistently, several studies reported that carriers of these non-wild-type alleles required lower mean daily warfarin dosage and were at a greater risk of over-anticoagulation and serious bleeding (Aithal *et al.*, 1999; Freeman *et al.*, 2000; Sanderson *et al.*, 2005). Those patients requiring low dose also had more difficulty with warfarin initiation (Aithal *et al.*, 1999; Higashi *et al.*, 2002; Veenstra *et al.*, 2005). Of note, up to 40% of Caucasians, while fewer Asians and Africans, carry one of these two variant alleles and hence are poor metabolizers (Daly and King, 2003). Thus, *CYP2C9* genotyping prior to warfarin initiation may provide useful information for prediction of the dose requirements as well as for reduction of the risk associated with over-anticoagulation in the carriers of *CYP2C9*2* and *CYP2C9*3* alleles.

CYP2D6 (cytochrome P450, subfamily 2D, polypeptide 6) variants. The metabolism of beta-blockers such as metoprolol, carvedilol, propranonol and antiarrhythmics such as propafenone, mexiletine and flecainide is catalyzed by the enzyme CYP2D6 (Johnson and Humma, 2002). For example, metabolism of metoprolol is primarily (~70–80%) carried out by CYP2D6. Accordingly, the polymorphisms in the *CYP2D6* gene have been well investigated. In Caucasians, 5–10% of the population lack CYP2D6 enzyme activity because of the inheritance of two nonfunctional alleles (e.g. *CYP2D6*3* or *CYP2D6*4* or *CYP2D6*5* or *CYP2D6*6*) of the *CYP2D6* gene and consequently these people are poor metabolizers (Bradford, 2002; Gaedigk *et al.*, 2008). On the other hand, subjects with two functional alleles (e.g. *CYP2D6*1*, *CYP2D6*2*) are extensive metabolizers, whereas heterozygous carriers of *CYP2D6* polymorphisms show large variability in their phenotype (Gaedigk *et al.*, 2008). Likewise, ultrarapid metabolizers have more than two functional copies of the *CYP2D6* gene and exhibit extremely high enzyme activity (Bijl *et al.*, 2009). However, the main polymorphism that leads to decreased enzyme activity is *CYP2D6*4*. This is a splice site substitution (G to A) mutation at the first nucleotide of exon 4 of the gene resulting in a shift of the splice site and introduction of a premature termination codon. It has been reported that the mutant protein had no residual activity (Gough *et al.*, 1990). Therefore, the plasma metoprolol concentrations in these patients having two copies of the *CYP2D6*4* allele can be as high as 5-fold over the normal level (Lennard *et al.*, 1983; McGourty *et al.*, 1985). Interestingly, poor metoprolol metabolizers did not experience significantly greater rates of toxicity from this drug in studies of hypertensives or heart failure patients (Johnson and Cavallari, 2005). However, a recent population-based cohort study of 1533 users of beta-blockers (mainly atenolol/metoprolol) established that in patients having *CYP2D6 *4/*4* genotype, the adjusted heart rate in metoprolol users was 8.5 beats/min lower than those with *1/*1 genotype, leading to an increased risk of bradycardia in the poor metabolziers (Bijl *et al.*, 2009).

CYP2D6 genetic polymorphism has also been reported to influence the cholesterol-lowering effect and tolerability of the HMG-CoA inhibitor simvastatin (Vermes and Vermes, 2004). *CYP2D6 *4* allele has also been associated with the adverse effect of atorvastatin such that the frequency of this allele was about 1.8-fold higher in atorvastatin-induced muscle patients as compared to the controls (Frudakis *et al.*, 2007).

PROCEDURE FOR DISCOVERY OF THE GENETIC ASSOCIATIONS WITH DRUG RESPONSE

Although much of the pharmacogenomics data available in the literature were generated without a systematic approach, any new project in this area should ideally involve the following steps.

Candidate Gene Selection

Pharmacogenomics researchers typically would start with a candidate gene approach in order to understand the variability in response to a drug among individuals. This is because there is prior knowledge of the genes/proteins that are important for pharmacokinetics or pharmacodynamics of the particular drug of interest. For example, if it is known that the drug is metabolized primarily by CYP2D6, then this metabolizing enzyme can be considered as a good candidate gene for pharmacogenomic study of that drug. Similarly, the drug target as well as all signal transduction proteins and upstream/downstream proteins should be included to select the candidate genes. For example, for pharmacogenomic study of an ACE inhibitor, besides ACE, other good candidate genes should be angiotensinogen, angiotensin type I receptor (AT1R) and bradykinin B2 (Johnson and Humma, 2002). Candidate genes may also be the genes coding for proteins involved in the physiological system that is interfered by the drug being studied. For example, in order to study the association of the response of lipid-lowering drugs (such as 'statins') to genetic variability, the candidate genes are not only those that code for the proteins directly involved in the drug response but also those involved in the lipid transport and metabolism (such as APOE, low-density lipoprotein receptor, lipoprotein lipase and CETP) (Johnson and Humma, 2002). Thus, selection of the candidate genes for pharmacogenomics research of a drug of interest should be based on the current knowledge about its metabolism, transport and mechanism of action as well as the physiological system in which the drug acts. Even a broader, more inclusive candidate gene approach may be taken into account because two or more systems may also be involved for the variable response to a drug. For example, the beta-adrenergic receptor system interacts with the renin–angiotensin system, as reflected by the association of an ACE gene polymorphism with beta-blocker response (McNamara *et al.*, 2001).

Discovery/Identification of Genetic Variations in the Candidate Genes

Once the candidate genes are selected, the pharmacogenomics researcher needs to know about the variability in the sequence of those genes. The investigator can get information about the known polymorphisms in the genes of interest from the NCBI SNP database (http://www.ncbi.nlm.nih.gov/SNP). Detection of those SNPs in the study population can be done by a number of methods such as polymerase chain reaction-restriction fragment length polymorphism (PCR-RFLP), denaturing high-performance liquid chromatography (DHLPC), pyrosequencing and others (see the section titled 'Genotyping techniques'). Alternatively, the investigator may undertake the SNP discovery approach to identify the variations in the sequence of the genes in the particular population of interest by re-sequencing the genes in a sufficient number of individuals (typically 100–200). In fact, the second approach may be better in view of the limitations (e.g. lack of validation and limited information on allele frequencies in diverse ethnic populations) on information in public databases. Typically, the proximal promoter (that contains binding sites for the transcription-regulatory proteins), the coding regions, intron/exon boundary regions as well the 5′- and 3′-UTRs (that contain elements interacting with specific translation-regulatory proteins) are sequenced (Wen *et al.*, 2004). However, the full intronic regions should also ideally be sequenced because intronic SNPs may also play important roles. For example, the intronic SNP rs1333049 near the cyclin-dependent kinase inhibitors *CDKN2A/2B* loci on chromosome 9p21 has been repeatedly associated with coronary artery disease in various populations in several independent studies (Hiura *et al.*, 2008; Meng *et al.*, 2008; Schunkert *et al.*, 2008).

Functional Studies of the Genetic Variants

After identification/discovery of the polymorphisms in a gene of interest, the pharmacogenomics researcher should carry out functional studies prior to clinical association studies. The functional significance of a particular SNP can often be explored by *in vitro* experiments as suggested below.

(1) Testing the function of promoter SNPs. To test whether a SNP located in the promoter of a gene has implication for gene expression, the wild-type (major allele SNP-containing) promoter as well the promoter containing the minor allele SNP from individual DNA samples (preferably homozygous to the SNP) are PCR-amplified and cloned into a promoter-less firefly luciferase vector (e.g. pGL3-basic; Promega, USA). Sequencing of the promoter–reporter constructs are done to ensure that the two types of constructs differ from each other only at the SNP position. If other variations are found between the two constructs, those are corrected by site-directed mutagenesis in order to specifically investigate role of the particular SNP. The constructs are utilized to transfect appropriate (determined on the basis of any tissue-specific expression of the concerned gene) cell lines, and the cell lysates are subjected to luciferase assay (Chen *et al.*, 2008). Reporter genes other than firefly luciferase may also be used to investigate the functional significance of a SNP discovered in the promoter region of the candidate gene. A significant difference in expression between the constructs would suggest that the SNP may be functional. Gel shift assays may also be done to test possible binding or alteration in the binding affinity of any transcription factor(s) at the site of SNP in the promoter under study (Mahapatra *et al.*, 2003, 2006).

(2) Testing the function of non-synonymous SNPs. This is typically done by expression of the wild-type and variant cDNAs in cell lines, followed by testing whether replacement with a particular amino acid causes enhancement or decrease or loss of function of the protein. Additionally, if the non-synonymous SNP alters an amino acid in a biologically active peptide, that peptide can be synthesized and its activity can be monitored by *in vitro* cell culture experiments. For example, as we have reported recently in the case of the endogenous peptide catestatin, the naturally occurring human variants displayed differential catecholamine-release-inhibitory potency (Mahata *et al.*, 2004; Mahapatra, 2008). Additionally, PANTHER database (that uses statistical models of protein families and subfamilies) is a good resource for assessing the likely functional effects of non-synonymous SNPs (Thomas *et al.*, 2006). This database (http://www.pantherdb.org/tools/csnpScoreForm.jsp) uses the patterns of sequence conservation and divergence found in related proteins from different organisms or other genes in the same organisms.

(3) Investigating the function of 5'- and 3'-UTR SNPs. The importance of UTRs in regulating gene expression is underlined by the finding that mutations that alter the UTR can have significant pathological implications (Conne *et al.*, 2000). Mechanistically, the post-transcriptional regulation of gene expression is mediated by *cis*-acting elements located in the 5′- and 3′-UTRs of mRNAs, which modulate the transport of mRNAs out of the nucleus, translation efficiency (van der Velden

and Thomas, 1999), subcellular localization (Jansen, 2001) and stability (Bashirullah *et al.*, 2001). Therefore, the pharmacogeomics researcher should investigate implication of any 5′- or 3′-UTR SNP. The experimental method involves PCR-amplification of UTR from genomic DNA samples (preferably homozygous to the wild-type and minor alleles), cloning at the upstream of SV40 promoter sequence (for 5′-UTR SNP) or downstream of the luciferase sequence (for 3′-UTR SNP) of the pGL3-promoter vector plasmid (Promega, USA; in which SV40 promoter drives the expression of firefly luciferase) and transfection into appropriate cell lines, followed by luciferase assay. It is noteworthy that similar plasmid vectors harboring other reporter genes may also be used to investigate the functional significance of the UTR SNPs. A time course experiment is done to investigate any influence of the SNP on message stability. A significant difference in luciferase activity between the constructs will suggest that the UTR SNP may be functional. Additionally, functional implication of any 3′-UTR SNP can be tested by investigating whether the SNP alters putative miRNA target sites and might be important effectors of phenotypic variation as in the case of G-to-A transition in the 3′-UTR of the myostatin (GDF8) gene creating a target site for mir1 and mir206, microRNAs that are highly expressed in skeletal muscle causing translational inhibition of the myostatin gene (Clop *et al.*, 2006). The 3′-UTR containing SNP may be analyzed to see whether it harbors any potential recognition motif of any microRNA using online algorithms (Rajewsky, 2006) such as PicTar (http://pictar.mdc-berlin.de) and RNA22 (http://cbcsrv.watson.ibm.com/rna22.html).

In vivo experimental approaches using transgenic mice can also be undertaken to test the functional significance of a SNP. For example, BAC transgenic mice models on a background of knockout of a locus of interest can be generated (Mahapatra *et al.*, 2005) in such as way that the 'humanized' transgenic strains express the human DNA variants. Such transgenic strains are then evaluated biochemically and physiologically. These experiments are technically more complex than above-mentioned *in vitro* cell culture experiments.

Clinical Association Studies

Once functional basis of a polymorphism in a candidate gene of interest for a particular drug is understood, clinical studies for possible association with any variation in drug response should be carried out. The clinical studies should have appropriate number of controls and patients to arrive at statistically significant conclusions because a study carried out with a small number of patients can give rise to false positive or false negative results. Indeed, to detect even relatively strong associations between genetic variants at a specific locus and variability in drug response, many cases and controls are necessary. For example, for detection of the effect of a gene variant that explains 5% of the total phenotypic variation in a quantitative response to a drug by genotyping 100 independent SNPs would require 500 patients to provide an 80% chance of detection, assuming an experiment-wide false-positive rate of 5% (Sham *et al.*, 2000; Goldstein *et al.*, 2003). Of note, the sample sizes for many of the reported pharmacogenomics studies are much smaller than required for this relatively modest aim. Thus, these studies are generally underpowered, even for detecting variants of relatively large effect (Goldstein *et al.*, 2003). Moreover, complications such as 'stratification' (Pritchard and Rosenberg, 1999; Reich and Goldstein, 2001) should be taken into account by the pharmacogenomics researcher. Stratification occurs when a patient population is genetically structured, and it can create spurious associations between genetic variations and drug responses (Goldstein *et al.*, 2003). Such false association can be detected and corrected as reported earlier (Siddiqui *et al.*, 2003). Another important issue regarding clinical association studies is lack of replication. Although ethnicity may account for the apparent anomaly between two studies (see the section titled 'Ethnicity and cardiovascular pharmacogenomics'), any clinical association should be investigated in independent populations for confirmation about the pharmacogenomics of the drug of interest.

Another approach that can be undertaken by pharmacogenomics researchers is the genome-wide approach. Polymorphisms in the study population can be discovered by using commercially available microarrays, as described in the subsection titled 'Genome-wide approach'. The next steps (*in vitro* and *in vivo* functional studies as well as clinical studies) should essentially be the same as discussed for candidate gene approach for association of drug response with genetic polymorphisms. Such systematically performed studies should potentially be important for clinical applications.

GENOTYPING TECHNIQUES

As discussed above, for pharmacogenomics studies, two approaches are taken to discover the genetic variation among individuals: candidate gene approach and genome-wide approach. In the first approach, the study is limited to one gene or a number of genes. On the other hand, the second approach involves looking for variations all over the genome; it has the potential to identify unsuspected genetic associations with drug response.

Candidate Gene Approach

A variety of techniques are used for determination of genetic variations in candidate genes. Researchers interested in SNP discovery carry out direct sequencing, which is the gold standard for genotyping. Typically, a DNA segment of interest is amplified from the genomic DNA of the patient/control population by PCR using sequence-specific primers, and the PCR product is sequenced by automated, fluorescence-based DNA sequencing. Then the sequences are aligned to detect the presence of SNPs. An example of SNP discovery using the chromatograms obtained by automated sequencing using fluorescent nucleotides is shown in Fig. 8.1. However, for those researchers who are interested in SNP genotyping (investigation to detect the presence or absence of previously reported SNPs in the patient/control populations) as opposed to SNP discovery (investigation to find out novel SNPs in the patient/control populations), DNA sequencing is rarely used as the primary genotyping method because of the limited availability of the sequencer equipment in every laboratory and higher expense per sample than other methods. Indeed, there are a number of other genotyping techniques available. Some of those commonly used methods are discussed below. The reader may go through the recently published reviews (Khripin, 2006; Kim and Misra, 2007; Wang *et al.*, 2007) for additional genotyping techniques.

(1) PCR-restriction fragment length polymorphism (PCR-RFLP). In this method, PCR is coupled with RFLP analysis (Shi, 2002). It involves PCR-amplification of a specific DNA segment containing the polymorphism of interest, followed by digestion of the PCR product with a specific restriction

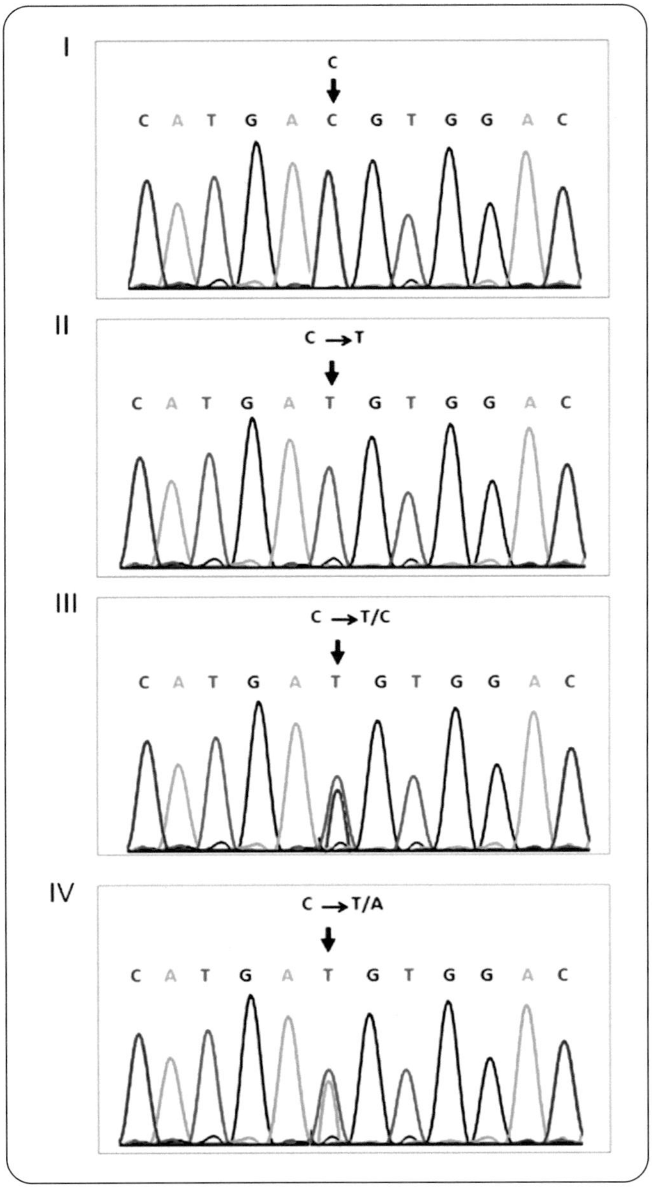

Fig. 8.1 ***Chromatograms of a Particular DNA Segment in Different Individuals (For color figure please see Plate 8)***

(The presence of nucleotide variations is discovered by comparing the DNA sequences. Screening of the chromatograms is particularly essential to detect the heterozygous alleles. *Panel I*, wild-type homozygous alleles (C); *Panel II,* homozygous mutant alleles (T); *Panel III,* a case of heterozygous mutant alleles (C to T/C representing substitution of the wild-type allele in one chromosome); *Panel IV*, another case of heterozygous mutant alleles (C to T/A representing substitution of the wild type alleles in both chromosomes). The polymorphic nucleotide position is indicated by downward arrow in each panel.)

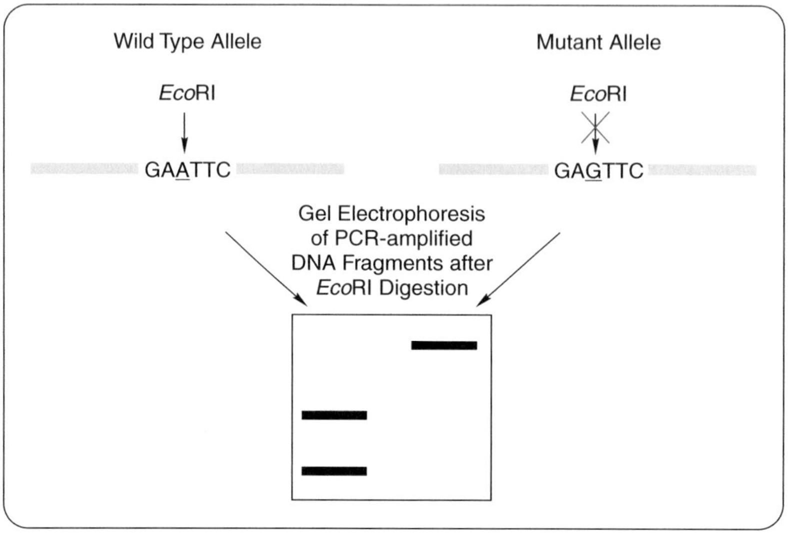

Fig. 8.2 *Schematic of PCR–RFLP Method for Detection of SNP*

(Genomic regions of interest are amplified by PCR and then the amplified DNA samples are digested with a specific restriction enzyme (e.g. *Eco*RI) and subjected to gel electrophoresis. The presence of a SNP alters the restriction endonuclease specificity and results in the different band pattern of the digested DNA fragments.)

enzyme that recognizes one polymorphic allele but not the other. The resulting DNA fragments are then separated by agarose gel electrophoresis and visualized by ethidium bromide staining (Fig. 8.2). This method has many advantages. It is cheap and does not require sophisticated instrumentation. Indeed, this method is widely used for the screening of limited number of known SNPs in a small number of samples. This method can also be utilized to ensure/complement the genotyping results of some samples that have been subjected to direct sequencing. However, this method has limitations too. First, a restriction enzyme that discriminates between the polymorphic alleles of interest may not always be commercially available. Second, this method is not automated and hence relatively time consuming and labor intensive. Therefore, it is not a feasible method for large-scale pharmacogenomic studies.

(2) Denaturing high-performance liquid chromatography (DHPLC). This method involves an ion-pair reversed-phase HPLC technique. It provides a useful platform for high-throughput mutation detection and SNP discovery required in candidate gene scanning projects (Xiao and Oefner, 2001). The method exploits the differential retention of homoduplex and heteroduplex DNA species that are generated by denaturation and annealing of PCR products under conditions of partial thermal denaturation. Homoduplexes are formed when both DNA strands have the same sequence, whereas heteroduplexes are formed by annealing of two strands with differing sequences. The heteroduplexes elute from the column earlier than the homoduplexes because of their reduced melting temperature. As the fragments elute, they are detected by ultraviolet (UV) light (typically at 254 or 260 nm). Analysis can be performed on individual samples to determine heterozygosity, or on mixed samples to identify

sequence variation between individuals. Indeed, efficient detection of single nucleotide variations including insertions and deletions in PCR-amplified DNA fragments can be achieved by DHPLC with a high level of automation (Yu *et al.*, 2006). The DHPLC results can be confirmed by direct sequencing. It is a cost-effective method to screen large numbers of crude PCR products for SNPs. DHPLC systems are available commercially from Cecil Instruments Ltd., UK, and Transgenomic WAVE System Instruments, USA.

(3) Pyrosequencing. This is a recently developed method for medium- to high-throughput determination of the nucleotide variations including deletions and insertions (Fakhrai-Rad *et al.*, 2002). The basic principle of pyrosequencing is that incorporation of each nucleotide by DNA polymerase into the DNA strand involves release of pyrophosphate, which is converted to ATP. The resultant ATP is utilized in the conversion of luciferin to oxyluciferin, which is accompanied by generation of light. The light thus produced is detected by a camera and displayed as a peak in a 'pyrogram'. Of note, the light signal (peak height) is indicative of the amount of ATP and hence it is proportional to the number of nucleotides incorporated. In the pyrosequencing reaction, each of the four dNTPs is added individually. If the added dNTP is complementary to the base in the template strand it is incorporated, giving rise to the light signal. The unincorporated dNTPs are degraded by the nucleotide-degrading enzyme Apyrase prior to addition of the next dNTP. Typically, the sequence of 20–30 nucleotides in the region of SNP is obtained by this method. This enables the user to verify the accuracy of the method. The major limitation of pyrosequencing is the cost of the instrument. However, technological advances to enhance the robustness of this technique as well as to reduce the cost and increase the throughput has made pyrosequencing as a genotyping method of choice to pharmacogenomics researchers (Ronaghi *et al.*, 2007). The instrument for pyrosequencing is commercially available from Biotage, Sweden.

(4) Single nucleotide primer extension (SNuPE). Single nucleotide primer extension followed by fluorescence detection technique can be used to rapidly detect SNPs for medium- to large-scale pharmacogenomic studies (Syvänen, 1999). A kit called 'SNaPshot', which utilizes the SNuPE technique, is commercially available from the Applied Biosystems, USA. The principle of the method is as follows. It first requires target amplification from genomic DNA, followed by purification of the amplified DNA. The SNaPshot primer targets a sequence immediately upstream of the SNP site and is extended by a single base in the presence of all four fluorescently labeled dideoxy nucleotides (ddNTPs). Each fluorescent ddNTP emits a different wavelength, which is translated into a specific color for each base. The size of the product is the size of the initial probe plus one fluorescent base. The genotypes are determined by the color and location of the peak that is generated from the emitted fluorescence. SNaPshot has been shown to be one of the best (considering accuracy, ease of use, throughput capability and cost-effectiveness) for genotyping large numbers of samples by virtue of its following useful features: nonradioactive, gel-free, able to genotype both alleles in a single reaction, does not require use of fluorescent oligonucleotide probes. Notably, this method can be multiplexed to detect up to 10 SNPs per sample by using differently sized primers, each of them designed to end one nucleotide upstream of the SNP position (Ben-Avi *et al.*, 2004; Pati *et al.*, 2004).

An alternative to fluorescent labeling to detect the appended nucleotide in SNuPE assays is based on the differences in molecular weights of the four nucleotides. In this method, mass (instead of color) of the resulting product after addition of the ddNTP (which is not fluorescently labeled) is measured by Mass Spectrometry through matrix-assisted laser desorption ionization-time of flight (MALDI-TOF) detectors to identify the polymorphic nucleotide (Griffin and Smith, 2000). This combination of SNuPE and MALDI-TOF can be fully automated for high-throughput genotype determination. Moreover, multiplexing to detect multiple SNPs in a single reaction is possible by using primers of different masses (Yang *et al.*, 2003). Indeed, the MassARRAY system from Sequenom, USA, can probe up to about 36 SNPs per sample using its iPLEX Gold assay kit.

In spite of such advantages, there is a major limitation of the SNuPE and MALDI techniques. These techniques are very sensitive to impurities that can affect the specificity of ddNTP incorporation by DNA polymerase during the SNuPE reaction and interfere with the mass spectrometry (Tost and Gut, 2002). Therefore, purification of the PCR product is required prior to the SNuPE reaction. The cost of a mass spectrometer is also quite high, limiting widespread use of this technique for pharmacogenomic studies. However, once the instrument is procured, the cost per sample is comparable to other methods.

Genome-Wide Approach

Identification of a large number of nucleotide variations across the genome can be done utilizing the several commercially available SNP microarrays. For example, the Genome-Wide Human SNP Array 6.0 developed by Affymetrix, USA, can test about 1 million SNPs at a time in a sample. The basic principle of this technique is hybridization of fluorescent-labeled allele-specific probes (generated from the genomic DNA) with oligos on microarrays (in which each array position corresponds to a particular genomic variant) followed by detection to record and interpret the hybridization signal. Similarly, Illumina, USA, offers BeadChip-based 'Infinium' products that can test up to 1.2 million genomic variations. In the 'Infinium' assay, genomic DNA is PCR-amplified, fragmented, hybridized to the array, and then extended by one base, which is fluorescently labeled. The allele is determined based on the resulting color. Given that there are an estimated 10 million SNPs in the genome, these arrays can capture only ~10% of the genetic variability. Nevertheless, these high-density microarrays are a significant improvement over their earlier versions, which could test only a few thousand SNPs at a time. Of note, although not for a pharmacogenomics project, such genotyping arrays (e.g. Human Mapping 500K Array Set from Affymetrix) were recently used to identify the SNPs associated with complex human diseases in large numbers of human samples, establishing the feasibility and reproducibility of genome-wide approaches (Fischer *et al.*, 2005; Samani *et al.*, 2007; The Wellcome Trust Case Control Consortium, 2007). These approaches are advantageous because of their potential to advance our understanding of the link between genes and health/diseases in a very short time span. However, the downsides of these methods include the difficulty to determine the true SNPs over false positives besides the high cost involved, although the expenses are declining gradually. Such genome-wide approach focusing on the overall variability within the genome has the greatest potential application in cardiovascular pharmacogenomics (Kennedy *et al.*, 2003).

It is hoped that genome-wide approaches will be perfected through the data from the International HapMap Project (http://www.hapmap.org). The HapMap project focuses on the finding that genetic variations often occur in blocks (called haplotypes). A haplotype is a group of genetic variants or genotypes closely linked in one chromosome and inherited together as a unit at a frequency higher than expected by chance. The HapMap catalogs the locations of common haplotypes throughout the genome and describes their distribution across populations. The major benefits associated with the identification of haplotypes rather than individual SNPs include the ability to reduce the amounts of tests necessary to find a genomic area of interest and to use a marker (tag) SNP to find a disease-causing SNP or an SNP associated with variable drug response (Skelding *et al.*, 2007). Of note, it is anticipated that the HapMap project might identify about 500,000 'tag' SNPs that could be the representative of the genetic variation across the entire human genome (Johnson and Cavallari, 2005). Besides HapMap, the 1000 Genomes Project <http://www.1000genomes.org> may also play significant roles in cardiovascular pharmacogenomics.

ETHNICITY AND CARDIOVASCULAR PHARMACOGENOMICS

Because people of different ethnicity are likely to have different genetic makeup, certain genetic variants may occur in higher or lower percentage in a particular ethnic group. Therefore, it is conceivable that a cardiovascular drug may have variable response in different populations: it may work better in one ethnic group as compared to another. Indeed, there are strong evidences for such ethnicity-specific effects, which have been summarized in a recent review (Johnson, 2008). The most notable differences were observed in response to beta-blockers, ACE inhibitors and angiotensin receptor blockers (ARBs). For example, 62% of people of European ancestry (Whites) and 54% of African ancestry (Blacks) achieved their blood pressure goal with propranolol, whereas such goal was attained with hydrochlorothiazide in 55% of Whites and 71% of Blacks (Veterans Administration Cooperative Study Group on Antihypertensive Agents, 1982). Similarly, atenolol and captopril were found to be less effective at lowering of blood pressure than hydrochlorothiazide and diltiazem, particularly in older Blacks (Materson *et al.*, 1993; Preston *et al.*, 1998). Many other studies also reported differential responses to antihypertensive drugs between Blacks and Whites. In general, Blacks respond slightly better than Whites to diuretics and calcium channel blockers, whereas Whites respond more favorably than Blacks to ACE inhibitors and beta-blockers (Brewster *et al.*, 2004; Evans and Johnson, 2001).

The influence of ethnicity on the warfarin dose required for maintaining a therapeutic international normalized ratio (INR) between 2 and 3 is another interesting example. Such difference is contributed by the variations in the *CYP2C9* gene among these ethnic groups (as discussed in the section titled 'Evidences of cardiovascular pharmacogenomics'). The average daily dose of the anticoagulant warfarin differs significantly among various ethnic groups: 3.4 mg in Asians, 5.1 mg in Whites and 6.1 mg in Blacks (Dang *et al.*, 2005). Given that the dosing algorithms typically recommend initiation of warfarin therapy at 5 mg/day, this is a reasonable starting dose in Whites but likely an excessive dose in Asians and an inadequate dose in Blacks.

Heart failure therapies have also associated with ethnicity-based differences, although with a lot of controversies. For example, the African American Heart Failure Trial (AHeFT), which enrolled only African Americans to test the efficacy of isosorbide dinitrate–hydralazine (I–H) and showed a 43% reduction in death compared to placebo, led to the FDA approval of I–H for treatment of African Americans with heart failure (Taylor *et al.*, 2004). Of note, the A-HeFT trial was stimulated by data from the V-HeFT (Vasodilator-Heart Failure Trial) I and V-HeFT II trials, which suggested that

Blacks derived greater benefit from I–H than Whites (Carson *et al.*, 1999). An explanation for better efficacy of I–H in Blacks than in Whites is that there might be a 'responsive' genotype that occurs more commonly in Blacks (Johnson, 2008).

Based on the findings on ethnic differences (including those highlighted above) in responses to cardiovascular drugs, one can speculate that pharmacogenomics may contribute to our understanding of ethnic differences in drug response and provide guidance during selection of drugs. However, besides the presumably different genetic makeup of the people from different ancestries, environmental (such as diet) as well as demographic differences may also contribute to the drug response variability. Additionally, for most drug responses, a variety of genes may be involved, thus making any calculation of the role of pharmacogenomics on ethnic differences more challenging. Moreover, accumulation of sufficient data to argue that the genetic information is predictive enough to be useful clinically as well as providing the necessary education to the clinicians for adoption to practice are challenging tasks (Johnson, 2008). It may be predicted that as more pharmacogenomics studies are carried out over the next few decades with advancement of genomic technologies, use of genetic and other patient-specific information, including environmental factors, may turn out to be superior to the ethnicity information to guide selections of cardiovascular drugs.

APPLICATION OF PHARMACOGENOMICS IN CARDIOVASCULAR DRUG DISCOVERY

The current drug discovery process (including that for cardiovascular drugs) is a lengthy, complicated and expensive exercise that usually requires several years of basic research (involving identification of a potential target gene and validation of the target), followed by establishment of effective screening assays allowing high-throughput screening of thousands of chemical entities (small organic molecules) to identify the 'hit' molecules, which affect the target protein. The hit molecules are then evaluated for their chemical properties, and potency in order to select 'lead' molecules, which are then subjected to further chemical modification (called 'lead optimization') for more effective drug function. Once a lead molecule is identified, preclinical studies including drug metabolism and toxicology in animal models are also undertaken. After the lead molecule displays safety and efficacy in animal studies, clinical trials in humans are done in various phases. In Phase I, the safety, metabolism and excretion of the molecule are tested in a small number of normal human volunteers using a small dose. Then the molecule enters the most crucial phase, Phase IIA, during which the efficacy (i.e. the desired clinical effect) as well as safety are tested in a relatively small number of patients (tens of patients). It has been estimated that even if ~100 patients participate in a Phase IIA study, the study would cost US $1 million (Roses, 2004). After the molecule passes the Phase IIA study, more extensive Phase IIB studies for safety, efficacy and dose ranging are done in a larger group of patients (hundreds of patients), which are followed by Phase III trials (randomized and controlled clinical studies for determination of comparative safety and efficacy) in a larger population (thousands of patients), requiring several hundreds of millions of dollars. Only those molecules that successfully pass these extensive trials are selected as drug molecules. As outlined below, pharmacogenomics principles can be applied at various stages of the drug discovery and drug development process.

As mentioned at the beginning of this section, the discovery of drug targets is the crucial step in supplying disease-relevant molecules to the drug development pipeline. The currently used drugs represent only about 500 different drug targets, majority of them belonging to target classes such as nuclear receptors, kinases and 7-transmembrane repeats (Drews, 2000). With the availability of human and mouse genome sequences, rapid analysis of the genes is now possible to discover addition target genes having similarity with the known targets (Roses, 2004). Indeed, there is a tremendous potential for increasing the number of novel drug targets because there could be up to 5000–10,000 potential drug targets, of which perhaps a few hundred might be relevant to the treatment of human diseases (Debouck and Metcalf, 2000; Searls, 2003; Johnson and Cavallari, 2005). Clearly, the prerequisite for this approach is an understanding of the molecular basis (the susceptibility genes and their molecular pathways) of the concerned diseases. The next step will be to discover the genetic variations (SNPs and haplotypes) among individuals by genomic techniques. Of note, it is unclear whether individual SNPs or the haplotypes in a particular gene represent most appropriate measures of genetic variability, because statistical algorithms indicate that there is no correct empirical choice and that both single SNPs and gene haplotypes could equally be suitable metrics for assessing correlations between genotype and clinical outcome (Gould Rothberg, 2001). Nevertheless, recent association studies on the responsiveness of B1- and B2-adrenergic receptors uncovered significant correlation between drug response and gene haplotypes, but not in individual SNPs suggesting the superiority of haplotypes over individual SNPs (Drysdale *et al.*, 2000; Small *et al.*, 2008). Thus, it may be important to perform SNP or haplotype assessment once the total number of candidate gene SNPs and their resulting haplotypes has been determined in order to find out the better predictor of genetic variability.

Pharmacogenomics information has typically been applied retrospectively to develop molecular diagnostics for optimization of drug selection as well as the dose of the drug (Dos Santos *et al.*, 2004; Paez *et al.*, 2004; Tantisira *et al.*, 2004). However, it is possible to apply the pharmacogenomics information related to drug efficacy in a prospective manner in order to reduce the attrition of effective drugs at an early stage (such as Phase IIA) of drug development. Indeed, most lead molecules fail in Phase IIA because the number of subjects (mixture of likely responders and likely nonresponders) at this stage is usually not large enough for convincing statistical significance (Roses, 2004). If the population of likely responders and likely nonresponders could be segmented on the basis of their genetic profiles early in Phase IIA, and only the potential responders are included, better outcome is expected. Reiterative studies can, anyway, be carried out to confirm whether or not the genetic variants identified in Phase IIA as being associated with efficacy are really useful for subsequent clinical studies. Thus, the pharmacogenomics approach (removing apparent nonresponders could enrich the remaining patient population) offers the possibility of reducing the size and expense of clinical trials (Shi *et al.*, 2001). Pharmacogenomic studies can also contribute to the safety issues, specifically ADRs, at two important stages in the development pipeline. First, during the early phases of clinical trials, if indications of a potential future ADR are observed in some participants, they present considerable risks to the drug development program. The second is after the launch of a drug, when thousands of patients consume the drug and ADRs are detected in some people (Roses, 2004). In both these stages, genomics information may be valuable to identify the genetic variations associated with the ADRs. The patients having the specific genetic variations that contribute to the

ADR should be excluded from the treatment with the particular drug. Thus, pharmacogenomics data can not only play a significant role during the clinical trials, but those can also improve the post-marketing surveillance system to address the safety issues related to the drug.

Another major advantage of utilization of pharmacogenomics data for segmentation of patients by therapeutic efficacy in the drug discovery process is the opportunity to develop multiple drug molecules for a particular disorder (Webster *et al.*, 2004). Some of the drug molecules may be useful for the patients belonging to a particular genomic subgroup (e.g. that harbors a particular allelic variant of the drug target) while some of these molecules may work in all subgroups (that have different allelic variants of the drug target, as may occur in people of different ethnicities). The lead molecules should extensively be tested to ensure their activity toward the allelic variants. Thus, pharmacogenomics can play important roles in various stages of the drug discovery pipeline. Essentially, application of the genetic variability information of drug (pharmacodynamics or pharmacokinetics) should make the drug discovery process more efficient and result in safer and more effective new medicines.

APPLICATION OF PHARMACOGENOMICS IN CARDIOVASCULAR CLINICS

Pharmacogenomics can play a tremendous role in the treatment of cardiovascular diseases. At present, all the patients diagnosed with a particular disease state (such as hypertension) are treated in the same way (with one or two drugs to reduce their blood pressure) although they will not respond similarly. As a result, the initial drug treatment is quite often abandoned because of a lack of response or ADR, and alternative drugs are administered. Of note, in the Antihypertensive and Lipid-Lowering Treatment to Prevent Heart Attack Trial (ALLHAT; the largest antihypertensive trial and the second largest lipid-lowering trial involving 42,418 patients), as many as 20% of the participants discontinued the initial treatment either due to ADR or drug failure (ALLHAT Officers and Coordinators for the ALLHAT Collaborative Research Group, 2002).

The existing (as detailed in the section titled 'Evidences of cardiovascular pharmacogenomics') and new knowledge that would be generated by pharmacogenomics research will find application in cardiovascular clinics. For example, apart from pravastatin and rosuvastatin, HMG-CoA reductase inhibitors are metabolized by the CYP superfamily of drug-metabolizing enzymes. Because CYP2D6 plays an important role in the metabolism of simvastatin and CYP2D6 genetic polymorphism influences the cholesterol-lowering effect and tolerability of this drug, determination of genetic variations in this gene may help to select the appropriate HMG-CoA reductase inhibitor as well as the optimal dose during the start of the statin treatment (Vermes and Vermes, 2004). Another example is the anticoagulant warfarin, its clinical outcome being influenced by the variations in the *CYP2C9* and *VKORC1* genes (discussed in the sections titled 'Evidences of cardiovascular pharmacogenomics' and 'Ethnicity and cardiovascular pharmacogenomics'). The CYP2C9 protein is involved in the metabolism of warfarin while the VKORC1 protein helps regulate the ability of warfarin to prevent blood from clotting. Patients with certain genetic variations are at an increased risk of bleeding with warfarin therapy and require a lower dose of warfarin doses than people without these genetic variations. Indeed, the initiation dose of warfarin may be determined on the basis of ethnicity and genetic varations in the patients. Although some people would argue that initiation of therapy with an inappropriate dose can be corrected quickly on the basis of close monitoring of INR, there is strong evidence suggesting that the risk of bleeding is highest in the first 30 days of therapy, when the appropriate dose is typically still being determined (White *et al.*, 1999). Therefore, a more accurate initial dosing of warfarin on the basis of pharmacogenomics data may reduce the early risk of bleeding and hence lead to better clinical management.

Pharmacogenomics has the potential to predict: (1) which hypertensive patients are likely to respond to particular antihypertensive drug(s), (2) which hypertensive patients are likely to have little or no benefit and (3) which hypertensive patients are at the risk of ADR. Therefore, clinicians can utilize pharmacogenomics information to choose a particular antihypertensive drug that is likely to produce the greatest blood pressure–lowering effect with the least risk of ADR for a particular patient. This approach is likely to minimize: (1) the period of time required to attain the required blood pressure, thereby reducing the risk for end organ damage due to sustained elevated blood pressure (for a relatively longer period of time as would be the case under current trial-and-error mode of treatment), (2) the expenses for unnecessary drugs and (3) the possibility of ADR. However, these health-care benefits of pharmacogenomics can only be realized by close collaboration between clinicians and scientists because pharmacogenomic associations cannot guide therapy without explicit clinical evaluations. Likewise, clinical assessments need to be carried out utilizing current information about the genetic variants and their influence on drug response (Goldstein *et al.*, 2003).

CONCLUSIONS AND PERSPECTIVES

The therapeutic management of cardiovascular diseases such as hypertension is currently done on a trial-and-error basis in spite of using a large arsenal of antihypertensive drugs since more than 50 years. Cardiovascular pharmacogenomics has the potential to take us to the era of 'personalized medicine', which will involve application of 'the right drug in the right dose to the right patient at the right time'. The first step toward this goal is to discover all the genes underlying the various cardiovascular disease states. Once we know all the susceptibility genes, novel drug molecules can be devised utilizing the important target molecules in the various pathways and taking the genetic variations across the populations into consideration.

Pharmacogenomics can impact various phases of drug development including clinical trial design. For example, during the clinical trials, selection of patients can be guided by their pharmacogenomics information to predict the potential responders and nonresponders. By selecting out the predicted nonresponders, clinical trials can be made smaller, faster as well as less expensive. Pharmacogenomics information can also be utilized for identifying the potential side effects before entering full clinical trials as well as for post-market pharmaco-vigilance to effectively manage the safety issues.

Ethnicity seems to play an important role in cardiovascular pharmacogenomics because several genetic variants affecting the metabolism of many common drugs may occur more often in a specific ethnic group. These pharmacogenomic findings can be utilized during the screening of novel drugs. If a new molecule is observed to use a pathway that is affected by a common gene variant, attempts should be made to modify the molecule or to develop another molecule, which exerts its effect via a less variable pathway. Thus, for a particular disease state, more than one molecule may be developed to cover most patients specifically instead of the current hit-or-miss approach of treatment with a series of drugs.

The effects of genetic variation on cardiovascular drugs are relatively better studied as compared to other drugs. Currently, there are strong evidences that genetic variations influence both the efficacy and toxicity of cardiovascular drugs. Such genomic information can be used to guide new drug design process as well as determining the suitability of a drug in a particular population or subpopulation. Indeed, pharmacogenomics might be utilized for treatment of cardiovascular diseases such as hypertension by prediction of likely response of a patient to various antihypertensive medications prior to drug initiation. Although it may take several decades before clinicians prescribe 'personalized medicine' for each patient, pharmacogenomics data may lead to the use of therapeutic options in segments of the human population predicted to respond to certain drugs in near future. Moreover, pharmacogenomics information can be utilized to minimize ADRs, which have been associated with cardiovascular drugs quite often.

A majority of the pharmacogenomic studies reported thus far were done retrospectively (i.e. the genetic studies were carried out after the responses had already been observed). Indeed, few genetic variants have been studied prospectively to assess how knowledge of the relevant genotype might be utilized to improve clinical outcomes, e.g. by adjusting doses or selecting the most appropriate drug as a function of the genotype (Goldstein *et al.*, 2003). Therefore, profound expansions of prospective studies are urgently needed for translation of pharmacogenomics research into improved therapies.

Although the area of pharmacogenomics is still in its infancy, it is evolving rapidly with extensive progress in genomics studies as the costs of genotyping are declining gradually. It is expected that continued research in this area, such as the 1000 Genomes Project (http://www.1000genomes.org) aiming to develop a new map of the human genome to provide a view of biomedically relevant DNA variations at an unprecedented resolution by sequencing the genomes of at least a thousand people from around the world, not only will play a significant role in guiding the drug therapy, but also will lead to the development of cardiovascular drugs with greater efficacy and fewer side effects, which in turn should result in a reduced number of cardiovascular events and lower the burden of health-care costs.

ACKNOWLEDGEMENTS

This work was supported in part by grants from the CSIR and DBT, Government of India, and a grant from the IC&SR, IIT Madras.

REFERENCES

Aithal, G.P., Day, C.P., Kesteven, P.J.L., Daly, A.K. (1999). Association of polymorphisms in the cytochrome P450 CYP2C9 with warfarin dose requirement and risk of bleeding complications. *Lancet* **353**:717–719.

ALLHAT Officers and Coordinators for the ALLHAT Collaborative Research Group. (2002). Major outcomes in high-risk hypertensive patients randomized to angiotensin-converting enzyme inhibitor or calcium channel blocker vs diuretic: The Antihypertensive and Lipid-Lowering Treatment to Prevent Heart Attack Trial (ALLHAT). *JAMA* **288**:2981–2997.

Bashirullah, A., Cooperstock, R.L., Lipshitz, H.D. (2001). Spatial and temporal control of RNA stability. *Proceedings of the National Academy of Sciences USA* **98**:7025–7028.

Baudin, B. (2005). Polymorphism in angiotensin II receptor genes and hypertension. *Experimental Physiology* **90**:277–282.

Ben-Avi, L., Durst, R., Shpitzen, S., Leitersdorf, E., Meiner, V. (2004). Apolipoprotein E genotyping: Accurate, simple, high throughput method using ABI Prism SNaPshot Multiplex System. *Journal of Alzheimer's Disease* **6**:497–501.

Bijl, M.J., Visser, L.E., van Schaik, R.H., Kors, J.A., Witteman, J.C., Hofman, A., Vulto, A.G., van Gelder, T., Stricker, B.H. (2009). Genetic variation in the CYP2D6 gene is associated with a lower heart rate and blood pressure in beta-blocker users. *Clinical Pharmacology and Therapeutics* **85**:45–50.

Bradford, L.D. (2002). CYP2D6 allele frequency in European Caucasians, Asians, Africans and their descendants. *Pharmacogenomics* **3**:229–243.

Brewster, L.M., van Montfrans, G.A., Kleijnen, J. (2004). Systematic review: antihypertensive drug therapy in black patients. *Annals of Internal Medicine* **141**:614–627.

Brodde, O.E. (2008a). Beta-1 and beta-2 adrenoceptor polymorphisms: Functional importance, impact on cardiovascular diseases and drug responses. *Pharmacology and Therapeutics* **117**:1–29.

Brodde, O.E. (2008b). Beta1- and beta2-adrenoceptor polymorphisms and cardiovascular diseases. *Fundamental and Clinical Pharmacology* **22**:107–125.

Cain, D., Hutson, S.M., Wallin, R. (1997). Assembly of the warfarin-sensitive vitamin K 2,3-epoxide reductase enzyme complex in the endoplasmic reticulum membrane. *Journal of Biological Chemistry* **272**:29068–29075.

Carson, P., Ziesche, S., Johnson, G., Cohn, J.N., Vasodilator-Heart Failure Trial Study Group (1999). Racial differences in response to therapy for heart failure: Analysis of the vasodilator-heart failure trials. *Journal of Cardiac Failure* **5**:178–187.

Cenarro, A., Artieda, M., Gonzalvo, C., Meriño-Ibarra, E., Arístegui, R., Gañán, A., Diaz, C., Sol, J.M., Pocoví, M., Civeira, F., ATOMIX Study Group (2005). Genetic variation in the hepatic lipase gene is associated with combined hyperlipidemia, plasma lipid concentrations, and lipid-lowering drug response. *American Heart Journal* **150**:1154–1162.

Chen, Y., Rao, F., Rodriguez-Flores, J.L., Mahapatra, N.R., Mahata, M., Wen, G., Salem, R.M., Shih, P.A., Das, M., Schork, N.J., Ziegler, M.G., Hamilton, B.A., Mahata, S.K., O'Connor, D.T. (2008). Common genetic variants in the chromogranin A promoter alter autonomic activity and blood pressure. *Kidney International* **74**:115–125.

Chiodini, B.D., Franzosi, M.G., Barlera, S., Signorini, S., Lewis, C.M., D'Orazio, A., Mocarelli, P., Nicolis, E., Marchioli, R., Tognoni, G., GISSI Investigators, SIBioC–GISSI Prevenzione Group (2007). Apolipoprotein E polymorphisms influence effect of pravastatin on survival after myocardial infarction in a Mediterranean population: The GISSI-Prevenzione study. *European Heart Journal* **28**:1977–1983.

Clop, A., Marcq, F., Takeda, H., Pirottin, D., Tordoir, X., Bibe, B., Bouix, J., Caiment, F., Elsen, J.M., Eychenne, F., Larzul, C., Laville, E., Meish, F., Milenkovic, D., Tobin, J., Charlier, C., Georges, M. (2006). A mutation creating a potential illegitimate microRNA target site in the myostatin gene affects muscularity in sheep. *Nature Genetics* **38**:813–818.

Conne, B., Stutz, A., Vassalli, J.D. (2000). The 3′ untranslated region of messenger RNA: A molecular 'hotspot' for pathology? *Nature Medicine* **6**:637–641.

Cusi, D., Barlassina, C., Azzani, T., Casari, G., Citterio, L., Devoto, M., Glorioso, N., Lanzani, C., Manunta, P., Righetti, M., Rivera, R., Stella, P., Troffa, C., Zagato, L., Bianchi, G. (1997). Polymorphisms of alpha-adducin and salt sensitivity in patients with essential hypertension. *Lancet* **349**:1353–1357.

Daly, A.K., King, B.P. (2003). Pharmacogenetics of oral anticoagulants. *Pharmacogenetics* **13**:247–252.

Dang, M.T., Hambleton, J., Kayser, S.R. (2005). The influence of ethnicity on warfarin dosage requirement. *Annals of Pharmacotherapy* **39**:1008–1012.

Darbar, D., Motsinger, A.A., Ritchie, M.D., Gainer, J.V., Roden, D.M. (2007). Polymorphism modulates symptomatic response to antiarrhythmic drug therapy in patients with lone atrial fibrillation. *Heart Rhythm* **4**:743–749.

Debouck, C., Metcalf, B. (2000). The impact of genomics on drug discovery. *Annual Review of Pharmacology and Toxicology* **40**:193–207.

Dos Santos, C., Essioux, L., Teinturier, C., Tauber, M., Goffin, V., Bougnères, P. (2004). A common polymorphism of the growth hormone receptor is associated with increased responsiveness to growth hormone. *Nature Genetics* **36**:720–724.

Drews, J. (2000). Drug discovery: A historical perspective. *Science* **287**:1960–1964.

Drysdale, C.M., McGraw, D.W., Stack, C.B., Stephens, J.C., Judson, R.S., Nandabalan, K., Arnold, K., Ruano, G., Liggett, S.B. (2000). Complex promoter and coding region beta 2-adrenergic receptor haplotypes alter receptor expression and predict *in vivo* responsiveness. *Proceedings of the National Academy of Sciences USA* **97**:10483–10488.

Evans, W.E., Johnson, J.A. (2001). Pharmacogenomics: The inherited basis for interindividual differences in drug response. *Annual Review of Genomics and Human Genetics* **2**:9–39.

Fakhrai-Rad, H., Pourmand, N., Ronaghi, M. (2002). Pyrosequencing: An accurate detection platform for single nucleotide polymorphisms. *Human Mutation* **19**:479–485.

Fischer, M., Broeckel, U., Holmer, S., Baessler, A., Hengstenberg, C., Mayer, B., Erdmann, J., Klein, G., Riegger, G., Jacob, H.J., Schunkert, H. (2005). Distinct heritable patterns of angiographic coronary artery disease in families with myocardial infarction. *Circulation* **111**:855–862.

Freeman, B.D., Zehnbauer, B.A., McGrath, S., Borecki, I., Buchman, T.G. (2000). Cytochrome P450 polymorphisms are associated with reduced warfarin dose. *Surgery* **128**:281–285.

Frudakis, T.N., Thomas, M.J., Ginjupalli, S.N., Handelin, B., Gabriel, R., Gomez, H.J. (2007). CYP2D6*4 polymorphism is associated with statin-induced muscle effects. *Pharmacogenetics and Genomics* **17**:695–707.

Gaedigk, A., Simon, S.D., Pearce, R.E., Bradford, L.D., Kennedy, M.J., Leeder, J.S. (2008). The CYP2D6 activity score: translating genotype information into a qualitative measure of phenotype. *Clinical Pharmacology and Therapeutics* **83**:234–242.

Gerdes, L.U., Gerdes, C., Kervinen, K., Savolainen, M., Klausen, I.C., Hansen, P.S., Kesäniemi, Y.A., Faergeman, O. (2000). The apolipoprotein epsilon4 allele determines prognosis and the effect on prognosis of simvastatin in survivors of myocardial infarction: A substudy of the Scandinavian simvastatin survival study. *Circulation* **101**:1366–1371.

Goldstein, D.B., Tate, S.K., Sisodiya, S.M. (2003). Pharmacogenetics goes genomic. *Nature Reviews Genetics* **4**:937–947.

Gough, A.C., Miles, J.S., Spurr, N.K., Moss, J.E., Gaedigk, A., Eichelbaum, M., Wolf, C.R. (1990). Identification of the primary gene defect at the cytochrome P(450) CYP2D locus. *Nature* **347**:773–776.

Gould Rothberg, B.E. (2001). Mapping a role for SNPs in drug development. *Nature Biotechnology* **19**:209–211.

Gratze, G., Fortin, J., Labugger, R., Binder, A., Kotanko, P., Timmermann, B., Luft, F.C., Hoehe, M.R., Skrabal, F. (1999), Beta-2 adrenergic receptor variants affect resting blood pressure and agonist-induced vasodilation in young adult Caucasians. *Hypertension* **33**:1425–1430.

Griffin, T.J., Smith, L.M. (2000). Single-nucleotide polymorphism analysis by MALDI–TOF mass spectrometry. *Trends in Biotechnology* **18**:77–84.

Gupta, R., Joshi, P., Mohan, V., Reddy, K.S., Yusuf, S. (2008), Epidemiology and causation of coronary heart disease and stroke in India. *Heart* **94**:16–26.

Higashi, M.K., Veenstra, D.L., Kondo, L.M., Wittkowsky, A.K., Srinouanprachanh, S.L., Farin, F.M., Rettie, A.E. (2002). Association between CYP2C9 genetic variants and anticoagulation-related outcomes during warfarin therapy. *JAMA* **287**:1690–1698.

Hingorani, A.D., Jia, H., Stevens, P.A., Hopper, R., Dickerson, J.E., Brown, M.J. (1995). Renin-angiotensin system gene polymorphisms influence blood pressure and the response to angiotensin converting enzyme inhibition. *Journal of Hypertension* **13**:1602–1609.

Hiura, Y., Fukushima, Y., Yuno, M., Sawamura, H., Kokubo, Y., Okamura, T., Tomoike, H., Goto, Y., Nonogi, H., Takahashi, R., Iwai, N. (2008). Validation of the association of genetic variants on chromosome 9p21 and 1q41 with myocardial infarction in a Japanese population. *Circulation Journal* **72**:1213–1217.

Hoit, B.D., Suresh, D.P., Craft, L., Walsh, R.A., Liggett, S.B. (2000). Beta2-adrenergic receptor polymorphisms at amino acid 16 differentially influence agonist-stimulated blood pressure and peripheral blood flow in normal individuals. *American Heart Journal* **139**:537–542.

Isaacs, A., Sayed-Tabatabaei, F.A., Njajou, O.T., Witteman, J.C., van Duijn, C.M. (2004). The -514 C->T hepatic lipase promoter region polymorphism and plasma lipids: A meta-analysis. *Journal of Clinical Endocrinology and Metabolism* **89**:3858–3863.

Jansen, R.P. (2001). mRNA localization: Message on the move. *Nature Reviews Molecular Cell Biology* **2**:247–256.

Jiang, X., Sheng, H.H., Lin, G., Li, J., Lu, X.Z., Cheng, Y.L., Huang, J., Xiao, H.S., Zhan, Y.Y. (2007). Effect of renin–angiotensin–aldosterone system gene polymorphisms on blood pressure response to antihypertensive treatment. *Chinese Medical Journal (English)* **120**:782–786.

Johnson, J.A. (2008). Ethnic differences in cardiovascular drug response: potential contribution of pharmacogenetics. *Circulation* **118**:1383–1393.

Johnson, J.A., Cavallari, L.H. (2005). Cardiovascular pharmacogenomics. *Experimental Physiology* **90**:283–289.

Johnson, J.A., Humma, L.M. (2002). Pharmacogenetics of cardiovascular drugs. *Briefings in Functional Genomics and Proteomics* **1**:66–79.

Joshi, P., Islam, S., Pais, P., Reddy, S., Dorairaj, P., Kazmi, K., Pandey, M.R., Haque, S., Mendis, S., Rangarajan, S., Yusuf, S. (2007). Risk factors for early myocardial infarction in South Asians compared with individuals in other countries. *JAMA* **297**:286–294.

Kathiresan, S., Melander, O., Anevski, D., Guiducci, C., Burtt, N.P., Roos, C., Hirschhorn, J.N., Berglund, G., Hedblad, B., Groop, L., Altshuler, D.M., Newton-Cheh, C., Orho-Melander, M. (2008). Polymorphisms associated with cholesterol and risk of cardiovascular events. *New England Journal of Medicine* **358**:1240–1249.

Kennedy, G.C., Matsuzaki, H., Dong, S., Liu, W.M., Huang, J., Liu, G., Su, X., Cao, M., Chen, W., Zhang, J., Liu, W., Yang, G., Di, X., Ryder, T., He, Z., Surti, U., Phillips, M.S., Boyce-Jacino, M.T., Fodor, S.P., Jones, K.W. (2003). Large-scale genotyping of complex DNA. *Nature Biotechnology* **21**:1233–1237.

Khripin, Y. (2006). High-throughput genotyping with energy transfer-labeled primers. *Methods in Molecular Biology* **335**:215–240.

Kim, S., Misra, A. (2007). SNP genotyping: Technologies and biomedical applications. *Annual Review of Biomedical Engineering* **9**:289–320.

King, B.P., Khan, T.I., Aithal, G.P., Kamali, F., Daly, A.K. (2004). Upstream and coding region CYP2C9 polymorphisms: Correlation with warfarin dose and metabolism. *Pharmacogenetics* **14**:813–822.

Kongkaew, C., Noyce, P.R., Ashcroft, D.M. (2008). Hospital admissions associated with adverse drug reactions: A systematic review of prospective observational studies. *Annals of Pharmacotherapy* **42**:1017–1025.

Kuivenhoven, J.A., Jukema, J.W., Zwinderman, A.H., de Knijff, P., McPherson, R., Bruschke, A.V., Lie, K.I., Kastelein, J.J. (1998). The role of a common variant of the cholesteryl ester transfer protein gene in the progression of coronary atherosclerosis. The Regression Growth Evaluation Statin Study Group. *New England Journal of Medicine* **338**:86–93.

Kurland, L., Melhus, H., Karlsson, J., Kahan, T., Malmqvist, K., Ohman, P., Nyström, F., Hägg, A., Lind, L. (2002). Polymorphisms in the angiotensinogen and angiotensin II type 1 receptor gene are related to change in left ventricular mass during antihypertensive treatment: Results from the Swedish Irbesartan Left Ventricular Hypertrophy Investigation versus Atenolol (SILVHIA) trial. *Journal of Hypertension* **20**:657–663.

Lazarou, J., Pomeranz, B.H., Corey, P.N. (1998). Incidence of adverse drug reactions in hospitalized patients: A meta-analysis of prospective studies. *JAMA* **279**:1200–1205.

Lennard, M.S., Tucker, G.T., Silas, J.H., Freestone, S., Ramsay, L.E., Woods, H.F. (1983). Differential stereoselective metabolism of metoprolol in extensive and poor debrisoquin metabolizers. *Clinical Pharmacology and Therapeutics* **34**:732–737.

Li, T., Lange, L.A., Li, X., Susswein, L., Bryant, B., Malone, R., Lange, E.M., Huang, T.-Y., Stafford, D.W., Evans, J.P. (2006). Polymorphisms in the VKORC1 gene are strongly associated with warfarin dosage requirements in patients receiving anticoagulation. *Journal of Medical Genetics* **43**:740–744.

Mahapatra, N.R. (2008). Catestatin is a novel endogenous peptide that regulates cardiac function and blood pressure. *Cardiovascular Research* **80**:330–338.

Mahapatra, N.R., Mahata, M., Ghosh, S., Gayen, J.R., O'Connor, D.T., Mahata, S.K. (2006). Molecular basis of neuroendocrine cell type-specific expression of the chromogranin B gene: Crucial role of the transcription factors CREB, AP-2, Egr-1 and Sp1. *Journal of Neurochemistry* **99**:119–133.

Mahapatra, N.R., Mahata, M., O'Connor, D.T., Mahata, S.K. (2003). Secretin activation of chromogranin A gene transcription. Identification of the signaling pathways in *cis* and in *trans*. *Journal of Biological Chemistry* **278**:19986–19994.

Mahapatra, N.R., O'Connor, D.T., Vaingankar, S.M., Hikim, A.P., Mahata, M., Ray, S., Staite, E., Wu, H., Gu, Y., Dalton, N., Kennedy, B.P., Ziegler, M.G., Ross, J., Mahata, S.K. (2005). Hypertension from targeted ablation of chromogranin A can be rescued by the human ortholog. *Journal of Clinical Investigation* **115**:1942–1952.

Mahata, S.K., Mahata, M., Wen, G., Wong, W.B., Mahapatra, N.R., Hamilton, B.A., O'Connor, D.T. (2004). The catecholamine release-inhibitory "catestatin" fragment of chromogranin A: Naturally occurring human variants with different potencies for multiple chromaffin cell nicotinic cholinergic responses. *Molecular Pharmacology* **66**:1180–1191.

Manunta, P., Burnier, M., D'Amico, M., Buzzi, L., Maillard, M., Barlassina, C., Lanella, G., Cusi, D., Bianchi, G. (1999). Adducin polymorphism affects renal proximal tubule reabsorption in hypertension. *Hypertension* **33**:694–697.

Mason, D.A., Moore, J.D., Green, S.A., Liggett, S.B. (1999). A gain-of-function polymorphism in a G-protein coupling domain of the human beta1-adrenergic receptor. *Journal of Biological Chemistry* **274**:12670–12674.

Materson, B.J., Reda, D.J., Cushman, W.C. (1995). Department of Veterans Affairs Single-Drug Therapy of Hypertension Study. Revised figures and new data. Department of Veterans Affairs Cooperative Study Group on Antihypertensive Agents. *American Journal of Hypertension* **8**:189–192.

Materson, B.J., Reda, D.J., Cushman, W.C., Massie, B.M., Freis, E.D., Kochar, M.S., Hamburger, R.J., Fye, C., Lakshman, R., Gottdiener, J., Ramirez, E.A., Henderson, W.G. (1993). Single-drug therapy for hypertension in men: A comparison of six antihypertensive agents with placebo. *New England Journal of Medicine* **328**:914–921.

Mathers, C.D., Loncar, D. (2006). Projections of global mortality and burden of disease from 2002 to 2030. *PLoS Med* **3**:e442.

McGourty, J.C., Silas, J.H., Lennard, M.S., Tucker, G.T., Woods, H.F. (1985). Metoprolol metabolism and debrisoquine oxidation polymorphism—Population and family studies. *British Journal of Clinical Pharmacology* **20**:555–566.

McNamara, D.M., Holubkov, R., Janosko, K., Palmer, A., Wang, J.J., MacGowan, G.A., Murali, S., Rosenblum, W.D., London, B., Feldman, A.M. (2001). Pharmacogenetic interactions between beta-blocker therapy and the angiotensin-converting enzyme deletion polymorphism in patients with congestive heart failure. *Circulation* **103**:1644–1648.

Mehta, U., Durrheim, D.N., Blockman, M., Kredo, T., Gounden, R., Barnes, K.I. (2008). Adverse drug reactions in adult medical inpatients in a South African hospital serving a community with high HIV/AIDS prevalence: Prospective observational study. *British Journal of Clinical Pharmacology* **65**:396–406.

Meng, W., Hughes, A.E., Patterson, C.C., Belton, C., Kee, F., McKeown, P.P. (2008). Chromosome 9p21.3 is associated with early-onset coronary heart disease in the Irish population. *Disease Markers* **25**:81–85.

Meyer, U.A. (2004). Pharmacogenetics—Five decades of therapeutic lessons from genetic diversity. *Nature Reviews Genetics* **5**:669–676.

Miller, J.A., Thai, K., Scholey, J.W. (1999). Angiotensin II type 1 receptor gene polymorphism predicts response to losartan and angiotensin II. *Kidney International* **56**:2173–2180.

Mohrschladt, M.F., van der Sman-de Beer, F., Hofman, M.K., van der Krabben, M., Westendorp, R.G., Smelt, A.H. (2005). TaqIB polymorphism in CETP gene: the influence on incidence of cardiovascular disease in statin-treated patients with familial hypercholesterolemia. *European Journal of Human Genetics* **13**:877–882.

Mukae, S., Aoki, S., Itoh, S., Iwata, T., Ueda, H., Katagiri, T. (2000). Bradykinin B(2) receptor gene polymorphism is associated with angiotensin-converting enzyme inhibitor-related cough. *Hypertension* **36**:127–131.

Muller-Nordhorn, J., Binting, S., Roll, S., Willich, S.N. (2008). An update on regional variation in cardiovascular mortality within Europe. *European Heart Journal* **29**:1316–1326.

Nebert, D.W. (1997). Polymorphisms in drug-metabolizing enzymes: What is their clinical relevance and why do they exist? *American Journal of Human Genetics* **60**:265–271.

Nemeth, A., Szakmary, K., Kramer, J., Dinya, E., Pados, G., Fust, G., Huettinger, M. (1995). Apolipoprotein E and complement C3 polymorphism and their role in the response to gemfibrozil and low fat low cholesterol therapy. *European Journal of Clinical Chemistry and Clinical Biochemistry* **33**:799–804.

Paez, J.G., Jänne, P.A., Lee, J.C., Tracy, S., Greulich, H., Gabriel, S., Herman, P., Kaye, F.J., Lindeman, N., Boggon, T.J., Naoki, K., Sasaki, H., Fujii, Y., Eck, M.J., Sellers, W.R., Johnson, B.E., Meyerson, M. (2004). EGFR mutations in lung cancer: Correlation with clinical response to gefitinib therapy. *Science* **304**:1497–1500.

Passarelli, M.C., Jacob-Filho, W., Figueras, A. (2005). Adverse drug reactions in an elderly hospitalised population: Inappropriate presciption is a leading cause. *Drugs and Aging* **22**:767–777.

Pati, N., Schowinsky, V., Kokanovic, O., Magnuson, V., Ghosh, S. (2004). A comparison between SNaPshot, pyrosequencing, and biplex invader SNP genotyping methods: Accuracy, cost, and throughput. *Journal of Biochemical and Biophysical Methods* **60**:1–12.

Preston, R.A., Materson, B.J., Reda, D.J., Williams, D.W., Hamburger, R.J., Cushman, W.C., Anderson, R.J. (1998). Age-race subgroup compared with renin profile as predictors of blood pressure response to antihypertensive therapy. *JAMA* **280**:1168–1172.

Pritchard, J.K., Rosenberg, N.A. (1999). Use of unlinked genetic markers to detect population stratification in association studies. *American Journal of Human Genetics* **65**:220–228.

Rajewsky, N. (2006) Micro RNA target predictions in animals. *Nature Genetics* **38(Suppl.)**:S8–13.

Reich, D.E., Goldstein, D.B. (2001). Detecting association in a case-control study while correcting for population stratification. *Genetic Epidemiology* **20**:4–16.

Rieder, M.J., Reiner, A.P., Gage, B.F., Nickerson, D.A., Eby, C.S., McLeod, H.L., Blough, D.K., Thummel, K.E., Veenstra, D.L., Rettie, A.E. (2005). Effect of VKORC1 haplotypes on transcriptional regulation and warfarin dose. *New England Journal of Medicine* **352**:2285–2293.

Rigat, B., Hubert, C., Alhenc-Gelas, F., Cambien, F., Corvol, P., Soubrier, F. (1990). An insertion/deletion polymorphism in the angiotensin I-converting enzyme gene accounting for half the variance of serum enzyme levels. *Journal of Clinical Investigation* **86**:1343–1346.

Roden, D. (2003). Cardiovascular pharmacogenomics. *Circulation* **108**:3071–3074.

Ronaghi, M., Shokralla, S., Gharizadeh, B. (2007). Pyrosequencing for discovery and analysis of DNA sequence variations. *Pharmacogenomics* **8**:1437–1441.

Rosamond, W., Flegal, K., Furie, K., Go, A., Greenlund, K., Haase, N., Hailpern, S.M., Ho, M., Howard, V., Kissela, B., Kittner, S., Lloyd-Jones, D., McDermott, M., Meigs, J., Moy, C., Nichol, G., O'Donnell, C., Roger, V., Sorlie, P., Steinberger, J., Thom, T., Wilson, M., Hong, Y., American Heart Association Statistics Committee and Stroke Statistics Subcommittee (2008). Heart disease and stroke statistics—2008 update: A report from the American Heart Association Statistics Committee and Stroke Statistics Subcommittee. *Circulation* **117**:e25–146.

Roses, A.D. (2004). Pharmacogenetics and drug development: The path to safer and more effective drugs. *Nature Reviews Genetics* **5**:645–656.

Samani, N.J., Erdmann, J., Hall, A.S., Hengstenberg, C., Mangino, M., Mayer, B., Dixon, R.J., Meitinger, T., Braund, P., Wichmann, H.E., Barrett, J.H., König, I.R., Stevens, S.E., Szymczak, S., Tregouet, D.A., Iles, M.M., Pahlke, F., Pollard, H., Lieb, W., Cambien, F., Fischer, M., Ouwehand, W., Blankenberg, S.,

Balmforth, A.J., Baessler, A., Ball, S.G., Strom, T.M., Braenne, I., Gieger, C., Deloukas, P., Tobin, M.D., Ziegler, A., Thompson, J.R., Schunkert, H., WTCCC, Cardiogenics Consortium (2007) Genomewide association analysis of coronary artery disease. *New England Journal of Medicine* **357**:443–453.

Sanderson, S., Emery, J., Higgins, J. (2005). CYP2C9 gene variants, drug dose, and bleeding risk in warfarin-treated patients: A HuGEnet systematic review and meta-analysis. *Genetics in Medicine* **7**:97–104.

Schmieder, R.E., Hilgers, K.F., Schlaich, M.P., Schmidt, B.M. (2007). Renin–angiotensin system and cardiovascular risk. *Lancet* **369**:1208–1219.

Schunkert, H., Götz, A., Braund, P., McGinnis, R., Tregouet, D.A., Mangino, M., Linsel-Nitschke, P., Cambien, F., Hengstenberg, C., Stark, K., Blankenberg, S., Tiret, L., Ducimetiere, P., Keniry, A., Ghori, M.J., Schreiber, S., El Mokhtari, N.E., Hall, A.S., Dixon, R.J., Goodall, A.H., Liptau, H., Pollard, H., Schwarz, D.F., Hothorn, L.A., Wichmann, H.E., König, I.R., Fischer, M., Meisinger, C., Ouwehand, W., Deloukas, P., Thompson, J.R., Erdmann, J., Ziegler, A., Samani, N.J., Cardiogenics Consortium (2008). Repeated replication and a prospective meta-analysis of the association between chromosome 9p21.3 and coronary artery disease. *Circulation* **117**:1675–1684.

Schunkert, H., Hense, H.W., Gimenez-Roqueplo, A.P., Stieber, J., Keil, U., Riegger, G.A., Jeunemaitre, X. (1997) The angiotensinogen T235 variant and the use of antihypertensive drugs in a population-based cohort. *Hypertension* **29**:628–633.

Schwarz, U.I., Ritchie, M.D., Bradford, Y., Li, C., Dudek, S.M., Frye-Anderson, A., Kim, R.B., Roden, D.M., Stein, C.M. (2008) Genetic determinants of response to warfarin during initial anticoagulation. *New England Journal of Medicine* **358**:999–1008.

Sciarrone, M.T., Stella, P., Barlassina, C., Manunta, P., Lanzani, C., Bianchi, G., Cusi, D. (2003). ACE and alpha-adducin polymorphism as markers of individual response to diuretic therapy. *Hypertension* **41**:398–403.

Scott, S.A., Edelmann, L., Kornreich, R., Desnick, R.J. (2008). Warfarin pharmacogenetics: CYP2C9 and VKORC1 genotypes predict different sensitivity and resistance frequencies in the Ashkenazi and Sephardi Jewish populations. *American Journal of Human Genetics* **82**:495–500.

Searls, D.B. (2003) Pharmacophylogenomics: Genes, evolution and drug targets. *Nature Reviews Drug Discovery* **2**: 613–623.

Sham, P.C., Cherny, S.S., Purcell, S., Hewitt, J.K. (2000). Power of linkage versus association analysis of quantitative traits, by use of variance-components models, for sibship data. *American Journal of Human Genetics* **66**:1616–1630.

Shi, M.M. (2002). Technologies for individual genotyping: Detection of genetic polymorphisms in drug targets and disease genes. *American Journal of PharmacoGenomics* **2**:197–205.

Shi, M.M., Bleavins, M.R., de la Iglesia, F.A. (2001) Pharmacogenetic application in drug development and clinical trials. *Drug Metabolism and Disposition* **29**:591–595.

Siddiqui, A., Kerb, R., Weale, M.E., Brinkmann, U., Smith, A., Goldstein, D.B., Wood, N.W., Sisodiya, S.M. (2003). Association of multidrug resistance in epilepsy with a polymorphism in the drug-transporter gene ABCB1. *New England Journal of Medicine* **348**:1442–1448.

Siest, G., Jeannesson, E., Visvikis-Siest, S. (2007). Enzymes and pharmacogenetics of cardiovascular drugs. *Clinica Chimica Acta* **381**:26–31.

Skelding, K.A., Gerhard, G.S., Simari, R.D., Holmes, D.R.J. (2007). The effect of HapMap on cardiovascular research and clinical practice. *Nature Clinical Practice Cardiovascular Medicine* **4**:136–142.

Small, K.M., Mialet-Perez, J., Liggett, S.B. (2008). Genetic variation within the beta1-adrenergic receptor gene results in haplotype-specific expression phenotypes. *Journal of Cardiovascular Pharmacology* **51**:106–110.

Stubbins, M.J., Harries, L.W., Smith, G., Tarbit, M.H., Wolf, C.R. (1996). Genetic analysis of the human cytochrome P450 CYP2C9 locus. *Pharmacogenetics* **6**:429–439.

Syvänen, A.C. (1999). From gels to chips: "Minisequencing" primer extension for analysis of point mutations and single nucleotide polymorphisms. *Hum Mutat* **13**:1–10.

Takahashi, H., Wilkinson, G.R., Nutescu, E.A., Morita, T., Ritchie, M.D., Scordo, M.G., Pengo, V., Barban, M., Padrini, R., Ieiri, I., Otsubo, K., Kashima, T., Kimura, S., Kijima, S., Echizen, H. (2006). Different contributions of polymorphisms in VKORC1 and CYP2C9 to intra- and inter-population differences in maintenance does of warfarin in Japanese, Caucasians and African-Americans. *Pharmacogenetics and Genomics* **16**:101–110.

Tantisira, K.G., Lake, S., Silverman, E.S., Palmer, L.J., Lazarus, R., Silverman, E.K., Liggett, S.B., Gelfand, E.W., Rosenwasser, L.J., Richter, B., Israel, E., Wechsler, M., Gabriel, S., Altshuler, D., Lander, E., Drazen, J., Weiss, S.T. (2004). Corticosteroid pharmacogenetics: Association of sequence variants in CRHR1 with improved lung function in asthmatics treated with inhaled corticosteroids. *Human Molecular Genetics* **13**:1353–1359.

Taylor, A.L., Ziesche, S., Yancy, C., Carson, P., D'Agostino, R.J., Ferdinand, K., Taylor, M., Adams, K., Sabolinski, M., Worcel, M., Cohn, J.N. (2004). Combination of isosorbide dinitrate and hydralazine in blacks with heart failure. *New England Journal of Medicine* **351**:2049–2057.

The Wellcome Trust Case Control Consortium (2007). Genome-wide association study of 14,000 cases of seven common diseases and 3,000 shared controls. *Nature* **447**:661–678.

Thomas, P.D., Kejariwal, A., Guo, N., Mi, H., Campbell, M.J., Muruganujan, A., Lazareva-Ulitsky, B. (2006). Applications for protein sequence-function evolution data: mRNA/protein expression analysis and coding SNP scoring tools. *Nucleic Acids Research* **34**:W645–650.

Tost, J., Gut, I.G. (2002). Genotyping single nucleotide polymorphisms by mass spectrometry. *Mass Spectrometry Reviews* **21**:388–418.

van der Velden, A.W., Thomas, A.A. (1999). The role of the 5′ untranslated region of an mRNA in translation regulation during development. *International Journal of Biochemistry and Cell Biology* **31**:87–106.

Veenstra, D.L., Blough, D.K., Higashi, M.K., Farin, F.M., Srinouanprachan, S., Rieder, M.J., Rettie, A.E. (2005). CYP2C9 haplotype structure in European American warfarin patients and association with clinical outcomes. *Clinical Pharmacology and Therapeutics* **77**:353–364.

Vermes, A., Vermes, I. (2004). Genetic polymorphisms in cytochrome P450 enzymes: Effect on efficacy and tolerability of HMG-CoA reductase inhibitors. *American Journal of Cardiovascular Drugs* **4**:247–255.

Veterans Administration Cooperative Study Group on Antihypertensive Agents (1982). Comparison of propranolol and hydrochlorothiazide for the initial treatment of hypertension, II: Results of long-term therapy. *JAMA* **248**:2004–2011.

Wang, L., Luhm, R., Lei, M. (2007). SNP and mutation analysis. *Advances in Experimental Medicine and Biology* **593**:105–116.

Webster, A., Martin, P., Lewis, G., Smart, A. (2004). Integrating pharmacogenetics into society: In search of a model. *Nature Reviews Genetics* **5**:663–669.

Wen, G., Mahata, S.K., Cadman, P., Mahata, M., Ghosh, S., Mahapatra, N.R., Rao, F., Stridsberg, M., Smith, D.W., Mahboubi, P., Schork, N.J., O'Connor, D.T., Hamilton, B.A. (2004). Both rare and common polymorphisms contribute functional variation at CHGA, a regulator of catecholamine physiology. *American Journal of Human Genetics* **74**:197–207.

White, R.H., Beyth, R.J., Zhou, H., Romano, P.S. (1999). Major bleeding after hospitalization for deep-venous thrombosis. *American Journal of Medicine* **107**:414–424.

Xavier, D., Pais, P., Devereaux, P.J., Xie, C., Prabhakaran, D., Reddy, K.S., Gupta, R., Joshi, P., Kerkar, P., Thanikachalam, S., Haridas, K.K., Jaison, T.M., Naik, S., Maity, A.K., Yusuf, S. (2008) Treatment and outcomes of acute coronary syndromes in India (CREATE): A prospective analysis of registry data. *Lancet* **371**:1435–1442.

Xiao, W., Oefner, P.J. (2001). Denaturing high-performance liquid chromatography: A review. *Human Mutation* **17**:439–474.

Yang, H., Wang, H., Wang, J., Cai, Y., Zhou, G., He, F., Qian, X. (2003). Multiplex single-nucleotide polymorphism genotyping by matrix-assisted laser desorption/ionization time-of-flight mass spectrometry. *Analytical Biochemistry* **314**:54–62.

Yu, B., Sawyer, N.A., Chiu, C., Oefner, P.J., Underhill, P.A. (2006). DNA mutation detection using denaturing high-performance liquid chromatography (DHPLC). *Current Protocols in Human Genetics* **Chapter 7** (Unit7):10.

9

Enzyme Inhibitors as Anti-Inflammatory Agents

P.M. Sivakumar and Mukesh Doble*

Department of Biotechnology, Indian Institute of Technology Madras, Chennai, India

INTRODUCTION

In the United States alone according to a 2000 census, 40 million people suffer from chronic recurrent headaches, 35 million from persistent back pains and 5 million from cancer-related pain, which are unresponsive to the most potent of painkillers, such as morphine (2000 data). Each year, it costs the US$4 billion work days, resulting in a $65 billion loss in work productivity. Annual sales for over-the-counter analgesics add up to $3 billion, and prescribed drugs account for another $100 billion a year. As demographics change and the mean age of the population rises, the incidence of chronic diseases such as diabetes, cardiovascular disease and rheumatoid arthritis is expected to increase, and with it the need for better anti-inflammatory drugs and analgesics. With the withdrawal of the popular drugs (cyclooxygenase-2 [COX-2] inhibitors) in the recent times, there is a need for an enhanced understanding of pain mechanisms, which will not only provide novel targets but also provide painkillers with minimal toxicities and side-effect profiles.

Inflammation is a defense reaction, and it is characterized by redness, swelling, heat and pain (Punchard *et al.*, 2004). Inflammatory pathways are regulated by various enzymes. Enzymes are induced by inflammatory stimuli, such as cytokines, and produce prostaglandins (PGs) that contribute to the pain and swelling or inflammation (Bindra and Bindra, 1977). Inflammatory cascades produce various chemicals (inflammatory mediators) that have a pathophysiological role; they are named as prostaglandins by von Euler. PGs were first identified from the human semen in the 1930s (Bindra and

* *mukeshd@iitm.ac.in*

Bindra, 1977). John Vane reported in 1971 the inhibition of PGs by nonsteroidal anti-inflammatory drugs (NSAIDs), which includes aspirin (the first anti-inflammatory agent, which has a structure analogous to that of salicylic acid). Aspirin is well known to inhibit COX enzymes as well (Vane, 1971), and the pathway that leads to the biosynthesis of leukotriene (which is also an important inflammatory mediator) mediated by 5-lipooxygenase (5-LOX) (Samuelsson, 1983). Three of the lipoxygenases can mediate the metabolism of arachidonic acid (AA). Leukotrienes are involved in asthmatic and certain allergic reactions. Another important biological messenger, nitric oxide (NO), can also play a role in inflammation. It has a potential role, as both a signaling molecule and a lethal effector molecule. Hence, researchers started paying attention to the inducible nitric oxide synthase pathway (iNOS) (Lincoln *et al.*, 1997). In phospholipase A2 (PLA2) pathway, AA is released from the phospholipid membrane disproportionately, which acts as a precursor/substrate for COX and 5-LOX pathways, and can be targeted to prevent the biosynthesis of AA. In addition, mitogen-activated protein kinase (MAPK), prostaglandin D_2 synthase and matrix metalloproteases are some of the important enzymes that are involved in inflammation and can be useful molecular targets for designing new anti-inflammatory agents. In this chapter, we report some of the important enzymatic pathways and their commercial inhibitors (drugs already in the market or under clinical trials) in the treatment of inflammation.

CYCLOOXYGENASE

Three different isoforms (COX-1, COX-2 and COX-3) of cyclooxygenases have been reported (Yamamoto *et al.*, 1998; Dannhardt and Laufer, 2000; Chandrasekharan *et al.*, 2002). All the three isoforms use AA as a common substrate. The isoform COX-1 is a constitutive and the isoform COX-2 is an inducible enzyme. Merlie *et al.* (1988) first cloned the constitutive isoform of COX in 1988, and COX-2 was discovered in 1989 by Simmons *et al.* (1989) and Rosen *et al.* (1989). Apart from inflammatory mediation, PGs are also involved in various pathophysiological conditions, which include cytoprotection in the gastrointestinal (GI) tract (PG production mediated by COX-1), vasodilation and constriction of pulmonary system and platelet aggregation. Hence, the inhibition of this isoform, COX-1, leads to ulcer and other consequences, including imbalance in bicarbonate and mucus secretion, and so on (Gustafson-Svard *et al.*, 1996). The inducible isoform, COX-2, is generated due to pro-inflammatory cytokines, interleukins (ILs), mitogens and endotoxins in the inflammatory cells such as monocytes and macrophages. Apart from inflammation, it is reported that COX-2 impacts on organs namely, reproductive system, kidney, brain, lungs and diseases like cancer'

Hence the inhibition of COX-2 enzyme has therapeutic potential in treating other diseases too. Table 9.1 compares COX-1, COX-2 and COX-3 enzymes.

BIOSYNTHESIS OF PROSTANOIDS

AA is converted into prostaglandin H_2 (PGH_2) in two steps (Fig. 9.1) by the isoforms of COX enzyme, and these isoforms are termed as PGH-synthase. In the first step, prostaglandin G_2 (PGG_2), a hydroperoxy-endoperoxide, is produced through double dioxygenation. This is mediated by the COX activity of the COX enzyme. The second step involves the conversion of PGG_2 to PGH_2, through the peroxidase activity of the same enzyme. The mechanism of utilization of AA is shown in Fig. 9.1. The exact mechanism of interaction of COX enzyme and its substrates has been given in detail in several

Table 9.1 *Comparison of COX isoforms*

Parameter	*COX-1*	*COX-2*	*COX-3*
Gene size (kb)	22	8.3	?
Chromosome	9	1	?
mRNA (kb)	2.8	4.1	5.2
mRNA regulation	Constitutive	Constitutive, inducible	Constitutive, inducible
Amino acids	599	604	633
Molecular weight (kDa)	70	70–72	ca. 65
Localization	Membrane.ER	Membrane.ER, cytoplasm	Membrane.ER
Glycolization	N-terminal	N-terminal	N-terminal
ASA acetylation site	Ser529	Ser516	?
Substrate specificity	AA Gamma-linolenic acid	AA Gamma-linolenic acid Alpha-linolenic acid	AA ? ?
Range of expression	2–4-fold	10–80-fold	–
Tissue expression	Platelets, endothelial cells, stomach, kidney, smooth muscle, most tissues	Most tissues, especially inflammatory cells Requires stimulation by growth factors, cytokines and hormones	?
Activity	23 mmol AA/mg/min	11 mmol AA/mg/min	–

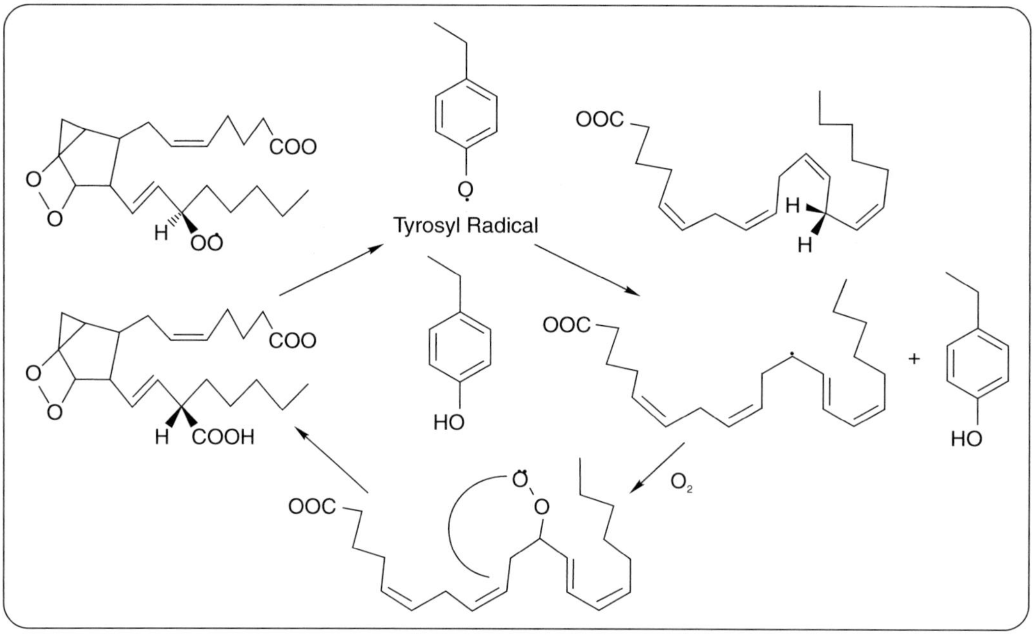

Fig. 9.1 *Biocatalytic Conversion of AA to PGG_2*

reviews (Smith *et al.*, 2000; Kurumbail *et al.*, 2001; Van der donk *et al.*, 2002; Rouzer and Marnett, 2003). PGG_2 and PGH_2 are the key intermediates in the AA cascade, and the latter is converted to prostaglandin E_2 (PGE_2), prostaglandin F_{2a} (PGF_{2a}), prostaglandin I_2 (PGI_2) and thromboxane A_2 (TXA_2) by the action of isoforms of PG synthases and TX synthases (Smith and Willis, 1971; Vane and Botting, 1992; Frolich, 1997). Fig. 9.2 shows the metabolic intermediates and end products in the prostanoid metabolic cascade.

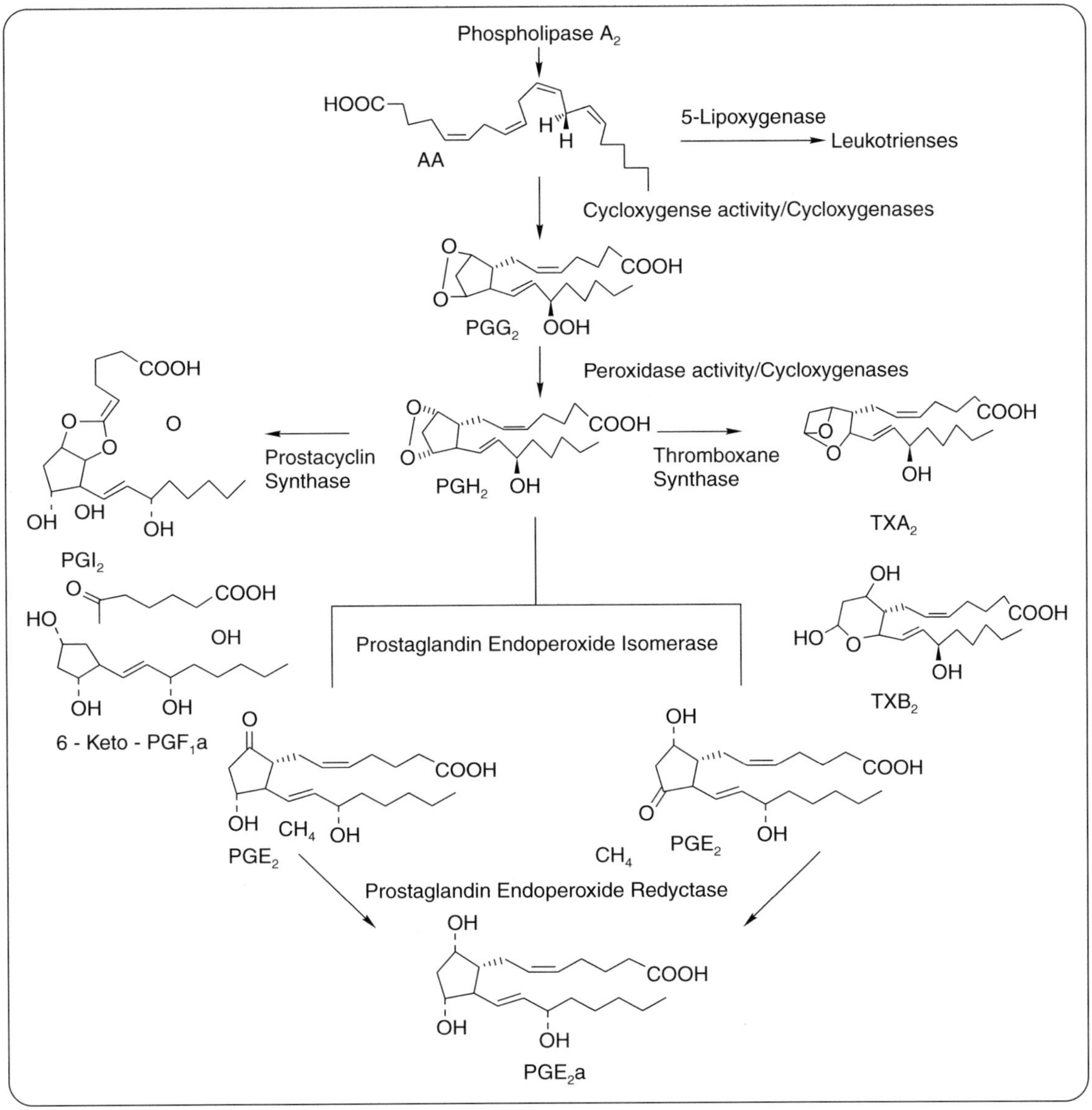

Fig. 9.2 ***Biosynthesis of Prostaglandins and Thromboxanes***

COMMERCIAL CYCLOOXYGENASE INHIBITORS

This class has been divided into nonselective and selective COX-2 inhibitors. As the name implies, the former inhibits all the COX isoforms and the latter inhibits only the COX-2 enzyme. The nonselective COX inhibitor ketoprofen (0.3 mg/kg) is one example that inhibits the biosynthesis of PGE_2 (Sommerauer *et al.*). Flurbiprofen, a NSAID belonging to the arylpropionic group of compounds, is effective as an analgesic for mild to moderate pain and is also an antipyretic (Valentovic, 2008). Ibuprofen is the most potent inhibitor of COX-1 rather than COX-2 in all the models tested (Mitchell *et al.*, 1993). Hence, an extended use of this drug leads to ulcer. The COX-1 inhibitor valeryl salicylate markedly reduces the level of PGE_2 in the plasma (Guerguerian *et al.*, 1998). Sulfasalazine (IC_{50} = 0.15 mM) inhibits the calcium ionophore–stimulated formation of contractile leukotriene activity (Nielsen *et al.*, 1998). It is increasingly becoming well established that NSAIDs such as flufenamic acid protect against tumors of the GI tract and may also protect against a variety of other tumors. These activities have been widely attributed to the inhibition of COXs, particularly COX-2 (Lovering *et al.*, 2004). The competitive inhibitor of COX-1, mefenamic acid, also displays competitive inhibition of COX-2. These results demonstrate the ability to generate selective NSAIDs, which could provide useful improvement therapeutically in the treatment of chronic inflammatory disease (Gierse *et al.*, 1995). All NSAIDs inhibit the COX isozymes to different extents, which accounts for their anti-inflammatory and analgesic activities and, in addition, their gastrointestinal side effects. Meclofenamic acid inhibits COX-2, and its esters are either inactive or nonselective (Kalgutkar *et al.*, 2000). Piroxicam is an NSAID that is widely used for the treatment of inflammatory arthritis. A major effect of NSAIDs is their ability to inhibit COX, the rate-limiting enzyme for conversion of AA to important signal molecules, including PGs, which profoundly affect the cellular functions in many tissues (Earnet *et al.*). Fig. 9.3 lists the structures of a few nonselective COX inhibitors. COX-2 has a larger secondary pocket in the active site when compared to COX-1, and thus it can accommodate compounds with a slightly larger volume. This was proved in our quantitative structure–activity relationship (QSAR) study, where we showed that volume has a positive correlation with COX-2 selectivity (correlation coefficient > 0.8) (Sivakumar and Doble, 2006). The major structural requirement for this group of compounds is the presence of two vicinal aryl moieties in the heterocyclic ring system. The heterocyclic ring is believed to position the inhibitor in the appropriate place. Presence of sulfonamide or methyl sulfonyl group at the fourth position in one of the aromatic groups is needed for selective COX-2 inhibition.

SELECTIVE COX-2 ENZYME INHIBITORS

Celecoxib (CELEBREX) and rofecoxib (VIOXX) are NSAIDs. These are the first members of a new class of drugs that preferentially inhibit the activity of COX-2 enzyme (Noble *et al.*, 2000). These are the first-generation orally active coxibs with diaryl pyrazole and diaryl furanone as scaffolds (Rahim *et al.*, 2002). Further attempts made to improve their bioavailability yielded newer analogues. Valdecoxib and deracoxib, the second-generation coxibs, and parecoxib prodrug, which was obtained from valdecoxib, are currently used as injectables. Parecoxib sodium is an injectable prodrug of the

COX-2-specific inhibitor valdecoxib, which has exhibited analgesic activity (Harris *et al.*, 2001). Fig. 9.4 lists the structures of a few selective COX-2 inhibitors.

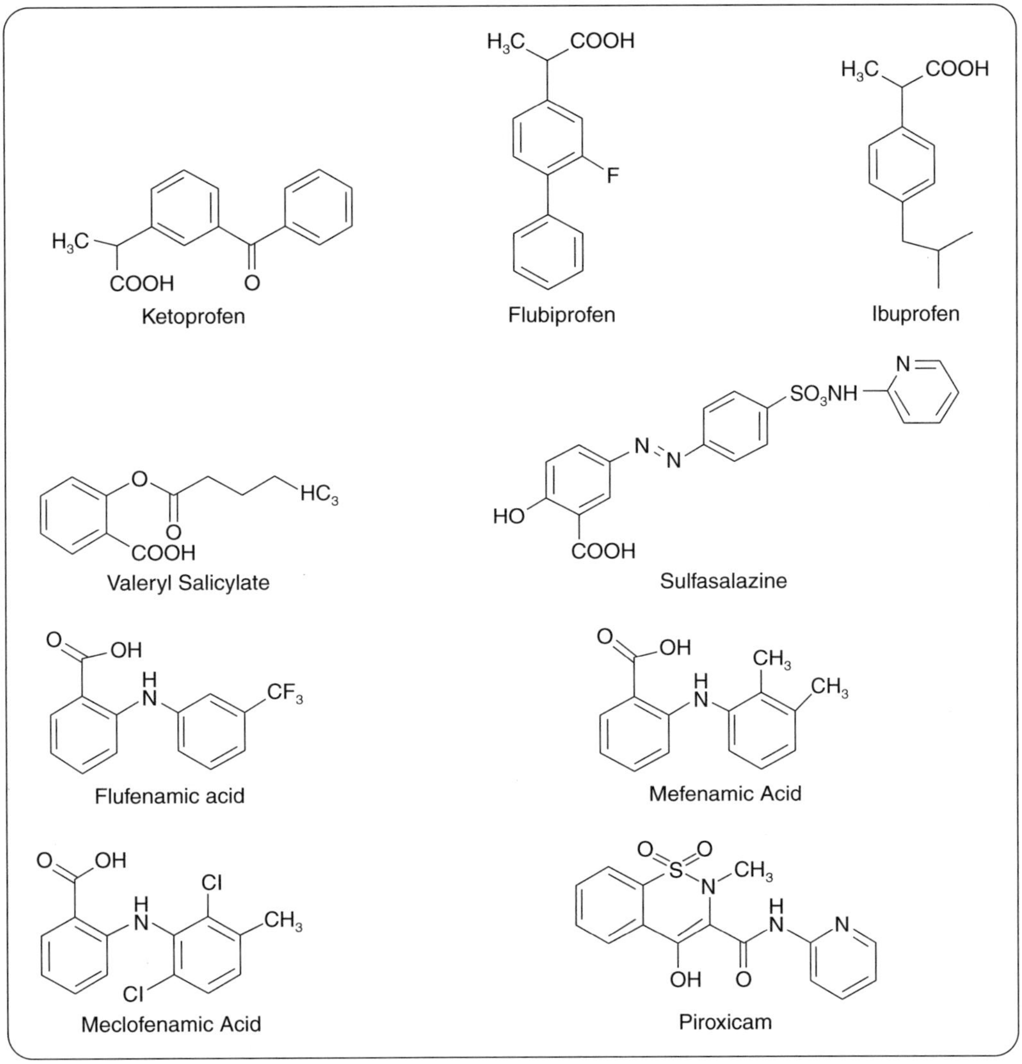

Fig. 9.3 *Nonselective COX-2 Enzyme Inhibitors*

The regular usage of diaryl heterocyclic COX-2 inhibitors has resulted in cardiovascular complications. Hence, research is being done to find newer COX-2 inhibitors that are free from side effects. Newer compounds are non-diaryl heterocyclic COX-2 inhibitors. Heterogenic chemical structures of COX-2 inhibitors added with substituted triaryl olefins and diaryl olefins (Murias *et al.*, 2004), aryl-substituted acetylenes (Chen *et al.*, 2005) and propenones (Jahng *et al.*, 2004) are newer non-diaryl heterocyclic COX-2 enzyme inhibitors.

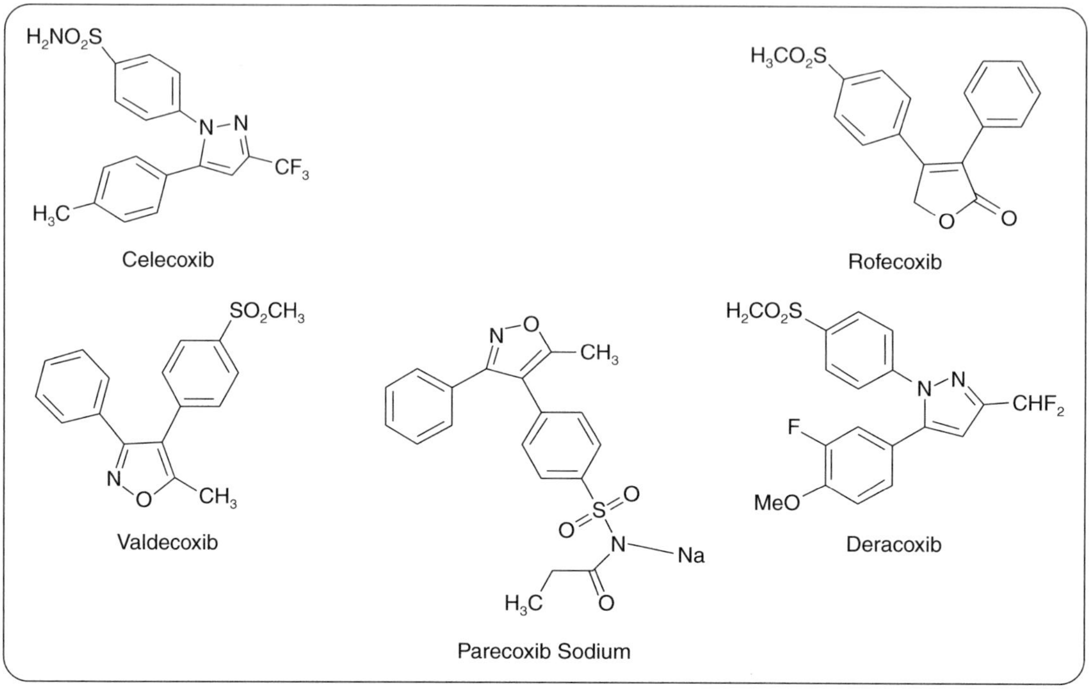

Fig. 9.4 *Various Structures of Selective COX-2 Enzyme Inhibitors*

5-LIPOXYGENASE PATHWAY

Lipoxygenase

5-LOX is a dioxygenase, the key enzyme in the biosynthesis of leukotriene. This enzyme dioxygenates polyunsaturated fatty acids at the regio- and stereoselective positions to produce a series of hydroperoxy fatty acids (Lehmann, 1994). 12-LOX and 15-LOX do not have a very significant biological role. In contrast, the biosynthesis of leukotriene by 5-LOX plays a major role in the inflammatory pathway (see Fig. 9.5).

Biosynthesis of Leukotrienes

5-LOXs utilize arachidonate as the primary substrate. When AA is liberated from phospholipids by the action of PLA2, 5-LOX converts AA to leukotriene A_4 (LTA_4), which is unstable in nature. The conversion of LTA_4 depends on the interaction between 5-lipoxygenase activating protein (FLAP) and 5-LOX (Reid *et al.*, 1990). Two different enzymes, namely LTA hydrolase and LTC synthase, act on LTA_4 and produce the dihydroxy acid leukotriene LTB_4 and the first cysteinyl leukotriene, LTC_4. Then LTC_4 is converted to LTD_4 and LTE_4 by the two ubiqutous enzymes, namely gamma glutamyl transpeptidase and dipeptidase. These cysteinyl leukotrienes bind to their receptors

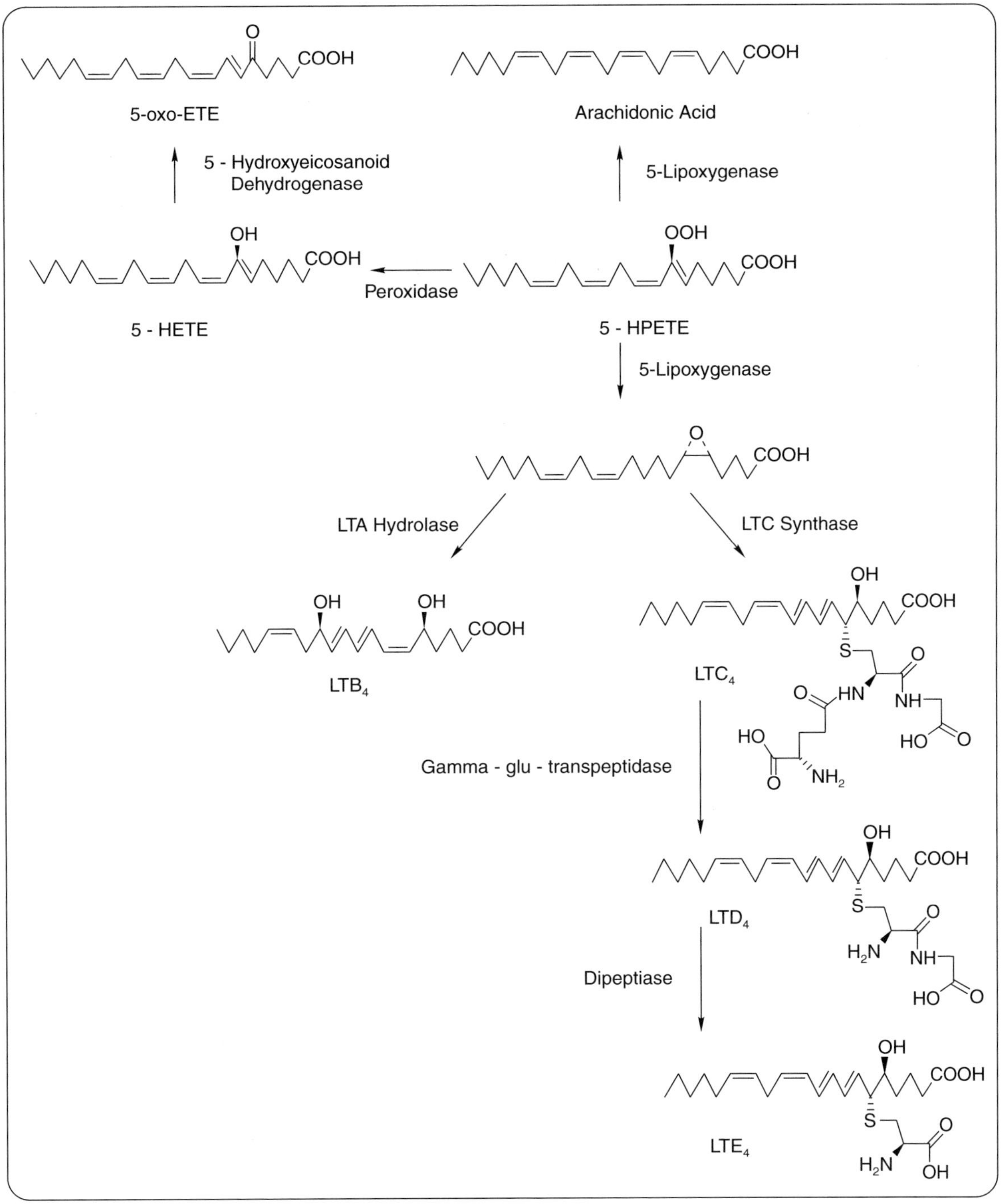

Fig. 9.5 *Biosynthesis of Leukotrienes*

CysLT1 and CysLT2 on the cell surface to induce pathophysiological functions. LTB_4 interacts with PPARα receptor, which indeed activates the genes involved in the lipid homeostasis (Funk, 2001). Leukotrienes LTB_4, LTC_4, LTD_4 and LTE_4 act as pro-inflammatory mediators and are also called cysteinyl leukotrienes due to the presence of the amino acid in the structure. Leukotrienes LTB_5, LTC_5, LTD_5 and LTE_5 are anti-inflammatory molecules. In addition, leukotrienes impact numerous other diseases like asthma and allergic and inflammatory disorders. So the inhibition of the biosynthesis of leukotriene through the inhibition of 5-LOX has also exhibited therapeutic potential toward asthma (Wenzel, 1998), allergy and inflammation (Brain and Williams, 1990; Drazen *et al.*, 1999), inhibiting the growth of cancer cells (Hayashi *et al.*, 2006) and induction of apoptosis (Hoque *et al.*, 2005), and so on.

Commercial 5-Lipoxygenase Inhibitors

Acetyl-11-keto-beta-boswellic acid (AKBA), a pentacyclic triterpene, is commercially available as a 5-LOX inhibitor (Fig. 9.6). AKBA has an IC_{50} value of 1.5 μM. Reduction or deacetylation of the acetoxy group in the molecule leads to a slight reduction in its activity (IC_{50} of 3 and 4.5 μM, respectively) (Sailer *et al.*, 1996). Licofelone is the first member of a new class of analgesic and anti-inflammatory drugs acting through a dual mechanism, namely inhibiting both COX and 5-LOX (Malhotra *et al.*, 2007). Zileuton is an active oral inhibitor of the enzyme 5-LOX. It is currently the only approved 5-LOX inhibitor in the market and is prescribed for the treatment of asthma. However, a growing body of investigations support its chemopreventive effects in cancer. 5-LOX inhibitors such as zileuton interfere with the activation of the catalytic site of 5-LOX, and cysteinyl receptor

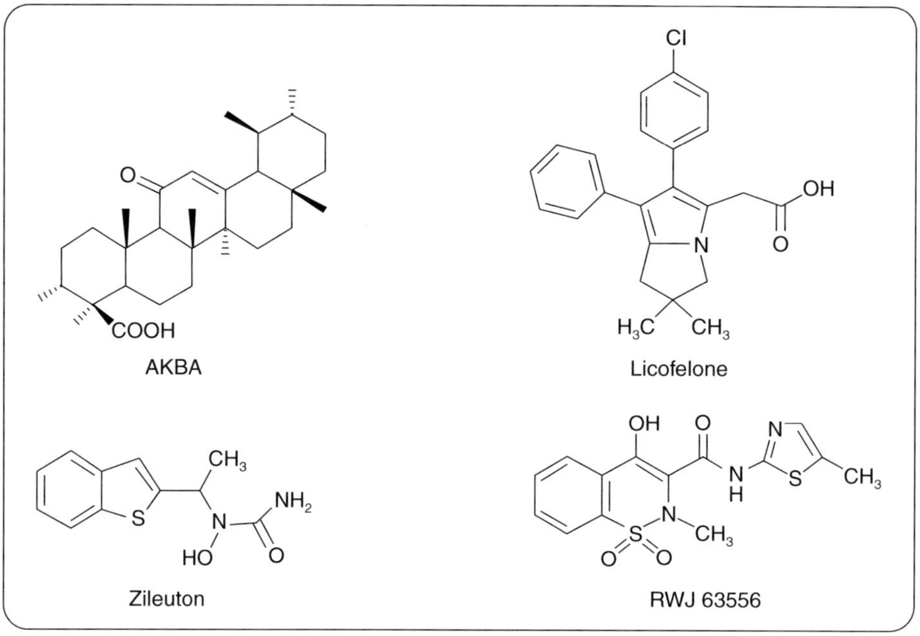

Fig. 9.6 *Various Classes of Natural 5-LOX Inhibitor*

antagonists act at their receptors (Singh *et al.*, 2005). RWJ 63556 is a potent, orally active COX-2-selective/5-LOX inhibitor and maintains its anti-inflammatory and LTB_4-inhibitory effects (Kirchner *et al.*, 1997).

INDUCIBLE NITRIC OXIDE SYNTHASE PATHWAY

The free radical NO, synthesized by the mammalian cells, can act as a physiological messenger and as a cytotoxic agent (Lincoln *et al.*, 1997). Nitric oxide synthesis is mediated in two ways: (1) nonenzymatic synthesis of NO and (2) enzymatic synthesis of NO through nitric oxide synthase (NOS) (Lincoln *et al.*, 1997).

NOS is widely spread in the activated macrophages, neurons in the brain and the endothelial cells. There are two types of NOS isoforms that are found in human body, namely constitutive (cNOS) and inducible (iNOS). In macrophages, NOS is expressed only after activation by endotoxin or cytokines. Another classification of NOS is made based on its origin in the cell, such as endothelial NOS and neuronal NOS.

Synthesis of Nitric Oxide

Arginine is converted to NO and citruline by NOS in a two-step process via the formation of the intermediate *N*-hydroxy-L-arginine (Nathan, 1992; Knowles and Moncada, 1994), and the pathway for the NO synthesis is given in Fig. 9.7. Tetrahydrobiopterin (BH_4) is required for the conversion of L-arginine to citruline and CO has the potential to inhibit the conversion of *N*-hydroxy-L-arginine, indicating that heme group is also involved in the process. INF-γ can also act at the posttranscriptional level to stabilize type II NOS mRNA. Transforming growth factor-beta (TGF-β), IL-4, IL-10 and corticosteroids have been shown to suppress the induction of iNOS. TGF-β is known to destabilize iNOS mRNA and decrease its translation. Cytokines IL-4 and IL-13 are known to be powerful inhibitors of the NO production from activated macrophages (Bogdan, Vodovotz, *et al.*, 1994; Bogdan, Thuring, *et al.*, 1999).

PHOSPOLIPASE A2

Phospholipases are a class of enzymes that play a crucial role in the metabolism of phospholipids (Divchev and Schieffer, 2008). PLA2 esterase catalyzes the cleavage of glycerophospholipids at the *sn-2* ester bond and releases the fatty acid and a lysophospholipid. The secretory PLA2 (sPLA2) are the oldest class of PLA2, typically the smallest (13–18 kDa), and they use histidine to hydrolyze the *sn-2* ester bond. In contrast, cytosolic PLA2 (cPLA2) and Ca^{2+}-independent PLA2 (iPLA2) are larger in size, typically 66–90 kDa, and the serine in their active site helps in hydrolyzing the *sn-2* ester bond (Hooks and Cummings, 2008). The PLA2 family of enzymes includes two types, viz. the calcium-dependent cPLA2 and the sPLA2 (Zhang *et al.*, 2009). Other types include the iPLA2 and the lipoprotein-associated PLA2 (lp-PLA2), also known as platelet-activating factor acetylhydrolase (PAF-AH). Phospholipases are commonly found in mammalian tissues as well as in insect and snake venom. Due to the increased presence and activity of PLA2 at the place of snake or insect bite, AA

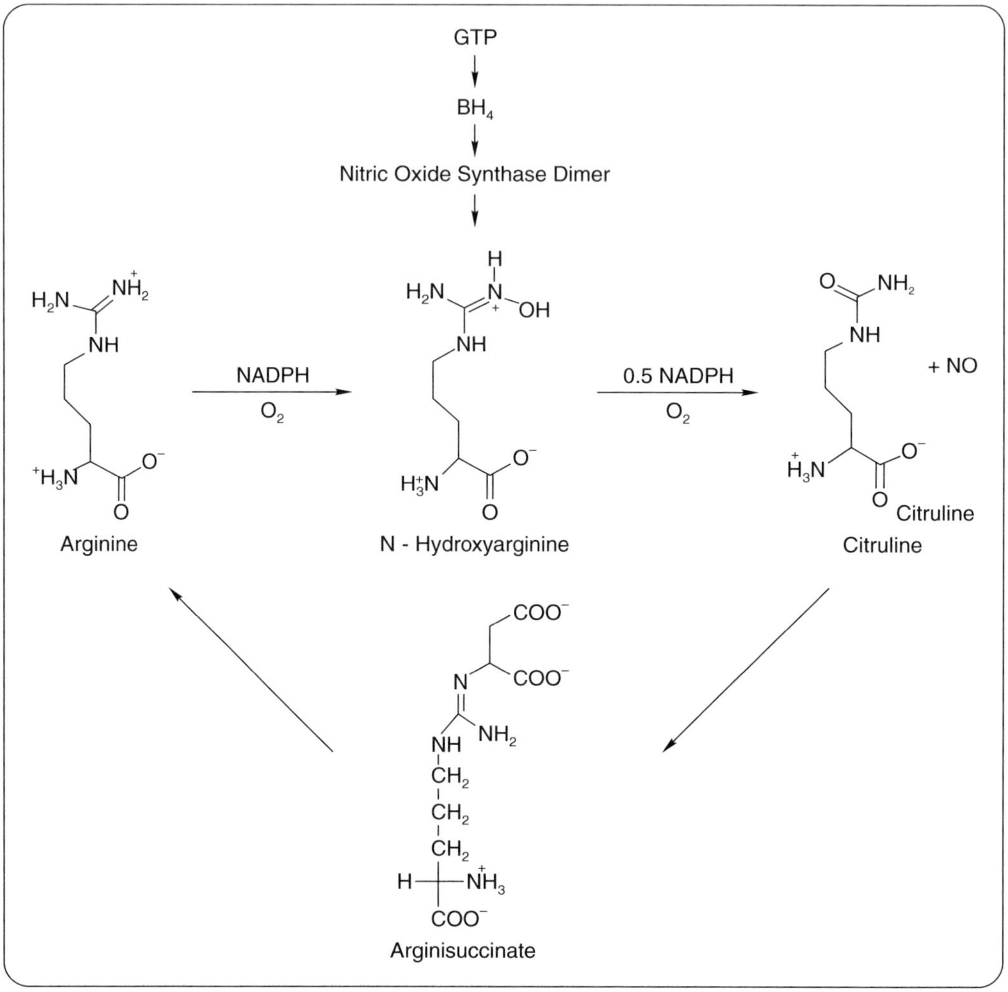

Fig. 9.7 *Enzymatic Synthesis of NO*

is released from the phospholipid membrane disproportionately, resulting in inflammation and pain at that site. PLA2-activating protein (PLAA) is a novel signaling molecule that regulates eicosanoid production and is also involved in the inflammatory responses.

Most of the cell types in the body can secrete sPLA2s; in particular, sPLA2-IIA is secreted by mesangial cell, vascular smooth muscle, endothelial cell, platelets, mast cells, neutrophils, macrophages and hepatic cells (Hooks and Cummings, 2008). Inflammatory processes include increased levels of extracellular PLA2 and cytokines such as IL-1 and tumor necrosis factor (TNF). The sequential induction, first by cytokines followed by PLA2, suggests that these cytokines may regulate the synthesis and secretion of PLA2 (Vadas *et al*., 1991). Activation of cPLA2 involves its translocation from the cytosol to the membrane, where it associates stably. cPLA2 binds to the membrane through a calcium-dependent lipid binding domain (Gijón *et al.*, 2000). Diacylglycerol (DAG) and PLA2 (with calcium) form a DAG–Ca–PLA2 complex, from which DAG is released. Addition of phosphoinositol 4,5-bisphosphate (PIP_2) to PLA2 leads to a PIP_2–PLA2 complex. PIP_2 is released during the biosynthesis of PLA2, as shown in Fig. 9.8.

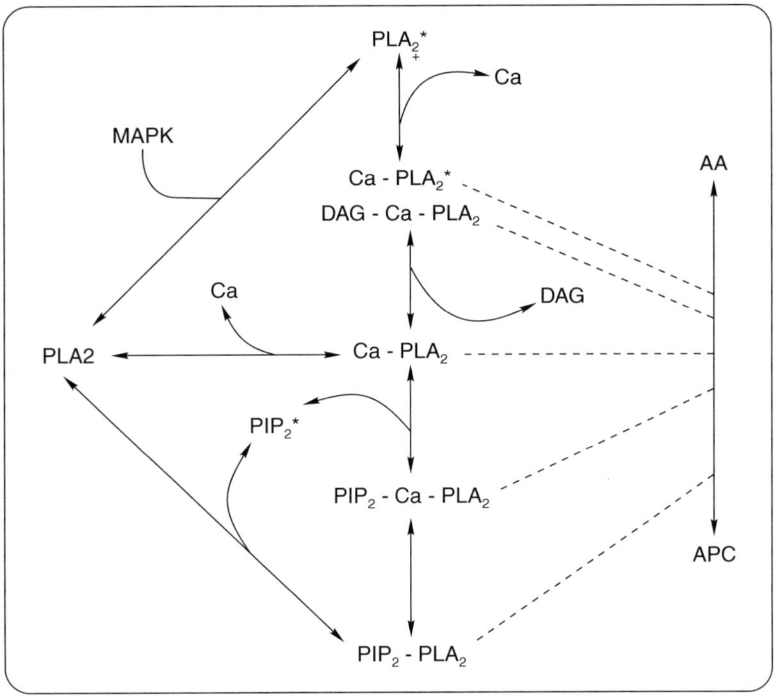

Fig. 9.8 ***Biosynthesis of Phospholipase A2***

The activation of PLA2 results immediately in hypersensitivity reactions (Marone *et al.*, 1981). Acute respiratory distress syndrome (ARDS) is a life-threatening lung injury characterized by arterial hypoxemia and noncardiogenic pulmonary edema. One of the features of ARDS is the alteration of a pulmonary surfactant, leading to an increase in surface tension at the air–liquid interface, resulting in alveolar collapse and impairment of gas exchange. The type II sPLA2 (sPLA2-II) plays a major role in the hydrolysis of surfactant phospholipids, and the presence of a surfactant inhibits its expression (Touqui and Arbibe, 1999). PLA2 in the central nervous system plays different roles in physiologic and pathologic states. Under physiologic conditions, PLA2 may be involved in many roles, such as phospholipid turnover, membrane remodeling, exocytosis, detoxification of phospholipid peroxides and neurotransmitter release. Under pathologic conditions, increased PLA2 activity may result in the loss of essential membrane glycerophospholipids, resulting in altered membrane permeability, ion homeostasis, increased free fatty acid release and accumulation of lipid peroxides. These processes, along with loss of ATP, may be responsible for the loss of membrane phospholipid and subsequent neuronal injury, which occurs during ischemia, spinal cord injury and other neurodegenerative diseases (*Farooqui et al., 1997*).

iPLA2 is involved in generating eicosanoids during inflammation. The inflammatory process consists of several discrete stages. The persistence of iPLA2 at the onset of inflammation generates eicosanoids, such as LTB_4, for recruiting inflammatory cells, leading to their influx. iPLA2 participates in eicosanoid generation and it is also activated at an appropriate stage of the inflammatory process by certain cell types, which does it through a specific and distinct mechanism (Hurley and McCormick, 2008). The cells that express iPLA2 routinely exhibit apoptosis under normal as well as inflammatory conditions. The association of elevated serum levels of sPLA2 in patients with cardiovascular disease and their presence in atherosclerotic lesions suggest that sPLA2 enzymes play a role in this disease. Its involvement in the atherosclerotic process is confirmed by the presence of more advanced atherosclerotic lesions that overexpress sPLA2 enzymes. Therefore, it can be concluded that the sPLA2 family of enzymes can provide reasonable targets for the prevention and treatment of atherosclerosis (Leite *et al.*, 2009).

Inhibition of these lipolytic enzymes is a highly challenging task because the enzymatic reaction occurs at the lipid/water interface (Gelb *et al.*). Mepacrine inhibits PLA2 activity in several tissues by a dose-dependent inhibition of histamine, which is released from human basophils by inducing several immunologic (i.e. antigen and anti-IgE) and nonimmunologic (i.e. formyl-methionine-containing peptide (f-met peptide) and the Ca^{2+} ionophore, A23187) stimuli (Marone *et al.*, 1981) (Fig. 9.9). cPLA2 plays a pivotal role in inflammation by catalyzing the release of AA (substrate for lipoxygenase and COX enzymes) from membrane phospholipids. Arachidonyl trifluoromethyl

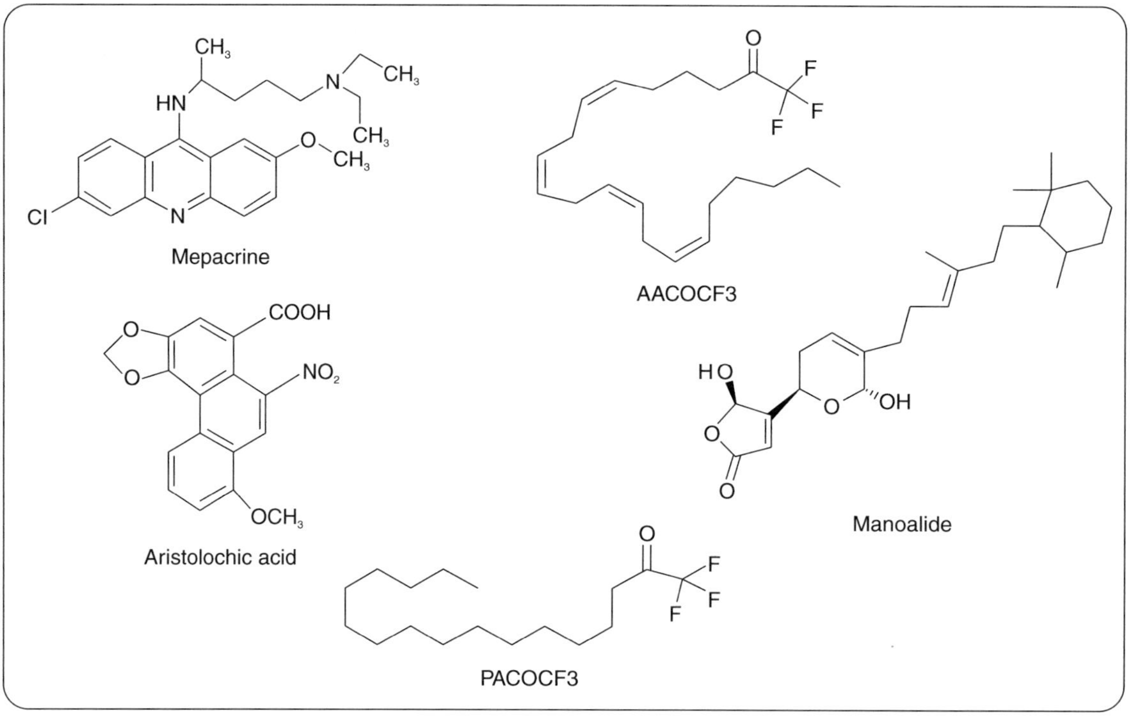

Fig. 9.9 *Commercial Inhibitors of Phospholipase A2*

ketone ($AACOCF_3$) is a specific inhibitor of the enzyme cPLA2. $AACOCF_3$ is an inhibitor of chronic but not acute inflammatory response. $AACOCF_3$ inhibits phorbol 12-myristate 13-acetate (PMA)-induced chronic ear edema (Malaviya *et al.*, 2006). Aristolochic acid is an inhibitor of the calcium-dependent, neutral-active PLA2, and it is isolated from the human neutrophils. The inhibition effect is dose dependent, with an IC50 value of 40 μM, and is rapid with near-maximal inhibition within 5 min. Aristolochic acid from human neutrophils is an effective inhibitor of A23187-stimulated PLA2 activity (Rosenthal *et al.*, 1989). Manoalide is a powerful anti-inflammatory marine natural product, directly inactivating the venom PLA2. Manoalide irreversibly inhibits PLA2 by correspondingly modifying a selective number of lysine residues (Glaser *et al.*, 1989).

PROSTAGLANDIN E SYNTHASE INHIBITOR

Upon stimulation, lipids are released from plasma membranes and metabolized into mediators capable of changing the cellular physiology. As these lipids are present at the first exposed site, they provide an ideal substrate for the synthesis of defensive mediators and homeostatic regulators. One such group of lipid mediators is the prostanoids, including the PGs and TXs. These mediators can act to both promote and inhibit the inflammation.

Prostanoids are produced when AA is released from the plasma membrane by phospholipases and metabolized by COXs to form PGH_2. PGH_2 forms a common substrate for a series of specific synthase/isomerase enzymes that produce PGs (PGD_2, PGE_2, $PGF_{2\alpha}$, PGI_2) and TXA_2 (Fig. 9.10).

The mechanism of action that permits the selective inhibition of the formation of PGE_2, an endogenous substance that has been shown to be central in inflammatory processes, has been discovered in recent years. The identification of the microsomal prostaglandin E synthase (mPGES) is the key to a new class of specific enzyme inhibitors, which leaves the formation of physiologically important PGs unchanged. Therefore, these drugs would be effective anti-inflammatory drugs but would have less problematic side effects. Currently, there are no commercial drugs in market for specific prostaglandin E synthase (PGES) inhibitors and receptor antagonists for all of the four PGE_2 receptor (EP) subtypes. This shows a potential field of study in inflammation and pain research.

PGESs is also like COXs exist in three isoforms: cytoplasmic PGES (cPGES), microsomal PGES-1 (mPGES-1) and microsomal PGES-2 (mPGES-2) (see Table 9.2).

Table 9.2 *Characteristics of PGES Isozymes*

	GSH (Cofactor) Requirement	*Subcellular Distribution*	*Gene Expression*	*Coupling with COXs*
cPGES	Yes	Cytosol	Constitutive	COX-1
mPGES-1	Yes	Perinuclear membrane	Inducible	COX-2
mPGES-2	No	Membrane	?	?

mPGES-1 is said to be mainly coupled with the inflammation-induced form of COX-2, whereas cPGES is coupled with COX-1 and is a constitutive enzyme. The role of mPGES-2 is still not very clear (Fig. 9.11).

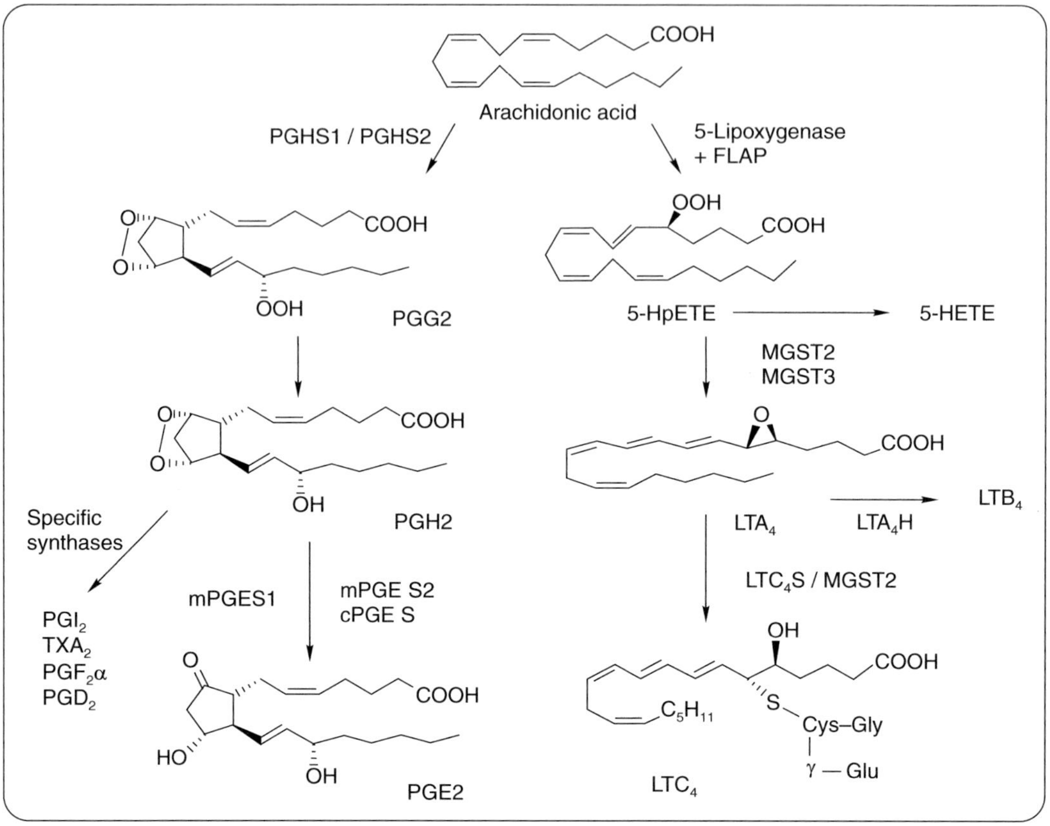

Fig. 9.10 *MAPEG Proteins in Arachidonic Acid Metabolism*

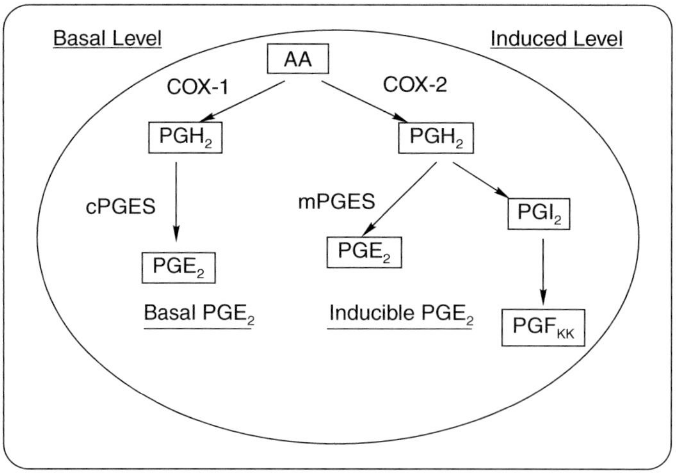

Fig. 9.11 *Coupling of COX and PGES Enzymes*

Two crystal structures of the mPGES-2 isoform are available in the Protein Data Bank (1Z9H with indomethacin as the ligand and 2PJB with Heme and glutathione (GSH) as cofactors). The other two isoforms, cPGES and mPGES-1, do not have either crystal or nuclear magnetic resonance (NMR) structures.

Very few inhibitors of mPGES-1, the inducible isoform are available in the literature. Table 9.3 gives the name, structure and activity values for a few reported inhibitors.

Table 9.3 *Reported mPGES-1 Inhibitors*

Name	*IC50 Values*	*Structure*	*Remark*
Indomethacin	The catalytic efficiency (k_{cat}/K_M) of the PGH_2 to PGE_2 reaction by mPGES-2 is 6.5×10^4 s^{-1} M^{-1} ($k_{cat} = 1.82$ s^{-1} and $K_M = 28\mu M$), which is a moderate rate, suggesting that tight binding of PGH_2 to the protein might not be required	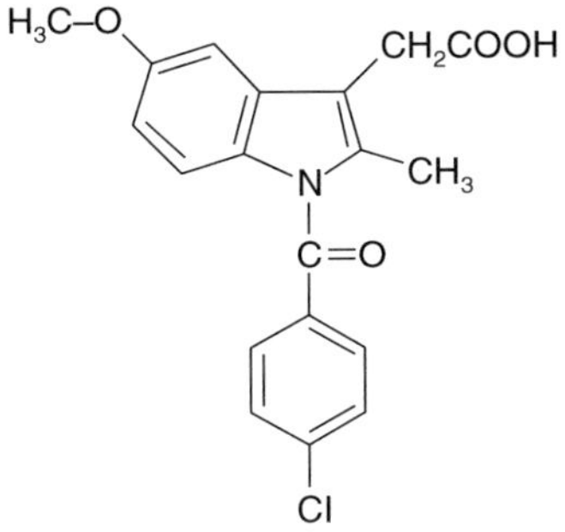	Crystal structure ligand for mPGES-2
15-Deoxy-D^{12,14}PGJ$_2$	0.3 mM	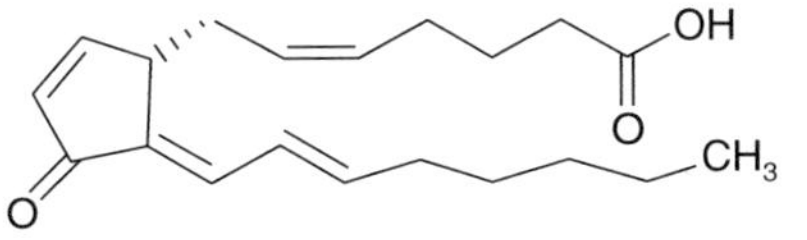 PGG2	Endogenous
Arachidonic acid	0.3 mM	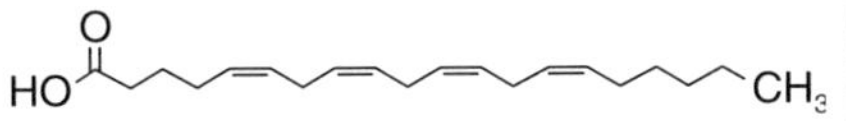	Endogenous
Docosahexaenoic acid	0.3 mM	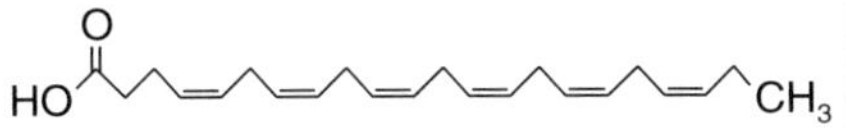	Endogenous
Eicosapentaenoic acid	0.3 mM	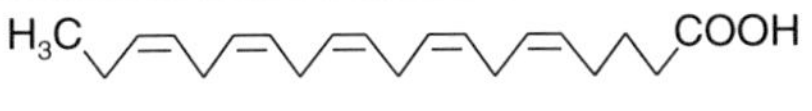	Endogenous
Exisulind (sulindac sulfone)	80 mM	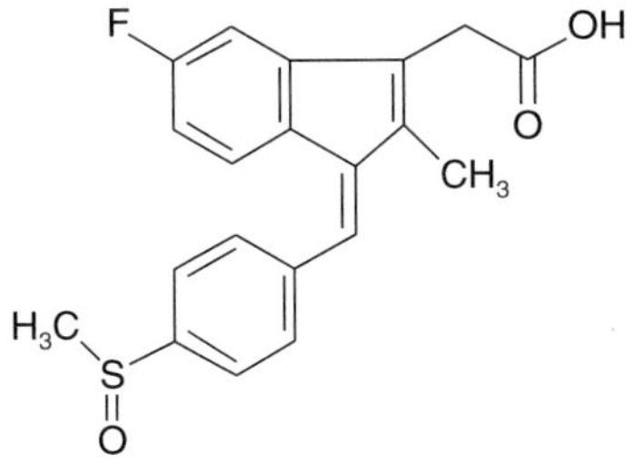	Development suspended in 2005 by OSI pharma

(Contd)

(Table 9.3 Contd)

Name	***IC50 Values***	***Structure***	***Remark***
NS-398	20 mM	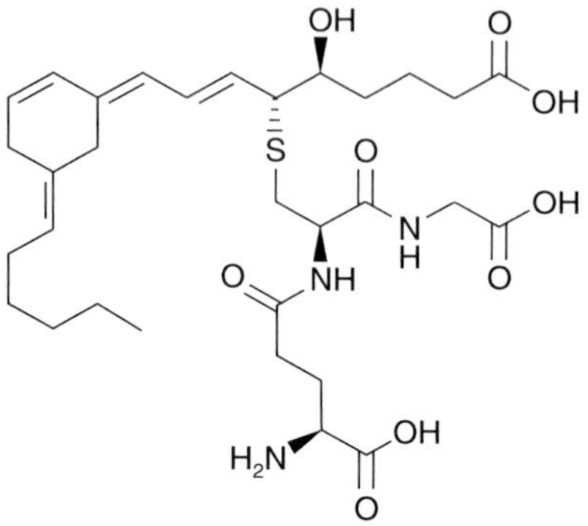	Development suspended in 2000 by Taisho Pharmaceutical
Leukotriene C_4	5 mM	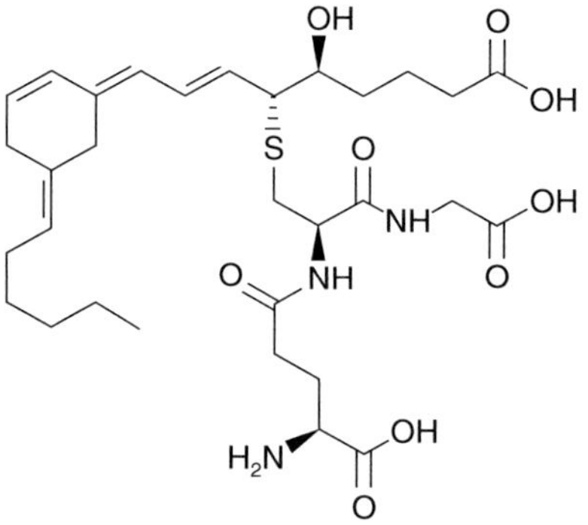	Endogenous
MK-886(potent indole FLAP inhibitor)	1.6 mM	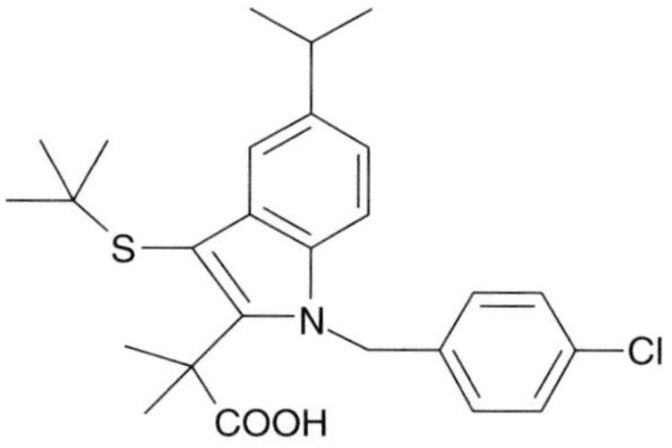	Development suspended in 1995 by Merck Pharma
Analog of MK-886; X = F, Y = Ph (belongs to a class of 5-phenylindoles)	3 nM		Using MK-886 as a lead structure, SAR studies were performed to identify more potent and selective inhibitors of mPGES-1

(Contd)

(Table 9.3 Contd)

Name	*IC50 Values*	*Structure*	*Remark*
Analog of MK-886; X = F, Y = 2-Me-Ph (belongs to a class of 5-phenylindoles)	7 nM	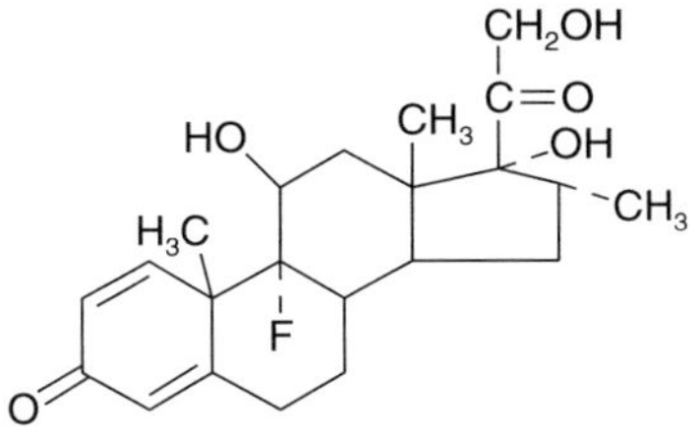	Same as above

REFERENCES

Bindra, J.S., Bindra, R. (1977). Prostaglandin Synthesis. New York: Academic Press.

Bogdan, C., Thuring, H., Dlaska, M., Rollinghoff, M., Weiss, G. (1997). Mechanism of suppression of macrophage nitric oxide release by IL-13: influence of the macrophage population. *The Journal of Immunology*, **159(9)**:4506–4513.

Bogdan, C., Vodovotz, Y., Paik, J., Xie, Q.W., Nathan, C. (1994). Mechanism of suppression of nitric oxide synthase expression by interleukin-4 in primary mouse macrophages. *Journal of Leukocyte Biology* **55(2)**:227–233.

Brain, S.D., Williams, T.J. (1990). Leukotrienes and inflammation. *Pharmacology and Therapeutics* **46(1)**:57–66.

Chandrasekharan, N.V., Dai, H., Roos, K.L., Evanson, N.K., Tomsik, J., Elton, T.S., Simmons, D.L. (2002). COX-3, a cyclooxygenase-1 variant inhibited by acetaminophen and other analgesic/antipyretic drugs: Cloning, structure, and expression, In: *Proceedings of the National Academy of Sciences of the United States of America*, **99(21)**:13926–13931.

Chen, Q.H., Rao, P.N.P., Knaus, E.E. (2005). Design, synthesis, and biological evaluation of linear 1-(4-, 3- or 2-methylsulfonylphenyl)-2-phenylacetylenes: A novel class of cyclooxygenase-2 inhibitors. *Bioorganic and Medicinal Chemistry* **13(23)**:6425–6434.

Dannhardt, G., Laufer, S. (2000). Structural approaches to explain the selectivity of COX-2 inhibitors: Is there a common pharmacophore? *Current Medicinal Chemistry* **7(11)**:1101–1112.

Divchev, D., Schieffer, B. (2008). The secretory phospholipase A_2 group IIA: A missing link between inflammation, activated renin–angiotensin system, and atherogenesis? *Vascular Health Risk Management* **4(3)**:597–604.

Drazen, J.M., Israel, E., O'Byrne, P.M. (1999). Treatment of Asthma with Drugs Modifying the Leukotriene Pathway. *The New England Journal of Medicine* **340(3)**:197–206.

Earnet, D.L., Hixson, L.J., Alberts, D.S. (2004). Piroxicam and other cyclooxygenase inhibitors: Potential for cancer chemoprevention. *Journal of Cellular Biochemistry* **50 (0)**:156–166.

Farooqui, Akhlaq A., Yang, Hsiu-Chiung, Rosenberger, Thad A., Horrocks, Lloyd A. (1997). Phospholipase A2 and its role in brain tissue. *Journal of Neurochemistry* **69(3)**:889–901.

Frolich, J.C. (1997). Prostaglandins, Arzneimittel-Forschung *Drug Research* **47(11)**:1289–96.

Funk, C.D. (2001). Prostaglandins and leukotrienes: *Advances in Eicosanoid Biology Science* **294(5548)**:1871–1875.

Gelb, M.H., Jain, M.K., Berg, O.G. (1994) Inhibition of phospholipase A2. *The FASEB Journal* **8(12)**:916–924.

Gierse, J.K., Hauser, S.D., Creely, D.P., Koboldt, C., Rangwala, S.H., Isakson, P.C., Seibert, K. (1995). Expression and selective inhibition of the constitutive and inducible forms of human cyclo-oxygenase. *Biochemical Journal* **305(Pt. 2)**:479–484.

Gijón, Miguel A., Spencer, Diane M., Siddiqi, Abdur R., Bonventre, Joseph V., Leslie, Christina C. (2000). Cytosolic phospholipase A_2 is required for macrophage arachidonic acid release by agonists that do and do not mobilize calcium. Novel role of mitogen-activated protein kinase pathways in cytosolic phospholipase A_2 regulation. *The Journal of Biological Chemistry* **275(26)**:20146–20156.

Glaser, K.B., de Carvalho, M.S., Jacobs, R.S., Kernan, M.R., Faulkner, D.J. (1989). Manoalide: Structure–activity studies and definition of the pharmacophore for phospholipase A_2 inactivation. *Molecular Pharmocology* **36(5)**:782–788.

Guerguerian, A.M., Hardy, P., Bhattacharya, M., Olley, P., Clyman, R.I., Fouron, J.C., Chemtob, S. (1998). Expression of cyclooxygenases in ductus arteriosus of fetal and newborn pigs. *American Journal of Obstetrics and Gynecology* **179(6)**:1618–1626.

Gustafson-Svard, C., Lilja, I., Hallbook, O., Sjodahl, R. (1996). Cyclooxygenase-1 and cyclooxygenase-2 gene expression in human colorectal adenocarcinomas and in azoxymethane induced colonic tumours in rats. *Gut* **38(1)**:79–84.

Harris, Stuart L, Kuss, Michael, Hubbard, Richard C., Goldstein, Jay L. (2001). Upper gastrointestinal safety evaluation of parecoxib sodium, a new parenteral cyclooxygenase-2-specific inhibitor, compared with ketorolac, naproxen, and placebo. *Clinical Therapeutics* **23(9)**:1422–1428.

Hayashi, T., Nishiyama, K., Shirahama, T. (2006). Inhibition of 5-lipoxygenase pathway suppresses the growth of bladder cancer cells. *International Journal of Urology* **13(8)**:1086–1091.

Hooks, S. B., Cummings, B. S. (2008). Role of Ca^{2+}-independent phospholipase as in cell growth and signaling. *Biochemical Pharmacology* **76(9)**:1059–1067.

Hoque, A., Lippman, S.M., Wu, T.T., Xu, Y., Liang, Z.D., Swisher, S., Zhang, H., Cao, L., Ajani, J.A., Xu, X.C. (2005). Increased 5-lipoxygenase expression and induction of apoptosis by its inhibitors in esophageal cancer: a potential target for prevention. *Carcinogenesis* **26(4)**:785–91.

Hurley, B.P., McCormick, B.A. (2008). Multiple roles of phospholipase A_2 during lung infection and inflammation. *Infection and Immunity* **76(6)**:2259–2272.

Jahng, Y., Zhao, L., Moon, Y., Basnet, A., Kim, E., Chang, H.W., Ju, H.K., Jeong, T.C., Lee, E. (2004). Simple aromatic compounds containing propenone moiety show considerable dual COX/5-LOX inhibitory activities. *Bioorganic and Medicinal Chemistry Letters* **14(10)**:2559–2562.

Kalgutkar, Amit S., Crews, Brenda C., Rowlinson, Scott W., Marnett, Alan B., Kozak, Kevin R., Remmel, Rory P., Marnett, Lawrence J. (2000). Biochemically based design of cyclooxygenase-2 (COX-2) inhibitors: Facile conversion of nonsteroidal antiinflammatory drugs to potent and highly selective COX-2 inhibitors. In: *Proceedings of the National Academy of Sciences of the United States of America* **97(2)**:925–930.

Kirchner, T., Argentieri, D.C., Barbone, A.G., Singer, M., Steber, M., Ansell, J., Beers, S.A., Wachter, M.P., Wu, W., Malloy, E., Stewart, A., Ritchie, D.M. (1997). Evaluation of the antiinflammatory activity of a dual cyclooxygenase-2 selective/5-lipoxygenase inhibitor, RWJ 63556, in a canine model of inflammation. *Journal of Pharmacology and Experimental Therapeutics* **282(2)**:1094–1101.

Knowles, R.G., Moncada, S. (1994). Nitric oxide synthases in mammals. *Biochemical Journal* **298(Pt 2)**:249–258.

Kurumbail, R.G., Kiefer, J.R., Marnett, L.J. (2001). Cyclooxygenase enzymes: catalysis and inhibition. *Current Opinion in Structural Biology* **11(6):**752–60.

Lehmann, W.D. (1994). Regio- and stereochemistry of the dioxygenation reaction catalyzed by (S)-type lipoxygenases or by the cyclooxygenase activity of prostaglandin H synthases. *Free Radical Biology and Medicine* **16(2)**:241–253.

Leite, J.O., Vaishnav, U., Puglisi, M., Fraser, H., Lincoln, J., Hoyle, C.H.V., Burnstock, G. (1997). Nitric Oxide in Health and Disease,United Kingdom, Cambridge University Press, pp. 1–3.

Lovering, A. L., Ride, J.P., Bunce, C.M., Desmond, J.C., Cummings, S. M., White, S.A. (2004). Crystal structures of prostaglandin D_2 11-ketoreductase (AKR1C3) in complex with the Nonsteroidal Anti-inflammatory drugs Flufenamic acid and Indomethacin. *Cancer Research* **64(5)**:1802–1810.

Malaviya, R., Ansell, J., Hall, L., Fahmy, M., Argentieri, R.L., Olini, G.C., Jr., Pereira, D.W., Sur, R., Cavender, D. (2006). Targeting cytosolic phospholipase A_2 by arachidonyl trifluoromethyl ketone prevents chronic inflammation in mice. *European Journal of Pharmacology* **539(3)**:195–204.

Malhotra, P., Gupta, O.P., Parihar, A., Bala, S., Gupta, G. (2007). Licofelone—A dual COX and 5-LOX inhibitor. *The Pharma Review* **31(6)**:207–208.

Marone, G., Kagey-Sobotka, A., Lichtenstein, L.M. (1981). Possible role of phospholipase A_2 in triggering histamine secretion from human basophils in vitro. *Clinical Immunology and Immunopathology* **20(2)**:231–239.

Merlie, J.P., Fagan, D., Mudd, J., Needleman, P. 1988, Isolation and characterization of the complementary DNA for sheep seminal vesicle prostaglandin endoperoxide synthase (cyclooxygenase). *The Journal of Biological Chemistry* **263(8):**3550–3553.

Mitchell, J.A., Akarasereenont, P., Thiemermann, C., Flower, R.J., Vane, J.R. (1993). Selectivity of nonsteroidal antiinflammatory drugs as inhibitors of constitutive and inducible cyclooxygenase. *Proceedings of the National Academy of Sciences of the United States of America* **90(24)**:11693–11697.

Murias, M., Handler, N., Erker, T., Pleban, K., Ecker, G., Saiko, P., Szekeres, T., Jager, W. (2004). Resveratrol analogues as selective cyclooxygenase-2 inhibitors: synthesis and structure-activity relationship. *Bioorganic and Medicinal Chemistry* **12(21)**:5571–5578.

Nathan, C. (1992). Nitric oxide as a secretory product of mammalian cells. *The FASEB Journal* **6(12)**:3051–3064.

Nielsen, S.T., Benignity, L., Buonato, C.B. (1988). Sulfasalazine and 5-aminosalicylic acid inhibit contractile leukotriene formation. *Scandinavian Journal of Gastroenterology* **23(3)**:272–276.

Noble, S.L., King, D.S., Olutade, J.I. (2000). Cyclooxygenase-2 enzyme inhibitors: Place in therapy. *Journal of AAFP*, **61(12)**:*3669*–3676.

Punchard, N.A., Whelan, C.J., Adcock, I. (2004). The Journal of Inflammation, *Journal of Inflammation (London)* **1:1**.

Rahim, M.A., Rao, P.N., Knaus, E.E. (2002). Isomeric acetoxy analogues of rofecoxib: A novel class of highly potent and selective cyclooxygenase-2 inhibitors. *Bioorganic and Medicinal Chemistry Letters* **12(19)**:2753–2756.

Reid, G.K., Kargman, S., Vickers, P.J., Mancini, J.A., Leveille, C., Ethier, D., Miller, D.K., Gillard, J.W., Dixon, R.A.F., Evans, J.F. (1990). Correlation between expression of 5-lipoxygenase-activating protein, 5-lipoxygenase, and cellular leukotriene synthesis. *Journal of Biological Chemistry* **265(32)**:19818–19823.

Rosen, G.D., Birkenmeier, T.M., Raz, A., Holtzman, M.J. (1989), Identification of a cyclooxygenase-related gene and its potential role in prostaglandin formation. *Biochemical and Biophysical Research Communications* **164(3):**1358–1365.

Rosenthal, M.D., Vishwanath, B.S., Franson, R.C. (1989). Effects of aristolochic acid on phospholipase A2 activity and arachidonate metabolism of human neutrophils. *Biochimica et Biophysica Acta* **1001(1)**:1–8.

Rouzer, C.A., Marnett, L.J. (2003). Mechanism of free radical oxygenation of polyunsaturated fatty acids by cyclooxygenases, *Chemical Reviews* **103(6):**2239–2304.

Sailer, E.R., Subramanian, L.R., Rall, B., Hoernlein, R.F., Ammon, H.P., Safayhi, H. (1996). Acetyl-11-keto-beta-boswellic acid (AKBA): structure requirements for binding and 5-lipoxygenase inhibitory activity. *British Journal of Pharmacology* **117(4)**:615–618.

Samuelsson, B. (1983). Leukotrienes: mediators of immediate hypersensitivity reactions and inflammation. *Science* **220(4597)**:568–575.

Simmons, D.L., Levy, D.B., Yannoni, Y., Erikson, R.L. (1989). Identification of a phorbol ester-repressible v-src-inducible gene. In: *Proceedings of the National Academy of Sciences of the United States of America* **86(4):**1178–1182.

Singh, V.P., Patil, Chandrashekhar S.P., Kulkarni, S.K. (2005). Differential effect of zileuton, a 5-lipoxygenase inhibitor, against nociceptive paradigms in mice and rats. Pharmacology. *Biochemistry and Behavior* **81(3)**:433–439.

Sivakumar, P.M., Doble, M. (2006). QSAR studies of COX-2 inhibitors of commercial interest. 10th International Conference of ISCB on Drug Discovery: Perspectives and Challenges, CDRI, Lucknow.

Smith, W.L., DeWitt, D.L., Garavito, R.M. (2000). CYCLOOXYGENASES: Structural, Cellular, and Molecular Biology. *Annual Review of Biochemistry* **69(1):**145–182.

Smith, J.B., Willis, A.L. (1971), Aspirin selectivity inhibits prostaglandin production in human platelets. *Nature—New Biology* **231(25)**:235–237.

Sommerauer, M., Ates, M., Gühring, H., Brune, K., Amann, R., Peskar, B.A. (2001) Ketoprofen-Induced Cyclooxygenase Inhibition in Renal Medulla and Platelets of Rats Treated with Caffeine. *Pharmacology* **63(4)** 234–239.

Touqui, L., Arbibe, L. (1999). A role for phospholipase A_2 in ARDS pathogenesis. *Molecular Medicine Today* **5(6)**:244–249.

Jose O.L., Ushma V., Michael P., Heather F., Trias, J., Fernandez, M.L. (2009). A-002 (varespladib), a phospholipase A2 inhibitor, reduces atherosclerosis in guinea pigs. *BMC Cardiovascular Disorders* **9(7)**.

Vadas, P., Pruzanski, W., Stefanski, E., Ellies, L.G., Aubin, J.E., Sos, A., Melcher, A. (1991). Extracellular phospholipase A2 secretion is a common effector pathway of interleukin-1 and tumour necrosis factor action. *Immunology Letters* **28(3)**:187–193.

Valentovic, M. (2008). Flurbiprofen. In: *xPharm: The Comprehensive Pharmacology Reference, pp. 1–6.*

Van der donk, W.A., Tsai, A.L., Kulmacz, R.J. (2002). The cyclooxygenase reaction mechanism. *Biochemistry* **41(52):**15451–15458.

Vane, J.R. (1971). Inhibition of prostaglandin synthesis as a mechanism of action for aspirin like drugs. *Nature—New Biology* **231(25)**:232–235.

Vane, J.R., Botting, R.M. The history of aspirin. In: Vane, J.R., Botting, R.M., editors. Aspirin and other salicylates. London:Chapman and Hall, 1992:3–16.

Wenzel, S.E. (1998). New approaches to anti-inflammatory therapy for asthma, *American Journal of Medicine* **104(3)**:287–300.

Yamamoto, S., Yamamoto, K., Kurobe, H., Yamashita, R., Yamaguchi, H., Ueda, N. (1998), Transcriptional regulation of fatty acid cyclooxygenases-1 and -2. *International Journal of Tissue Reactions* **20(1)**:17–22.

Zhang, F., Suarez, G., Sha, J., Sierra, J.C., Peterson, J.W., Chopra, A.K. (2009). Phospholipase A2-activating protein (PLAA) enhances cisplatin-induced apoptosis in HeLa cells. *Cellular Signalling* **21(7)**:1085–1099.

10

Cardiotonics

Padma Priya P.V. and Mukesh Doble*

Department of Biotechnology, IIT Madras, Chennai, India

INTRODUCTION

Congestive heart failure (CHF) is an increasingly prevalent problem in cardiology associated with the final stages of various cardiovascular disorders. The annual mortality rate of patients who have CHF remains high regardless of therapy with a variety of drugs (Consensus Recommendations for Heart Failure, 1999). Therapeutic interventions may improve the performance of the failing heart in three ways. First, drugs may increase ejection fraction of the failing left ventricle by directly stimulating cardiac contractility. This approach, utilized by positive inotropic agents, can produce immediate hemodynamic benefits in the short term. Long-term treatment with these drugs may increase morbidity and mortality (Packer *et al*., 1991; Cowley and Skene 1994; Hampton *et al*., 1997). Second, drugs may increase ejection fraction by decreasing impedance to left ventricular ejection through the relaxation of peripheral blood vessels. These vasodilator interventions again may relieve symptoms in the short term, but do not produce clinical benefits in the long term (Packer, Narahara, *et al*.; 1993, Packer, Rouleau, *et al*. 1993; Califf *et al*., 1997). Third, drugs may improve ejection fraction by affecting the process of cardiac remodeling. This approach is utilized by neurohormonal antagonists such as angiotensin-converting enzyme (ACE) inhibitors, beta-adrenergic receptor blockers (Konstam *et al*., 1993; Australia–New Zealand Heart Failure Research Collaborative Group, 1995) and vasodilators/growth inhibitors, such as nitrates (Jugdutt *et al*., 1994). They may not produce immediate symptomatic benefits, but long-term treatment with these drugs can improve clinical status and decrease the risk of major cardiac events (Garg and Yusuf 1995; Lechat *et al*., 1998).

**mukeshd@iitm.ac.in*

The primary symptom or defect in CHF is the loss of cardiac contractile function, which leads to reduced organ perfusion and hypotension. In association with the therapies mentioned in the second and third methods, an attempt to ameliorate cardiac contractile dysfunction by means of positive inotropic cardiotonic agents as mentioned in the first approach has played a central role in the pharmacological therapy of CHF and is the focus of this chapter.

CARDIOTONICS

Cardiotonics are cardio-stimulatory drugs, which improve the cardiac function by increasing the pumping ability of the heart. They enhance the cardiac function by positive inotropy (myocardial contractility) and positive chronotropy (increased heart rate), which in turn increases the cardiac output and arterial pressure. The improvement in cardiac function is also due to reducing afterload and increasing preload. These effects have life-saving potential and hence cardiotonic drugs are suitable for treatment of CHF, cardiogenic shock and hypotension.

Based on their mechanism of action, which mainly involves mobilizing Ca^{2+} into the cardiac myocytes and making it more accessible for myocyte contraction, three different classes of cardiotonics are available in clinical practice for the treatment of hemodynamic crisis in CHF. They are: (1) cardiac glycosides (also known as digitalis compounds), (2) sympathomimetic catecholamines (also known as beta-agonists) and (3) phosphodiesterase-3 (PDE3) inhibitors.

Cardiac Glycosides or Digitalis Compounds

Cardiac glycosides represent a family of compounds that are derived from the foxglove plant (*Digitalis purpurea*). William Withering published his treatment of heart patients with cardiotonic foxglove plant extract, also known as digitalis, in 1785 and described its therapeutic benefits (Aronson, 1985). This research led to the discovery of digoxin, marketed as the brand Lanoxin (GlaxoSmithKline, Research Triangle Park, North Carolina) (Smith, 1930). It has been used to treat arrhythmia and CHF ever since.

Mechanism of Action for Positive Inotropic Effects of Cardiac Glycosides

The mechanisms through which digitalis causes its therapeutic and toxic actions have been studied for nearly half a century (Fig. 10.1). The regulation of cardiac cell by intracellular ions via the sodium–potassium (Na^+/K^+) adenosine triphosphatase (ATPase) and how it is altered by cardiac glycosides have also been understood (Andrew and Gary, 2005).

The digitalis glycosides exert their primary effects in patients with heart failure by virtue of their ability to inhibit Na^+–K^+-ATPase (NKA). Inhibition of this enzyme in cardiac cells results in an increase in the contractile state of the heart (Akera *et al.*, 1973).

The Na^+/K^+ pump is identified as a membrane-bound ATP-hydrolyzing enzyme system, which is activated by the combined effect of Na^+ on the cytoplasmic side and K^+ on the extracellular side of the membrane. Most mammalian cells have the Na^+/K^+ pump in their membranes, which pumps Na^+ ions out of and K^+ ions into the cell, thereby creating an electrochemical gradient. The pumping requires energy, and the Na^+/K^+ pump is an energy transducer, which converts chemical energy from the hydrolysis of ATP to an electrochemical gradient of the cations (Skou, 1988). The

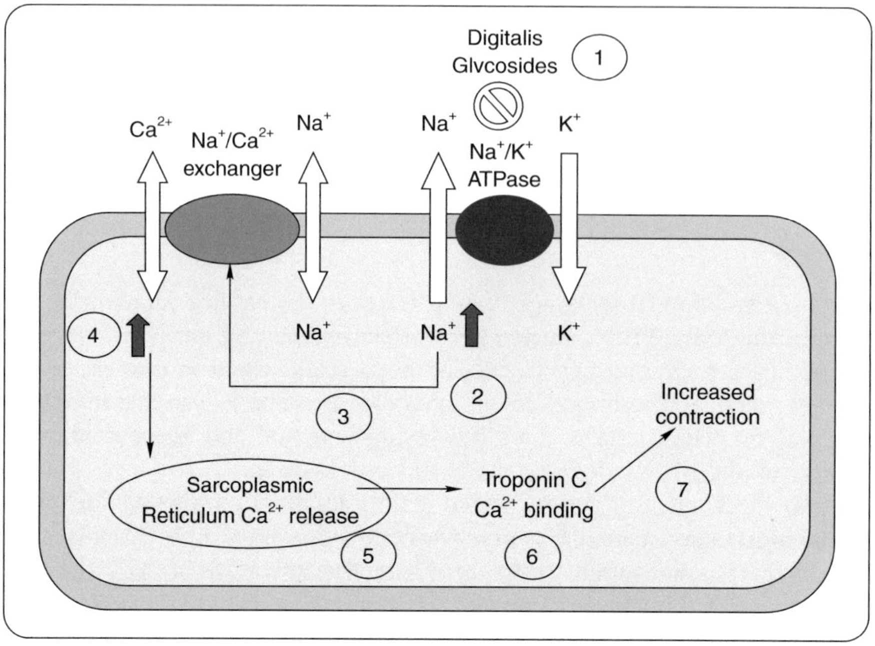

Fig. 10.1 *A Schematic Illustrating the 'Na Pump Lag Hypothesis' for Digitalis Glycoside in a Heart Muscle Cell*

transport is electrogenic, i.e. for each ATP molecule hydrolyzed three Na^+ ions are transported out of the cell and two K^+ ions into the cell. The net movement of positive charges to the outside of the membrane adds a few millivolts to the membrane potential. In 1953 it was observed that active Na^+/K^+ transport is inhibited by cardiac glycosides by binding to the extracellular side of the system (Skou, 1988). The Na^+ pump lag theory (Langer, 1970; Woodbury, 1963) was proposed to explain the physiological mechanism underlying the positive inotropic action. At nontoxic concentrations all cardiac glycosides specifically bind to and inhibit the sarcolemmal Na^+/K^+ ATPase, causing a partial inhibition of the ion-pumping function in the cardiac myocytes. Once glycoside has bound to and inhibited the enzyme, the intracellular Na^+ ion concentration increases in proportion to the new balance between influx and diminished extrusion. This accumulation of Na^+ causes a secondary increase in free intracellular Ca^{2+} concentration via Na^+/Ca^{2+} exchange (NCX). The resulting increase in Ca^{2+} uptake or Ca^{2+} mobilization into the cardiac myocyte is directly available for binding to troponin C, leading to contraction of the cardiac muscle; This is responsible for the positive inotropic and therapeutic action of cardiac glycosides (Andrew and Gary, 2005).

However, the benefits of digitalis may in part be related to enzyme inhibition in noncardiac tissues. Inhibition of Na^+/K^+ ATPase in vagal afferents acts to sensitize cardiac baroreceptors, which may in turn decrease sympathetic outflow from the central nervous system (Thames, 1979; Ferguson *et al.*, 1989). In addition, by inhibiting Na^+/K^+ ATPase in the kidney, digitalis decreases the renal tubular reabsorption of sodium (Torretti *et al.*, 1972). The resulting increase in the delivery of sodium to the distal tubules leads to the suppression of renin secretion from the kidneys (Covit *et al.*, 1983). These observations have led to the hypothesis that digitalis acts in heart failure primarily by attenuating the activation of neurohormonal systems, and not as a positive inotropic drug (Gheorghiade and Ferguson1991).

Although a variety of digitalis glycosides (Table 10.1) have been used in the treatment of heart failure during the last 200 years, the most commonly used preparation is digoxin. It is the only glycoside that has been evaluated in placebo-controlled trials, and has been reviewed by FDA and deemed effective for the treatment of patients with CHF (Andrew and Gary 2005).

Table 10.1 *List of Cardiac Glycosides and Their Structures*

Cardiac Glycoside	*Structure*
Digitoxin	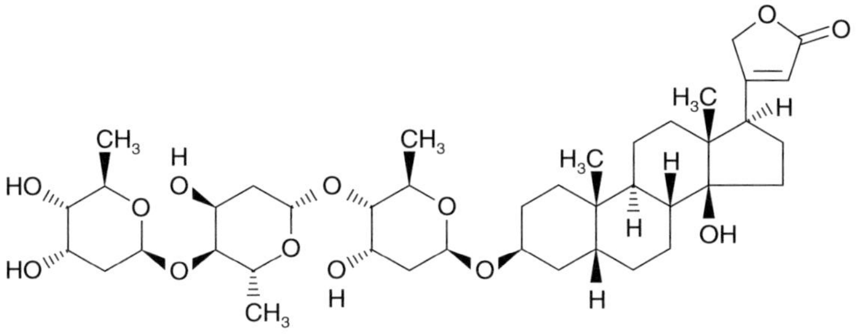 D00297
Digoxin	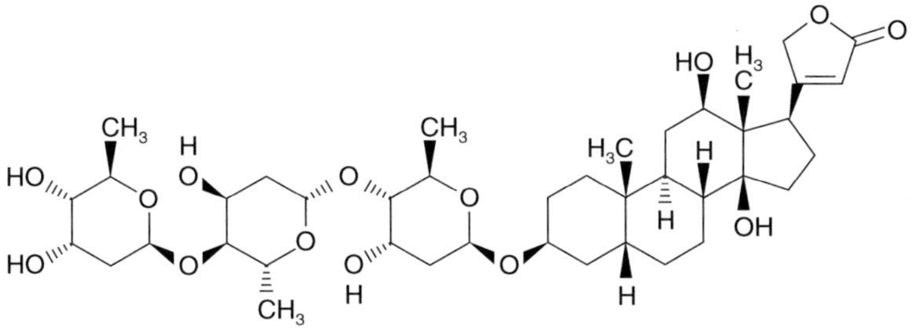 D00298
Deslanoside	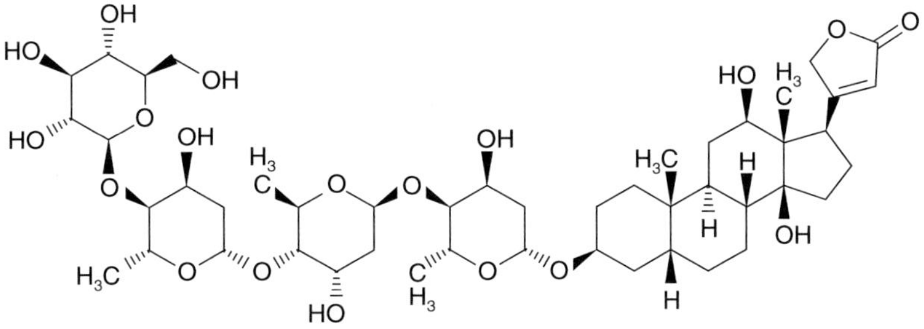 D01240

(Contd)

(Table 10.1 Contd)

Cardiac Glycoside	***Structure***
Lanatoside C	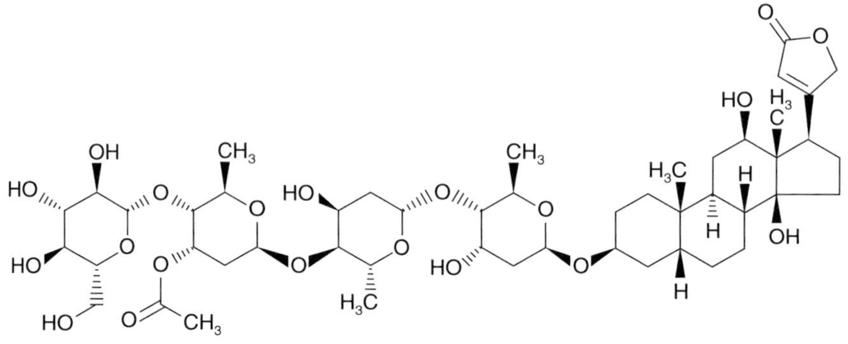 D01972
Metildigoxin	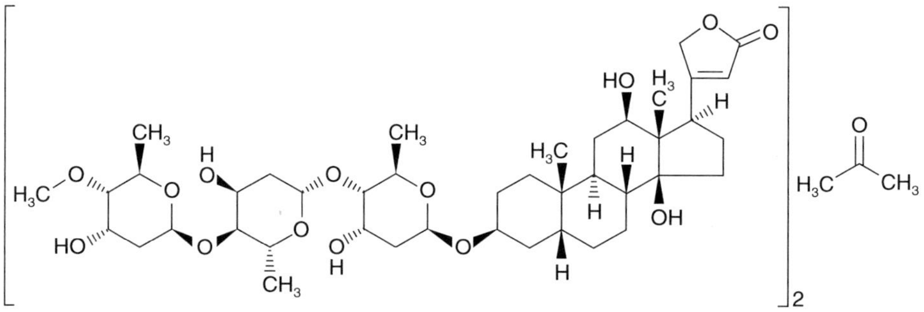 D02587

Source: Structures have been taken from the KEGG Database.

Side Effects

Digoxin poisoning is quite common because of the narrow therapeutic range in which the drug acts. The heart can start beating abnormally leading to arrhythmias if the usual level of digoxin is only doubled or tripled. Depending on the severity of the toxicity, its use needs to be stopped. Potassium supplements and antiarrhythmic drugs can also help, and in very severe cases doctors administer antibody fragments that work specifically against digoxin (Smith, 1991).

The principal adverse effects of digoxin toxicity include: (1) cardiac arrhythmias, (2) gastrointestinal symptoms such as anorexia, nausea and vomiting, and (3) neurologic complaints such as visual disturbances, disorientation and confusion. These side effects are commonly associated with serum digoxin levels of 0.2 ng/ml. But digitalis toxicity may occur with lower digoxin levels, especially if hypokalemia, hypomagnesemia or hypothyroidism also coexists (Fogelman *et al.*, 1971; Ingelfinger and Goldman 1976). The concomitant use of drugs such as quinidine, verapamil, spironolactone, flecainide, propafenone and amiodarone can increase serum digoxin levels and may increase the likelihood of digitalis toxicity (Hager *et al.*, 1979; Moysey *et al.*, 1981; Klein *et al.*, 1982; Paladino *et al.*, 1984; Weeks *et al.*, 1986, Bizjak and Mauro1997; Woodland *et al.*, 1997).

Beta-Adrenergic Receptor Agonists

Beta-adrenergic receptor (βAR) agonists are sympathomimetic catecholamine drugs that bind to beta-adrenoceptors located in cardiac nodal tissue, the conducting system and contracting myocytes. There are several cardiac receptor systems that are involved in the regulation of contractility and/or heart rate (Bylund *et al.*, 1998). In the human heart the beta-adrenergic receptor–G-protein–adenylyl cyclase system is the most powerful physiological mechanism to acutely increase contractility and/or heart rate. Three βAR subtypes have been identified in mammals, viz. $\beta 1$, $\beta 2$ and $\beta 3$. In the human heart, $\beta 1$ and $\beta 2$ coexist, whereby $\beta 1$ AR predominates. In general, the ratio of $\beta 1$:$\beta 2$AR is about 70%:30% in the atria and 80%:20% in the ventricles. On the other hand, total βAR number appears to be equally distributed over atria and ventricles (Brodde and Michel 1999).

Mechanism of Action of Beta-Adrenergic Receptor Agonists

It is well documented that in heart failure βAR changes play an important role (Fig. 10.2) (Brodde *et al.*, 2006). βARs that couple to the heterotrimeric guanine nucleotide binding protein (G_s) are the major determinants of cardiac contractility. Under normal physiological conditions in the heart, βARs

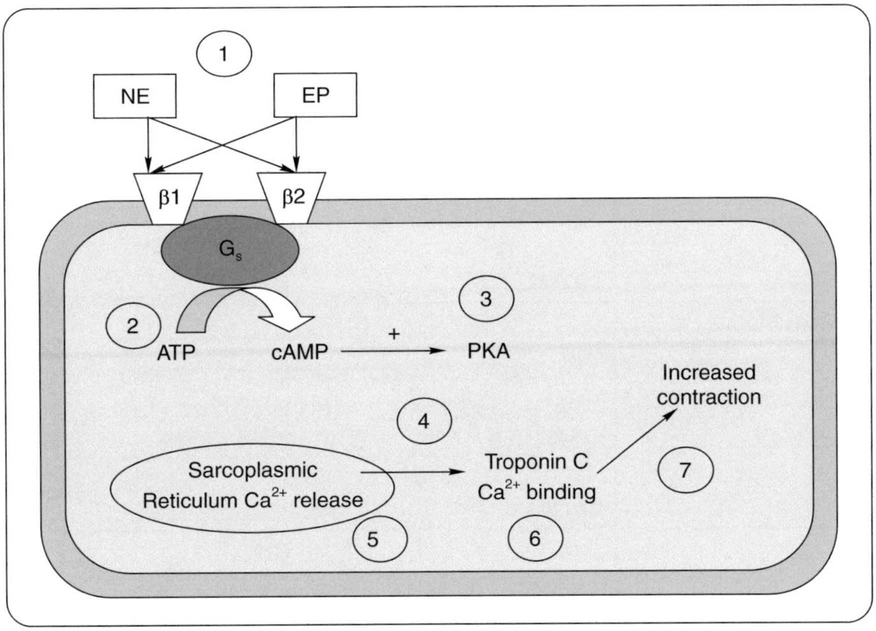

Fig. 10.2 *A Schematic of the Mechanism of Action of β-Agonists in a Heart Muscle Cell*

(NE—Norepinepherin, EP—Epinepherin, $\beta 1$—Beta-1 adrenoreceptor, $\beta 2$—Beta-2 adrenoreceptor, PKA—Protein kinase A, AC—Adenylyl cyclase.)

are targets for catecholamines such as the sympathetic neurotransmitter norepinephrine and the adrenal hormone epinephrine (Table 10.2). The catecholamine stimulation of myocardial βARs triggers a series of transmembrane signaling events through G_s protein, which lead to the increased production

Table 10.2 *List of β-Agonists and Their Structures*

β-Agonist	*Structure*
Epinephrine	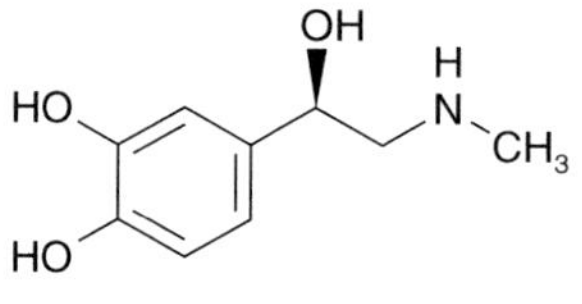 D00095
Norepinephrine	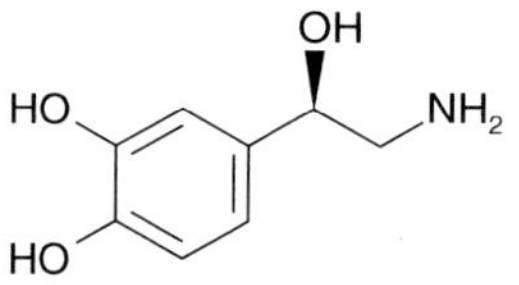 D00076
Dopamine hydrochloride	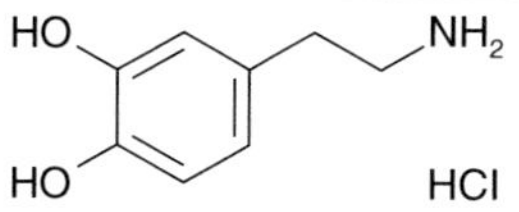 D00633
Dobutamine hydrochloride	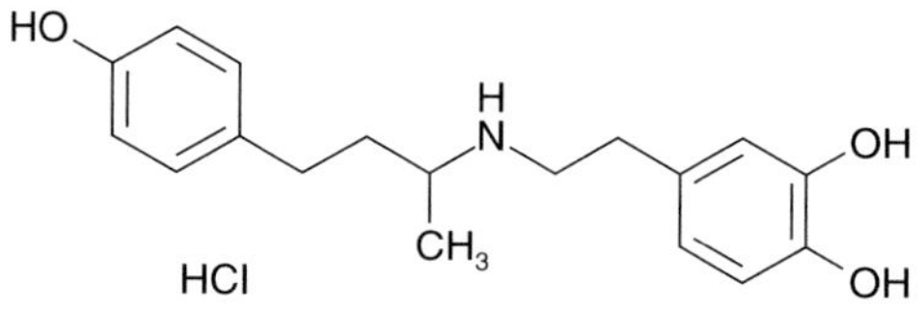 D00632
Isoproterenol hydrochloride	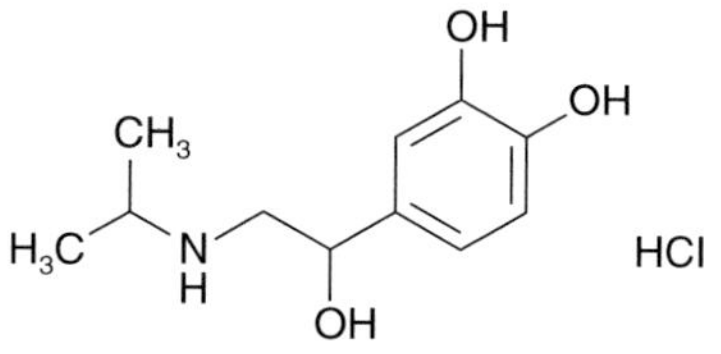 D01390
Denopamine	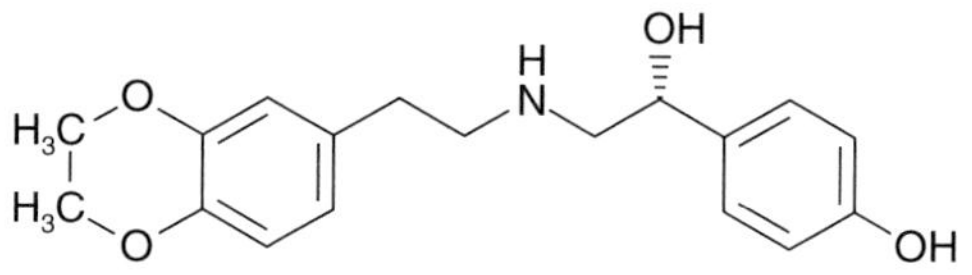 D02614

Source: Structures have been taken from the KEGG Database.

of cAMP. This increase activates a cAMP-dependent protein kinase (PKA) that phosphorylates L-type calcium channels, which causes increased calcium entry into the cells. This leads to enhanced release of calcium by SR in the heart. This provides more calcium for binding to troponin C, which enhances contractility. In the myocyte, this results in positive inotropy, dromotropy and chronotropy (Brodde, 1993; Guido *et al.*, 1998; Stiles and Lefkowitz, 1984). Acute agonists mimic this action in failing heart, thereby increasing its contractility. There are several different β-agonists that are used clinically for the treatment of heart failure or circulatory shock, all of which are either natural catecholamines or analogues.

Side Effects

A major side effect of β-agonists is cardiac arrhythmia. Because these drugs increase myocardial oxygen demand, they can precipitate angina in patients with coronary artery disease. Headache and tremor are also common. The β-agonists are associated with hemodynamic and clinical improvements in patients with CHF; however, they increase the risk of mortality, especially when taken on a long-term basis. In the failing human myocardium β1AR number is decreased. This is also accompanied by a reduced β1AR-mediated positive inotropic effect. The cardiac β2AR number may or may not decrease. However, β2AR-mediated positive inotropic effects are also reduced, possibly because the functional activity of myocardial Gi is increased, thereby inhibiting the formation of cyclic AMP. In patients with chronic heart failure, cardiac βAR function is decreased, and this decrease is related to the degree of heart failure. However, both cardiac β1AR and β2AR adrenoceptors seem to be differentially affected depending on the type of heart failure and its etiology. β1AR function decreases in all forms of chronic heart failure. β2AR function, on the other hand, decreases in mitral valve disease, tetralogy of Fallot and end-stage ischaemic cardiomyopathy. It seems to be unaltered or only mildly uncoupled in end-stage dilated cardiomyopathy, and possibly in aortic valve disease. Since the human heart has few spare beta-adrenoceptors and these declines with increasing degree of heart failure, β-agonists may be of therapeutic use only if the heart needs acute inotropic support. Under these conditions, treatment with β-agonists seems to be of limited use as it might further downregulate cardiac βAR, resulting finally in a loss of therapeutic efficacy (Brodde, 1991).

Acute agonist exposure also triggers a series of counter-regulatory mechanisms that lead to the functional uncoupling of βARs, a process known as desensitization [40]. So drugs acting by the stimulation of ß1AR and/or ß2AR such as dopamine, dobutamine, prenalterol, pirbuterol, salbutamol, terbutaline and fenoterol have initial beneficial effects but seem to be ineffective after prolonged treatment. Therefore, their use should be limited to the short-term management of acute exacerbations of CHF (Hilleman, 1993).

Phosphodiesterase-3 Inhibitors

Cyclic nucleotide phosphodiesterases are enzymes that convert cAMP or cGMP (second messengers), which activate cAMP- and cGMP-dependent protein kinases (PKA and PKG, respectively), to their inactive counterparts AMP and GMP. Eleven families of these enzymes have been described. Those in the PDE3 family, which hydrolyze both cAMP and cGMP, are especially important in regulating cyclic nucleotide–mediated responses in cardiac and vascular smooth muscle myocytes (Conti and Jin 1999; Movsesian 2003).

Mechanism of Action of Phosphodiesterase-3 inhibitors

Drugs that inhibit these enzymes have inotropic and vasodilatory actions (Fig. 10.3) (Movsesian 1999, 2003). The inotropic action results from the inhibition of cAMP hydrolysis, and increase in intracellular cAMP content and PKA activity in cardiac myocytes. Among the many PKA substrates, there are those whose phosphorylation may contribute to the inotropic action of PDE3 inhibitors; those whose phosphorylation increases Ca^{2+} sequestration by the SR during diastole (Simmerman and Jones 1998; James *et al.*, 1989; Movsesian 2003); ryanodine-sensitive Ca^{2+} channels, whose phosphorylation increases Ca^{2+} release by the SR during systole (Seiler *et al.*, 1984; Takasago *et al.*, 1989; Movsesian 2003); and dihydropyridine-sensitive Ca^{2+} channels, whose phosphorylation increases Ca^{2+} influx during systole (Sculptoreanu *et al.*, 1993; Movsesian 2003).

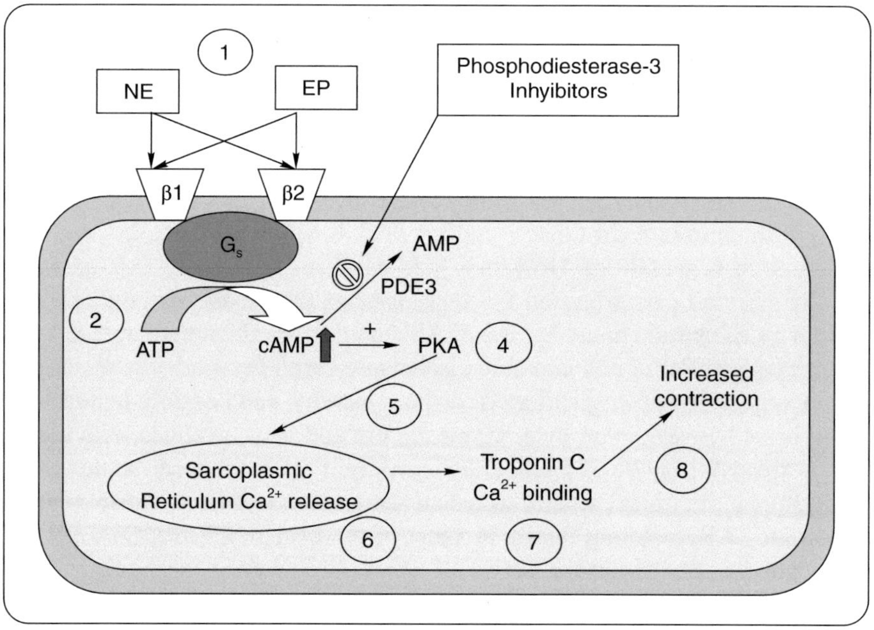

Fig. 10.3 ***A Schematic Illustrating the Mechanism of Action of PDE3 Inhibitors in a Heart Muscle Cell***

(NE—Norepinepherin, EP—Epinepherin, *β*1—Beta-1 adrenoreceptor, *β*2—Beta-2 adrenoreceptor, PKA—Protein kinase A, AC—Adenylyl cyclase, PDE3—Phosphodiesterase-3.)

Side Effects

The inotropic and vasodilatory actions of PDE3 inhibitors would seem desirable in the treatment of dilated cardiomyopathy. PDE3 inhibitors were shown to have beneficial effects on myocardial contraction and vascular relaxation in clinical applications (Benotti *et al.*, 1978; Baim *et al.*, 1983; Sinoway *et al.*, 1983; Uretsky *et al.*, 1983; Jaski *et al.*, 1985; Movsesian 2003). Subsequent clinical trials, however, showed that significant increase in mortality (up to 2–3-fold in some studies and >40% in 1 meta-analysis) occurred when these drugs were used chronically to treat patients with dilated cardiomyopathy (Uretsky *et al*., 1990; Packer *et al*., 1991; Feldman *et al*., 1993; Nony *et al*., 1994; Cohn *et al*., 1998; Movsesian 2003). These observations are consistent with the notion that increase in intracellular cAMP content in cardiac myocytes have favorable effects on cardiac function in the short term but have adverse effects in the long term. This notion is also consistent with other studies that show that βAR antagonists, which lower intracellular cAMP content in cardiac myocytes, have beneficial effects on survival in patients with dilated cardiomyopathy. The mechanisms through which PDE3 inhibition increases mortality in patients with dilated cardiomyopathy have not been identified and are apparently related to their arrhythmogenic effect (Movsesian 2003).

Among the drugs inhibiting phosphodiesterases, sulmazole, amrinone, milrinone and fenoximone have been shown to improve cardiac performance in patients with CHF in the short term (Table 10.3). However, results of long-term treatment with most of these drugs seem less encouraging.on the myocardium (Andersson, 1986).

Calcium Sensitizers

Attempts to ameliorate cardiac contractile dysfunction by Ca^{2+} mobilizers, such as sympathomimetic catecholamines, phosphodiesterase (PDE) inhibitors and digitalis, play an important role in pharmacotherapy for CHF. These agents in the long run cause Ca^{2+} overload resulting in arrhythmogenicity and damage to cardiomyocytes. In addition they possess poor pharmacokinetic properties (Endoh, 2003).

Since the early 1980s, extensive efforts have been made to develop novel cardiotonic agents to replace these drugs. More recently, a newer class of drug called calcium sensitizer has been introduced (Endoh, 2003).

Mechanism of Action of Calcium Sensitizers

Calcium-sensitizing agents are a heterogeneous group of positive inotropic agents that mediate their cardiovascular actions by increasing the sensitivity of the contractile elements to calcium. This increased sensitivity may be related to changes in calcium binding to troponin C, or to the direct effects on the actin–myosin complex. Ca^{2+} sensitizers that act directly on contractile proteins are free from the risk of Ca^{2+} overload. They could also improve hemodynamic parameters with minimum increase in energy expenditure even under pathological conditions, including acidosis and stunned myocardium (Lehmann *et al*., 2003). Calcium sensitizers may enhance myocardial performance without increasing myocardial oxygen consumption and without provoking fatal arrhythmias (Lehmann *et al*., 2003).

Two calcium sensitizers are currently available for the treatment of cardiac failure. Pimobendan is a drug with positive inotropic effects that additionally inhibits the production of pro-inflammatory cytokines. However, it exerts a significant inhibition of PDE3 at clinically relevant doses. Levosimendan is a calcium sensitizer with no major inhibition of PDE3 at clinically relevant doses. It opens ATP-dependent potassium channels and thus has vasodilating and cardioprotective effects

Table 10.3 *List of PDE3 Inhibitors and Their Structures*

Phosphodiesterase-3 Inhibitor	*Structure*
Milrinone	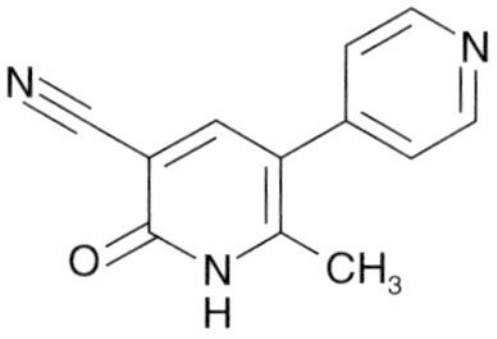 D00417
Amrinone	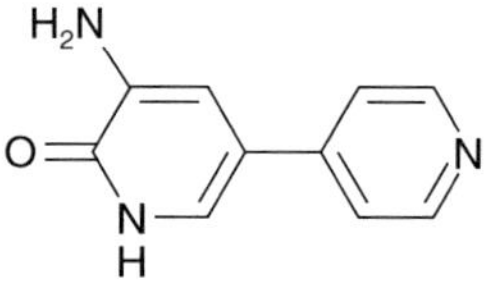 D00231
Pimobendan	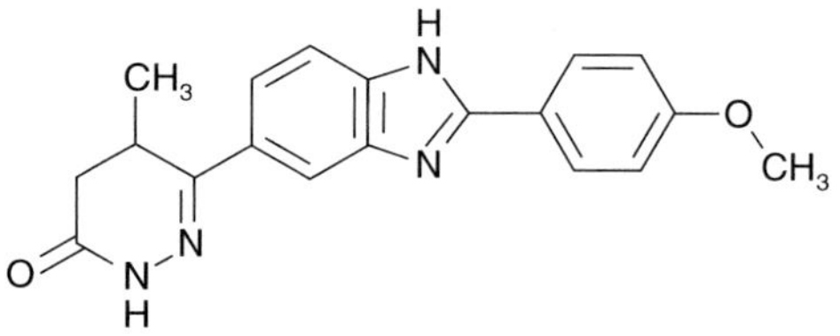 D01133
Vesnarinone	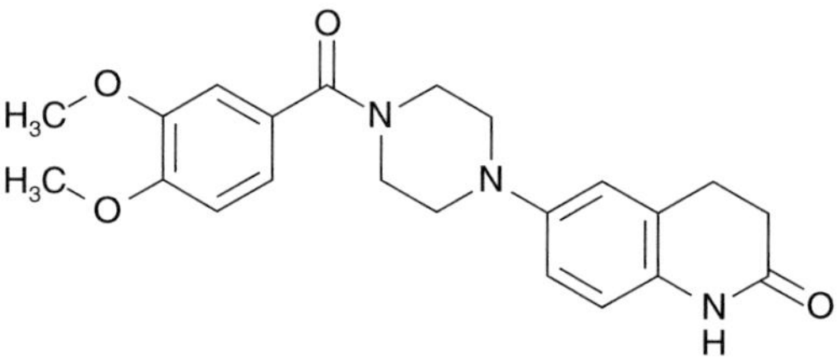 D01690
Olprinone hydrochloride hydrate	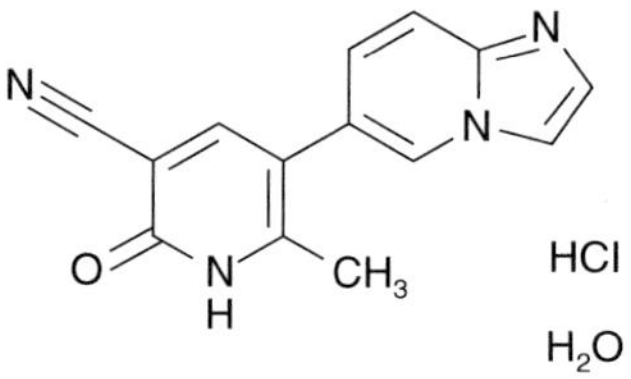 D02042

Source: Structures have been taken from the KEGG Database.

(Mathew and Katz 1998). Levosimendan, a myofilament Ca^{2+} sensitizer with inotropic effects, increases the myocardial performance without substantial changes in oxygen consumption and with neutral effects on heart rhythm. In addition, it has vasodilatory effects, which are achieved by the stimulation of ATP-dependent potassium channels. This action may be of specific interest in the setting of myocardial ischemia. To date, this drug is approved in 31 countries worldwide (Toller and Stranz 2006).

Side Effects

Because many of the calcium-sensitizing agents also inhibit PDE3 activity, the long-term safety of these agents is uncertain. Large-scale survival trials are required to determine the long-term safety and efficacy of these agents before their role in the treatment of CHF can be defined (Mathew *et al.*, 1998).

CONCLUSIONS

The most effective means of decreasing the risk of hospitalization and death in patients with CHF is to address the primary mechanisms that contribute to disease progression rather than to stimulate the contractility of the failing left ventricle (Consensus Recommendations for Heart Failure, 1999).

Clinically available cardiotonic agents, such as beta-adrenoceptor agonists and selective PDE3 inhibitors, act mainly via cAMP/PKA-mediated facilitation of Ca^{2+} mobilization (upstream mechanism). These agents are associated with the risk of Ca^{2+} overload, leading to arrhythmias, myocardial cell injury and premature cell death. In addition, they are energetically disadvantageous because of an increase in activation energy and metabolic effects. Cardiac glycosides also act via an upstream mechanism and readily elicit Ca^{2+} overload with a narrow safety margin. More data are needed for agents that act primarily via an increase in the myofilament sensitivity to Ca^{2+} ions (central and/or downstream mechanisms). Novel Ca^{2+} sensitizers currently being researched may deserve clinical trials to examine the therapeutic potential to replace currently employed agents in acute and chronic heart failure patients.

REFERENCES

Akera, T., Baskin, S.I., Tobin, T., Brody, T.M. (1973). Ouabain: Temporal relationship between the inotropic effect and the *in vitro* binding to, and dissociation from (Na^+–K^+)-activated ATPase. *Naunyn-Schmiedeberg's Archives of Pharmacology* **277**:151–162.

Andersson, K.E. (1986). Some new positive inotropic agents. *Acta Medica Scandinavica, Supplementum* **707**:65–73.

Andrew, J.W., Gary, L.A. (2005). Digitalis: New actions for an old drug. *American Journal of Physiology—Heart and Circulatory Physiology* **289**:1781–1793.

Aronson, J.K. (1985). *An Account of the Foxglove and Its Medical Uses 1785–1985*. Oxford: Oxford Uni. Press.

Australia–New Zealand Heart Failure Research Collaborative Group. (1995). Effects of carvedilol, a vasodilator-b-blocker, in patients with congestive heart failure due to ischemic heart disease. *Circulation* **92**:212–218.

Baim, D.S., McDowell, A.V., Cherniles, J., Monrad, E.S., Parker, J.A., Edelson, J., E Braunwald, E.,and Grossman, W. (1983). Evaluation of a new bipyridine inotropic agent—milrinone—in patients with severe congestive heart failure. *New England Journal of Medicine* **309**:748–756.

Benotti, J.R., Grossman, W., Braunwald, E., Davolos, D.D., Alousi, A.A. (1978). Hemodynamic assessment of amrinone. *New England Journal of Medicine* **299**:1373–1377.

Bizjak, E.D., Mauro, V.F. (1997). Digoxin–macrolide drug interaction. *Annals of Pharmacotherapy* **31**:1077–1099.

Brodde, O.E. (1991). Beta1 and beta2-adrenoceptors in the human heart: Properties, function, and alterations in chronic heart failure. *Pharmacological Reviews* **43(2)**: 203–242.

Brodde, O.E. (1993). Beta-adrenergic receptors in failing human myocardium. *Basic Research in Cardiology* **91**:35–40.

Brodde, O.E., Bruck, H., Leineweber, K. (2006). Cardiac adrenoceptors: Physiological and pathophysiological relevance. *Journal of Pharmacological Sciences* **100**:323–337.

Brodde, O.E., Michel, M. (1999). Adrenergic and muscarinic receptors in the human heart. *Pharmacological Reviews* **51**:651–689.

Bylund, D.B., Bond, R.A., Clarke, D.E., Eikenburg, D.C., Hieble, J.P., Langer, S.Z., Lefkowitz, R.J., Minneman, K.P., Molinof, P.B., Ruffolo, R.R., Strosberg, A.D., Trendelenburg, U.G (1998). Adrenoceptors. *The IUPHAR Compendium of Receptor Characterization and Classification*, pp. 58–74. London: IUPHAR Media.

Califf, R.M., Adam, K.F., McKenna, W.J., Gheorgiade, M., Uretsky, B.F., McNulty, S.E., Darius, H., Schulman, K., Zannad, F., Handberg-Thurmond, E., Harrell, F.E., Jr., Wheeler, W., Soler-Soler, J., Swedberg, K. (1997). A randomized controlled trial of epoprostenol therapy for severe congestive heart failure: The Flolan International Randomized Survival Trial (FIRST). *American Heart Journal* **134**:44–54.

Cohn, J.N., Goldstein, S.O., Greenberg, B.H., Lorell, B.H., Bourge, R.C., Jaski, B.E., Gottlieb, S.O, McGrew, F. 3rd, DeMets, D.L., White, B.G. (1998). A dose-dependent increase in mortality with vesnarinone among patients with severe heart failure. *New England Journal of Medicine* **339**:1810–1816.

Consensus Recommendations for Heart Failure (1999). *American Journal Of Cardiology* **83(2A)**:1–38.

Conti, M., Jin, S.L. (1999). The molecular biology of cyclic nucleotide phosphodiesterases. *Progress in Nucleic Acid Research and Molecular Biology* **63**:1–38.

Covit, A.B., Schaer, G.L., Sealey, J.E., Laragh, J.H., Cody, R.J. (1983). Suppression of the renin–angiotensin system by intravenous digoxin in chronic congestive heart failure. *American Journal of Medicine* **75**:445–447.

Cowley, A.J., Skene, A.M. (1994). Treatment of severe heart failure: Quantity or quality of life? A trial of enoximone. *British Heart Journal* **72**:226–230.

Endoh, M. (2003). The therapeutic potential of novel cardiotonic agents. *Expert Opinion on Investigational Drugs* **12(5)**:735–750.

Feldman, A.M., Bristow, M.R., Parmley, W.W., Carson, P.E., Pepine, C.J., Gilbert, E.M., Bristow, M.R., Powers, E.R., Parmley, W.W., Hendrix, G.H., Carson, P.E., Strobeck, J.E., Bain, R.P., White, B.G., for

The Vesnarinone Study Group.(1993). Effects of vesnarinone on morbidity and mortality in patients with heart failure. *New England Journal of Medicine* **329**:149–155.

Ferguson, D.W., Berg. W.J., Sanders, J.S., Roach, P.J., Kempf, J.S., Kienzle, M.G. (1989). Sympathoinhibitory responses to digitalis glycosides in heart failure patients: Direct evidence from sympathetic neural recordings. *Circulation* **80**:65–77.

Fogelman, A.M., La Mont, J.T., Finkelstein, S., Rado, E., Pearce, M.L. (1971). Fallibility of plasma-digoxin in differentiating toxic from non-toxic patients. *Lancet* **2**:727–729.

Garg, R., Yusuf, S. (1995). Overview of randomized trials of angiotensin-converting enzyme inhibitors on mortality and morbidity in patients with heart failure. *JAMA* **273**:1450–1456.

Gheorghiade, M., Ferguson, D. (1991). Digoxin. A neurohormonal modulator in heart failure? *Circulation* **84**:2181–2186.

Guido, I., Eric, D.T., Robert, J.L., Walter, J.K. (1998). Reciprocal *in vivo* regulation of myocardial G protein–coupled receptor kinase expression by β-adrenergic receptor stimulation and blockade. *Circulation* **98**:1783–1789.

Hager, W.D., Fenster, P., Mayersohn, M., Perrier, D., Graves, P., Marcus, F.I., Goldman, S. (1979). Digoxin–quinidine interaction: Pharmacokinetic evaluation. *New England Journal of Medicine* **300**:1238–1241.

Hampton, J.R., van Veldhuisen, D.J., Kleber, F.X., Cowley, A.J., Ardia, A., Block, P., Cortina, A., Cserhalmi, L., Follath, F., Jensen, G., Kayanakis, J., Lie, K.I., Mancia, G., Skene, A.M. (1997). Randomised study of effect of ibopamine on survival in patients with advanced severe heart failure. *Lancet* **349**:971–977.

Hilleman, D.E. (1993). Assessing the treatment of congestive heart failure: Inotropic agents and calcium channel blockers. *Pharmacotherapy* **5(2)**:88S–93S.

Ingelfinger, J.A., Goldman, P. (1976). The serum digitalis concentration—Does it diagnose digitalis toxicity? *New England Journal of Medicine* **294**:867–870.

James, P., Inui, M., Tada, M., Chiesi, M., Carafoli, E. (1989). Nature and site of phospholamban regulation of the Ca^{2+} pump of the sarcoplasmic reticulum. *Nature* **342**:90–92.

Jaski, B.E., Fifer, M.A., Wright, R.F., Braunwald, E., Colucci, W.S. (1985). Positive inotropic and vasodilator actions of milrinone in patients with severe congestive heart failure. Dose–response relationships and comparison to nitroprusside. *Journal of Clinical Investigation* **75**:643–649.

Jugdutt, B.I., Khan, M.I. (1994). Effect of prolonged nitrate therapy on left ventricular remodeling after canine myocardial infarction. *Circulation* **89**:2297–2307.

Klein, H.O., Lang, R., Weiss, E., Di Segni, E., Libhaber, C., Guerrero, J., Kaplinsky, E. The influence of verapamil on serum digoxin concentration. *Circulation* **65**:998–1003.

Konstam, M.A., Kronenberg, M.W., Rousseau, M.F., Udelson, J.E., Melin, J., Stewart, D., Dolan, N., Edens, T.R., Ahn, S., Kinan, D., Howe, D.M., Kilcoyne, L., Metherall, J., Benedict, C., Yusuf, S., Pouleur, H. (1993). Effects of the angiotensin converting enzyme inhibitor enalapril on the long-term progression of left ventricular dilatation in patients with asymptomatic systolic dysfunction. *Circulation* **88**:2277–2283.

Langer, G.A. (1970). The role of sodium ion in the regulation of myocardial contractility. *Journal of Molecular and Cellular Cardiology* **1**:203–207.

Lechat, P., Packer, M., Chalon, S., Cucherat, M., Arab, T., Boissel, J.P. (1998). Clinical effects of β-adrenergic blockade in chronic heart failure. A meta-analysis of double-blind, placebo-controlled, randomized trials. *Circulation* **98**:1184–1191.

Lehmann, A., Boldt, J., Kirchner, J. (2003). The role of Ca++-sensitizers for the treatment of heart failure. *Current Opinion in Critical Care* **9(5)**:337–344.

Mathew, L., Katz, S.D. (1998). Calcium sensitising agents in heart failure. *Drugs and Aging* **12(3)**:191–204.

Movsesian,M.A. (1999). Beta-adrenergic receptor agonists and cyclic nucleotide phosphodiesterase inhibitors: Shifting the focus from inotropy to cAMP. *Journal of the American College of Cardiology* **34**:318–324.

Movsesian,M.A. (2003). PDE3 inhibition in dilated cardiomyopathy: Reasons to reconsider. *Journal of Cardiac Failure* **9(6)**: 475–480.

Moysey, J.O., Jagga Rao, N.S., Grundy, E.N., Chamberlain, D.A. (1981). Amiodarone increases plasma digoxin concentrations.*BMJ* **282**:272 (Abstract).

Nony, P., Boissel, J.P., Lievre, M., Leizorovicz, A., Haugh, M.C., Fareh, S., de Breyne, B. (1994). Evaluation of the effect of phosphodiesterase inhibitors on mortality in chronic heart failure patients. A meta-analysis. *European Journal of Clinical Pharmacology* **46**:191–196.

Packer, M., Carver, J.R., Rodeheffer, R.J., Ivanhoe, R.J., DiBianco, R., Zeldis, S.M., Hendrix, G.H., Bommer, W.J., Elkayam, U., Kukin, M.L., Mallis, G.I., Sollano, J.A., Shannon, J., Tandon, P.K., DeMets, D.L. (1991). Effect of oral milrinone on mortality in severe chronic heart failure. *New England Journal of Medicine* **325**:1468–1475.

_____, Narahara, K.A., Elkayam, U., Sullivan, J.M., Pearle, D.L., Massie, B.M., Creager, M.A. (1993). Doubleblind, placebo-controlled study of the efficacy of flosequinan in patients with chronic heart failure. *Journal of the American College of Cardiology* **22**:65–72.

_____, Rouleau, J.L., Swedberg, K., Pitt, B., Fisher, L., Klepper, M. (1993). Effect of flosequinan on survival in chronic heart failure: Preliminary results of the PROFILE study. *Circulation* **88(I)**:301.

Paladino, J.A., Davidson, K.H., McCall, B.B. (1984). Influence of spironolactone on serum digoxin concentration. *JAMA* **251**:470–471.

Sculptoreanu, A., Rotman, E., Takahashi, M., Scheuer, T., Catterall, W.A. (1993). Voltage-dependent potentiation of the activity of cardiac L-type calcium channel alpha 1 subunits due to phosphorylation by cAMP-dependent protein kinase. *Proceedings of the National Academy of Sciences USA* **90**:10135–10139.

Seiler, S., Wegener, A.D., Whang, D.D., Hathaway, D.R., Jones, L.R. (1984). High molecular weight proteins in cardiac and skeletal muscle junctional sarcoplasmic reticulum vesicles bind calmodulin, are phosphorylated, and are degraded by Ca^{2+}-activated protease. *Journal of Biological Chemistry* **259**:8550–8557.

Simmerman, H.K., Jones, L.R. (1998). Phospholamban: Protein structure, mechanism of action, and role in cardiac function. *Physiological Reviews* **78**:921–47.

Sinoway, L.S., Maskin, C.S., Chadwick, B., Forman, R., Sonnenblick, E.H., Le Jemtel, T.H. (1983). Long-term therapy with a new cardiotonic agent, WIN 47203: Drug-dependent improvement in cardiac performance and progression of the underlying disease. *Journal of the American College of Cardiology* **2**:327–331.

Skou, J.C. The Na-K Pump, *Physiology.*1992; 7: 95–100

Smith, S. (1930). Digoxin, a new digitalis glucoside. *Journal of the Chemical Society* 72:508–510.

Smith, T.W. (1991). Review of clinical experience with digoxin immune Fab (ovine). *American Journal of Emergency Medicine* **9**:1–6.

Stiles, G.L., Lefkowitz, R.J. (1984). Cardiac adrenergic receptors. *Annual Review of Medicine* **35**:149–164.

Takasago, T., Imagawa, T., Shigekawa, M. (1989). Phosphorylation of the cardiac ryanodine receptor by cAMP-dependent protein kinase. *Journal of Biochemistry (Tokyo)* **106**:.872–877.

Thames, M.D. (1979). Acetylstrophanthidin-induced reflex inhibition of canine renal sympathetic nerve activity mediated by cardiac receptors with vagal afferents. *Circulation Research* **44**:8–15.

Toller, W.G., Stranz, C. (2006). Levosimendan, a new inotropic and vasodilator agent. *Anesthesiology* **104(3)**:556–569.

Torretti, J., Hendler, E., Weinstein, E., Longnecker, R.E., Epstein, F.H. (1972). Functional significance of Na-K-ATPase in the kidney: Effects of ouabain inhibition. *American Journal of Physiology* **222**:1398–1405.

Uretsky, B.F., Generalovich, T., Reddy, P.S., Spangenberg, R.B., Follansbee, W.P. (1983). The acute hemodynamic effects of a new agent, MDL 17,043, in the treatment of congestive heart failure. *Circulation* **67**:823–828.

Uretsky, B.F., Jessup, M., Konstam, M.A., Dec, G.W., Leier, C.V., Benotti, J., Murali, S. Herrmann, H.C., Sandberg, J.A. (1990). Multicenter trial of oral enoximone in patients with moderate to moderately severe congestive heart failure. Lack of benefit compared with placebo. *Circulation* **82**:774–780.

Weeks, C.E., Conard, G.J., Jvam, D.C., Fox, J.M., Chang, S.F., Paone, R.P., Lewis, G.P. (1986). The effect of flecainide acetate, a new antiarrhythmic, on plasma digoxin levels. *Journal of Clinical Pharmacology* **26**:27–31.

Woodbury, J.W. (1963). Interrelationships between ion transport mechanisms and excitatory events. *Federation Proceedings* **22**:31–35.

Woodland, C., Varjee, Z., Giesbrecht, E., Koren, G., Ito, S. (1997). The digoxin propafenone interaction: Characterization of a mechanism using renal tubular cell monolayers. *Journal of Pharmacology and Experimental Therapeutics* **283**:39–45.

11

Inositides as Potential Therapeutic Agents

Alexis Traynor-Kaplan

ISM Therapeutics, Seattle, WA

INTRODUCTION

Inositides (inositol polyphosphates and phosphoinositides) are a class of cytosolic and membrane-bound compounds containing key intracellular messengers that regulate processes affecting carcinogenesis, ion channel function, inflammation and immunity. Recent studies suggest that selected inositides and/or their derivatives may have therapeutic utility in cystic fibrosis and cancer while having characteristics making them suitable for drug development. Advances in the therapeutic development of these molecules are discussed along with factors impacting their utility as drugs.

Binding proteins for inositides number in the hundreds and comprise a growing category of therapeutic targets for diverse disorders ranging from cancer to high blood pressure to diabetes (Itoh and Takenawa, 2002; Balla, 2005; Lemmon, 2007, 2008; Sasaki *et al.*, 2007). In fact, one such protein class, that of pleckstrin homology (PH) domain–containing proteins (the 11th most common domain in the human genome), has recently become the subject of a therapeutic patent (Lemmon, 2008). Inositides are a body of cellular inositol phosphate–containing compounds consisting of both hydrophilic cytosolic compounds (inositol polyphosphates) and amphipathic membrane-bound phospholipids (phosphoinositides), which are interconverted and metabolized through the activities of multiple phosphatases and kinases. In many cases, both the precursor and product are distinct intracellular signals, one of the many unique features of this set of signaling entities (Fleischer *et al.*, 1994; Seeds *et al.*, 2005; Huang *et al.*, 2007; Miller *et al.*, 2008). Inositides as a group impact every aspect of cell function, so that a comprehensive review of inositide signaling is not possible here but we refer the reader to selected reviews (Balla, 2005; Irvine, 2005; Michell, 2007; Alcazar-Roman and Wente, 2008). In the current document we will focus on the potential for the utilization of specific inositides for the development of therapeutic agents to address specific diseases such as cystic fibrosis

(CF) and cancer. Finally we will speculate on the future potential for inositides and their analogues as therapeutic agents and discuss the practical aspects of their utility.

CYSTIC FIBROSIS

CF is one of the most common single-gene defects and the largest genetic killer of children of European descent. It is characterized by unusually thick and sticky mucus primarily affecting membranes lining the throat, nasal passages, sinuses, bronchial passages, lungs, gall bladder, sweat glands, pancreas and intestines (Davis, 1987; Neijens *et al.*, 1990; Drumm and Collins, 1993; Boucher, 2007; Saeed *et al.*, 2007; Elizur *et al.*, 2008). Over time, the abnormally thick mucus associated with CF leads to infections and inflammation that can cause chronic pulmonary disease, pancreatic insufficiency, liver disease, intestinal obstructions and ultimately death, most often due to lung failure.

CF stems from a genetic defect in the cystic fibrosis transmembrane regulator (CFTR), a protein found in mucosal epithelial cells (Collins, Riordan *et al.*, 1990). While the CFTR acts as a chloride channel, its regulation of other ion channels including the outwardly rectifying chloride channel (ORCC), calcium-activated chloride conductance and the sodium channel, ENaC, may be equally as relevant to CF pathophysiology as the absence of CFTR conductance (Devidas and Guggino, 1997; Kunzelmann, Kiser *et al.*, 1997; Kunzelmann, Mall *et al.*, 1997). In mouse CFTR knockout models of CF, the lack of lung pathology has been attributed to the extraordinary activity of the calcium-activated Cl^- channel (Clarke *et al.*, 1994; Grubb *et al.*, 1994; Grubb and Boucher, 1997; Tarran *et al.*, 2002), suggesting that modulation of alternate ion channels might be therapeutic in CF. Sodium hyper-absorption is another hallmark of CF that by itself could result in disease manifestation. A lack of the inhibitory effect of the properly functioning CFTR on Na^+ absorption through ENaC disables the maintenance of adequate mucosal hydration necessary to permit normal mucociliary clearance, making dysregulated sodium absorption a key factor in CF pathophysiology (Boucher, 2007). In fact, Mall and co-workers (Mall *et al.*, 2004) describe an ENaC-overexpressing mouse model that replicates CF symptomatology, including reduced mucus transport, mucus plugs, neutrophil infiltration and pulmonary infections. Moreover, activation of other Cl^- channels may also be able to substitute for the CFTR in regulating ENaC (Bachhuber *et al.*, 2005).

Without adequate airway hydration and mucociliary clearance, mucus stagnates, bacteria proliferate and infection and inflammation ensue. Agents that can improve Na^+, Cl^- and fluid movement to apical mucosal surfaces are expected to remediate the underlying pathophysiology that leads to morbidity and mortality in CF. Most current therapies for CF are palliative, focusing on controlling infections or mucus buildup. Of the several strategies currently being put forward to deal directly with ion channel dysfunction in CF, one is a membrane-permeant inositol tetrakisphosphate analogue, INO-4995.

Inositides Regulate Ion Channel Function

The most widely recognized inositide, *myo*-inositol 1,4,5-trisphosphate ($InsP_3$), is a second messenger modulator of intracellular calcium levels $[Ca^{++}]_i$ (Berridge, 1986). Other inositides are also turning out to be important regulators of ion channels (Eckmann *et al.*, 1997; Jiang *et al.*, 1998;

Irvine and Schell, 2001; Hilgemann, 2004; Ma and Eaton, 2005; Ma *et al*., 2007; Pochynyuk *et al*., 2008). Three out of four of the most commonly occurring inositol tetrakisphosphates modulate ion channel activities including Cl^- and K^+ channels (Vajanaphanich *et al*., 1994; Eckmann *et al*., 1997; Jiang *et al*., 1998; Irvine and Schell, 2001). One of these, inositol 3,4,5,6-tetrakisphosphate (Ins(3,4,5,6)P_4), inhibits the calcium-activated chloride channel activity in mammalian systems (Kachintorn *et al*., 1993; Vajanaphanich *et al*., 1993; Ismailov *et al*., 1996; Carew *et al*., 2000; Ho *et al*., 2001) as well as a 4,4′-diisothiocyanostilbene disulphonic acid (DIDs) sensitive oscillatory Cl^- efflux in pollen tubes (Zonia *et al*. 2002). Furthermore, rationally designed Ins(3,4,5,6)P_4 analogues reversed the Ins(3,4,5,6)P_4-mediated inhibition of calcium-activated chloride secretion in T_{84} colonic epithelial cells (Rudolf *et al*., 2003).

INO-4995

INO-4995 is a membrane-permeant Ins(3,4,5,6)P_4 analogue, which was originally designed as a possible Ins(3,4,5,6)P_4 antagonist. However, there is no evidence that INO-4995 antagonizes the Ins(3,4,5,6)P_4 inhibition of calcium-activated chloride secretion in T_{84} colonic epithelia as do other Ins(3,4,5,6)P_4 analogues (Rudolf *et al*., 2003; Shears, 2005).

Although its Ins(3,4,5,6)P_4 antagonism is in question, INO-4995 unexpectedly inhibits the epithelial sodium channel, ENaC, and improves the mucosal apical surface liquid volume over human CF airway epithelia, establishing it as a potential CF therapeutic (Moody *et al*., 2005). The primary target of INO-4995 accounting for its affects on ENaC may be ENaC itself. ENaC has been found to be directly regulated by phosphoinositides (Ma and Eaton, 2005; Ma *et al*., 2007; Pochynyuk *et al*., 2008), raising the possibility that INO-4995 might be acting on an inositide binding site in the ENaC protein. INO-4995 inhibits ENaC in excised outside out patches within 1.5 min of exposure (Moody *et al*., 2005) a time frame similar to the time course of action reported for other inositides on ENaC (Pochynyuk *et al*., 2007).

Inositol polyphosphate regulation of phosphoinositide signaling is not unprecedented. We have previously demonstrated the antagonist effects of membrane-permeant Ins(1,4,5,6)P_4 on PIP_3-mediated inhibition of K^+ channel activity (Eckmann *et al*., 1997; Jiang *et al*., 1998) in T_{84} cells. Others have subsequently observed the Ins(1,4,5,6)P_4 antagonism of PIP_3 signaling in COS cells, providing data suggesting that Ins(1,4,5,6)P_4 can directly antagonize PIP_3 signaling through the PH domain–containing protein, Akt (Razzini *et al*., 2000). More recently, Ins(1,3,4,5)P_4 has been demonstrated to allosterically regulate PIP_3-mediated interleukin-2 tyrosine kinase (ITK) signaling in T cells (Huang *et al*., 2007). Further studies would be required to determine if INO-4995 similarly regulates phosphoinositide effects on ENaC.

Although no effect is seen with a single dose, repeated administration of INO-4995 also potentiates ATP-triggered calcium-activated Cl^- secretion in human CF airway epithelia in the presence of amiloride (Traynor-Kaplan *et al*., 2010), suggesting INO-4995 acts on another channel in addition to ENaC. The mechanism of this effect is unknown but patch clamp data with both INO-4995 in perforated patch and de-esterified forms of INO-4995 in ruptured patches indicate this Cl^- channel effect may be linked to stimulation of outwardly rectifying chloride channels with characteristics of calcium-activated chloride channels (Duerson *et al*., 2000, 2004).

Prolonged Duration of Action

CF patients are burdened with multiple medications, many of which are administered via nebulizer up to three times per day. Therefore, dose, ease of administration and duration of action are critical factors impacting the delivery mode and ultimately the compliance and patient fatigue. INO-4995 characteristics and activity appear suited to address these needs.

Basal short circuit current (I_{sc}) is abnormally elevated in CF epithelia due to the excess ENaC activity (Boucher *et al.*, 1988; Ismailov *et al.*, 1997; Kunzelmann, Kiser *et al.*, 1997; Mall *et al.*, 1999). In cultured CF epithelia, INO-4995 acts within 30 min after cell application and is effective at inhibiting the abnormally elevated basal I_{sc} for up to 48 h after the compound (5 μM) is washed off the cells (Traynor-Kaplan *et al.*, 2005). This time frame is consistent with the rate of INO-4995 uptake, de-esterification and half-life of the de-esterified active product (Traynor-Kaplan, Nur *et al.*, 2007). A prolonged inhibition of basal I_{sc} in CF epithelial cells lasting up to 4 days is observed when cells are treated with 100 μM INO-4995 for 2 h followed by a washout, with no apparent effect on cell viability or tight junction integrity (Moody *et al.*, 2005). These uptake parameters coupled with the prolonged duration of action suggest that daily or alternate daily dosing may be possible.

Dose

INO-4995 inhibition of basal I_{sc} is observed 24 h after a 2-h exposure to concentrations as low as 1 μM (Moody *et al.*, 2005). However, repeated daily administration lowered the effective concentration for inhibition of fluid absorption and amiloride-sensitive I_{sc} in cultured cells and reduced the nasal potential difference (NPD) to nearly control levels in CF mice with a dose of 0.8 μg/kg (Traynor-Kaplan *et al.*, 2008; Traynor-Kaplan *et al.*, 2010) administered daily for 4 days. Furthermore, safety studies in mice demonstrated that an acute intraperitoneal or intravenous dose of INO-4995 of 0.15–150 mg/kg had no adverse effect on survival, weight gain or blood chemistries when measured immediately after or on Day 14 following dosing (Traynor-Kaplan *et al.*, 2003). This coupled with the ability to be formulated for a metered dose inhaler suggests that a safe and effective dosing strategy is possible.

Bioavailability

Bioavailability could be an issue with inositol polyphosphate–based therapeutics. Inositol polyphosphates contain polar phosphate groups that can prevent them from crossing cellular membranes. Furthermore, phosphate groups are subject to hydrolysis in biological compartments containing phosphatases. While a number of inositide phosphatases have considerable substrate specificity, inositides are also potential substrates for nonspecific alkaline phosphatases that are active at both alkaline and physiological pH levels (McPherson, 1990; Picher *et al.*, 2003). Although a number of studies have depicted the effects of unprotected inositides in cell-based as well as *in vivo* assays (Berrie and Falasca, 2000; Razzini *et al.*, 2000; Vucenik and Shamsuddin, 2003, 2006; Piccolo, Vignati *et al.*, 2004; Maffucci, Piccolo *et al.*, 2005), large doses are required and questions of whether the actions were direct effects of the delivered compound or a metabolite remain (Grases, Simonet *et al.*, 2001, 2002; Vucenik and Shamsuddin, 2006; Letcher *et al.*, 2008). Thus, it is probable that inositide-based drugs of the future will benefit from modifications that facilitate targeting and cell entry and prevent premature metabolism to be practical. One technique to improve bioavailability is to shield phosphate groups with bioactivatable ester groups such as acyl (alkyl) esters. The resulting prodrug analogues permit passive diffusion across the plasma membrane to the interior of the cell, where intracellular esterases cleave the protecting groups and liberate the biologically active molecule (Vajanaphanich *et al.*, 1994; Li *et al.*, 1997; Rudolf *et al.*, 1998; Schultz, 2003). These membrane-permeant inositol polyphosphate analogues modulate ion channel activities from inside the cell and thus have a greater potential for prolonged activity than extracellularly active compounds that are rapidly eliminated from the airway surface liquid. Similar protecting group strategies are currently employed with a number of drugs and drug candidates (Schultz, 2003; Hatfield *et al.*, 2008).

The CF mucosal epithelia are covered by excess mucus, creating a physical barrier to pulmonary drug delivery. In addition, mucus contains carboxylesterases, which could hydrolyze INO-4995 protecting groups and thereby impede its entrance into cells (Satoh and Hosokawa, 2006; Hatfield *et al.*, 2008; Hosokawa, 2008). To evaluate the possible effect of mucus on INO-4995 bioavailability we tested the effect of mucus on INO-4995 penetration to human CF tracheal sheets where the naturally occurring mucus was either left intact or removed with repeated washing. The presence of mucus reduced [^{3}H]INO-4995 penetration by 50% (Traynor-Kaplan, Madhumitha *et al.*, 2007). Thus, although mucus clearly inhibited the INO-4995 access to target tissue, quantities adequate to obtain a therapeutic effect were able to penetrate the mucosal layer. These data suggest that mucus, although an impeding factor, can be circumvented with appropriate formulation and dosing. Furthermore, large mucus plugs blocking airway branches in CF patients are expected to migrate, so that with daily administration of compound it should be possible to reach the majority of target tissue over time.

Summary

By positively affecting electrolyte imbalance, INO-4995 has the therapeutic potential for treating the underlying defect of CF. INO-4995 effects on bioelectrics are noticeable within 30 min of application and persist for 24–96 h depending on the dose (Moody *et al.*, 2005). It inhibits sodium absorption and improves fluid hydration. The effective concentration is substantially reduced with repeated dosing, leading to restoration of normal NPD in a CF mouse model at a dose of 0.8 μg/kg. Due to its low effective dose, prolonged duration of action and solubility profile, INO-4995 could be conveniently dosed once per day via metered dose inhaler. This is well below the dose of 150 mg/kg that showed no adverse effects in safety studies. The mechanism of action as an ion channel modulator, the effect on mucosal hydration, inhibition of I_{sc} and convenient formulation make INO-4995 a viable candidate therapy for CF, attesting to the therapeutic potential of inositide analogues.

BREAST CANCER

General Rationale

Phosphatidylinositol 3,4,5-triphosphate (PIP_3) is a phosphoinositide product of phosphatidylinositol-3-kinase (PI3K). The PI3K/Akt signaling pathway is now recognized as the signaling pathway (Fig. 11.1) most often deviated in human cancer (Powis *et al.*, 2006), having been implicated in *all* aspects of tumor biology including genomic instability, angiogenesis, metastases, protection from apoptosis and cancer stem cells (Janzen and Scadden, 2006; Shaw and Cantley, 2006). Four proteins in this pathway are most frequently subject to mutation or anomalous expression and vary according to tissue: (1) the p110α gene product of PIK3CA, (2) the p85 regulatory subunit of PI3K, (3) phosphatase and tensin homologue deleted from chromosome 10 (PTEN) and (4) Akt (Levine, Bogomolniy *et al.*, 2005). PI3K (including p85 and PIK3CA), PTEN and Akt are all linked by the major product of PI3K, PIP_3. The PIK3CA gene product, p110alpha, is the catalytic subunit of Class 1 PI3K, which phosphorylates phosphatidylinositol 4,5-bisphosphate (PIP_2) on the D-3 position of the *myo*-inositol ring to generate PIP_3. PIP_3 attracts PH domain–containing proteins such as PDK1, Akt and multiple Akt substrates to the membrane enabling activation of this signaling pathway. PIK3CA mutations are unusual because they typically enhance enzymatic activity of the gene product by upregulating downstream effectors such as Akt. Over 80% of somatic PIK3CA mutations are missense gain-of-function mutations, which can lead to increased PIP_3 levels in affected cells (Ikenoue *et al.*, 2005; Kang *et al.*, 2005; Samuels and Ericson, 2006). In contrast PTEN, an enzyme that hydrolyzes PIP_3, is a tumor suppressor with reduced expression in a variety of cancers (Carnero *et al.*, 2008; Yuan and Cantley, 2008).

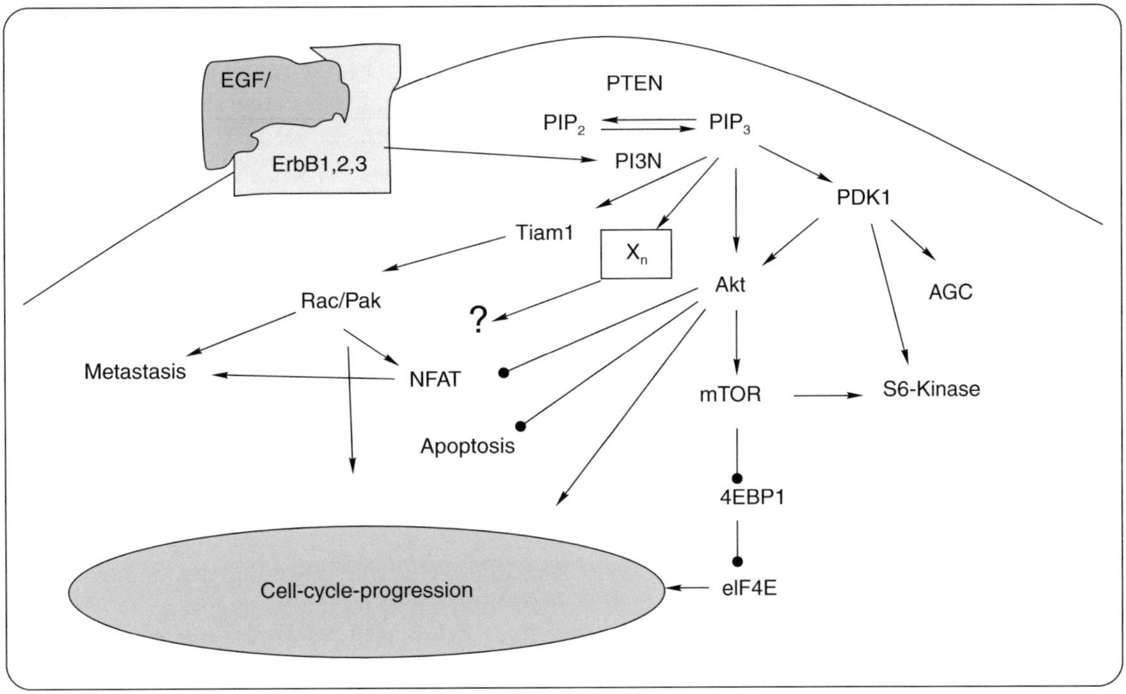

Fig. 11.1 ***Selected Signaling Elements Relevant to Cancer.***

(A number of proteins in the PI3K/PIP_3 signaling pathway are abnormal in cancer. Several PIP_3 targets relevant to oncogenesis such as Akt, PDK1 and Tiam1 have been identified while other targets (X_n) are yet to be characterized. Drugs targeting PI3K, Akt and mTor are currently in development for the treatment of various cancers.)

Inositides in Breast Cancer

Breast cancer may be particularly receptive to intervention in inositide signaling. Herceptin (trastuzumab), an antibody drug targeting the erbB2 (HER2/neu) receptor, has been successful in prolonging the lives of breast cancer patients overexpressing erbB2 (Garrison *et al.*, 2007; Iwata, 2007; Lin and Rugo, 2007; Lazaridis *et al.*, 2008). The proposed mechanism of action of erbB2 involves triggering the PI3K/Akt pathway and phosphorylation of Akt substrates such as p27kip, a regulator of cell cycle progression. All four of the cancer-linked proteins described above have been found to be aberrant in a significant fraction of breast cancer specimens and are either a cause or consequence of elevated PIP_3 levels. Anomalous elevation of PIP_3 levels, whether through activation of PI3K or suppression of PTEN, tends to be tumorigenic and correspond to cancer aggressiveness, whereas decreased PIP_3 levels suppress tumor formation (Depowski *et al.*, 2001; Panigrahi *et al.*, 2004; Saal *et al.*, 2007).

In a recent meta-analysis the p110alpha gene, PIK3CA, was found to contain point mutations in approximately 30% of somatic colon and breast cancer samples (Bader *et al.*, 2006). Overall, separate studies have estimated the fraction of PIK3CA somatic mutations in breast cancer ranging from 18% to 40%. Although PIK3CA mutations are somewhat more common in ER+ tumors (34%) versus ER tumors (19%), there is no association with HER2/neu (erbB2) expression (Saal *et al.*, 2005). In contrast, the tumor suppressor PTEN, although seldom mutated in breast cancer biopsy studies, was underexpressed in up to 48% of tumor specimens (Depowski *et al.*, 2001; Panigrahi *et al.*, 2004; Saal *et al.*, 2005; Shaw and Cantley, 2006; Saal *et al.*, 2007). Furthermore, reduced PTEN transcript levels in stage II breast cancer specimens were reflective of reduced protein levels (Saal *et al.*, 2007), which would result in an elevated PIP_3. It is significant that there is very little overlap between specimens with PIK3CA mutations and PTEN underexpression, *suggesting that PIP_3 levels are elevated either through PI3KCA mutation or PTEN underexpression in at least 70–88% of breast cancer cases.*

This is consistent with Akt activity observed in breast cancer tumor specimens. Akt acts as a decision point downstream of PIP_3, leading to accelerated metabolism, proliferation and suppression of apoptosis through multiple mediators (Fig. 11.1), many of which rely on PIP_3 for purposeful membrane localization. Akt is seldom mutated in breast cancer and accordingly Akt protein expression anomalies are rarely associated with breast cancer (Zinda *et al.*, 2001) (see Table 11.1). Nevertheless, Akt protein *activity* is upregulated, presumably due to elevated PIP_3 levels resulting from dysregulation of upstream proteins PI3K and PTEN (Nakatani *et al.*, 1999; Sun, Paciga *et al.*, 2001; Sun, Wang *et al.*, 2001). Consequently, there is ample rationale suggesting that agents disrupting PIP_3 binding with downstream effectors such as Akt, PDK, etc., may have therapeutic potential in breast as well as other forms of cancer. In fact, the development of inhibitors targeting the PI3K/Akt pathway including the downstream effector mTOR has become a major effort engaging academia, industry and government. As a result a number of drug candidates targeting this pathway are making their way through clinical trials, being tested for treatment of a range of cancers. Currently, there are five different PI3K inhibitors, viz. PX-866, GSK1059615, CAL-101, BGT226 and BEZ235, in Phase I or Phase I/II clinical trials (http://www.clinicaltrials.gov) (McMullen and Jay, 2007) and over 400 patent applications for PI3K inhibitors filed with the US Patent and Trademark Office. Other compounds targeting this pathway downstream of PIP_3 that have been tested in clinical trials include lipid-based Akt inhibitors such as perifosine and mitelfosine, PDK inhibitors and mTOR inhibitors. Progress with these approaches has been mixed but generally encouraging (Granville *et al.*, 2006; LoPiccolo *et al.*, 2007, 2008; Garcia-Echeverria and Sellers, 2008; Marone *et al.*, 2008; van Blitterswijk and Verheij, 2008; Yap *et al.*, 2008; Yuan and Cantley, 2008). Gastrointestinal and cardiac toxicities have occurred, and in some cases in early trials with perifosine, gastrointestinal side effects resulted in cessation of the trial.

Table 11.1 *Level of Deviation in Regulation in Breast Specimens in PI3K/AKT Signaling Path*

	DNA Mutation	*RNA Transcript*	*Protein Expression*	*Protein Activity*
PI3KCa	18–40%			
p85			79% increased	
PTEN	Not common	48% underexpressed	48% underexpressed	
Akt	Not common		Unchanged	80% increased

Sources: Philp *et al.*, 2001; Bachman *et al.*, 2004; Campbell *et al.*, 2004; Levine *et al.*, 2005; Saal *et al.*, 2005; Maruyama *et al.*, 2007; Rojo *et al.*, 2007; Saal *et al.*, 2007.

INOSITIDE ANALOGUES CURRENTLY IN DEVELOPMENT

There are currently no inositide analogues in clinical trials for the treatment of cancer. However, rationally designed phosphatidylinositol (PtdIns) analogues that interfere with Akt signaling have been identified (Kozikowski *et al.*, 2003; Van Meter *et al.*, 2006; Castillo *et al.*, 2004; Meuillet *et al.*, 2004) and the effects of specific analogues on Akt signaling in cancer cells have been characterized. In these studies ether-linked 3-deoxy PtdIns analogues (PIAs) inhibited Akt signaling at low micromolar doses while stimulating the stress kinase p38α (Gills *et al.*, 2007), two actions the authors demonstrated contributed to the apoptosis of the tumor cell lines that were tested. In intact cells PIAs interfered with Akt recruitment to membranes and phosphorylation of downstream substrates of Akt without inhibiting PI3K or PDK-1 or numerous other upstream kinases (Castillo *et al.*, 2004). However, PIAs also inhibited other targets not associated with the PI3K/Akt/mTOR pathway, suggesting that they are biologically distinct from other agents targeting this pathway (Gills *et al.*, 2006).

Proposed Use of Inositol Polyphosphate Derivatives to Differentially Inhibit Signaling through Select PIP_3 Binding Proteins

Current drugs in development that target single proteins such as PI3K, mTOR and Akt have drawbacks that limit their potency and/or safety profile (LoPiccolo *et al.*, 2008; Yap *et al.*, 2008). Targeting individual entities in signaling pathways with complex feedback loops can be problematic due to circumvention via recursive or redundant pathways. Therefore, an approach that regulates a wider range of coordinated targets may be more effective, such as a drug that targets a subset of PIP_3 binding proteins most relevant to cell proliferation (Fig. 11.2). Although we do not yet know whether such a drug could exist, there is evidence suggesting that individual inositol tetrakisphosphate analogues can differentially modulate the distinct PIP_3 signaling branches. For instance, while a membrane-permeant Ins(1,4,5,6)P_4 analogue antagonized the PIP_3 electrophysiological actions (Eckmann *et al.*, 1997), it mimicked the inhibitory effect of PIP_3 on NADPH oxidase (Traynor-Kaplan *et al.*, 2001).

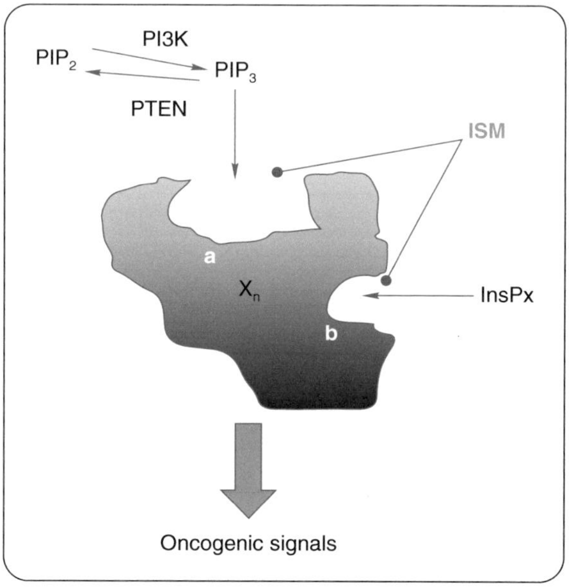

Fig. 11.2 ***Therapeutic Inositol Signaling Molecule (ISM) Analogue Targets in Cancer.***

(PIP_3 levels are increased in cancer cells either through overproduction due to gain-of-function mutations in PI3K or through loss-of-function mutations in the tumor suppressor PTEN. Therapeutic inositide analogues can target either the PIP_3 binding pocket 'a' or the $InsP_x$ binding pocket 'b' (or both) in oncogenic proteins (X_n) stimulated by PIP_3, thus interfering with oncogenic signal transduction. Inositol polyphosphate analogues that can target specific subsets of PIP_3 binding proteins, either enhancing or inhibiting PIP_3 actions in regulating proliferation, apoptosis and metastases, may be more effective than the agents developed thus far.)

As described above, overproduction of PIP_3 is implicated as a common denominator in a high percentage of breast cancers as well as other cancers. While inhibitors of two of its immediate downstream effectors, Akt1 and PDK, are in drug development, there are many other PIP_3 binding proteins that may als o play a role in cancer to varying degrees (Balla, 2005; Minard *et al.*, 2006; Sasaki *et al.*, 2007). Akt and PDK are members of a group of over 80 proteins containing PH domains, the 11th most common domain in the human proteome. Proteins (including Akt and PDK) bind to PIP_3 via their PH domains, anchoring them in the membrane adjacent to upstream activators and downstream effectors. PH domains are one of the several PIP_3 binding domains that have been identified (Sasaki *et al.*, 2007). PH domains display a considerable degree of heterogeneity and have differential binding affinities for various inositides *in vitro* (Kavran *et al.*, 1998). However, only 10% of the PH domain–containing proteins bind to inositides with great affinity, showing a preference for inositides with two adjacent phosphates (Lemmon, 2007).

Inositol Polyphosphates may be Endogenous Regulators of Tumorigenic PIP_3 Effectors

Inositides constitute a large body of diverse molecules, some of which are continuously present in the intracellular milieu at micromolar concentrations, while others such as PIP_3 are typically only formed transiently at very low levels. This mixture makes it very difficult to extrapolate from *in vitro* binding studies to predict the effect of inositides on inositide binding proteins in intact cells, especially when other as yet uncharacterized intracellular molecules could also modulate access or binding affinity. While it has been difficult to determine the *in vivo* binding behavior of inositides, cleverly designed studies have recently established that inositol polyphosphates co-regulate a PH domain protein together with PIP_3, demonstrating co-regulation by dual intracellular signals, an inositol polyphosphate and a phosphoinositide (Irvine, 2004, 2007; Huang *et al.*, 2007). In these studies, Ins(1,3,4,5)P_4 binding to a separate binding site allosterically augments PIP_3 binding to the interleukin-2-inducible tyrosine kinase (Itk) PH domain in T cells. This hints that other PIP_3 binding proteins may be similarly regulated by Ins(1,3,4,5)P_4 or one of the many other inositol polyphosphates present in the cytosol. This type of interaction could explain our earlier observations of Ins(1,4,5,6)P_4 modulation of PIP_3 signaling in colonic epithelia (Eckmann *et al.*, 1997) and subsequent observations by Razzini and co-workers in COS-7 cells (Razzini *et al.*, 2000). Furthermore, since inositol polyphosphate analogues can antagonize the function of endogenous compounds (Rudolf *et al.*, 2003), this would indicate that similar inhibition of PH domain proteins (or proteins containing one or more of the several other PIP_3 binding domains) could be accomplished with appropriately engineered inositol polyphosphate derivatives. It has previously been proposed that inositol polyphosphate modulation of green fluorescent protein (GFP)–labelled inositide binding proteins can be used to identify cancer targets, which can then be used to screen for potential drugs (Berrie and Falasca, 2000). However, inositol polyphosphates themselves are endogenous regulators of PIP_3 signaling and may be suitable starting points for cancer drug development. Structural modifications of inositol polyphosphate analogues could broaden or narrow specificity, so that analogues would modulate a delimited subset of PIP_3 binding proteins that are the most relevant to tumorigenesis. In one scenario, inositol polyphosphate analogues could affect PIP_3 targets by enhancing/inhibiting association with one target relative to another.

Targeting Signal Integration

The diversity of inositol polyphosphates along with the potential for dual signals suggest that ratios of two inositides in the vicinity of a particular protein may be more pertinent to inositide signaling than absolute levels of a specific inositide. Titration of dual signals enables greater fine-tuning with fewer signals than a one-signal, one-target system. Inositol polyphosphate analogues that can target specific subsets of PIP_3 binding proteins, either enhancing or inhibiting actions in regulating proliferation, apoptosis and metastases, may be safer and more effective than the agents developed thus far.

DRUGGABILITY OF INOSITIDE ANALOGUES

Inositides clearly have activities that make them relevant drug candidates. However, other factors such as safety and practicality of formulation and manufacturing can limit the feasibility of successful drug development. One question that arises when contemplating inositide-based therapeutics is whether a compound that affects such key elements in signaling as inositol polyphosphates and phosphoinositides can have sufficient specificity to be therapeutically useful with minimal side effects. Although no red flags have emerged from early safety studies with INO-4995, ultimately we would not know the answer to the safety question until more extensive studies have been performed and it has been tested in thousands of people. Another means of mitigating safety concerns are through use of targeted delivery. In the case of INO-4995, it can be formulated for aerosol delivery to the pulmonary epithelia via use of a metered dose inhaler to reduce systemic exposure. Membrane-permeant alkyl (acyl) ester inositide analogues share a number of physical chemical properties with one another. Therefore, a formulation that works for one compound (e.g. INO-4995) would be expected to work for others in this category. The INO-4995 synthetic route has been optimized and manufacturing costs are anticipated to be moderate.

Potential advantages of inositide analogues for therapeutic development include the following:

- Expected to differentially regulate diverse inositide/PIP_3 binding proteins through selective binding to PH and other inositide/PIP_3 lipid binding domains
- Act on key decision switches in cells
- Emulate endogenous regulators
- Potential for greater specificity/fine-tuning through titrating two signals, e.g. inositol polyphosphate versus PIP_3
- Potential to trigger multiple sites with coordinated activity through interacting with homologous domains on a group of proteins
- Can be converted to membrane-permeant prodrugs
- Amenable to further modifications to optimize binding selectivity/effect
- Can be engineered to be metabolized intracellularly to products indistinguishable from native molecules, thus avoiding problems associated with overwhelming liver and kidney detoxification pathways

THE FUTURE OF INOSITIDE-BASED THERAPEUTICS

Our understanding of disease is changing. Chronic inflammatory diseases, autoimmune diseases and cancer are all categories where less target specificity of a drug may be preferable. Drugs that have only one target are subject to circumvention through feedback processes inherent in all biological systems at every level. Inositides and inositide derivatives may provide the appropriate level of specificity to address this need. However, we will not fully realize this potential without a concerted effort to unravel the complexities of inositide signaling utilizing systems approaches.

The balance of cellular phosphoinositides and inositol phosphates direct global cellular events. For instance, recent data suggest that it is not sufficient to only know the levels of PIP_3

to predict a particular cellular decision, but rather to subtend the relative levels of a number of inositol polyphosphates and phosphoinositides that can modify its actions. Our understanding of inositide signaling has been constricted by our snapshot perspective of relative chemical levels at discreet points in time in a particular cell line. Inositol polyphosphates and phosphoinositides are rapidly and continuously interconverted and compete with one another at multiple binding sites. Inositol polyphosphates can allosterically regulate phosphoinositide signaling at specific targets. Some inositides turn over within seconds and milliseconds, while others turn over within the course of days.

Thus, it may be more useful to see the 30+ body of inositides as a type of cellular alphabet. It is not the individual letters that matter as much as the combination of letters occurring at a particular point in space, articulating a command to a receptive protein or set of proteins.

From this perspective we have only begun to decipher the language of inositides. What is the most relevant measurement to gain understanding of this language? Is it chemical levels of inositides, their rate of turnover, the relative amounts of various inositides, levels or activity of enzymes, oscillation frequency of inositide levels or the amplitude of those oscillations? Whatever the answer, one thing is clear: understanding the dynamics/language of these molecules holds enormous potential for future inositide-based drug design. We could exploit this potential by initiating a systems biology approach to cataloging inositide behavior. Meanwhile, educated guesses have yielded promising candidates, e.g. INO-4995.

REFERENCES

Alcazar-Roman, A.R., Wente, S.R. (2008). Inositol polyphosphates: A new frontier for regulating gene expression. *Chromosoma* **117(1)**:1–13.

Bachhuber, T., Konig, J., *et al.* (2005). Cl^- interference with the epithelial Na+ channel ENaC. *Journal of Biological Chemistry* **280(36)**:31587–31594.

Bachman, K.E., Argani, P., Samuels, Y., Silliman, N., Ptak, J., Szabo, S., Konishi, H., Karakas, B., Blair, B. G., Lin, C. (2004). The PIK3CA gene is mutated with high frequency in human breast cancers. *Cancer Biology and Therapy* **3(8)**:772–775.

Bader, A.G., Kang, S., Vogt, P.K. (2006). Cancer-specific mutations in PIK3CA are oncogenic *in vivo*. *Proceedings of the National Academy of Sciences USA* **103(5)**:1475–1479.

Balla, T. (2005). Inositol–lipid binding motifs: Signal integrators through protein–lipid and protein–protein interactions. *Journal of Cell Science* **118(Pt. 10)**:2093–2104.

Berridge, M.J. (1986). Inositol trisphosphate and calcium mobilization. *Journal of Cardiovascular Pharmacology* **8(Suppl. 8)**:S85–90.

Berrie, C.P., Falasca, M. (2000). Patterns within protein/polyphosphoinositide interactions provide specific targets for therapeutic intervention. *FASEB Journal* **14(15)**:2618–2622.

Boucher, R.C. (2007a). Airway surface dehydration in cystic fibrosis: Pathogenesis and therapy. *Annual Review of Medicine* **58**:157–170.

Boucher, R.C. (2007b). Cystic fibrosis: A disease of vulnerability to airway surface dehydration. *Trends in Molecular Medicine* **13(6)**:231–240.

Boucher, R.C., Cotton, C.U., Gatzy J.T, Knowles M.R, Yankaskas J.R. (1988). Evidence for reduced Cl^- and increased Na^+ permeability in cystic fibrosis human primary cell cultures. Journal of Physiology **405**:77–103.

Campbell, I.G., Russell, S.E., (2004). Mutation of the PIK3CA gene in ovarian and breast cancer. *Cancer Research* **64(21)**:7678–7681.

Carew, M.A., Yang, X., Schultz, C. and Shears, S. B. (2000). *myo*-Inositol 3,4,5,6-tetrakisphosphate inhibits an apical calcium-activated chloride conductance in polarized monolayers of a cystic fibrosis cell line. *Journal of Biological Chemistry* **275(35)**:26906–26913.

Carnero, A., Blanco-Aparicio, C., Renner, O., Link, W. and Leal, J. F. (2008). The PTEN/PI3K/AKT signalling pathway in cancer, therapeutic implications. *Current Cancer Drug Targets* **8(3)**:187–198.

Castillo, S.S., Brognard, J. Petukhov, C. Zhang, J. Tsurutani, C.A. Granville, M. Li, M. Jung, K.A. West, J.G. Gills, A.P. Kozikowski, and P.A. Dennis,. (2004). Preferential inhibition of Akt and killing of Akt-dependent cancer cells by rationally designed phosphatidylinositol ether lipid analogues. *Cancer Research* **64(8)**:2782–2792.

Clarke, L.L., Grubb, B.R., J.R. Yankaskas, C.U. Cotton, A. McKenzie, and R.C. Boucher. (1994). Relationship of a non-cystic fibrosis transmembrane conductance regulator-mediated chloride conductance to organ-level disease in Cftr(-/-) mice. In: *Proceedings of the National Academy of Sciences USA* **91(2)**:479–483.

Collins, F.S., Riordan, J.R., L.C. Tsui. (1990). The cystic fibrosis gene: Isolation and significance. *Hospital Practice (Office Edition)* **25(10)**:47–57.

Davis, P.B. (1987). Pathophysiology of cystic fibrosis with emphasis on salivary gland involvement. *Journal of Dental Research* **66**:667–671.

Depowski, P.L., Rosenthal, S.I., J.S. Ross. (2001). Loss of expression of the PTEN gene protein product is associated with poor outcome in breast cancer. *Modern Pathology* **14(7)**:672–676.

Devidas, S., Guggino, W.B. (1997). CFTR: domains, structure, and function. *Journal of Bioenergetics and Biomembranes* **29(5)**:443–451.

Drumm, M.L., Collins, F.S. (1993). Molecular biology of cystic fibrosis. *Molecular Genetic Medicine* **3**:33–68.

Duerson, K., Moody, M., A. Schnaars, C. Schultz, and A. Traynor-Kaplan *l*. (2000). Patch clamp analysis of a Cl^- current stimulated by a membrane-permeant inositol polyphosphate analogue in CF nasal epithelial cells. *Pediatric Pulmonology* **30(S20)**:199–200.

Duerson, K., Moody, M., C. Schultz, and A. Traynor-Kaplan. (2004). A deesterified form of INO-4995, (INO-4913) stimulates whole cell Cl^- currents in CF human nasal epithelial cells. *Pediatric Pulmonology* **38(S27)**:241–242.

Eckmann, L., Rudolf, M.T., A. Ptasznik, C. Schultz, T. Jiang, N. Wolfson, R. Tsien, J. Fierer, S.B. Shears, M.F. Kagnoff, and A.E. Traynor-Kaplan. (1997). D-*myo*-Inositol 1,4,5,6-tetrakisphosphate produced in human intestinal epithelial cells in response to *Salmonella* invasion inhibits phosphoinositide 3-kinase signaling pathways. In: *Proceedings of the National Academy of Sciences USA* **94(26)**:14456–14460.

Elizur, A., Cannon, C.L., T.W. Ferkol. (2008). Airway inflammation in cystic fibrosis. *Chest* **133(2)**:489–495.

Fleischer, B., Xie, J., Mayrleitner, M., Shears,S.B., Palmer, D.J. and S. Fleischer. (1994). Golgi coatomer binds, and forms K(+)-selective channels gated by, inositol polyphosphates. *Journal of Biological Chemistry* **269(27)**:17826–17832.

Garcia-Echeverria, C., Sellers, W.R. (2008). Drug discovery approaches targeting the PI3K/Akt pathway in cancer. *Oncogene* **27(41)**:5511–5526.

Garrison, L.P., Jr., Lubeck, D. Lalla, D., Paton, V., Dueck, A., and Perez, E.A. (2007). Cost-effectiveness analysis of trastuzumab in the adjuvant setting for treatment of HER2-positive breast cancer. *Cancer* **110(3)**:489–498.

Gills, J.J., Castillo, S.S., Zhang, C., Petukhov, P.A., Memmott, R.M., Hollingshead, M., Warfel, N., Han, J., Kozikowski, A.P., and Dennis, P.A. (2007). Phosphatidylinositol ether lipid analogues that inhibit AKT also independently activate the stress kinase, p38alpha, through MKK3/6-independent and -dependent mechanisms. *Journal of Biological Chemistry* **282(37)**:27020–27029.

Gills, J.J., Holbeck, S., Hollingshead, M., Hewitt, S.M., Kozikowski, A.P., and Dennis, P.A. (2006). Spectrum of activity and molecular correlates of response to phosphatidylinositol ether lipid analogues, novel lipid-based inhibitors of Akt. *Molecular Cancer Therapeutics* **5(3)**:713–722.

Granville, C.A., Memmott, R.M., Gills, J.J., and Dennis, P.A. (2006). Handicapping the race to develop inhibitors of the phosphoinositide 3-kinase/Akt/mammalian target of rapamycin pathway. *Clinical Cancer Research* **12(3 Pt. 1)**:679–689.

Grases, F., Simonet, B.M., Vucenik, I., Perello, J., Prieto, R.M., and Shamsuddin, A.M. (2002). Effects of exogenous inositol hexakisphosphate (InsP(6)) on the levels of InsP(6) and of inositol trisphosphate (InsP(3)) in malignant cells, tissues and biological fluids. *Life Sciences* **71(13)**:1535–1546.

Grases, F., Simonet, B.M., Vucenik, I., Prieto, R.M., Costa-Bauza, A., March, J.G., and Shamsuddin, A.M. (2001). Absorption and excretion of orally administered inositol hexaphosphate (IP(6) or phytate) in humans. *Biofactors* **15**(1):53–61.

Grubb, B.R., Boucher, R.C. (1997). Enhanced colonic Na^+ absorption in cystic fibrosis mice versus normal mice. *American Journal of Physiology* **272(2 Pt. 1)**:G393–400.

Grubb, B.R., Vick, R.N., Boucher, R.C. (1994). Hyperabsorption of Na^+ and raised $Ca^{(2+)}$-mediated Cl^- secretion in nasal epithelia of CF mice. *American Journal of Physiology* **266(5 Pt. 1)**:C1478–1483.

Hatfield, J.M., Wierdl, M., Wadkins, R.M., and Potter, P.M. (2008). Modifications of human carboxylesterase for improved prodrug activation. *Expert Opinion on Drug Metabolism and Toxicology* **4(9)**:1153–1165.

Hilgemann, D.W. (2004). Biochemistry. Oily barbarians breach ion channel gates. *Science* **304(5668)**:223–224.

Ho, M.W., Kaetzel, M.A., Armstrong, D.L., and Shears, S.B. (2001). Regulation of a human chloride channel. a paradigm for integrating input from calcium, type II calmodulin-dependent protein kinase, and inositol 3,4,5,6-tetrakisphosphate. *Journal of Biological Chemistry* **276(22)**:18673–18680.

Hosokawa, M. (2008). Structure and catalytic properties of carboxylesterase isozymes involved in metabolic activation of prodrugs. *Molecules* **13(2)**: 412–431.

Huang, Y.H., Grasis, J.A., Miller, A.T., Xu, R., Soonthornvacharin, S., Andreotti, A.H., Tsoukas, C.D., Cooke, M.P., and Sauer, K. (2007). Positive regulation of Itk PH domain function by soluble IP4. *Science* **316(5826)**:886–889.

Ikenoue, T., Kanai, F., Hikiba, Y., Obata, T., Tanaka, Y., Imamura, J., Ohta, M., Jazag, A., Guleng, B., Tateishi, K.*et al.* (2005). Functional analysis of PIK3CA gene mutations in human colorectal cancer. *Cancer Research* **65(11)**:4562–4567.

Irvine, R. (2004). Inositol lipids: To PHix or not to PHix? *Current Biology* **14(8)**:R308–310.

Irvine, R. (2007). Cell signaling. The art of the soluble. *Science* **316(5826)**: 845–846.

Irvine, R.F. (2005). Inositide evolution—Towards turtle domination? *Journal of Physiology* **566(Pt. 2)**:295–300.

Irvine, R.F., Schell, M.J. (2001). Back in the water: The return of the inositol phosphates. *Nature Reviews Molecular Cell Biology* **2(5)**:327–338.

Ismailov, I.I., Berdiev, B.K., Shlyonsky, V.G., Fuller, C.M., Prat, A.G., Jovov, B., Cantiello, H.F., Ausiello, D.A., and Benos, D.J. (1997). Role of actin in regulation of epithelial sodium channels by CFTR. *American Journal of Physiology* **272(4 Pt. 1)**:C1077–1086.

Ismailov, I.I., Fuller, C.M., Berdiev, B.K., Shlyonsky, V.G., Benos, D.J., and Barrett, K.E. (1996). A biologic function for an "orphan" messenger: D-*myo*-Inositol 3,4,5,6-tetrakisphosphate selectively blocks epithelial calcium-activated chloride channels. In: *Proceedings of the National Academy of Sciences USA* **93(19)**:10505–10509.

Itoh, T., Takenawa, T. (2002). Phosphoinositide-binding domains: Functional units for temporal and spatial regulation of intracellular signalling. *Cellular Signalling* **14(9)**:733–743.

Iwata, H. (2007). Perspective of trastuzumab treatment. *Breast Cancer* **14(2)**:150–155.

Janzen, V., Scadden, D.T. (2006). Stem cells: good, bad and reformable. *Nature* **441(7092)**:418–419.

Jiang, T., Sweeney, G., Rudolf, M.T., Klip, A., Traynor-Kaplan, A., and Tsien, R.Y. (1998). Membrane-permeant esters of phosphatidylinositol 3,4,5-trisphosphate. *Journal of Biological Chemistry* **273(18)**:11017–11024.

Kachintorn, U., Vajanaphanich, M., Barrett, K.E., and Traynor-Kaplan, A.E. (1993). Elevation of inositol tetrakisphosphate parallels inhibition of $Ca^{(2+)}$-dependent Cl^- secretion in T84 cells. *American Journal of Physiology* **264(3 Pt. 1)**:C671–676.

Kang, S., Bader, A.G., Vogt, P.K. (2005). Phosphatidylinositol 3-kinase mutations identified in human cancer are oncogenic. In: *Proceedings of the National Academy of Sciences USA* **102(3)**:802–807.

Kavran, J.M., Klein, D.E., Lee, A., Falasca, M., Isakoff, S.J., Skolnik, E.Y., and Lemmon, M.A. (1998). Specificity and promiscuity in phosphoinositide binding by pleckstrin homology domains. *Journal of Biological Chemistry* **273(46)**:30497–30508.

Knowles, M.R., Boucher, R.C. (2002). Mucus clearance as a primary innate defense mechanism for mammalian airways. *Journal of Clinical Investigation* **109(5)**:571–577.

Kozikowski, A.P., Sun, H., Brognard, J., and Dennis, P.A. (2003). Novel PI analogues selectively block activation of the pro-survival serine/threonine kinase Akt. *Journal of the American Chemical Society* **125(5)**:1144–1145.

Kunzelmann, K., Kiser, G.L., Schreiber, R., and Riordan, J.R. (1997). Inhibition of epithelial Na^+ currents by intracellular domains of the cystic fibrosis transmembrane conductance regulator. *FEBS Letters* **400(3)**:341–344.

Kunzelmann, K., Mall, M., Briel, M., Hipper, A., Nitschke, R., Ricken, S., and Greger, R (1997). The cystic fibrosis transmembrane conductance regulator attenuates the endogenous Ca^{2+} activated Cl^- conductance of *Xenopus* oocytes. *Pflügers Archiv* **435(1)**:178–181.

Lazaridis, G., Pentheroudakis, G., Pavlidis, N. (2008). Integrating trastuzumab in the neoadjuvant treatment of primary breast cancer: Accumulating evidence of efficacy, synergy and safety. *Critical Reviews in Oncology/Hematology* **66(1)**:31–41.

Lemmon, M.A. (2007). Pleckstrin homology (PH) domains and phosphoinositides. *Biochemical Society Symposia* **(74)**:81–93.

Lemmon, M.A. (2008). Membrane recognition by phospholipid-binding domains. *Nature Reviews Molecular Cell Biology* **9(2)**:99–111.

Lemmon, M.A., Ferguson, K.M., Sigler, P.B., Schlessinger, J. (2008).US Patent 7,314,620. Methods for diagnosis and Treatment of PH Domain Signal Transduction Disorders. New York University: New York.

Letcher, A.J., Schell, M.J., Irvine, R,F. (2008). Do mammals make all their own inositol hexakisphosphate? *Biochemical Journal*. 416(2):263–70

Levine, D.A., Bogomolniy, F., Yee, C.J., Lash, A., Barakat, R.R., Borgen, P.I., and Boyd, J.*l*. (2005). Frequent mutation of the PIK3CA gene in ovarian and breast cancers. *Clinical Cancer Research* **11(8)**:2875–2878.

Li, W., Schultz, C., Llopis, J., and Tsien, R.Y. (1997). Membrane Permeant esters of inositol polyphosphates, chemical synthesis and biological applications. *Tetrahedron* **53(35)**:12017–12040.

Lin, A., Rugo, H.S. (2007). The role of trastuzumab in early stage breast cancer: Current data and treatment recommendations. *Current Treatment Options in Oncology* **8(1)**:47–60.

LoPiccolo, J., Blumenthal, G.M., Bernstein, W.B., and Dennis, P.A. (2008). Targeting the PI3K/Akt/mTOR pathway: Effective combinations and clinical considerations. *Drug Resistance Updates* **11(1–2)**:32–50.

LoPiccolo, J., Granville, C.A., Gills, J.J., and Dennis, P.A. (2007). Targeting Akt in cancer therapy. *Anticancer Drugs* **18(8)**:861–874.

Ma, H.P., Chou, C.F., Wei, S.P., and Eaton, D.C. (2007). Regulation of the epithelial sodium channel by phosphatidylinositides: Experiments, implications, and speculations. *Pflügers Archiv* **455(1)**:169–180.

Ma, H.P., Eaton, D.C. (2005). Acute regulation of epithelial sodium channel by anionic phospholipids. *Journal of the American Society of Nephrology* **16(11)**:3182–3187.

Maffucci, T., Piccolo, E., Cumashi, A., Iezzi, M., Riley, A.M., Saiardi, A., Godage, H.Y., Rossi, C., Broggini, M., Iacobelli, S. Potter BV, Innocenti P, Falasca M. (2005). Inhibition of the phosphatidylinositol 3-kinase/Akt pathway by inositol pentakisphosphate results in antiangiogenic and antitumor effects. *Cancer Research* **65(18)**:8339–8349.

Mall, M., Bleich, M., Kuehr, J., Brandis, M., Greger, R., and Kunzelmann, K. (1999). CFTR-mediated inhibition of epithelial Na^+ conductance in human colon is defective in cystic fibrosis. *American Journal of Physiology* **277(3 Pt. 1)**:G709–716.

Mall, M., Grubb, B.R., Harkema, J.R., O'Neal, W.K., and Boucher, R.C. (2004). Increased airway epithelial Na^+ absorption produces cystic fibrosis-like lung disease in mice. *Nature Medicine* **10(5)**:487–493.

Marone, R., Cmiljanovic, V., Giese, B., and Wymann, M.P. (2008). Targeting phosphoinositide 3-kinase: moving towards therapy. *Biochimica et Biophysica Acta* **1784(1)**:159–185.

Maruyama, N., Miyoshi, Y., Taguchi, T., Tamaki, Y., Monden, M., and Noguchi, S. (2007). Clinicopathologic analysis of breast cancers with PIK3CA mutations in Japanese women. *Clinical Cancer Research* **13(2 Pt. 1)**:408–414.

McMullen, J.R., Jay, P.Y. (2007). PI3K(p110alpha) inhibitors as anti-cancer agents: Minding the heart. *Cell Cycle* **6(8)**:910–913.

McPherson, G.A. (1990). Paradoxical digestion of *myo*-inositol phosphates by alkaline phosphatase at low pH. *Life Sciences* **47(17)**:1569–1577.

Meuillet, E.J., Ihle, N., Baker, A.F., Gard, J.M., Stamper, C., Williams, R., Coon, A., Mahadevan, D., George, B.L., Kirkpatrick, L., Powis, G. (2004). *In vivo* molecular pharmacology and antitumor activity of the targeted Akt inhibitor PX-316. *Oncology Research* **14(10)**:513–527.

Michell, R.H. (2007). Evolution of the diverse biological roles of inositols. *Biochemical Society Symposia* **(74)**:223–246.

Miller, A.T., Chamberlain, P.P., Cooke, M.P. (2008). Beyond IP3: Roles for higher order inositol phosphates in immune cell signaling. *Cell Cycle* **7(4)**:463–467.

Minard, M.E., Ellis, L.M., Gallick, G.E (2006). Tiam1 regulates cell adhesion, migration and apoptosis in colon tumor cells. *Clinical and Experimental Metastasis* **23(5–6)**:301–313.

Moody, M., Pennington, C., Schultz, C., Caldwell, R., Dinkel, C., Rossi, M.W., McNamara, S., Widdicombe, J., Gabriel, S., and Traynor-Kaplan, A.E. (2005). Inositol polyphosphate derivative inhibits Na^+ transport and improves fluid dynamics in cystic fibrosis airway epithelia. *American Journal of Physiology—Cell Physiology* **289(3)**:C512–520.

Nakatani, K., Thompson, D.A., Barthel, A., Sakaue, H., Liu, W., Weigel, R.J., and Roth, R.A. (1999). Up-regulation of Akt3 in estrogen receptor-deficient breast cancers and androgen-independent prostate cancer lines. *Journal of Biological Chemistry* **274(31)**:21528–21532.

Neijens, H.J., Sinaasappel, M., de Groot, R., de Jongste, J.C., and Overbeek, S.E. (1990). Cystic fibrosis, pathophysiological and clinical aspects. *European Journal of Pediatrics* **149(11)**:742–751.

Panigrahi, A.R., Pinder, S.E., Chan, S.Y., Paish, E.C., Robertson, J.F., and Ellis, I.O. (2004). The role of PTEN and its signalling pathways, including AKT, in breast cancer; an assessment of relationships with other prognostic factors and with outcome. *Journal of Pathology* **204(1)**:93–100.

Philp, A.J., Campbell, I.G., Leet, C., Vincan, E., Rockman, S.P., Whitehead, R.H., Thomas, R.J., and Phillips, W.A. (2001). The phosphatidylinositol 3′-kinase p85alpha gene is an oncogene in human ovarian and colon tumors. *Cancer Research* **61(20)**:7426–7429.

Piccolo, E., Vignati, S., *Maffucci, T., Innominato, P.F., Riley, A.M., Potter, B.V., Pandolfi, P.P., Broggini, M., Iacobelli, S., Innocenti, P., Falasca M.* (2004). Inositol pentakisphosphate promotes apoptosis through the PI 3-K/Akt pathway. *Oncogene* **23(9)**:1754–1765.

Picher, M., Burch, L.H., Hirsh, A.J., Spychala, J., and Boucher, R.C. (2003). Ecto 5′-nucleotidase and nonspecific alkaline phosphatase. Two AMP-hydrolyzing ectoenzymes with distinct roles in human airways. *Journal of Biological Chemistry* **278(15)**:13468–13479.

Pochynyuk, O., Bugaj, V., Stockand, J.D. (2008). Physiologic regulation of the epithelial sodium channel by phosphatidylinositides. *Current Opinion in Nephrology and Hypertension* **17(5)**:533–540.

Pochynyuk, O., Tong, Q., Staruschenko, A., and Stockand, J.D. (2007). Binding and direct activation of the epithelial Na^+ channel (ENaC) by phosphatidylinositides. *Journal of Physiology* **580(Pt. 2)**:365–372.

Powis, G., Ihle, N., Kirkpatrick, D.L. (2006). Practicalities of drugging the phosphatidylinositol-3-kinase/Akt cell survival signaling pathway. *Clinical Cancer Research* **12(10)**:2964–2966.

Razzini, G., Berrie, C.P., Vignati, S., Broggini, M., Mascetta, G., Brancaccio, A., and Falasca, M. (2000). Novel functional PI 3-kinase antagonists inhibit cell growth and tumorigenicity in human cancer cell lines. *FASEB Journal* **14(9)**:1179–1187.

Rojo, F., Najera, L., Lirola, J., Jimenez, J., Guzman, M., Sabadell, M.D., Baselga, J., and Ramon y Cajal, S (2007). 4E-binding protein 1, a cell signaling hallmark in breast cancer that correlates with pathologic grade and prognosis. *Clinical Cancer Research* **13(1)**:81–89.

Rudolf, M.T., Dinkel, C., Traynor-Kaplan, A.E., and Schultz, C. (2003). Antagonists of *myo*-inositol 3,4,5,6-tetrakisphosphate allow repeated epithelial chloride secretion. *Bioorganic and Medicinal Chemistry* **11(15)**:3315–3329.

Rudolf, M.T., Traynor-Kaplan, A.E., Schultz, C. (1998). A membrane-permeant, bioactivatable derivative of Ins(1,3,4)P3 and its effect on $Cl^{(-)}$-secretion from T84 cells. *Bioorganic and Medicinal Chemistry Letters* **8(14)**:1857–1860.

Saal, L.H., Holm, K., Maurer, M., Memeo, L., Su, T., Wang, X., Yu, J.S., Malmstrom, P.O., Mansukhani, M., Enoksson, J. Hibshoosh H, Borg A, Parsons R. (2005). PIK3CA mutations correlate with hormone receptors, node metastasis, and ERBB2, and are mutually exclusive with PTEN loss in human breast carcinoma. *Cancer Research* **65(7)**:2554–9.

Saal, L.H., Johansson, P., Holm, K., Gruvberger-Saal, S.K., She, Q.B., Maurer, M., Koujak, S., Ferrando, A.A., Malmstrom, P., Memeo, L Isola J, Bendahl PO, Rosen N, Hibshoosh H, Ringnér M, Borg A, Parsons R. (2007). Poor prognosis in carcinoma is associated with a gene expression signature of aberrant PTEN tumor suppressor pathway activity. *Proceedings of the National Academy of Sciences USA* **104(18)**:7564–7569.

Saeed, Z., Wojewodka, G., Marion, D., Guilbault, C., and Radzioch, D. (2007). Novel pharmaceutical approaches for treating patients with cystic fibrosis. *Current Pharmaceutical Design* **13(31)**:3252–3263.

Samuels, Y., Ericson, K. (2006). Oncogenic PI3K and its role in cancer. *Current Opinion in Oncology* **18(1)**:77–82.

Sasaki, T., Sasaki, J., Sakai, T., Takasuga, S., and Suzuki, A (2007). The physiology of phosphoinositides. *Biological and Pharmaceutical Bulletin* **30(9)**:1599–1604.

Satoh, T., Hosokawa, M. (2006). Structure, function and regulation of carboxylesterases. *Chemico-Biological Interactions* **162(3)**:195–211.

Schultz, C. (2003). Prodrugs of biologically active phosphate esters. *Bioorganic and Medicinal Chemistry* **11(6)**:885–898.

Seeds, A.M., Bastidas, R.J., York, J.D. (2005). Molecular definition of a novel inositol polyphosphate metabolic pathway initiated by inositol 1,4,5-trisphosphate 3-kinase activity in *Saccharomyces cerevisiae*. *Journal of Biological Chemistry* **280(30)**:27654–27661.

Shaw, R.J., Cantley, L.C. (2006). Ras, PI(3)K and mTOR signalling controls tumour cell growth. *Nature* **441(7092)**:424–430.

Shears, S.B. (2005). Can intervention in inositol phosphate signalling pathways improve therapy for cystic fibrosis? *Expert Opinion on Therapeutic Targets* **9(6)**:1307–1317.

Sun, M., Paciga, J.E., Feldman, R.I., Yuan, Z., Coppola, D., Lu, Y.Y., Shelley, S.A., Nicosia, S.V., and Cheng, J.Q. (2001). Phosphatidylinositol-3-OH Kinase (PI3K)/AKT2, activated in breast cancer, regulates and is induced by estrogen receptor alpha (ERalpha) via interaction between ERalpha and PI3K. *Cancer Research* **61(16)**:5985–5991.

Sun, M., Wang, G., Paciga, J.E., Feldman, R.I., Yuan, Z.Q., Ma, X.L., Shelley, S.A., Jove, R., Tsichlis, P.N., Nicosia, S.V. Cheng, J.Q. (2001). AKT1/PKB alpha kinase is frequently elevated in human cancers and its constitutive activation is required for oncogenic transformation in NIH3T3 cells. *American Journal of Pathology* **159(2)**:431–437.

Tarran, R., Loewen, M.E., Paradiso, A.M., Olsen, J.C., Gray, M.A., Argent, B.E., Boucher, R.C., and Gabriel, S.E. (2002). Regulation of murine airway surface liquid volume by CFTR and Ca^{2+}-activated Cl^- conductances. *Journal of General Physiology* **120(3)**:407–418.

Traynor-Kaplan, A., Madhumitha, R., Widdicombe, J. (2007). [^{3}H]INO-4995 crosses mucus to enter airway epithelia but does not traverse epithelial sheets. *Pediatric Pulmonology* **42(S30)**:308.

Traynor-Kaplan, A., Moody, M., Pennington, C., and Langton-Webster, B. (2003). Preclinical profile of an inositol polyphosphate analog, INO-4995, a candidate therapeutic for cystic fibrosis. *Pediatric Pulmonology* **25(Supplement)**:248.

Traynor-Kaplan, A., Moody, M., Schultz, C. (2005). An inositol phosphate analog, INO-4995 normalizes electrophysiology in CF airway epithelia. *Advances in Experimental Medicine and Biology* **558**:115–127.

Traynor-Kaplan, A., Moody, M., Nur,M. Gabriel, S. Majerus,P.W. Drumm, M.L. and Langton-Webster, B. INO-4995 Therapeutic Efficacy is Enhanced with Repeat Dosing in CF KO Mice and Human Epithelia. (2010). *American Journal of Respiratory Cell and Molecular Biology*. Jan;42(1):105–12 Epub 2009 Apr 3.

Traynor-Kaplan, A., Nur, M., Wilson, M., and Majerus, P.W. (2007). Uptake of the pro-drug, INO-4995 and half-life of its active metabolite, INO-4913. *Pediatric Pulmonology* **42(S30)**:308.

Traynor-Kaplan, A., Schultz, C., Rudolf, M.T. (2001). Inositol derivatives for inhibiting superoxide anion production. US Patent 6,221,856North Bend, WA, and Oakland, CA: Inologic, Inc. and Regents of the University of California.

Vajanaphanich, M., Kachintorn, U., *Barrett, K.E., Cohn, J.A., Dharmsathaphorn, K., and Traynor-Kaplan, A.* (1993). Phosphatidic acid modulates Cl^- secretion in T84 cells: Varying effects depending on mode of stimulation. *American Journal of Physiology* **264(5 Pt. 1)**:C1210–1218.

Vajanaphanich, M., Schultz, C., Rudolf, M.T., Wasserman, M., Enyedi, P., Craxton, A., Shears, S.B., Tsien, R.Y., Barrett, K.E., and Traynor-Kaplan, A. (1994). Long-term uncoupling of chloride secretion from intracellular calcium levels by Ins(3,4,5,6)P4. *Nature* **371(6499)**:711–714.

van Blitterswijk, W.J., Verheij, M. (2008). Anticancer alkylphospholipids: mechanisms of action, cellular sensitivity and resistance, and clinical prospects. *Current Pharmaceutical Design* **14(21)**:2061–2074.

Van Meter, T.E., Broaddus, W.C., Cash, D., and Fillmore, H. (2006). Cotreatment with a novel phosphoinositide analogue inhibitor and carmustine enhances chemotherapeutic efficacy by attenuating AKT activity in gliomas. *Cancer* **107(10)**:2446–2454.

Vucenik, I., Shamsuddin, A.M. (2003). Cancer inhibition by inositol hexaphosphate (IP6) and inositol: From laboratory to clinic. *Journal of Nutrition* **133(11 Suppl. 1)**:3778S–3784S.

Vucenik, I., Shamsuddin, A.M. (2006). Protection against cancer by dietary IP6 and inositol. *Nutrition and Cancer* **55(2)**:109–125.

Yap, T.A., Garrett, M.D., Walton, M.I., Raynaud, F., de Bono, J.S., and Workman, P. (2008). Targeting the PI3K–AKT–mTOR pathway: Progress, pitfalls, and promises. *Current Opinion in Pharmacology* **8(4)**:393–412.

Yuan, T.L., Cantley, L.C. (2008). PI3K pathway alterations in cancer: variations on a theme. *Oncogene* **27(41)**:5497–5510.

Zinda, M.J., Johnson, M.A., Paul, J.D., Horn, C., Konicek, B.W., Lu, Z.H., Sandusky, G., Thomas, J.E., Neubauer, B.L., Lai, M. (2001). AKT-1, -2, and -3 are expressed in both normal and tumor tissues of the lung, breast, prostate, and colon. *Clinical Cancer Research* **7(8)**:2475–2479.

Zonia, L., Cordeiro, S., Tupy, J., and Feijo, J.A. (2002). Oscillatory chloride efflux at the pollen tube apex has a role in growth and cell volume regulation and is targeted by inositol 3,4,5,6-tetrakisphosphate. *Plant Cell* **14(9)**:2233–2249.

Editor's Profile

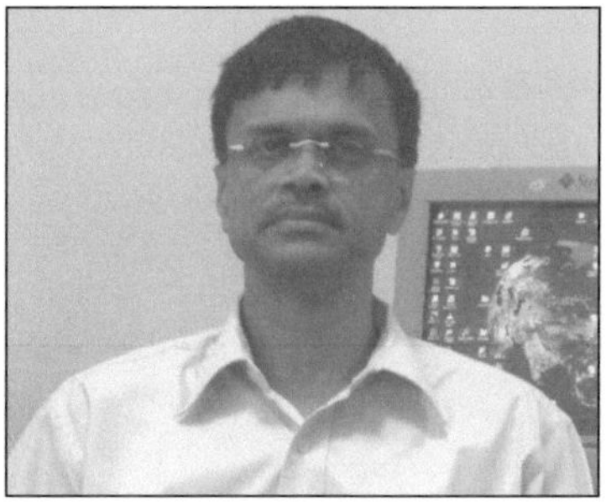

MUKESH DOBLE is Professor with the Department of Biotechnology at IIT Madras. Before joining IITM, he worked for 20 years in Imperial Chemical Industries (ICI) and General Electric (GE) Technology centers. His areas of interest are drug design, molecular modelling, biomaterials, bioreactors, and bioremediation. His other specialisations include hazard analysis, six sigma, and statistical process control. Prof. Doble holds B Tech and M Tech degrees in Chemical Engineering from IIT Madras and a PhD from University of Aston, Birmingham, UK and postdoctoral from University of Cambridge, UK, and Texas A&M, USA. He has authored or co-authored 170 technical papers: five books, including *Green Chemistry and Processes* (Elsevier); *Biochemical Engineering* (Prentice Hall); *Biotreatment of Industrial Effluents* (Elsevier); *Biotransformations & Bioprocesses* (Marcell Dekker: New York); and *Homogeneous Catalysis: Mechnanisms & Industrial Applications* (John Wiley & Sons), and filed 4 patents.

He is a recipient of the Herdillia Award for "Excellence in Basic Research" from Indian Institute of Chemical Engineers. He is a Fellow of Royal Society of Chemistry, England. He is in the editorial board of the journal *Chemical Engineering* (a McGraw-Hill publication) and a member of the American and Indian Institute of Chemical Engineers.

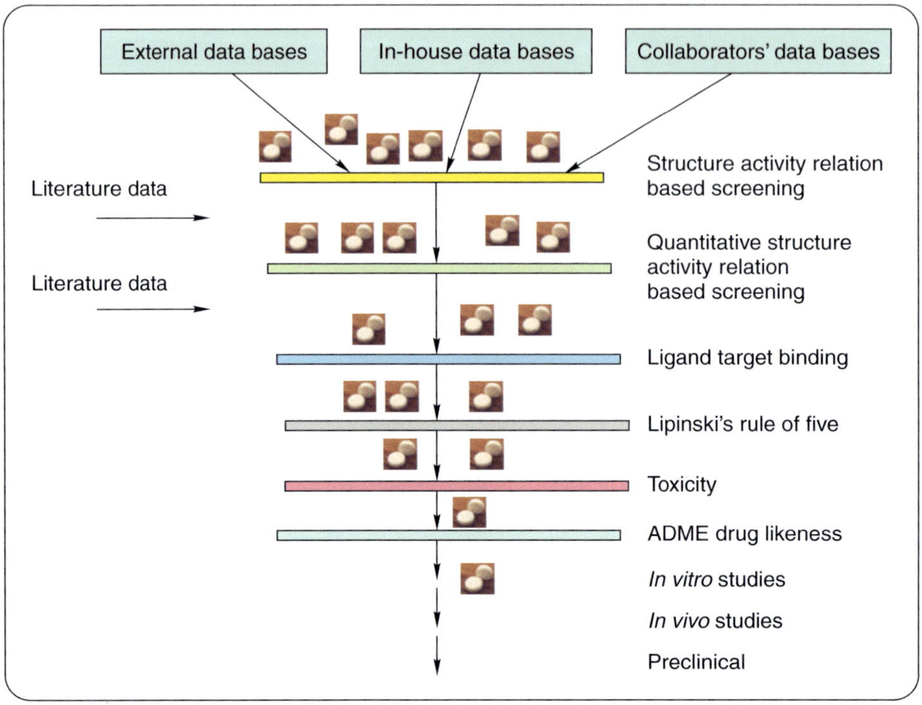

Fig 1.3 In Silico *Screening of Possible Lead Molecules*

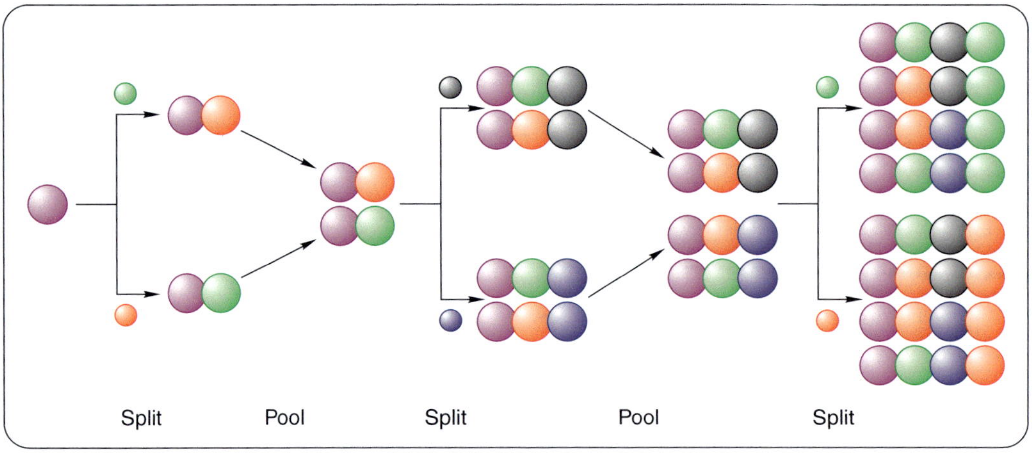

Fig 1.4 *Schematic of Split Pool Synthesis*

Plate 2

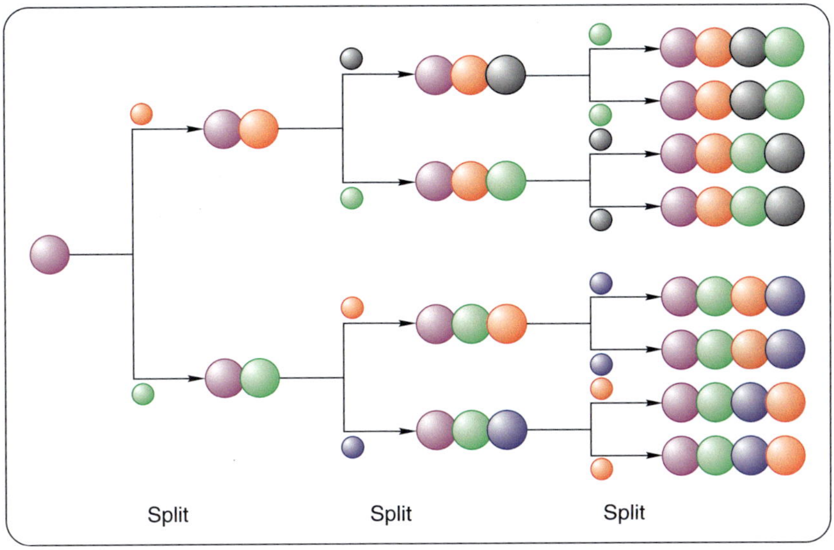

Fig 1.5 *Schematic of Parallel Synthesis*

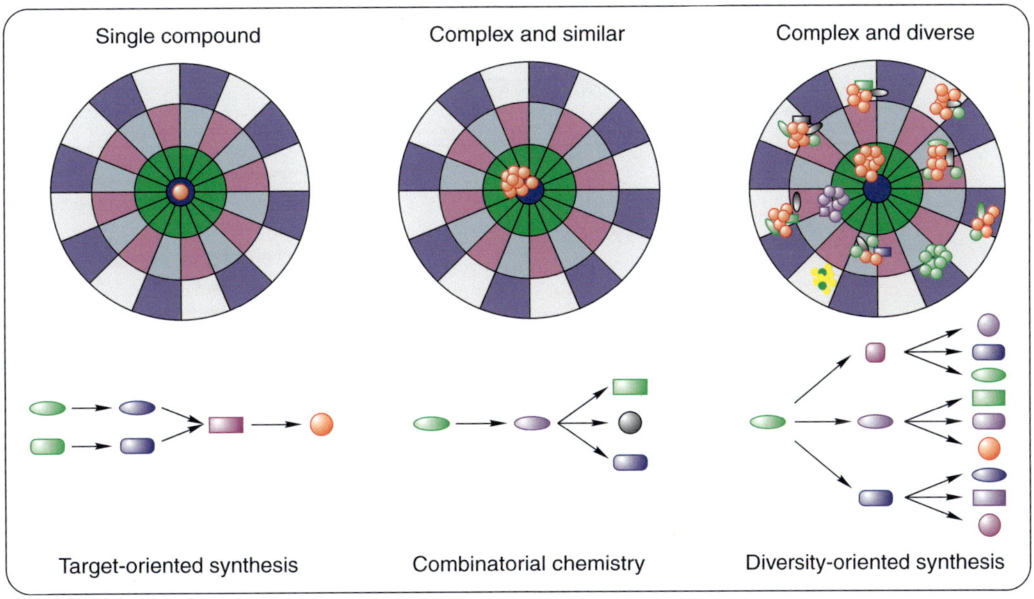

Fig 1.6 *Target-Oriented Synthesis, Combinatorial Chemistry and Diversity-Oriented Synthesis*

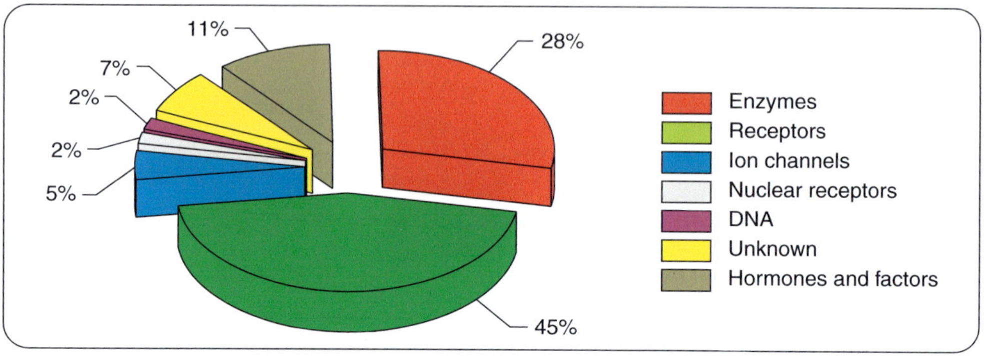

Fig 2.4 *Distribution of Targets by Biochemical Criteria*

Source: Potential Drug Target Database.

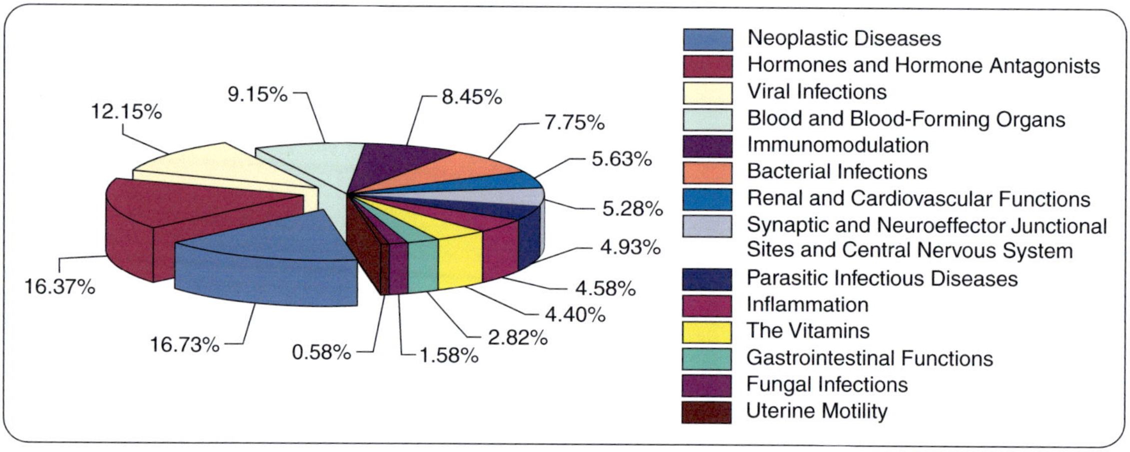

Fig 2.5 *Distribution of Targets in Therapeutic Areas*

Source: Potential Drug Target Database.

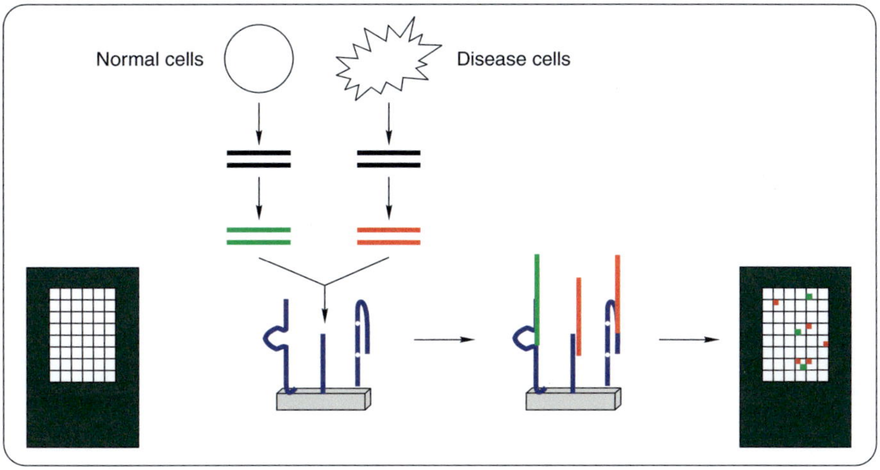

Fig 2.6 *DNA Microarray Technology*

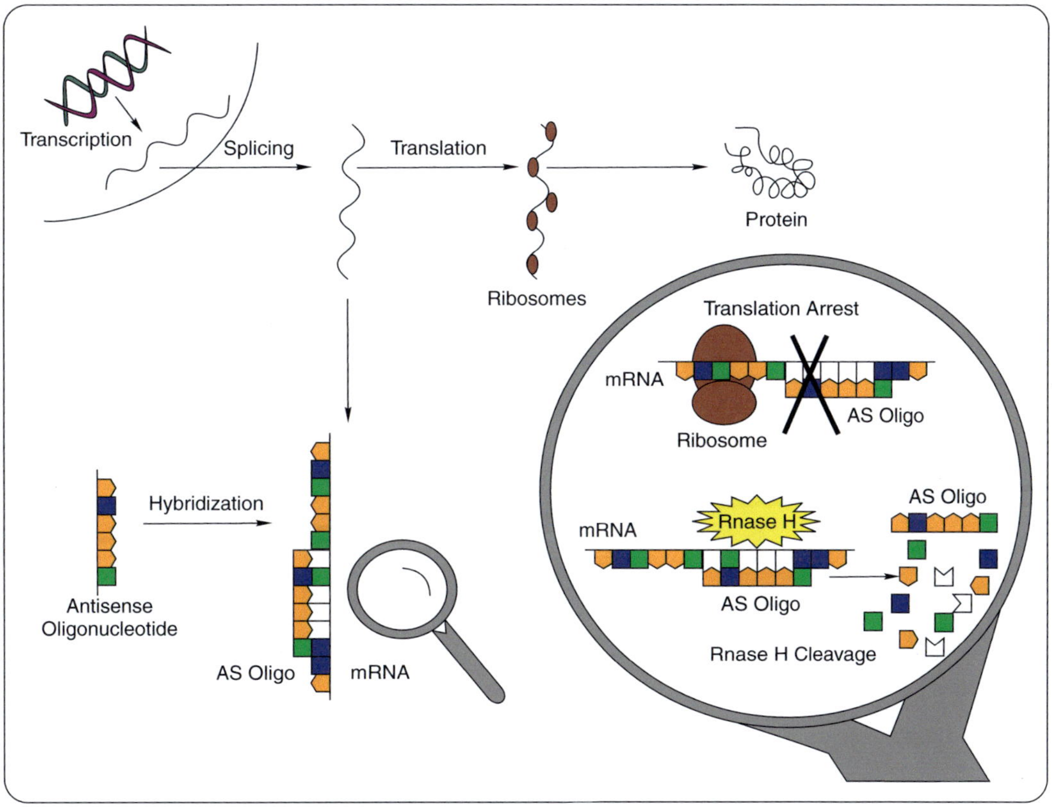

Fig 2.7 *Schematic Representation of Antisense Mechanisms*

Source: Rayburn *et al*. (2005).

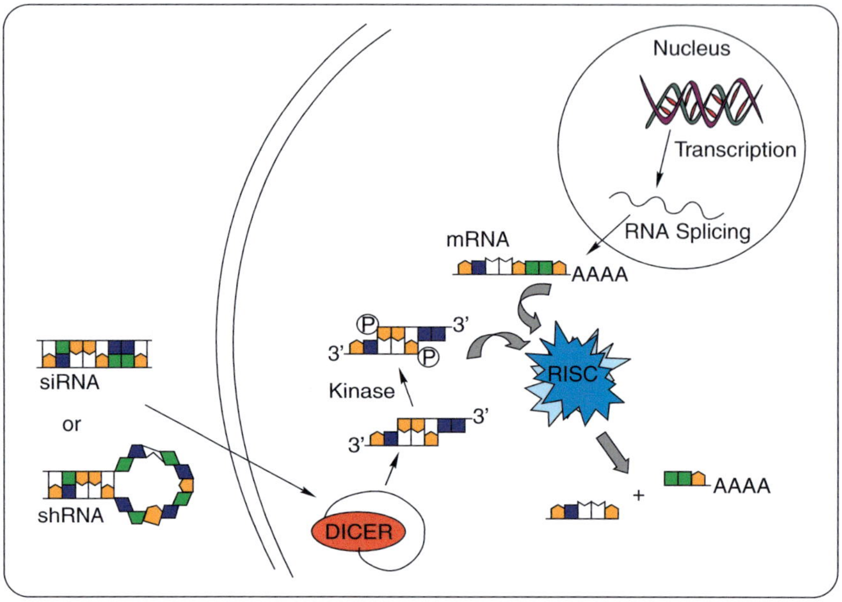

Fig 2.8 *Schematic Representation of RNAi Mechanisms. The Interfering RNA Molecule is Processed by the Dicer Enzyme Complex, which Cleaves RNA Strands into Smaller Nucleotide Fragments, which go on to Bind to the RISC. The RISC also Binds the Complementary Target mRNA Sequence, which is then Degraded, Blocking Gene Expression. si/shRNA: Small Interfering/Short Hairpin RNA, RISC: RNA-induced Silencing Complex.*

Source: Owino *et al*. (2008).

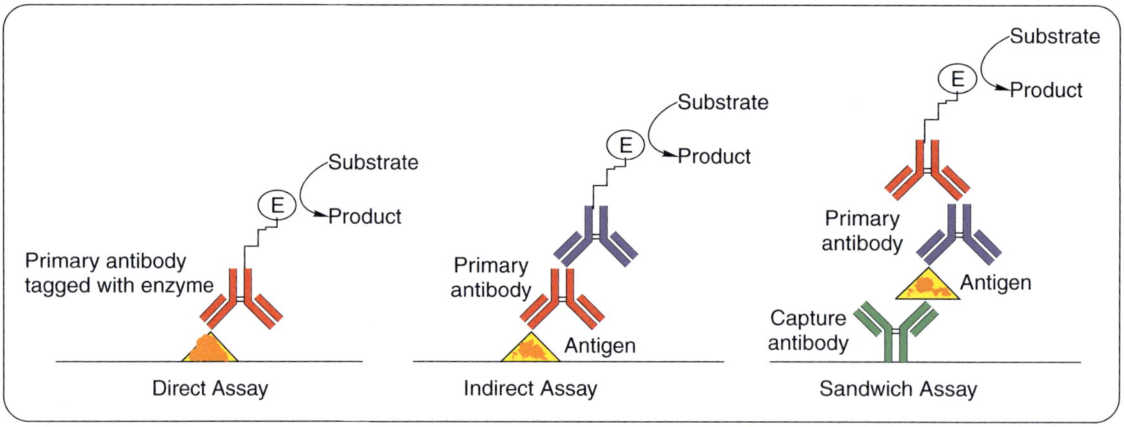

Fig 3.6 *Formats of ELISA*

Plate 6

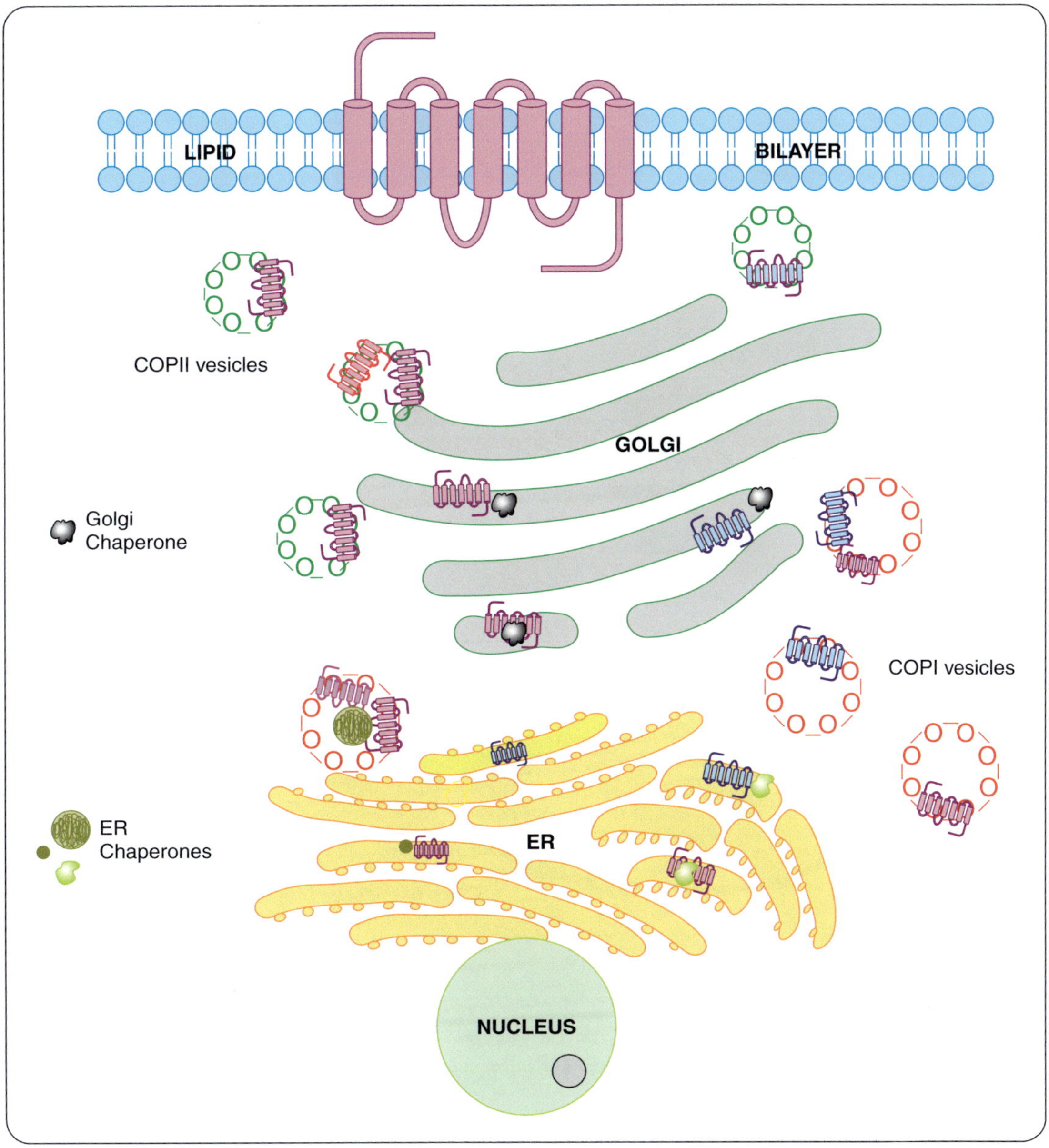

Fig 7.3 *Biogenesis of GPCR from ER to Plasma Membrane through Golgi with the Help of Various Chaperones, RAMPs and Clathrin-Coated Pits Proteins involved in the Trafficking are also Potential Drug Targets.*

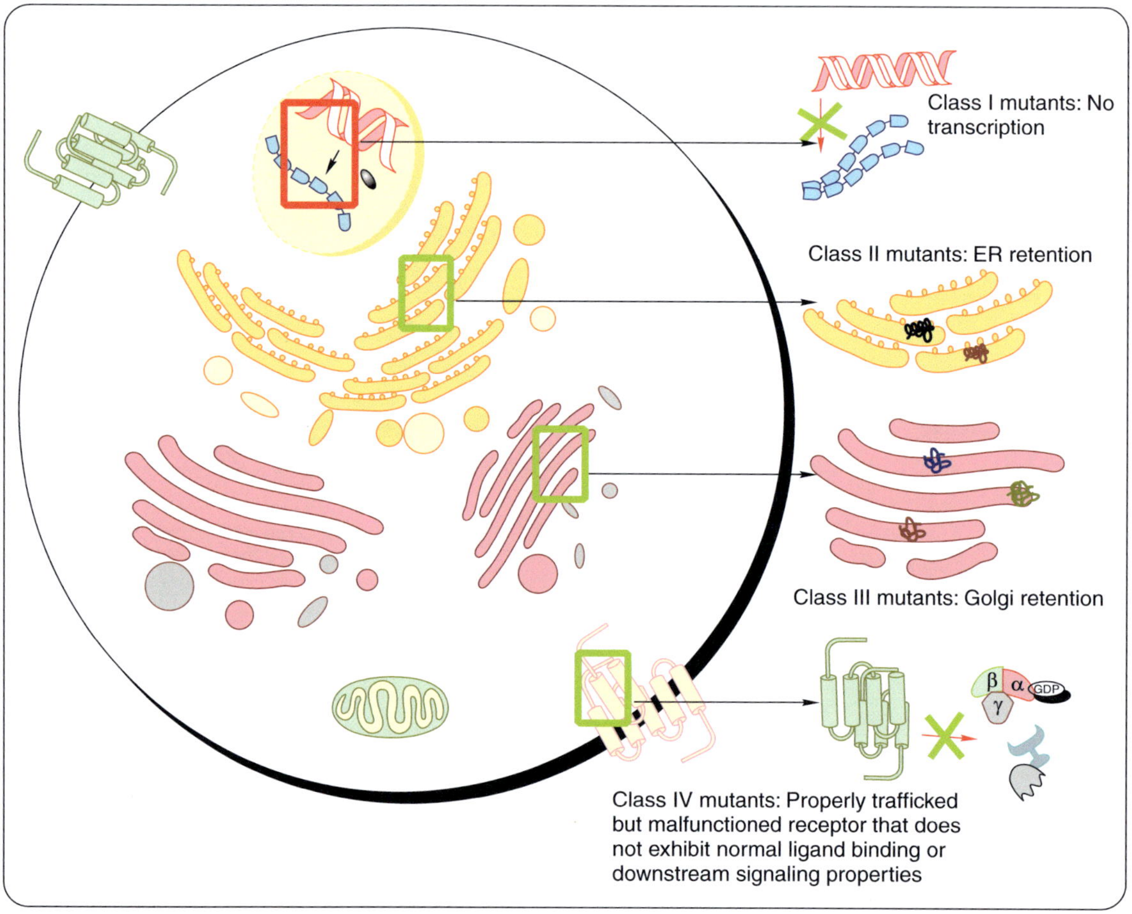

Fig 7.6 *Defects in GPCR Functioning Can Be because of Many Mutations in GPCR-Encoding Gene. Various Classes of Defects in GPCRs, which Lead to Their Dysfunction, have been Elucidated.*

Plate 8

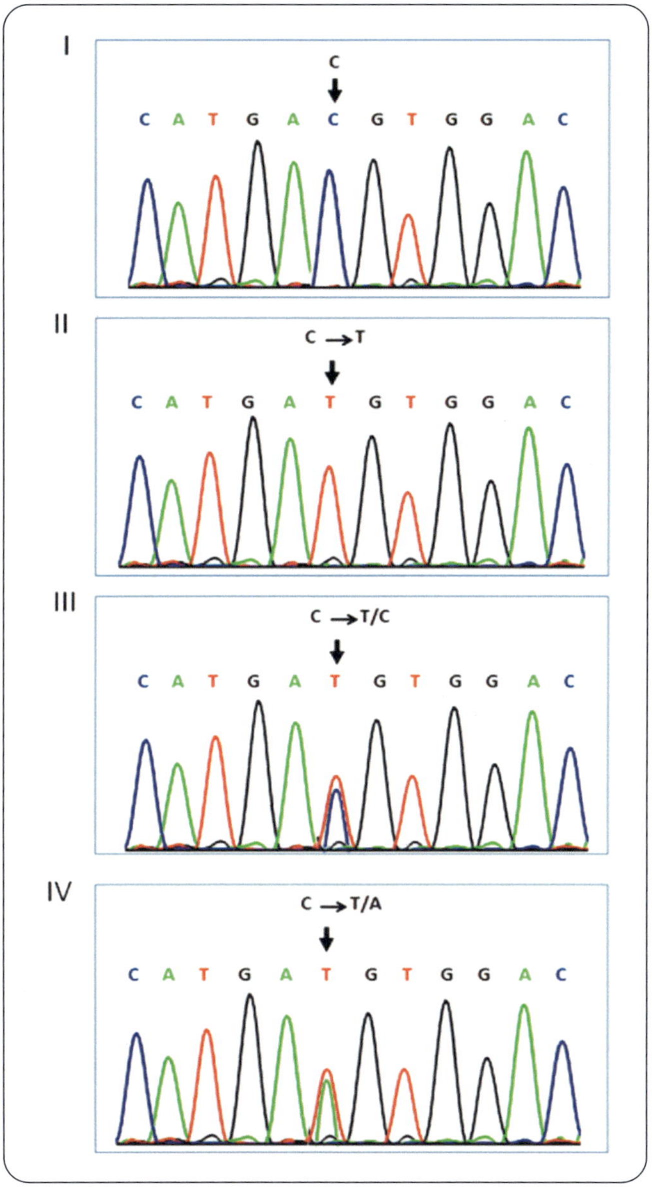

Fig 8.1 *Chromatograms of a Particular DNA Segment in Different Individuals*

(The presence of nucleotide variations is discovered by comparing the DNA sequences. Screening of the chromatograms is particularly essential to detect the heterozygous alleles. *Panel I*, wild-type homozygous alleles (C); *Panel II,* homozygous mutant alleles (T); *Panel III,* a case of heterozygous mutant alleles (C to T/C representing substitution of the wild-type allele in one chromosome); *Panel IV*, another case of heterozygous mutant alleles (C to T/A representing substitution of the wild type alleles in both chromosomes). The polymorphic nucleotide position is indicated by downward arrow in each panel.)

Made in the USA
Las Vegas, NV
03 November 2026

57423687R00233